Nutrition Handbook

for
Nursing Practice

THIRD EDITION

Susan G. Dudek, RD, CDN, BS

Part-time Assistant Professor
Dietetic Technology Program
Erie Community College
Williamsville, New York

Consultant Dietitian
Chaffee Hospital and Home
Springville, New York

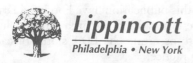

Lippincott
Philadelphia • New York

Sponsoring Editor: Susan M. Keneally
Project Editor: Barbara Ryalls
Production Manager: Helen Ewan
Production Coordinator: Patricia McCloskey
Design Coordinator: Melissa Olson
Indexer: Victoria Boyle

Edition 3

9 8 7 6 5 4 3 2 1

Library of Congress Cataloging in Publications Data

Dudek, Susan G.
    Nutrition handbook for nursing practice / Susan G. Dudek. — 3rd ed.
        p.   cm.
    Includes bibliographical references and index.
    ISBN 0-397-55364-1 (alk. paper)
    1. Diet therapy.   2. Nutrition.   3. Nursing.   I. Title.
    [DNLM: 1. Diet Therapy—handbooks.   2. Diet Therapy—nurses'
instruction.   3. Nutrition—nurses' instruction.   4. Nutrition—
handbooks.   WB 39 D845n 1997]
    RM216.D863   1997
    615.8'54—dc20
    DNLM/DLC
    for Library of Congress   96-26302
                                                                                    CIP

Care has been taken to confirm the accuracy of the information presented and to
describe generally accepted practices. However, the authors, editors, and publisher
are not responsible for errors or omissions or for any consequences from application
of the information in this book and make no warranty, express or implied, with
respect to the contents of the publication.

The authors, editors and publisher have exerted every effort to ensure that drug
selection and dosage set forth in this text are in accordance with current recommendations and practice at the time of publication. However, in view of ongoing
research, changes in government regulations, and the constant flow of information
relating to drug therapy and drug reactions, the reader is urged to check the package
insert for each drug for any change in indications and dosage and for added warnings and precautions. This is particularly important when the recommended agent is
a new or infrequently employed drug.

Some drugs and medical devices presented in this publication have Food and Drug
Administration (FDA) clearance for limited use in restricted research settings. It is
the responsibility of the health care provider to ascertain the FDA status of each
drug or device planned for use in their clinical practice.

*For Joseph, Christopher, Kaitlyn, and Kara—
who so patiently waited for me to finish my "story."*

Reviewers

Elaine Rooney, RN, MS
Assistant Professor of Nursing
University of Pittsburgh at Bradford
Bradford, Pennsylvania

Andrea Dillaway-Huber, PhD, RD
Adjunct Faculty
Allen Center for Nutrition
Department of Nutrition
Cedar Crest College
Allentown, Pennsylvania

Patricia M. Olsen, RN, MSN, MAEd
Assistant Professor
Department of Nursing
Walsh University
North Canton, Ohio

Andrea Koepke, BSN, MA, DNS
Professor of Nursing
Anderson University
Anderson, Indiana

Laura Filippelli, MS, RD, LDN
Instructor of Nutrition and Diet Therapy
Clinical Staff Dietician
St. Joseph Hospital—School of Nursing
North Providence, Rhode Island

Fran Hammerly, RNCS, MS
Instructor
Stark Technical College
Canton, Ohio

Preface

Because nutrition is a basic human need, ever-changing throughout the life cycle and along the wellness–illness continuum, it is a vital and integral component of nursing care. Knowledge of nutrition principles and the ability to apply that knowledge are required of nurses, whether they are involved in home health, community wellness, outpatient settings, or acute or long-term care. Today, more than ever, health care providers are expected to do more with less; often the constraints of time and resources challenge nurses to "be all things to all people." With the movement of health care toward wellness and primary prevention, the significance of nutrition becomes more evident.

Like its two predecessors, this third edition of **Nutrition Handbook for Nursing Practice** is intended to be used as a core or supplemental text by students from a variety of educational backgrounds, or as a reference manual by practicing nurses. Using the nursing process format, it provides easily accessible, practical information to facilitate the integration of nutrition into nursing care plans. Tables and displays are used extensively throughout the book to present concise yet comprehensive information. Current and sometimes controversial topics are featured under the heading *Food for Thought*. *Drug Alerts* highlight possible adverse nutritional side effects of commonly used medications and specify appropriate actions to alleviate those effects. *Menus* allow the reader to see at a glance how recommendations and guidelines translate into everyday food choices. Modified diets are presented in tabular form and emphasize potential problems, the rationale, nursing interventions, and client teaching to enable the nurse to not only convey information, but to facilitate change, which is the purpose of nutritional counseling. Appendices provide a wealth of useful reference material such as food composition tables, the American Diabetes Association/American Dietetic Association Exchange Lists for Meal Planning, a composite of selected adult enteral formulas and supplements, and generalizations about drug and nutrient interactions.

Section One: Principles of Nutrition presents the fundamentals of nutrition. Topics covered include carbohydrates, protein, lipids, vitamins, minerals, fluid and electrolytes, and metabolism. Background data on nutrient functions, sources, and requirements are augmented by brief overviews of nutrient or body metabolism. Potential adverse side effects of deficient and excessive intakes, and current intake recommendations are discussed. Consumption trends and future areas of research are presented where applicable.

Section Two: Nutrition in Health Promotion begins with planning a diet that is adequate but not excessive. Cultural, personal, and food safety considerations are also discussed. The chapter on nutritional assessment criteria and interpretation is followed by optimal nutrition for the "well" population at various stages of the life cycle. Where appropriate, alterations in health that commonly occur only at certain stages of the life cycle (i.e., during pregnancy, infancy, and childhood) are discussed, along with recommended dietary interventions.

Building on the foundation laid in Sections One and Two, Section Three: Nutrition in Clinical Practice combines the knowledge and application for nutrition in clinical practice. Alterations in health are presented, ranging from obesity to oncology. For each particular disorder, background information regarding etiology, complications, treatment, and nutrition intervention objectives is reviewed. Assessment data follows; note that the focus of this information is on the nutritional and dietary implications of each specific disorder, and therefore, should not be viewed as a complete nursing assessment guide. A sample, or generic, nursing diagnosis is given for each clinical disorder to illustrate how nutrition can be incorporated into nursing care plans. It should be noted that in practice, actual nursing diagnoses are formulated only after all pertinent assessment data is gathered and analyzed. For any given individual, the sample diagnoses may be incomplete or inappropriate. Although, in practice, Planning and Implementation are two distinct steps, they are grouped together for the sake of written presentation. As with the assessment data, client goals and nursing interventions, including Diet Management, Client Teaching, and Monitoring, focus only on nutrition. Evauation projects optimal client outcomes.

In retrospect, I am surprised at the number of changes and additions to this edition; clearly, the "science" and "art" of nutrition are evolving at a rapid pace. New to this edition are Women's Health Issues, information on antioxidants, and nutrition interventions for chronic obstructive pulmonary disease. A chapter on metabolism has been added, and the topic of AIDS has been expanded and incorporated into the oncology chapter. Other expanded topics include vegetarian meal planning, artificial fats, the impact of culture on food choices, and dysphagia diets. Eating disorders are grouped with obesity and presented in the section on clinical practice. The labeling regulations implemented in 1994 are included, as is the 1995 edition of the Dietary Guidelines for Americans. The newest edition of the Exchange Lists for Meal Planning reflects the change in philosophy and nutrition therapy recommendations put forth by the American Diabetic Association in 1994.

Format changes include the addition of *Key Terms* at the beginning of each chapter; key terms appear in boldface in the text where they are defined. At the end of each chapter are *Key Concepts* that summarize the chapter's most important ideas. Throughout the sections on Health Promotion and Clinical Practice, *Focus on Critical Thinking Exercises* have been included to help the student assimilate nutrition information.

New to this edition is a supplemental *Instructor's Manual*, which provides a brief overview of each chapter, student objectives, classroom teaching strategies, clinical activities (where appropriate), and test questions.

Acknowledgments

I am grateful for the support and help of all the people whose efforts contributed to the development and production of this book, and feel honored to be associated with the dedicated and creative professionals at JB Lippincott.

I thank:

Donna L. Hilton and Mary Gyetvan for directing and nurturing this project.

Susan M. Keneally, Assistant Editor, my "slave driver" who was always ready, willing, and able to lend a kind word and helping hand.

Barbara Ryalls, Project Editor, for her conscientious attention to detail, skillful editing, and much-appreciated sense of humor.

All the behind-the-scenes design and production professionals at JB Lippincott whose combined efforts work magic.

The readers of the second edition and reviewers of the third edition, whose thoughtful comments and suggestions helped guide the evolution of this text into a new and improved edition.

Gary Maedl, for sharing his technical resources with me.

And special thanks to:

Jeanne Scherer, author and editor of nursing textbooks, who has been my mentor and inspiration. I am forever indebted to her for believing in me.

My parents, Charles and Annie Maedl, for a lifetime of love and support.

My family, Joseph, Christopher, Kaitlyn, and Kara, for their support and encouragement, and all the sacrifices they made for this book.

Contents

Appendices   *721*

Index   *812*

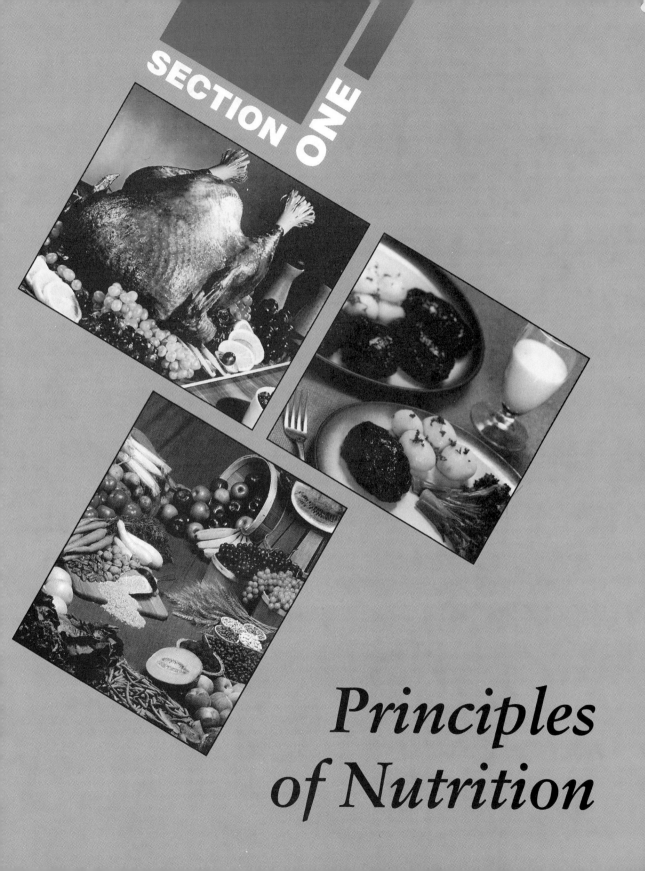

SECTION ONE

*Principles
of Nutrition*

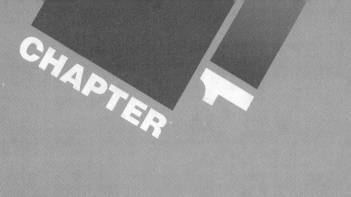

CHAPTER

Carbohydrates

Chapter Outline

Key Terms

Carbohydrates

Dietary fiber

Disaccharides

Fiber

Fructose

Glucose

Glycogen

Lactose

Monosaccharides

Non-nutritive sweetener

Nutritive sweetener

Polysaccharides

Starch

Sucrose

Sugar alcohols

*C*arbohydrates (CHO), commonly known as sugars and starches, provide the major source of energy in almost all human diets. Although Americans 20 years of age and older consume approximately 50% of their total calories from carbohydrates (CDC, 1994), leading governmental and health agencies recommend that up to 60% of total calories should be from CHO. People in developing countries may obtain as much as 80% to 90% of total calories from CHO.

Carbohydrates are found mainly in plants. Compared to the complexities of raising animals for food, plants are easy to grow, have a high energy yield per unit of land, are easy to store after harvesting, and are therefore relatively inexpensive. As such, CHO intake and income have an inverse relationship—as income goes up, CHO intake decreases, and the intake of protein and fat (more expensive forms of energy) increases.

SYNTHESIS

Through the process of photosynthesis, all green plants trap energy from the sun, water from the soil, and carbon dioxide from the air to make CHO. Plants store CHO as either sugar (ie, fruit and sugar beets) or starch (ie, root and tuber vegetables, dried peas and beans, and cereal grains). As some plants ripen and mature, they become less sweet as sugar is converted to starch (ie, peas, corn, and carrots). Conversely, fruit becomes more sweet as it ripens because starch is converted to sugar.

Chemically, all CHO are composed of the elements carbon (C), hydrogen (H), and oxygen (O). Like water (H_2O), CHO have twice as many hydrogen atoms as oxygen atoms. Because each particular CHO has a distinct chemical arrangement, sweetness and other physical properties vary.

CLASSIFICATIONS

The two major classifications of carbohydrates are simple carbohydrates (sugars) and complex carbohydrates (starches and fiber). *Simple carbohydrates* are composed of one or two sugar, or saccharide, molecules; they are known as **monosaccharides** and **disaccharides**, respectively. This group includes naturally occurring sugars that do not taste sweet (eg, lactose, maltose), as well as sugar sweeteners, like sucrose and fructose, which are known as **nutritive sweeteners** because they provide calories (Figure 1-1). (**Non-nutritive** sweeteners, like aspartame and saccharin, are considered noncaloric, high-intensity, or alternative sweeteners; they are not true carbohydrates.)

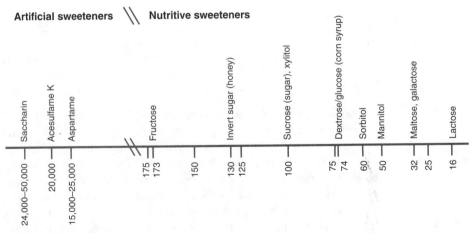

Figure 1-1
Sweetness scale of sugar and other sweetners.

Complex carbohydrates, or **polysaccharides**, are made of long chains of many (poly) sugar (saccharide) molecules. Because of the way their sugar molecules are arranged, polysaccharides do not taste sweet. Starch, dextrins, glycogen, and fiber belong to this category.

Monosaccharides: Simple Sugars

Monosaccharides are the simplest type of CHO because they cannot be hydrolyzed (broken down) into smaller molecules; instead, they are absorbed directly into the bloodstream without undergoing digestion. Depending on the number of carbon atoms contained in each sugar molecule, monosaccharides may be classified as trioses, tetroses, pentoses, or hexoses (atoms of three, four, five, or six carbons, respectively). The hexoses, specifically glucose, fructose, and galactose, are the only monosaccharides that are abundant in food and nutritionally significant (Table 1-1). Mannose is a hexose of limited nutritional importance.

GLUCOSE: D-GLUCOSE, DEXTROSE, GRAPE SUGAR, BLOOD SUGAR

Glucose is the major fuel of the body and the form of CHO to which all other CHO are converted in order to be transported through the blood or utilized for energy. Because of this, glucose is the only sugar found in the body in significant amounts. Normal blood glucose levels range from 70 mg/dl to 110 mg/dl and are regulated by hormones (Table 1-2).

FRUCTOSE: FRUIT SUGAR, LEVULOSE

Fructose, the sweetest simple sugar, is found naturally in fruits, as an added sugar in a crystalline form, and as a component of high-fructose corn syrup (HFCS). Pure crystalline fructose, produced from cornstarch through a process called isomerization, is a granulated substance that looks and tastes like sucrose. It is particularly effective at sweetening high-acid and cold foods, such as citrus drinks. When it is used in combination with other sweeteners, a synergistic effect increases the sweetening power of both sweeteners (ADA, 1993a). HFCS generally contains 42%, 55%, or 90% fructose; it is used by manufacturers in soft drinks, canned fruits, and jams. Like other sugars, fructose is converted to glucose in the liver. Large amounts of fructose can cause osmotic diarrhea (ADA, 1993a). Fructose is widely used both in the pharmaceutical industry and in food processing.

Table 1-1
The Common Hexoses and Their Sources

Hexose	Sources
Glucose	Fruits, vegetables, honey, and corn syrup; made commercially from the hydrolysis of starch or corn through the action of heat, acid, or enzymes
Fructose	Fruits, honey; crystalline fructose is produced commercially from cornstarch; high-fructose corn syrup (HFCS) is made commercially from dextrose in corn
Galactose	Not found freely in food, but is combined with glucose to form the disaccharide lactose
Mannose	Found in small amounts in peaches, apples, and oranges

Table 1-2
The Effect of Hormones on Blood Glucose Levels

Hormone	Effect on Blood Glucose Level	Mechanism
Insulin: produced by the β cells of the islets of Langerhans in the pancreas	Decrease	Enhances the uptake of glucose by muscle and adipose cells
		Promotes the conversion of glucose to glycogen in the liver and muscle cells (glycogenesis)
		Enhances the conversion of glucose to fat in the liver and adipose cells (lipogenesis)
Glucagon: produced by the α cells of the islets of Langerhans in the pancreas	Increase	Stimulates the synthesis of glucose from non-CHO sources (gluconeogenesis)
		Promotes the breakdown of glycogen to release glucose (glycogenolysis)
Epinephrine: produced by the adrenal medulla	Increase	Stimulates glycogenolysis
		Decreases the release of insulin
Glucocorticoids: produced by the adrenal medulla	Increase	Stimulate gluconeogenesis
		Cause the tissue to be insensitive to the action of insulin
Thyroxine: produced by the thyroid gland	Increase	Stimulates glycogenolysis in the liver
		Stimulates gluconeogenesis
		Increases the rate of intestinal absorption of the hexoses

GALACTOSE

Galactose is not found freely in food but is combined with glucose in the disaccharide lactose. It is also converted to glucose in the liver.

Monosaccharide Derivatives: Sugar Alcohols

Sugar alcohols, of which sorbitol, mannitol, and xylitol are the most common, are produced when an aldehyde group is changed to an alcohol. Although references list sugar alcohols as calorically equivalent to other sugars (4 cal/g), studies indicate that their calorie content cannot be precisely determined and may vary with the mode of consumption and other individual variables (ADA, 1993a). Sugar alcohols are found naturally in some foods, but are used most commonly as sugar substitutes in dietetic products because they are slowly absorbed and produce less of an effect on blood glucose levels and insulin secretion than sucrose. However, sorbitol is not recommended for use in large amounts, because it can cause abdominal gas, discomfort, and osmotic diarrhea. Sources of sugar alcohols appear in Table 1-3.

Disaccharides

Disaccharides are double sugars made from the chemical union of one molecule of glucose and one other monosaccharide (Table 1-4).

Table 1-3
Sugar Alcohols and Their Sources

Sugar Alcohol	Sources
Sorbitol	Apples, cherries, pears, and plums
	Hard candy, sugarless gum, jams, jellies
	Made commercially from glucose and used as a sweetener in many dietetic products
Mannitol	Pineapples, olives, asparagus, carrots, and sweet potatoes
	Used as a drying agent in some foods
Xylitol	Raspberries, strawberries, spinach, cauliflower, cereals, and seaweed
	Made commercially from birch tree chips and used in dietetic chewing gum and other dietetic products

SUCROSE: SUGAR, TABLE SUGAR

Sucrose, commonly known as "sugar," is the least expensive and most common sweetener in the diet. Daily sucrose consumption in the United States ranges from 14 to 60 g, with an average of 41 g/day (1/4 cup) (ADA, 1993a). Sucrose provides, on average, approximately 7% to 11% of total calorie intake. As sucrose intake has declined over the last decade, the intake of corn-derived sweeteners and non-nutritive sweeteners has increased. It is estimated that the average daily intake of added sugars for the total U.S. population is 53g/day (ADA, 1993a). Unfortunately, there is no difference in caloric or nutritional value between sucrose and all other nutritive sweeteners (see display, The Many Tastes of "Sugar"), so that no particular one is any healthier than another.

LACTOSE: "MILK SUGAR"

Lactose, also known as milk sugar, is insoluble in water, is not very sweet, and is more slowly digested than sucrose. Lactose promotes the growth of friendly intestinal

Table 1-4
Disaccharides: Their Composition and Common Food Sources

Disaccharide	Composition	Sources
Sucrose	Glucose + fructose	Sugar cane, sugar beets, molasses, maple syrup, bananas, dates, ripe pineapple, peas, and sweet potatoes
Lactose	Glucose + galactose	Milk and milk products
Maltose	Glucose + glucose	Produced in the malting and fermentation of grains (*ie,* present in malted food products and beer)
		Insignificant as a dietary source of CHO

The Many Tastes of "Sugar"

Blackstrap molasses: the syrup remaining after the third and final extraction of sugar from the boiled juice of sugar cane or beets. It is very dark and bitter and is barely sweet.

Brown sugar ("sugar with a suntan"): partly purified white sugar (sucrose) that contains molasses. The lighter the color, the more purified the sugar.

Cane sugar: a concentrated syrup of mixed sugars made by boiling cane sap.

Corn syrup: a syrup produced by hydrolyzing cornstarch with acids. Glucose is the major sugar.

Date sugar: ground dates, which are high in natural sugars and very sweet.

High-fructose corn syrup (HFCS): a commercially made sweetener made by treating regular corn syrup with enzymes to break down the glucose to fructose, which is much sweeter; HFCS is used extensively in soft drinks, canned foods, and other processed foods because it is cheaper than sucrose. It is estimated that the average American consumes about 39 lb of HFCS yearly.

Honey: the nectar of flowers that is collected, modified, and concentrated by bees. Contains mostly glucose and fructose, and small amounts of sucrose. Honey containing more than 8% sucrose is considered adulterated.

Invert sugar: a mixture of equal amounts of glucose and fructose that forms when sucrose is hydrolyzed by enzymes or by being heated in water. It is sweeter than white sugar.

Lump sugar: sucrose pressed into a cube or tablet form.

Maple syrup: made from the concentrated sap of maple trees. May be boiled down into maple sugar.

Molasses: the residue that remains after sucrose crystals have been removed from the juices of the sugar cane or beet. Contains mostly sucrose, with smaller amounts of glucose and fructose.

Powdered sugar: made from white granulated sugar that has been machine-ground. Powdered sugar ranges in texture from coarse to extrafine: Generally the more ×s on the label, the finer the powder (*ie,* 10× is finer than 6×). Cornstarch is usually added to prevent caking.

Raw sugar: coarse granulated sugar made by the evaporation of sugar cane juice. By law, impurities must be removed before raw sugar can be sold in the United States.

Sorghum: a syrup made from sorghum cane that looks like molasses. Sorghum has about the same sugar content as cane syrup.

Turbinado sugar: produced by separating raw sugar crystals and washing them with steam to remove impurities and most of the molasses contained in raw sugar. It has a slight molasses flavor and is coarser than white sugar.

Unsulfured molasses: made directly from sugar cane juice before any sugar crystals have been extracted. It is the sweetest type of molasses and is free of sulfur dioxide.

bacteria that produce vitamin K and enhances the absorption of calcium. It is added to infant formulas and is used by food processing and pharmaceutical industries.

MALTOSE: "MALT SUGAR"

Maltose is not found free in food but is produced as an intermediate in starch digestion and also through the processes of malting (malted milk drinks) and brewing (beer). It is used in some infant formulas, instant foods, and bakery products in the form of maltodextrin.

Complex Carbohydrates: Polysaccharides

Polysaccharides are complex compounds that are each composed of 10 or more glucose units. Polysaccharides are not sweet and are usually insoluble (Table 1-5).

STARCH

Starch is the storage form of glucose for plants; it is composed of hundreds to thousands of glucose molecules, which may be arranged in one long chain (amylose) or in a branched chain (amylopectin). Different sources of starch (potatoes, rice, corn, and wheat) have different physical properties (solubility, thickening power, and flavor) based on the ratio of amylose to amylopectin. Other good sources of starch include barley, dried peas and beans, and lentils.

Plants store starch in microscopic granules that swell and rupture when moist heat is applied. Cooking makes starch more digestible and slightly sweeter.

Modified food starches are natural starches that are commercially treated to improve their viscosity, stability, clarity, or solubility. They are used extensively in commercially prepared sauces, frozen fruit pies, infant foods, canned and instant puddings, and gum drops.

DEXTRINS

Dextrins are polysaccharide fragments, or intermediates, that form when starch is subjected to enzymes (digestion) or heat (cooking or toasting). They are more soluble and slightly sweeter than starch but do not have the thickening power of starch.

Table 1-5
Polysaccharides: Their Composition and Sources

Polysaccharide	Composition	Sources
Starch	Hundreds to thousands of glucose molecules	Grains and grain products, legumes, potatoes and other root vegetables, and unripe fruit
Dextrin	Fragments of starch	Leaves of starch-forming plants
		Also formed as an intermediate in the breakdown of starch by the action of heat (ie, cooking and toasting) or enzymes
Glycogen	30 to 60 thousand glucose molecules	Not considered a significant form of CHO in the diet. After animals are slaughtered, the glycogen in their muscles quickly breaks down and virtually disappears.
		Oysters, scallops, and lobsters do contain some glycogen, but they are not eaten in large enough quantities to be considered significant.
Cellulose	Many glucose molecules arranged in a way that they cannot be digested by the enzymes present in the human GI tract	Skins of fruit, shells of corn kernels, the fibers of plants, the coverings of seeds, and the structural part of plants

GLYCOGEN: ANIMAL STARCH

Glycogen, the only form of CHO that animals and humans can store, is found in the liver and muscles. It is not considered a significant form of carbohydrate in the diet because only small amounts are contained in meat, and most of that is converted to lactic acid at the time of slaughter. However, it has great physiologic importance.

A typical adult can store up to three quarters of a pound of glycogen (the primary and most readily available source of glucose and energy) or about 1400 calories—enough calories for half a day of moderate activity. Glycogen that is stored in the liver can be broken down quickly into glucose to maintain normal blood glucose levels between meals and to provide fuel for tissues. Glycogen that is stored in the muscle is used primarily as a source of energy. Athletes can almost double their storage of glycogen to increase their energy reserve for long-distance events by practicing "glycogen loading" (see Chapter 11).

FIBER

The precise definition of fiber has yet to be universally agreed on. Most commonly, **fiber** is defined as the portion of plant cell walls that is resistant to digestion by human enzymes; a large percentage of fibers are broken down in the large intestine by colonic bacteria to produce fatty acids and gas (ADA, 1993b). Although only cellulose is truly fibrous, **dietary fiber** is the accepted group name for roughage or residue that includes cellulose, hemicellulose, pectins, lignin, gums, mucilages, and polysaccharides from algae and seaweed. Methylcellulose is a cellulose derivative that absorbs large amounts of water. It is used in low-calorie foods such as imitation syrups and salad dressings and in bulk-forming laxatives.

Because fiber is defined physiologically, it is difficult to obtain accurate measurements. In the past, *crude fiber* was used to describe what was left after a plant was treated with dilute acids and dilute alkalis, but it has been found that this method greatly underestimated dietary fiber content and was not relevant to human nutrition. *Dietary fiber*, which is what remains after a food is digested, is difficult to measure, but is estimated to be two to three times greater than the crude fiber content of food. Unfortunately, data on fiber content are not available for all food sources.

Fiber is commonly classified according to its solubility in water because insoluble and soluble fibers have different physiologic effects (Table 1-6). Although specific sources are listed for either insoluble or soluble fibers, most plant foods are composed of various amounts and types of both kinds of fiber. The most consistent benefit from fiber is the relief from constipation that it provides; however, only insoluble fibers, like hemicellulose in wheat bran, actually increase stool weight and promote regularity. Soluble fibers, like gums found in oatmeal, have little effect on elimination but have been shown to lower serum cholesterol and stabilize or reduce blood glucose levels in diabetics.

Because of the variable physiologic effects of fiber, it is difficult to define precise need. Current evidence suggests that 20 to 35 g of fiber daily, combined with a high-carbohydrate, low-fat intake, may be optimal for health promotion and may reduce the risk of certain diseases (see display, To Get at Least 25 g of Fiber Daily . . .).

Table 1-6
Major Types of Fiber: Their Sources and Physiologic Effects

Types of Fiber	Physiologic Effects	Sources

Water-soluble fibers
    gums
    pectins
    mucilages
    some hemicelluloses
	Delay gastric emptying and intestinal transit time
	Lower serum cholesterol levels
	Delay glucose absorption, which helps improve glucose tolerance in diabetics
		Oats
		Legumes
		Apples
		Citrus fruits

Water-insoluble fibers
    lignin
    cellulose
    remaining hemicelluloses
	Accelerate intestinal transit
	Increase fecal weight
	Slow starch hydrolysis
	Delay glucose absorption
		Wheat bran
		    and other whole
		    grain bread and
		    cereals

According to the Third National Health and Nutrition Examination Survey for 1988–1991, the median daily fiber intake for adults were 12 to 14g (CDC). Except for use in relief of constipation, fiber supplements are not recommended.

CARBOHYDRATE FUNCTIONS

Provide Energy

The primary function of carbohydrates in the diet is to provide the major source of energy for the body. Under normal conditions, the nervous system and lung tissue rely on glucose as their sole source of energy. Glucose is also the major fuel used by

To Get at Least 25 g of Fiber Daily . . .

Sources of Fiber	g Fiber/Svg	Eat
Bread, cereal, rice, and pasta group		
white bread, rice, pasta	1	6–11 servings/day for 12–16 g fiber or more/day
whole grain breads,	2–5	
cereals with adequate fiber,	2–5	
high-fiber cereals	7–11	PLUS
Fruits	about 2	2–4 servings for 4–8 g fiber/day
		PLUS
Vegetables	about 2	3–5 servings for 6–10 g fiber/day
		PLUS
Dried peas and beans	about 5	3 servings/week for average of 2 g fiber/day
		EQUALS
		At least 25 g fiber/day

muscles. Unlike protein and fat, glucose is burned efficiently and completely and does not leave a toxic end-product that the kidneys must eliminate.

Regardless of the source, all carbohydrates supply 4 cal/g, with the exception of undigestible fibers, which are essentially calorie free because they cannot be broken down and absorbed. Because the amounts of stored glycogen and circulating glucose are limited, carbohydrates should be eaten at frequent and regular intervals to meet the body's energy needs.

A common misconception is that CHO are "fattening," even though ounce-for-ounce they have the same number of calories as protein and less than half the calories of fat. Depending on the amount eaten, any food can be considered "fattening" or "nonfattening." And, as was stated earlier in the Chapter, excess calories from any source—CHO, protein, or fat—are converted to fat and stored in the body, so CHO do not have a greater tendency to "turn to fat" than other sources of calories.

Spare Protein

For protein to be used most efficiently (ie, to carry on its specific functions such as repairing and replacing tissue), the diet must contain enough CHO calories to meet the body's energy requirements. An adequate CHO intake is particularly important any time protein requirements increase, such as after surgery or trauma, and during periods of rapid growth like infancy, pregnancy, and lactation.

If CHO intake is inadequate, the body will convert dietary protein—or break down and convert its own protein tissue—into glucose to be used for energy (gluconeogenesis). If protein is used for energy, it cannot be used to repair and replace tissue; also, the kidneys are overburdened with excretion of the nitrogenous wastes that remain after protein is degraded.

Prevent Ketosis

Some carbohydrates are needed to oxidize fat completely. When CHO intake is inadequate to meet energy needs, fat is inefficiently and incompletely broken down into ketones. The accumulation of ketones in the bloodstream leads to nausea, fatigue, loss of appetite, and ketoacidosis. Dehydration and sodium depletion may follow as the body tries to rid itself of ketones through the kidneys (ketonuria). The rapid weight loss characteristic of low-CHO fad diets is related to loss of body fluids resulting from the use of protein and fat for energy.

Combine With Other Compounds To Form Important Body Constituents

One example of such a combination is mucopolysaccharides, a group of complex compounds that occur in various body secretions and structures. They are composed of polysaccharides combined with protein and amino sugars. The following are common mucopolysaccharides:

- Hyaluronic acid, found in the fluid that lubricates the joints and the vitreous humor of the eyeball

- Chondroitin sulfate, found in cartilage, skin, and bone
- Heparin, the naturally occurring anticoagulant in blood
- Keratan sulfate, present in hard structures like fingernails
- Dermatan sulfate, present in the skin

HOW THE BODY HANDLES CARBOHYDRATES

Digestion

Carbohydrates are digested more quickly and completely than protein and fat (Fig. 1-2). In most diets, more than 90% of the CHO is digested; the remainder is excreted in the feces. Diets that are high in cellulose and other fibers are less well digested.

Cooked starch begins to undergo digestion in the slightly alkaline medium of the mouth by the action of salivary amylase, or ptyalin. Virtually no chemical digestion of starch occurs in the stomach. Some sucrose may be hydrolyzed to fructose and glucose in the presence of hydrochloric acid (HCl).

The principal site of CHO digestion is the slightly alkaline medium of the small intestine. In the duodenum, pancreatic amylase hydrolyzes complex CHO into maltose. The intestinal disaccharidases, located within the brush border of the intestine, break down the disaccharides into monosaccharides, which are the end-products of CHO digestion.

Absorption

The monosaccharides (glucose, fructose, and galactose) are absorbed through the intestinal mucosa and transported to the liver through the portal blood circulation.

The physical structure of the food, its nutrient content (protein, fat, and fiber), and food processing and preparation methods used can all affect the rate and extent of CHO absorption (Morgan [ed], 1994). Although it was once believed that macronutrients, including CHO, are 95% absorbed, studies have indicated that 2% to 20% of the starch in wheat flour, rice, beans, bananas, and potatoes is not absorbed in the small intestine and passes into the colon with dietary fiber (Morgan [ed], 1994).

Metabolism

In the liver, fructose and galactose are converted readily to glucose. Normally, blood glucose levels are held fairly constant by the action of hormones (see Table 1-2). As blood glucose levels rise after eating, insulin is secreted to move glucose out of the bloodstream and into the cells. Muscle cells may convert glucose to glycogen to maintain their stores. Through a complex series of metabolic reactions, cells oxidize (burn) glucose to produce energy, carbon dioxide, and water. Depending on calorie intake and energy requirements, the time period between CHO consumption and the release of energy may vary from minutes to hours to months.

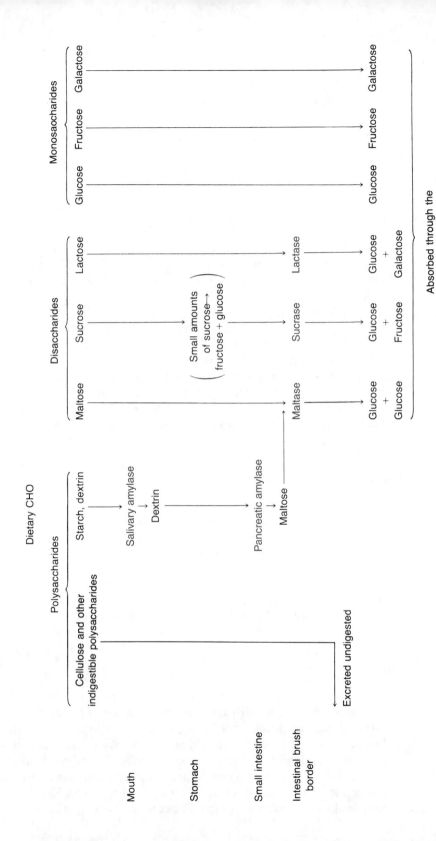

Figure 1-2
CHO digestion.

As cells take glucose out of the blood serum and use it for energy or storage, liver glycogen is broken down continually to maintain serum glucose levels (glycogenolysis). Even a slight drop in serum glucose triggers hunger, a signal for the body to replenish its supply of glucose. If eating is not resumed and fasting is prolonged, the body will synthesize glucose from amino acids and glycerol (glyconeogenesis). Table 1-7 lists the signs and symptoms and possible etiology of altered blood glucose levels.

Glucose that is not needed as an immediate source of energy or to replace glycogen (glycogenesis) may be converted in the liver to other essential carbohydrates like ribose, a component of ribonucleic acid (RNA) and deoxyribonucleic acid (DNA). The liver may also break down glucose to provide a carbon stem that the body uses to make nonessential amino acids (if nitrogen and other necessary components are available).

Table 1-7
Altered Blood Glucose Levels: Signs, Symptoms, and Possible Etiology*

	Hyperglycemia	**Hypoglycemia**
BLOOD GLUCOSE LEVEL	>140 mg/dl	<70 mg/dl
SIGNS AND SYMPTOMS	Polyphagia, polyuria, polydipsia, dehydration, glucosuria, ketonuria, blurred vision, changes in vision, weight loss, recurrent or persistent infections, weakness, fatigue, muscle wasting, and cramps	Fatigue, weakness, confusion, headache, psychosis, irritability, anxiety, rapid, shallow breathing, hunger, nausea, tingling, pallor, slurred speech, ataxia, marked personality changes, diaphoresis, dizziness, convulsions, coma, and death if untreated
POSSIBLE ETIOLOGY	Diabetes mellitus related to a relative or absolute deficiency of insulin (see Chap. 18) Excessive CHO intake, such as concentrated TPN solutions Hormone imbalances Stress Liver disease Head injuries Anesthesia Toxemia of pregnancy	Excessive insulin secretion, such as hypoglycemia secondary to postgastrectomy Excessive exogenous insulin or oral antidiabetic agents Deficient glucose production related to certain drugs Deficiency of hormones that increase blood glucose levels (*ie,* glucagon, epinephrine) Increased glucose utilization related to exercise, fever, renal glycosuria, and pregnancy Decreased glucose production related to diffuse liver disease

* Alterations in blood glucose levels are symptoms of underlying problems, not diseases themselves. Numerous claims that allergies, depression, hyperactivity in children, substance abuse, and criminal behavior are caused by hypoglycemia are unproven, as is the assumption that hypoglycemia is a common malady caused by eating a high-CHO diet.

Finally, any glucose that remains can be converted by liver and adipose cells to fatty acids and stored as triglycerides (fat). Calories eaten in excess of need, regardless of the source, are converted to fat, and unfortunately, the body has an unlimited capacity to store fat. The body cannot rid itself of an excess carbohydrate intake through excretion.

The many reactions involved in the metabolism of CHO require adequate amounts of B vitamins, particularly thiamine, riboflavin, and niacin, which act as coenzymes.

SOURCES OF CARBOHYDRATES

Carbohydrates are found almost exclusively in plants. Complex CHO are found in grains and vegetables, including dried peas and beans. Fruits and sugar (by all its names) are sources of simple CHO. The only significant source of animal CHO is lactose, which is found in milk and dairy products.

The exchange system, developed by the American Diabetic Association and the American Dietetic Association, is a fairly simple and accurate method of estimating CHO intake, as well as the amount of protein, fat, and calories consumed. Each exchange group contains foods with similar CHO, protein, and fat content per amount specified (see Appendix 11). The five groups that contain CHO are listed in Table 1-8. Not listed is pure sugar, which contains 4 g of CHO and 16 calories per teaspoon.

Sweets and other desserts appear in the exchange list under a group named "Other Carbohydrates." Studies show that when CHO intake is held constant, its source (ie, sugar or starch) does not appear to be a major factor in determining the effect of the food on blood glucose levels; therefore, moderate amounts of sucrose can be used for part of the total CHO requirement for most people with diabetes.

The new food label, "Nutrition Facts" lists the grams of sugar provided in each serving. Because this number includes both natural and added sugars, some "healthy" foods, like milk and fruit juice, appear high in sugar. Also, it is impossible to tell how much added sugar is contained in products that contain both natural and added sugar. Generally, if sugar is one of the first ingredients listed on the label, it is likely that the item is a high-sugar food, unless of course, there are only a few ingredients in the product. On the other hand, a product may be a high-sugar food even if sugar is listed as the last ingredient, if other sweeteners appear high on the ingredient list. It is required that sugars not be added to a food labeled "no added sugar," "without added sugar," or "no sugar added." No % Daily Value has been set for sugar, thus this space on the label is always blank. Percent daily value for carbohydrates is based on the standard value of 300 g (ie, 60% of calories in a 2000-calorie diet).

CARBOHYDRATE REQUIREMENTS AND AVERAGE INTAKES

A recommended dietary allowance (RDA) for CHO has not been established because the body can synthesize glucose from amino acids and the glycerol com-

Table 1-8
Sources of Carbohydrate Based on the American Diabetic Association/American Dietetic Association Exchange Lists

Source	CHO (g)	Protein (g)	Fat (g)	Calories per Serving
CARBOHYDRATE GROUP				
Starch	15	3	1 or less	80
1 slice bread				
½ c cooked cereal				
¾ c unsweetened ready-to-eat cereal				
½ c pasta				
½ c potato				
½ c corn				
½ c legumes				
6 saltines				
Fruit	15	—	—	60
1 small to medium fresh fruit				
½ c canned fruit				
½ c fruit juice				
¼ c dried fruit				
Milk				
1 c skim	12	8	0–3	90
1 c low-fat	12	8	5	120
1 c whole	12	8	8	150
Other Carbohydrates	15	Varies	Varies	Varies
(mainly sweets and desserts)				
Vegetables	5	2	—	25
1 c raw vegetables				
½ c juice				
½ c cooked vegetables				
GROUPS WITHOUT CARBOHYDRATES				
Meat and Meat Substitutes				
very lean	—	7	0–1	35
lean	—	7	3	55
medium fat	—	7	5	75
high fat	—	7	8	100
Fat Group	—	—	5	45

ponent of fat. However, carbohydrate is an essential component of the diet. According to the 10th edition of *Recommended Dietary Allowances*, adults need 50 to 100 g of CHO per day to prevent the effects of a low-CHO diet, which can include ketoacidosis, muscle protein breakdown, sodium depletion, and dehydration. However, 100 g of CHO supplies only 400 calories or about 20% of the total calories needed by most adults. Most experts agree that 50% to 60% of total calories consumed should be supplied by CHO, and most of those in the form of complex CHO.

According to data from the third National Health and Nutrition Examination Survey, CHO provided approximately 50% of total calories in the overall population during the survey period of 1989 to 1991, compared to 46% of calories during 1980. Carbohydrate intake was highest in men from 16 to 19 years of age, with an average intake of 381 g/day. Data from the USDA's "Food Consumption, Prices, and Expenditures, 1970–93" indicated that in 1990 grain products contributed the largest number of carbohydrate calories, followed by sugars and sweeteners, then vegetables (Fig. 1-3).

Currently, the average daily intake of total sugars (both natural and added sugars, with the exception of lactose) is 80 g/day (320 calories) for the total population, or approximately 18% of total calories (Gibney et al, 1995). Thirty-nine percent of sugar consumed is obtained from the "Others" category at the peak of the Food Guide Pyramid (Gibney et al, 1995). Since the 1970s, sucrose consumption has declined while intake of corn sweeteners (namely high fructose corn syrup) has increased, with the shift away from the sugar bowl to soft drinks and sweetened processed foods. However, with the increased popularity of sugar substitutes (see Food for Thought, Non-Nutritive Sweeteners: Tasty or Toxic?) and low-sugar foods, sugar intake has begun to decline.

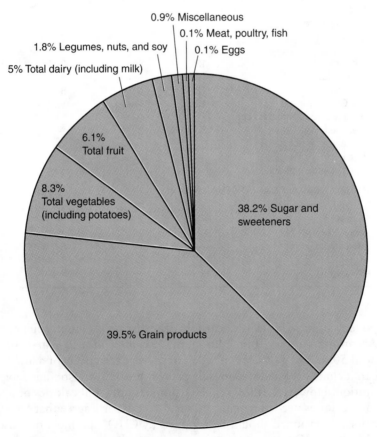

Figure 1-3
Carbohydrate contributed from major food groups to the U.S. food supply, 1990.

FOOD *for* THOUGHT

Non-Nutritive Sweeteners: Tasty or Toxic?

Non-nutritive sweeteners, also called intense sweeteners, alternative sweeteners, and very low calorie sweeteners, are manmade products intended to provide the sweet taste of sugar without the calories—a popular idea with diet-conscious Americans. Since they were first introduced into the U.S. food supply, their use has increased dramatically as more sweeteners are approved for use and the number of products they are used in continues to grow. Currently, three non-nutritive sweeteners are approved for use in the United States, and approval of three others is being sought.

Beginning with aspartame, the FDA began setting an acceptable daily intake (ADI) for non-nutritive sweeteners (ADA, 1993b). ADI is defined as the amount of a food additive that can safely be consumed on a daily basis over a person's lifetime without an adverse effect. Because the ADI includes a 100-fold safety factor, it is not harmful to consume the ADI on a daily basis, even though it is unlikely anyone would achieve that intake.

APPROVED NON-NUTRITIVE SWEETENERS

Saccharin ("Sprinkle Sweet," "Sweet 10," "Sugar Twin," and "Sweet 'n Low")

Saccharin, the oldest non-nutritive sweetener, is produced from a purified petroleum product that occurs naturally in grapes. It is 300× sweeter than sugar, is heat stable, has a long shelf-life, and does not promote cavities. Saccharin does have a slightly bitter or metallic aftertaste. Saccharin is not digested by humans, is rapidly excreted in the urine, and does not accumulate in body tissues.

In 1977, saccharin was banned because of numerous reports that it may contribute to bladder cancer. At that time, Congress enacted the Saccharin Study and Labeling Act, which requires that foods containing saccharin have warning labels and that establishments selling saccharin-containing products display warning signs. How-

ever, because safety issues remain unresolved and consumer demand is widespread, Congress has imposed numerous extensions to prevent the withdrawal of saccharin from the market. The current moratorium extension will expire May 1, 1997. However, studies indicate that saccharin is probably not a human carcinogen. At current levels of intake, saccharin is assumed to be safe for the general public and is approved for use in more than 90 countries. Some industry experts believe that the ban on saccharin will eventually be repealed.

Aspartame ("NutraSweet," "Equal," "NutraTaste")

Aspartame, made by combining the two amino acids aspartic acid and phenylalanine, was discovered in 1965. It has a clean, sweet taste, no aftertaste, and is 200× sweeter than sugar. Although it provides 4 cal/g, its caloric contribution is negligible because such small amounts are needed. When digested, aspartame yields its two component amino acids and methanol; amounts generated are very small compared to amounts obtained from the normal diet.

Initially, aspartame was approved for use as a tabletop sweetener and in dry foods in 1981. Today it appears in more than 150 food product categories. The average aspartame content of a 12-oz diet soft drink is 170 mg, 80 mg per 4-oz diet gelatin, and 35 mg per one packet of tabletop sweetener.

Studies show that aspartame can be safely used by healthy adults, children, adolescents, pregnant and lactating women, and people with diabetes; it is not associated with any adverse health effects. Warnings on all products that contain aspartame are intended to alert people with phenylketonuria (PKU) to the presence of phenylalanine, although aspartame is thought to pose only a small risk.

The ADI for aspartame is 50 mg/kg or body weight, the equivalent of 20 12-oz cans of diet

(continued)

FOOD *for* THOUGHT   (Continued)

soft drinks or 97 packets of tabletop sweeteners for a 150 pound adult. Actual intake in the general population is 2–3 mg/kg per day. Ninety percent of users consume less than 5 mg/day. Aspartame is approved for use by more than 90 countries.

Acesulfame K ("Sweet One")

Acesulfame is an organic salt composed of carbon, nitrogen, oxygen, hydrogen, sulphur, and potassium atoms. In 1988, the FDA granted approval for its use as a sugar substitute in powder (Sunette) and tablet form, and also for use in numerous food products. It is 200× sweeter than sucrose, has a synergistic sweetening effect when combined with other sweeteners, and is heat stable. It has no aftertaste and, because it is excreted through the GI tract unchanged, it provides no calories.

Long-term and animal studies conclude that acesulfame is safe. The ADI of 15 mg/kg/day is the equivalent of a 132-pound person consuming approximately 36 tsp of sugar daily. It is approved for use in more than 40 countries.

NON-NUTRITIVE SWEETENERS NOT YET APPROVED

Sucralose

Sucralose, a chlorinated sucrose product, tastes 400 to 800× sweeter than sugar, and has a high-quality flavor. Most of it is excreted unchanged. The limited amount that is absorbed by the body is not metabolized for energy; therefore, it is noncaloric. It has no effect on insulin secretion or CHO metabolism in healthy people. In more than 100 animal and human studies, sucralose has not been found to pose any health problems. Although it is approved for use in Canada, the FDA has not yet approved its use in the United States.

Alitame

Alitame, formed from two amino acids and a novel amide, is 2000× sweeter than sucrose and has a clean taste. It is well absorbed, and provides a maximum of 1.2 cal/g. More than 15 studies have shown that alitame is safe. Because it is stable at high temperatures and over a wide pH range, and is highly soluble in water, alitame would be suitable in a wide variety of products.

Cyclamates

Cyclamates were removed from the Generally Recognized As Safe (GRAS) list in 1969 after an experiment linked use of cyclamates, at doses of 2500 mg/kg/day, to bladder tumors in rats. Subsequent studies have failed to show a relationship between cyclamates and cancer, and the National Academy of Sciences has concluded that neither cyclamates nor its major metabolites are carcinogenic. Although the FDA has approved the use of cyclamates in beverages, it is not yet a legal food additive.

RECOMMENDATIONS FOR CARBOHYDRATE INTAKE

The Fourth Edition of *Dietary Guidelines for Americans*, issued by the United States Department of Agriculture (USDA) and the United States Department of Health and Human Services (USDHHS), makes two recommendations concerning carbohydrate intake.

Choose a Diet With Plenty of Grain Products, Vegetables, and Fruits

Americans are urged to eat plenty of grains, vegetables, and fruits because they provide vitamins, minerals, complex CHO (starch and fiber), and other substances that are important for good health; also, dried peas and beans from the Meat Group provide the same nutrients. More specifically, the Guidelines recommend (as depicted in the Food Guide Pyramid) a daily intake of 6 to 11 servings of grain products, 3 to 5 servings of various vegetables and vegetable juices, and 2 to 4 servings of various fruits and fruit juices (see display, For a Diet Rich in Complex CHO and Fiber).

BENEFITS OF A HIGH–COMPLEX CHO DIET

Diets high in complex CHO are proportionately low in fat, and studies suggest that high-fat diets increase the risk of certain chronic disorders that occur frequently in the United States. Because fats are a concentrated source of energy (9 cal/g compared to 4 cal/g for CHO), a high-fat diet increases the risk of obesity and its complications, such as type II diabetes, hypertension, and increased surgical complications. A high-fat diet is also implicated in the development of coronary heart disease and certain types of cancer, especially of the colon. Conversely, diets high in complex CHO are not associated with any adverse health effects. In his 1988 *Report on Nutrition and Health,* the Surgeon General recommends increasing complex carbohydrate intake as the best alternative to eating fats and cholesterol (USDHHS, 1988).

For a Diet Rich in Complex CHO and Fiber

Eat:

6–11 SERVINGS OF GRAIN PRODUCTS (BREADS, CEREALS, PASTA, AND RICE)*

- Eat products made from a variety of whole grains, such as wheat, rice, oats, corn, and barley.
- Eat several servings of whole-grain breads and cereals daily.
- Prepare and serve grain products with little or no fats and sugars.

3–5 SERVINGS OF VARIOUS VEGETABLES AND VEGETABLE JUICES*

- Choose dark green leafy and deep yellow vegetables often.

- Eat dry beans, peas, and lentils often.
- Eat starchy vegetables, such as potatoes and corn.
- Prepare and serve vegetables with little or no fats.

2–4 SERVINGS OF VARIOUS FRUITS AND FRUIT JUICES*

- Choose citrus fruits or juices, melons, or berries regularly.
- Eat fruits as desserts or snacks.
- Drink fruit juices.
- Prepare and serve fruits with little or no added sugars.

*(From USDA, USDHHS, 1995)

Another benefit of complex carbohydrates, especially whole grains and cereals, is that they are often a rich source of vitamins, minerals, and fiber. With the exception of vitamin B_{12}, which is found only in animal products or fortified foods, *whole grains* provide significant amounts of the B vitamins, several minerals, protein, and fiber. *Refined grains* are whole grains with most of the germ and bran removed; consequently, they are still high in complex carbohydrates, but many nutrients and fiber are lost (see display, Low Fiber/High Fiber). The Food and Drug Administration (FDA) has set minimum levels of iron, thiamine, riboflavin, and niacin to be attained by product enrichment; however, the other vitamins, minerals, and fiber that are removed during refining are not replaced. Although enrichment is credited with virtually eliminating once-common thiamine-, riboflavin-, and niacin-deficiency diseases, enriched products are not nutritionally equivalent to their whole grain counterparts (Table 1-9).

BENEFITS OF INCREASING FIBER INTAKE

Many leading health organizations urge Americans to increase their intake of fiber by eating whole grain breads and cereals, and greater quantities of fruits and vegetables. Potential benefits include the following:

The prevention or relief of constipation. Insoluble fibers draw water into the gut, which increases fecal bulk, stimulates peristalsis, and reduces transit time (see Chapter 16). The related decrease in pressure within the intestinal lumen may help prevent or alleviate both diverticular disease and hemorrhoids.

Low Fiber/High Fiber

Low Fiber "Refined"	Moderate Fiber "Whole grain"	High Fiber "Bran"
WHEAT		
White flour	Whole wheat flour	Wheat bran
Pasta	Whole wheat pasta	
Cream of Wheat	Shredded Wheat cereal	
OAT		
Oat flour	Oatmeal	Oat bran
	Rolled oats	
CORN		
Cornstarch	Cornmeal	Corn bran
Cornflakes		
RICE		
White rice	Brown rice	Rice bran
Rice Krispies		

Table 1-9

Nutritional Comparison Between Whole Wheat and Enriched White Bread (per slice)

	Whole Wheat Bread	Enriched White Bread
CHO (g)	11.4	11.7
Protein (g)	2.4	2.0
Fat (g)	1.1	0.9
Fiber (g)	1.6	<1.0
NUTRIENTS ENRICHED BY LAW		
Iron (mg)	0.86	0.68
Thiamine (mg)	0.09	0.11
Riboflavin (mg)	0.05	0.07
Niacin (mg)	1.0	0.9
NUTRIENTS NOT REPLACED WITH ENRICHMENT		
Vitamin B_6 (µg)	0.05	0.01
Folacin, total (µg)	14	8
Pantothenic acid (mg)	0.18	0.10
Calcium (mg)	18	30
Magnesium (mg)	23	5
Potassium (mg)	44	27
Zinc (mg)	0.40	0.15

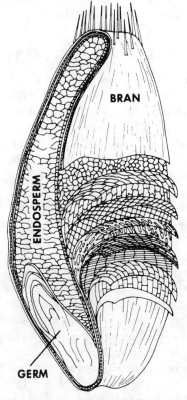

Endosperm . . . about 83% of the kernel
Source of white flour. Of the nutrients in the whole kernel the endosperm contains about

- 70–75% of the protein
- 43% of the pantothenic acid
- 32% of the riboflavin   } B-complex vitamins
- 12% of the niacin
- 6% of the pyridoxine
- 3% of the thiamine

Enriched flour products contain added quantities of riboflavin, niacin, and thiamine, plus iron, in amounts equal to or exceeding whole wheat—according to a formula established on the basis of popular need of those nutrients.

Bran . . . about 14½% of the kernel
Included in whole wheat flour. Of the nutrients in whole wheat, the bran, in addition to indigestible cellulose material contains about

86% of the niacin	42% of the riboflavin
73% of the pyridoxine	33% of the thiamine
50% of the pantothenic acid	19% of the protein

Germ . . . about 2½% of the kernel
The embryo or sprouting section of the seed, usually separated because it contains fat, which limits the keeping quality of flours. Available separately as human food.
Of the nutrients in whole wheat, the germ contains about:

64% of the thiamine	8% of the protein
26% of the riboflavin	7% of the pantothenic acid
21% of the pyridoxine	2% of the niacin

From Pennington, J.A.T.: Bowes and Church's Food Values of Portions Commonly Used, 16th ed. Philadelphia: JB Lippincott, 1993.

A decrease in serum cholesterol levels. By one or more poorly understood mechanisms, soluble fiber lowers serum cholesterol levels, which corresponds to a lower risk of coronary heart disease.

A reduction in fasting blood glucose levels and decreased insulin requirements in diabetics.

A decreased risk of colon cancer. However, both animal and epidemiologic studies have yielded inconsistent results. Further research is needed to determine the relationship between fiber and cancer.

Facilitation of weight reduction. Fiber delays gastric emptying time and provides a feeling of fullness, or satiety. Studies have shown that eating a high-fiber breakfast causes people to eat fewer calories for lunch. Fiber can also help control weight by displacing calorie-dense foods. For instance, when a high-fiber cereal is chosen over bacon and eggs, fiber intake increases at the expense of fat and cholesterol intake.

A reduced incidence of dental caries when fiber replaces sugars in the diet. Fiber may also help clean the teeth.

Choose a Diet That is Moderate in Sugars

Moderation in sugar intake is recommended to maintain a nutritious diet and healthy weight, while minimizing the risks of dental caries.

POTENTIAL BENEFITS OF MODERATE SUGAR INTAKE

Fermentable carbohydrates (which include both sugars and starches) + susceptible teeth + oral bacteria = tooth decay from an increase in acid production

Bacteria that reside in the mouth can ferment carbohydrates, especially sugars, which produces an acid that eats away at tooth enamel, resulting in dental caries. Although sticky sweets have been viewed traditionally as the major culprit, experts now believe that frequency of CHO consumption and whether they are eaten alone or with meals is just as important, or perhaps more important, than their consistency (see Chapter 11 for more on diet and dental health).

Except for its contribution to dental caries, studies indicate that there is no health hazard to the general public from sugar at the current level of consumption (IFIC, 1995c). In fact, there appears to be an inverse relationship between sugar and fat intake: As sugar intake declines, fat intake rises. The potential risks from a high-fat diet exceed those associated with a diet that is high in sugar.

In theory, high-sugar foods may displace the intake of other foods that are nutrient dense. Sugars are called *empty calories* because they provide few or no nutrients other than calories. The more empty calories in the diet, the harder it is to eat a nutritionally adequate diet without exceeding calorie requirements. For instance, a child who eats half of his or her daily calorie requirement in the form of high-sugar foods (which is common) has relatively few calories remaining to meet all requirements for essential nutrients like protein, vitamins, and minerals. The child may, therefore, not meet his or her nutritional requirements, or may have to exceed calorie requirements to consume enough nutrients. However, limiting sugar intake alone does not guarantee a nutritionally adequate diet, nor does high sugar intake necessarily indicate a poor diet (IFIC, 1995c).

Despite popular misconceptions, sugar consumption is not an independent risk factor for any particular disease, including obesity, impaired glucose tolerance, diabetes mellitus, or heart disease (ADA, 1993a). Nor is there evidence that sugar or other sweeteners are related to behavioral changes. Sugars are toxic only to the few people who have genetic abnormalities of CHO metabolism, such as galactosemia and hereditary fructose intolerance (Glinsmann and Park, 1995).

Obesity is caused by excessive calorie intake; it is not necessary that the excess calories be consumed in the form of sugars for obesity to occur. People can become obese by eating too much "good" food as well as too much "junk" food. Studies indicate that overweight people do not eat more sugar than thin people, and may even eat less, although sugar intake may decline after obesity is established.

Type II diabetes, commonly called *sugar diabetes*, also is related to an excessive calorie intake, not to an overconsumption of sweets. People who have diabetes have been treated traditionally with low-sugar diets, based on the premise that simple CHO raise blood glucose levels too rapidly and too high. Research indicates, however, that some simple sugars actually may have less of an effect on blood glucose levels than some sources of complex CHO, and that the amount of protein and fat in the meal (both of which slow the rise in blood glucose levels) may be as important as the form of CHO eaten. Because of this, as was pointed out earlier in the Chapter, controlled amounts of sugar are now allowed in the diets of most diabetics (see Chapter 18 for more information on diabetes).

Heart disease has been shown to be clearly related to diets that are high in total calories, fat, and cholesterol. No relationship between sugar intake and heart disease is apparent.

Hyperactivity in children is blamed frequently on sugar. However, sucrose does not cause aggressive behavior in children, nor does it negatively influence mental performance (IFIC, 1995c) (see Chapter 11 for additional discussion of hyperactivity).

ALCOHOL, A CARBOHYDRATE DERIVATIVE

Ethyl alcohol (ethanol) is produced from the fermentation of CHO (glucose) by the enzymes in yeast. Other than providing 7 cal/g, or 5.6 cal/ml, alcohol has no nutritional value and therefore is not considered a nutrient.

Absorption, Metabolism, and Utilization

Alcohol is absorbed rapidly and completely from the stomach and small intestine. The presence of food in the stomach slows the rate of alcohol absorption from the stomach but does not decrease the rate of absorption from the small intestine. Because it is water soluble, alcohol is evenly dispersed throughout the body fluids. The greater the water content of a tissue, the greater the concentration of alcohol (ie, a large amount of absorbed alcohol is found in the blood, whereas very little is present in bone and adipose tissue).

About 10% of absorbed alcohol is excreted in the urine and expired through exhalations; the remaining 90% is oxidized by the liver at a fixed rate of about 10 ml/hour. Exercise, food, caffeine, vitamin supplements, and cold showers do not increase the rate of alcohol metabolism.

In the liver, several enzyme systems work to oxidize alcohol into acetyl-CoA, a form of energy that all tissues and muscles use. Skeletal muscles cannot initiate the metabolism of alcohol because they lack the necessary enzymes.

The liver preferentially oxidizes alcohol over glucose and fatty acids until alcohol is removed from the circulation. Because glucose and fatty acids are spared, alcohol can contribute to a positive calorie balance (see Table 1-10 for the calorie content of selected alcoholic beverages).

Alcohol abuse can lead to multiple nutritional deficiencies by several different mechanisms. Most obvious is that food intake may be inadequate—alcoholics may consume up to 50% of their calories in the form of alcohol. In addition, alcohol intake can interfere with eating by altering the senses of taste and smell, and by caus-

Table 1-10
Alcoholic Beverages: Calorie, CHO, and Alcohol Content

Beverage	Serving Size	Calories	CHO (g)	Alcohol (g)
DISTILLED LIQUORS				
Gin, rum, vodka, whisky (rye/scotch)				
94 proof	1½ oz	116	0	16.7
100 proof	1½ oz	124	0	17.9
WINES				
Table, red	3.5 oz	72	1.4	9.6
Table, rose	3.5 oz	73	1.5	9.6
Table, white	3.5 oz	70	0.8	9.6
MALT LIQUORS (AMERICAN)				
Ale	12 oz	157	11.1	15.5
Beer, light	12 oz	100	4.8	11.3
Beer	12 oz	146	13.2	12.8
COCKTAILS				
Daiquiri	1 cocktail	111	4.1	13.9
Manhattan	1 cocktail	128	1.8	17.4
Martini	1 cocktail	156	0.2	22.4
Pina colada	4.5 oz	262	39.9	14.0
Screwdriver	7 oz	174	18.4	14.1
Tequila sunrise	5.5 oz	189	14.7	18.7
Tom Collins	7.5 oz	121	3.0	16.0
Whiskey sour	3 oz	123	5.0	15.1

From Pennington, J.A.T., Church, H.N.: Bowes and Church's Food Values of Portions Commonly Used, 16th ed. Philadelphia: JB Lippincott, 1993.

ing gastrointestinal upset. Nutrients that are consumed may be less well absorbed because of the toxic effect of alcohol on the intestinal mucosa. The metabolism of alcohol requires the use of nutrients, especially the B vitamins; nutrients that are "wasted" on the metabolism of alcohol cannot be used to perform other necessary metabolic functions. Finally, alcohol can alter nutrient metabolism by decreasing storage, increasing nutrient catabolism, and increasing nutrient excretion.

Chronic alcohol abuse can affect every organ system of the body, especially the nervous system (polyneuritis, Wernicke-Korsakoff syndrome) and the liver (fatty liver → hepatitis → cirrhosis; see Chapter 16).

KEY CONCEPTS

- Carbohydrates (CHO), found almost exclusively in plants, provide the major source of energy in almost all human diets.
- Simple carbohydrates (sugars) and complex carbohydrates (polysaccharides) are the two major types of carbohydrates (CHO).
- Monosaccharides and disaccharides are simple sugars composed of one or two sugar molecules, respectively. Simple sugars vary in their sweetness.
- Polysaccharides, namely, starch, dextrin, glycogen, cellulose, and other fibers, are made of 10 or more glucose molecules. They are not sweet.
- Fiber, the portion of plant cell walls that is resistant to digestion, is commonly classified as either water soluble or water insoluble; each has different physiologic effects.
- The major functions of CHO are to provide energy, spare protein, and prevent ketosis.
- CHO are digested more quickly and completely than protein and fat. Diets high in fiber are less well digested.
- The end products of CHO digestion are monosaccharides. Monosaccharides consumed in the diet do not undergo digestion before being absorbed.
- Because the body can make glucose from amino acids (protein) and glycerol (fat), an RDA has not been established. Most experts recommend CHO provide 50% to 60% of total calories consumed, with an emphasis on complex CHO.
- Americans are eating less sucrose (sugar) as the use of corn sweeteners (high fructose corn sweeteners) increases. Although sugars, as well as other CHO, contribute to dental decay, no other health hazards exist for the general public at current levels of sugar intake.
- Alcohol is a CHO derivative produced by the fermentation of glucose. It supplies calories but has no other nutritional value.
- Alcohol is metabolized in the liver at a fixed rate that is not influenced by exercise, caffeine, or a cold shower.
- Alcohol abuse has profound effect on nutritional status by altering nutrient intake, absorption, metabolism, storage, and excretion.

REFERENCES

American Diabetes Association, American Dietetic Association (1995). Exchange Lists for Meal Planning.

American Dietetic Association (1993a). Position of The American Dietetic Association: Use of nutritive and non-nutritive sweeteners. J Am Diet Assoc, 93(7), 816–820.

American Dietetic Association (1993b). Position of The American Dietetic Association: Health implications of dietary fiber. J Am Diet Assoc, 93(12), 1446–1447.

Anderson, J., Smith, B., and Gustafson, N. (1994). Health benefits and practical aspects of high-fiber diets. Am J Clin Nutr, 59(suppl), 1242S–1247S.

Centers for Disease Control and Prevention/National Center for Health Statistics (1994). Advance Data. Energy and macronutrient intakes of persons ages 2 months and over in the United States: Third National Health and Nutrition Examination Survey, Phase 1, 1988–1991. DHHS Publication No. (PHS) 95-1250.

Gibney, M., Sigman-Grant, M., Stanton, J., and Keast, D. (1995). Consumption of sugars. Am J Clin Nutr, 62(suppl), 178–194S.

Glinsmann, W. and Park, Y. (1995). Perspective on the 1986 Food and Drug Administration assessment of the safety of carbohydrate sweeteners: Uniform definitions and recommendations for future assessments. Am J Clin Nutr, 62(suppl), 161S–169S.

International Food Information Council (1995a). Carbohydrates. Fueling up. Food Insight, Jan/Feb, 1, 4.

International Food Information Council (1995b). Spotlight on fructose. Food Insight, Jan/Feb, 5.

International Food Information Council (1995c). Sweet facts about sugars and health. IFIC Review, August.

Morgan, K (ed) (1994). Carbohydrates and the Food Guide Pyramid. Nutrition Update, Summer, 2–4.

National Research Council (1989). Recommended Dietary Allowances (10th ed). Washington, DC: National Academy Press.

United States Department of Agriculture, United States Department of Health and Human Services (1995). Nutrition and Your Health: Dietary Guidelines for Americans (4th ed). Home and Garden Bulletin No. 232.

United States Department of Health and Human Services (1988). The Surgeon General's Report on Nutrition and Health: Summary and Recommendations. DHHS (PHS) Publication No. 88-50211.

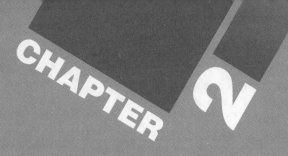

CHAPTER 2

Protein

Chapter Outline

Key Terms

Anabolism
Biologic value
Catabolism
Complementary proteins
Complete proteins
Conjugated proteins
Essential amino acids
High biologic value (HBV)
Incomplete proteins

Kwashiorkor
Lacto-ovo vegetarian
Lacto-vegetarian
Limiting amino acid
Metabolic pool
Negative nitrogen balance
Net protein utilization
Nitrogen balance
Nitrogen equilibrium

Nonessential amino acids
Positive nitrogen balance
Proteases
Proteins
Simple proteins
Turnover
Vegans

*I*n Greek, *protein* means "to take first place," and indeed, life could not exist without protein. Protein is a component of every living cell: plant, animal, and even microorganism. The human body contains more than a thousand different proteins, which carry out a variety of essential functions. In the adult, protein accounts for 20% of total weight. Almost half of the body's protein is in muscle, one fifth in bone and cartilage, one tenth in skin, and the rest in other tissues and body fluids. With the exception of bile and urine, every tissue and fluid in the body contains some protein.

COMPOSITION AND STRUCTURE

Proteins are large, complex molecules composed of at least 100 individual chemical building blocks known as amino acids (Fig. 2-1). Like carbohydrates and fats, amino acids contain carbon, hydrogen, and oxygen atoms. Protein also contains 16% nitrogen, which distinguishes it from the other energy nutrients. Because amino acids contain both a basic amino group (NH_2) and an acidic carboxylic group (COOH) attached to a carbon atom, they can act as buffers to neutralize either acids or bases.

The body needs amino acids, and not protein *per se*, to build its own proteins. Of the 22 known amino acids, 9 must be supplied in the diet because they cannot be synthesized in the body. These are known as indispensable or **essential amino acids**. The remaining amino acids are no less important, but because they can be manufactured in the body from nitrogen and carbohydrate or fat, they are **nonessential amino acids**, or dispensable, in terms of dietary intake (Table 2-1).

Just as the 26 letters of the alphabet can be arranged to make an almost infinite number of words, the amino acids can be joined together by peptide bonds to form a virtually limitless variety of proteins. Based on their composition, proteins in the body may be classified as **simple** (proteins composed only of amino acids or their deriva-

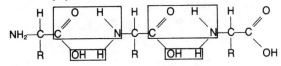

Generic amino acid

C: carbon stem
H: hydrogen
NH_2: basic amino group
COOH: acid carboxylic group
R: radical group, the chemical variable that distinguishes one amino acid from another

Generic peptide chain

COHN: peptide bond
H_2O: water formed from the peptide bond

Figure 2-1
Amino acid and peptide structures.

Table 2-1
Amino Acids

Essential	Nonessential
Histidine	Alanine
Isoleucine	Arginine
Leucine	Asparagine
Lysine	Aspartic acid
Methionine	Cystine (cysteine)
Phenylalanine	Glutamic acid
Threonine	Glutamine
Tryptophan	Glycine
Valine	Hydroxyproline
	Hydroxylysine
	Proline
	Serine
	Tyrosine

tives) or **conjugated** (simple proteins combined with a nonprotein substance) (Tables 2-2a and 2-2b). The wide variations in physical characteristics and functions among different types of protein are related to differences in any of the following factors:

- The total number of amino acids contained in the protein
- The particular amino acids that are present in the protein molecule and how frequently they occur
- The order in which the amino acids are joined
- The actual shape of the protein molecule; that is, whether it is coiled, folded, or straight

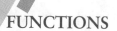

FUNCTIONS

The major function of protein in the diet is to supply adequate amounts and proportions of amino acids for the synthesis of body proteins.

In the body, proteins are used to repair body tissues that break down from normal "wear and tear," to support growth through the synthesis of new tissues, and to

Table 2-2A
Simple Proteins

Example	Occurrence
Albumin	Plasma protein
Insulin	Hormone produced by the pancreas
Histones	Cell nuclei
Globulins	Myosin, a muscle protein

Table 2-2B
Conjugated Proteins

Type	Example	Composition
Nucleoproteins	DNA (deoxyribonucleic acid) in cell nuclei	Protein + nucleic acid
Glycoproteins, mucoproteins	Mucin in mucous membrane secretions	Protein + CHO
Phosphoproteins	Casein in milk	Protein + phosphorus-containing substances other than phospholipid or nucleic acids
Chromoproteins	Hemoglobin	Protein + a nonprotein pigment
Lipoproteins	HDL (high-density lipoproteins)	Protein + a triglyceride or other lipid
Metalloproteins	Ferritin, the storage form of iron	Protein + a metal

provide a framework for the body. Bones, muscles, tendons, blood vessels, skin, hair, and nails are all protein-containing structures.

Protein is also used to synthesize many essential body secretions and fluids, such as hormones (eg, insulin, thyroxine, and epinephrine), plasma proteins (eg, albumin, hemoglobin), neurotransmitters (eg, serotonin, acetylcholine), all enzymes, breast milk, mucus, sperm, bile acids, and histamine. Antibodies (immunoglobins), which help the body resist infection and disease, are also made from protein.

Protein is included in numerous body compounds such as opsin, the light-sensitive visual pigment in the eye, and thrombin, a protein necessary for normal blood clotting.

Specific amino acids have specific functions within the body. For instance, tryptophan is a precursor of the vitamin niacin, and tyrosine is the precursor of melanin, the pigment that colors hair and skin.

Protein has a role in regulating fluid balance by maintaining oncotic pressure. Plasma proteins, particularly albumin, help maintain proper water balance between the bloodstream and the fluid surrounding the blood vessel. A decrease in serum albumin leads to edema. Protein also helps regulate acid–base balance by buffering excess acids or bases, and works to detoxify harmful foreign substances.

Another function of protein is to transport other substances through the blood. For instance, lipoproteins transport triglycerides, cholesterol, phospholipids, and the fat-soluble vitamins; transferrin transports iron; protein-bound iodine transports iodine; and albumin transports free fatty acids, bilirubin, and many drugs.

Protein also can be oxidized to provide energy. Like CHO, protein supplies 4 cal/g. However, using protein for energy is a physiologic and economic waste, because when amino acids are used for energy, they cannot be used to synthesize protein, a function unique to amino acids. Protein oxidation is most likely to occur when protein is consumed in excess of need or when protein intake is of poor quality (ie, one or more essential amino acids are present in inadequate amounts), and is therefore unable to support protein synthesis. When this occurs, amino acids that are present in the body can be used only for energy. In addition, whenever protein-sparing calorie intake from carbohydrates is inadequate, protein is converted to energy to meet the body's calorie requirements.

Another disadvantage of using protein for energy is that proteins are not as efficiently and completely burned for energy as carbohydrates. The nitrogenous wastes resulting from protein metabolism burden the kidneys and require energy for excretion. Protein is also more expensive to buy than CHO, and rich sources of protein are often high in fat.

Before amino acids can be used for energy, the amino group (NH_2) must be removed from the carbon stem (see Fig. 2-1). Although the amino group may be used to synthesize other compounds, most of it is converted to urea in the liver and then excreted in the urine. After the amino group is removed, the body can convert the remaining carbon stem to an intermediate to be used by the peripheral tissues for immediate energy. It can also be converted to glucose or fat and used for immediate energy, or converted to fat and stored in adipose tissue.

SOURCES OF PROTEIN

According to the American Diabetic Association and American Dietetic Association exchange lists, protein is found in milk, vegetables, meats, and starches (Table 2-3). Fruits contain only trace amounts of protein, and pure fats (eg, oils, butter, shortening, and so forth) contain none.

CLASSIFICATION OF FOOD PROTEINS

With the exception of gelatin, all dietary proteins contain some of each of the known amino acids. Because different proteins have different amounts, types, and ratios of amino acids, they are not all equal in terms of quality. Although most sources of protein in the diet contain all the essential amino acids, they may not all be present in adequate amounts to meet the body's needs.

Complete Proteins

Based on the relative quantities of amino acids present, dietary proteins can be classified as **complete proteins**, or high-quality proteins, if they provide all the essential amino acids in adequate amounts and proportions needed by the body for growth and tissue maintenance. With the exception of gelatin, all animal sources of protein (meat, fish, poultry, eggs, and dairy products) are complete proteins.

Incomplete Proteins

Dietary proteins can be classified as **incomplete proteins**, or low-quality proteins, if they are deficient in one or more essential amino acids. The essential amino acid present in the smallest amount is known as the **"limiting amino acid"** because it limits protein synthesis to the extent of its availability. Once it is used up, protein synthesis cannot continue, and the remaining amino acids are broken down and wasted as a source of energy.

Table 2-3
Sources of Protein Based on the American Diabetic Association/American Dietetic Association Exchange Lists

Group	Serving Size	CHO (g)	Protein (g)	Fat (g)	Calories
EXCHANGE LISTS CONTAINING COMPLETE PROTEIN					
Meat					
Very lean	1 oz	—	7	0–1	35
Lean	1 oz	0	7	3	55
Medium-fat	1 oz	0	7	5	75
High-fat	1 oz	0	7	8	100
Milk					
Skim	1 cup	12	8	0–3	90
Low-fat	1 cup	12	8	5	120
Whole	1 cup	12	8	8	150
EXCHANGE LISTS CONTAINING INCOMPLETE PROTEIN					
Starch		15	3	1 or less	80
Examples:					
Bread	1 slice				
Cereal, cooked	½ cup				
Most ready-to-eat					
unsweetened cereal, dry	¾ cup				
Starchy vegetable, pasta	½ cup				
Rice	⅓ cup				
Vegetable	½ cup cooked or 1 cup raw	5	2	0	25
EXCHANGE LISTS CONTAINING NO PROTEIN					
Fruit	Varies	15	0	0	60
Fat	Varies	0	0	5	45

Plant proteins (legumes, grains, nuts, and seeds) are incomplete proteins when they are eaten alone. However, because different plant proteins lack different essential amino acids, they can be combined in certain ways, or "complemented," to provide sufficient quantities and proportions of all the essential amino acids (Table 2-4). Over the course of a day, different **complementary proteins** provide adequate amounts of all essential amino acids to support protein synthesis. Another method of complementing proteins is to consume a small amount of a complete protein with an incomplete protein. Because complete proteins supply adequate amounts of all the essential amino acids, any complete protein (ie, milk, eggs, and meat) may be used to complement any plant protein.

EVALUATING PROTEIN QUALITY

The terms *complete* and *incomplete* are nonspecific with regard to actual protein quality. For instance, even though eggs and meat are both complete proteins, they differ in their relative amino acid composition and pattern, as well as in their

Table 2-4
Complementary Proteins

Food Group	Limiting Amino Acids	Abundant Amino Acids	Complementary Proteins

Grains	Lysine
	Isoleucine
	Threonine
		Methionine
		Tryptophan
			Grains + legumes
			  Rice + Kidney beans
			  Rice + soybeans
			  Brown bread + baked beans
			  Wheat bread + peanut butter*
			  Corn tortillas + black bean soup
			  Toast + pea soup
			  Rice + lentil curry
			Grains + milk products
			  Bread pudding
			  Rice pudding
			  Cereal + milk
			  Cheese sandwich
			  Macaroni + cheese
			  Rice + cheese

Legumes	Methionine
	Tryptophan
		Lysine
		Threonine
		Isoleucine
			Legumes + grains (see above)
			Legumes + milk products
			  Lentils + cheese
			  Garbanzo beans + cheese
			  Bean soup + milk

Nuts, seeds	Lysine
	Isoleucine
		Methionine
		Tryptophan
			Nuts (seeds) + legumes
			  Sesame seeds + black-eyed peas
			  Sesame seeds + bean soups or
			    casseroles
			Nuts (seeds) + milk products
			  Sesame seeds + milk
			  Sunflower seeds + cheese

Vegetables	Methionine
	Isoleucine
		Lysine
		Tryptophan
			Vegetables + milk products
			  Broccoli + cheese
			  Cream of cauliflower soup
			  Corn pudding

* Peanuts are actually legumes.

digestibility. Such factors influence the extent to which proteins can be used by the body for tissue maintenance and growth. The next sections discuss more specific measurements of protein quality (Table 2-5).

Biologic Value

Biologic value refers to the percentage of absorbed nitrogen that is retained by the body; the higher the proportion of nitrogen supplied by the essential amino acids, the higher the biologic value (BV) of that food. Proteins with biologic values greater than 70% are considered to be **high–biologic value (HBV) proteins** and are able to support growth if calorie needs are met. Generally, complete proteins have a high biologic value and incomplete proteins have a low biologic value.

Table 2-5
Measurements of Protein Quality

Protein Source	Biologic Value (BV) (%)	Net Protein Utilization (NPU) (%)	Protein Efficiency Ratio (PER)
Egg	100	94	3.92
Cow's milk	93	82	3.09
Wheat germ	75	71	2.90
Fish	75	—	3.55
Beef	75	67	2.30
Soybeans	73	61	2.32
Corn	72	36	—
Whole wheat	65	49	1.53
Oats	65	—	2.19
Peas	64	55	1.57
Polished rice	64	57	2.18
Sesame seeds	62	53	1.77
Peanuts	55	55	1.65

From Williams, S.R.: Nutrition and Diet Therapy, 5th ed. St Louis: Times Mirror/Mosby, 1985.

Net Protein Utilization (NPU)

Net protein utilization is the amount of protein that is actually available for the body to use; therefore, it is a more useful measurement than biologic value. It differs from biologic value in that the digestibility of a protein is considered. That is, the biologic value and NPU are the same for proteins that are completely digested; proteins that are less well digested have NPU values that are lower than the biologic value.

Protein Efficiency Ratio (PER)

Protein efficiency ratio is the measure of grams of body weight gained by a test animal per gram of protein food eaten in an adequate diet over a specific test period.

HOW THE BODY HANDLES PROTEIN

Digestion

Chemical digestion of protein begins in the stomach, where HCl converts pepsinogen to the active enzyme pepsin (Fig. 2-2). Pepsin breaks down protein into smaller units called polypeptides.

The principal site of protein digestion is the small intestine, where protein hydrolysis continues under the action of pancreatic **proteases** (a generic term for enzymes that break down protein).

Mouth:

Stomach:

Small intestine:
   Pancreatic proteases:

Intestinal wall secretions:

End products for absorption:

Dietary Protein
↓
Pepsin
↓
Polypeptides
↓
Trypsin, chymotrypsin, carboxypeptidase
↓
Polypeptides, dipeptides, amino acids
↓
Aminopeptidase
↓
Dipeptides, amino acids
↓
Dipeptidase
↓
Amino acids

Figure 2-2
Protein digestion.

Three major proteases (trypsin, chymotrypsin, carboxypeptidases) break down peptones into polypeptides, dipeptides, and free amino acids.

Two more proteases (aminopeptidase, dipeptidase), which are secreted by glands in the intestinal wall, complete the breakdown of protein into free amino acids.

Absorption

Free amino acids are absorbed through the mucosa of the small intestine by active transport, which is an energy-requiring process. Amino acid absorption also requires vitamin B_6 and the mineral manganese. Once absorbed, amino acids are transported through the portal blood circulation to the liver. Some dipeptides may be absorbed and may enter the portal bloodstream.

Newborns are able to absorb whole proteins. This allows breast-fed infants to absorb the protein antibodies in colostrum, thus receiving immunity from the mother.

Some amino acids remain in the intestinal mucosa, where they are used to synthesize intestinal enzymes and new intestinal cells.

Normally, only about 1% of ingested protein is excreted in the feces. Although urine contains nitrogenous wastes that are derived from protein metabolism, it normally is protein free.

Metabolism

In the liver, amino acids may be used to synthesize specific proteins, that is, to make liver cells, nonessential amino acids, or specialized proteins such as plasma albumin.

The liver also releases amino acids into the bloodstream for transport to tissues and cells where protein synthesis can occur. If amino acids are needed for energy, or if amino acids are consumed in excess of protein need, they are metabolized (after the nitrogen is removed) to produce energy. Amino acids that are not needed for protein synthesis or energy can be converted to fat and stored.

PROTEIN SYNTHESIS

Like all body constituents, body proteins are in a constant state of flux. New proteins are continuously synthesized (**anabolism**) to replace old proteins that break down (**catabolism**) from normal "wear and tear." Red blood cells, for example, are broken down and replaced every 60 to 120 days, and gastrointestinal cells are replaced every 2 to 3 days. Enzymes that are used in the digestion of food are continuously replenished. The synthesis of new proteins also occurs during periods of tissue growth and development—pregnancy and lactation, infancy, childhood, and adolescence.

The arrangement of amino acids for each particular type of protein is determined by the genetic code located within each cell nucleus.

The amino acids that are needed for protein synthesis may come either from dietary proteins (exogenous) or from the catabolism of tissue protein (endogenous). Following an "all or none" rule, protein synthesis proceeds only when all the needed amino acids are present simultaneously and in the proper ratio or pattern. When the supply of the limiting amino acid is used up, the remaining amino acids cannot be used to build proteins; thus, they are broken down for energy.

PROTEIN CATABOLISM

Catabolism, the opposite reaction of anabolism, is the ongoing process of breaking down old, worn-out tissues. Normal catabolism occurs regardless of the amount of protein in the diet; however, a low-calorie or low-protein diet, as well as certain diseases, trauma, and stress, can accelerate protein catabolism.

METABOLIC POOL

Amino acids, which are obtained from either protein digestion or tissue catabolism, are used to synthesize new proteins. Although the body cannot truly store excess amino acids for future use, a limited quantity of amino acids is available in a so-called **metabolic pool**. These amino acids exist in a dynamic state of equilibrium because of the constant buildup and breakdown of body tissues.

Turnover refers to the cycle of anabolism and catabolism of body proteins. Although the body cannot store amino acids as protein, it can use tissue proteins to supply amino acids during a time of need. For instance, the turnover of proteins in the liver, pancreas, and small intestine is rapid, and during starvation, these tissues supply amino acids for protein synthesis or energy. The turnover of muscle proteins is slower, but because muscle mass is so large, a considerable quantity of amino acids is derived from muscle during starvation. The turnover in the brain and nervous system is negligible.

NITROGEN BALANCE

Nitrogen balance is a measure of the degree of both protein anabolism and catabolism. Although protein synthesis and breakdown occur simultaneously and continuously within every cell, the net effect of these processes determines the state of nitrogen balance. Hormones that influence protein metabolism are outlined in Table 2-6.

Nitrogen Intake

Protein, the only energy nutrient that contains nitrogen, is approximately 16% nitrogen by weight. Therefore, 1 g of nitrogen equals 6.25 g of protein. Nitrogen intake can be determined by dividing the grams of protein consumed by 6.25.

Nitrogen Excretion

Nitrogen is lost continuously through the urine (urine–urea nitrogen), feces, hair, nails, and skin. To account for the nitrogen that is lost in the feces, hair, nails, and skin, a coefficient of 4 is usually added to the amount of urea collected in a 24-hour urine sample.

States of Nitrogen Balance

NITROGEN EQUILIBRIUM

Nitrogen equilibrium exists when nitrogen intake equals nitrogen excretion, which indicates that protein buildup is occurring at approximately the same rate as protein breakdown (Fig. 2-3). Healthy adults who consume a diet that is adequate in calories and all the essential amino acids are in a state of nitrogen equilibrium.

Table 2-6
Hormonal Influences on Protein Metabolism

ANABOLIC HORMONES
(Stimulate Protein Synthesis)
Growth hormone (GH)
Insulin
Testosterone (stimulates protein synthesis during growth only)
Thyroxine (in normal amounts; excess thyroxine stimulates protein catabolism)

CATABOLIC HORMONES
(Stimulate Protein Breakdown)
Glucocorticoids

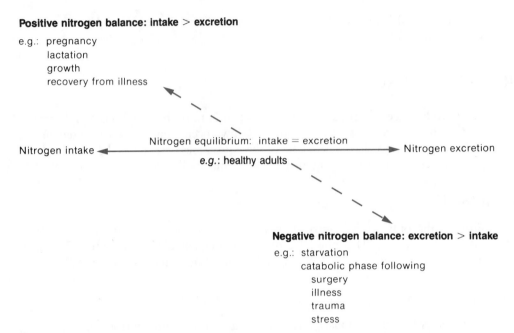

Positive nitrogen balance: intake > excretion

e.g.: pregnancy
        lactation
        growth
        recovery from illness

Nitrogen intake ◄————————— Nitrogen equilibrium: intake = excretion —————————► Nitrogen excretion
                                    e.g.: healthy adults

Negative nitrogen balance: excretion > intake

e.g.: starvation
        catabolic phase following
          surgery
          illness
          trauma
          stress

Figure 2-3
States of nitrogen balance.

POSITIVE NITROGEN BALANCE (NITROGEN INTAKE > NITROGEN EXCRETION)

A **positive nitrogen balance** results when the rate of tissue synthesis exceeds the rate of tissue breakdown, reflecting the growth of tissue. This occurs during periods of rapid growth, such as during infancy, childhood, adolescence, pregnancy, and lactation (if the protein content of the breast milk is considered). A positive nitrogen balance also occurs during the anabolic or recovery phase after surgery, burns, trauma, and stress, when tissue is being replaced.

NEGATIVE NITROGEN BALANCE (NITROGEN EXCRETION > NITROGEN INTAKE)

A negative nitrogen balance occurs when the rate of tissue breakdown exceeds the rate of tissue synthesis, reflecting body wasting and the loss of body protein. This is an undesirable state and is most likely to occur during any of the following:

- Periods of inadequate calorie and protein intake, resulting in the use of dietary and tissue protein for energy
- Starvation, infection, prolonged immobility, and stress
- Catabolic phase immediately after surgery and crush injuries

PROTEIN REQUIREMENTS
AND RECOMMENDATIONS

Nitrogen balance studies are used to determine amino acid requirements and minimum total protein needs. The estimated minimum level of protein that is required to maintain nitrogen equilibrium in the healthy adult is 0.6 g/kg of ideal body weight, if calorie needs are met (National Research Council, 1989). However, the recommended dietary allowance (RDA) is set substantially higher, at 0.8 g/kg/day for both sexes, to account for wide variations in need among individuals. These differences in need are related to numerous factors (Table 2-7). Another reason why the RDA is higher than the estimated minimum is because the average American diet, which consists of both animal and plant proteins, has a protein utilization efficiency of 75%.

The RDA for protein for various age groups and conditions are listed in Table 2-8. For any age, protein needs increase when calorie intake is inadequate or marginal, or when protein intake is of poor quality (eg, when there is a low percentage of net protein utilization, or when not all of the essential amino acids are supplied at the same time). Ideally, a high-quality protein or two complementary plant proteins should be consumed at every meal to supply the tissues adequately with all the essential amino acids needed for tissue synthesis. Table 2-9 lists conditions that may require adjustments in protein intake.

Most leading health organizations (eg, American Heart Association, American Diabetes Association) recommend that protein contribute 10% to 20% of total calorie intake.

Table 2-7
Factors Influencing Individual Protein Requirements

Factor	Effect on Protein Requirements
Body size	The greater the size and weight of the body, the greater the protein requirements.
Age	Protein requirements per unit of body weight decrease from infancy through adulthood; however, the elderly may require more protein than younger adults to maintain nitrogen equilibrium.
Sex	Although the RDA lists protein allowances for all adults at 0.8 g/kg of body weight, women actually need less protein than men of the same age and weight because of differences in body composition: Women have smaller muscle masses and a larger percentage of body fat.
Nutritional status	Undernutrition increases protein requirements.
Stress, infection, and heat	Emotional or physical stress, infection, and high environmental temperatures all increase nitrogen losses and therefore increase protein requirements.
Physical training	Physical training → increased muscle mass → increased protein requirements.

Table 2-8
RDA for Protein

Category	Age (years) or Condition	Weight (kg)	Recommended Dietary Allowance (g/kg)*	(g/day)
Both sexes	0–0.5[1]	6	2.2	13
	0.5–1	9	1.6	14
	1–3	13	1.2	16
	4–6	20	1.1	24
	7–10	28	1.0	28
Men	11–14	45	1.0	45
	15–18	66	0.9	59
	19–24	72	0.8	58
	25–50	79	0.8	63
	51+	77	0.8	63
Women	11–14	46	1.0	46
	15–18	55	0.8	44
	19–24	58	0.8	46
	25–50	63	0.8	50
	51+	65	0.8	50
Pregnancy	1st trimester			+10
	2nd trimester			+10
	3rd trimester			+10
Lactation	1st 6 months			+15
	2nd 6 months			+12

* Amino acid score of typical U.S. diet is 100 for all age groups, except young infants. Digestibility is equal to reference proteins. Values have been rounded upward to 0.1 g/kg.
Source: National Research Council.

Recommendations regarding protein intake, per se, are not addressed in the Fourth Edition of *Dietary Guidelines for Americans* (see Chapter 8). However, the Food Guide Pyramid, which is the tool devised to teach the Dietary Guidelines, recommends that Americans consume 2 to 3 servings daily (approximate total of 5–7 oz per day) from the Meat, Poultry, Fish, Dry Beans, Eggs, and Nuts Group, and generally 2 servings from the Milk, Yogurt, and Cheese Group (USDA, 1992). From both groups, lean or low-fat varieties are emphasized.

CONSUMPTION TRENDS IN THE UNITED STATES

According to data from the third National Health and Nutrition Examination Survey, Phase 1, 1988–1991, among adults 20 years of age and older, protein contributed 15.5% of total calories in the diet (CDC, 1994). Mean protein intakes were similar among different racial and ethnic groups at 88 to 92 g for men and 63 to 66 g in women. In men, protein intake was higher among adolescents and young adults and declined thereafter. Women showed a similar pattern, although intakes were

Table 2-9
Conditions Requiring Alterations in Protein Intake

Alteration	Indications
Increase total protein intake	Pregnancy and lactation
	Hypermetabolic conditions, such as burns, sepsis, and major trauma
	Protein-energy malnutrition
	Cancer cachexia
	Major surgery
	Peritoneal dialysis
	Multiple fractures
	Protein-losing renal diseases
	Hepatitis
	Malabsorption syndromes, including protein-losing enteropathy, short-bowel syndrome, inflammatory bowel diseases, and celiac disease
Maintain normal total protein intake but reduce or eliminate specific protein substances:	
Gluten-free diet	Celiac disease (see Chap. 16)
Low-phenylalanine diet	Phenylketonuria (see Chap. 11)
Low-purine diet	Gout (see Chap. 20)
Low-tyramine diet	People taking monoamine oxidase (MAO) inhibitors (see Appendix 5)
Decrease total protein intake	Chronic renal failure not treated with dialysis
	Cirrhosis of the liver with signs of impending coma

generally lower than those of men in the same age group. Although the percentage of calories from protein in the diet and the total amount of protein intake have remained fairly constant over the last 70 to 80 years, the source of protein has changed significantly. Today, approximately two thirds of protein intake is derived from animal sources, whereas plant and animal sources contributed almost equally to the total protein intake during 1909 to 1913. This change can be attributed to the increase in meat, poultry, and fish consumption and the decline in the intake of grain products: Meat is the largest contributor of protein in the diet for all age–sex groups (Fig. 2-4).

America's love of protein, especially meat, is centered around several common myths and attitudes, such as:

- Protein builds muscle. Although muscle tissue is composed of protein, protein consumed in excess of need is not magically converted to muscle. Instead, excess protein, like excess CHO or fat, is converted to and stored as body fat. The only way to increase the size of muscles is by repeated use of them.
- Protein is nonfattening. At 4 cal/g, pure protein is just as fattening, or nonfattening, as pure CHO. But pure protein does not exist in the diet: Protein foods also contain CHO (grains, vegetables, and milk) or fat (meat, whole and low-fat milk and milk products). Some supposedly high-protein foods actually provide more calories from fat than from protein (Table 2-10).

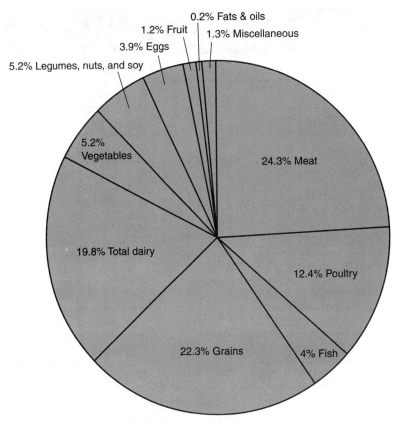

Figure 2-4
Protein contributed from major food groups to the U.S. food supply, 1990.

- Protein aids in weight reduction. It is true that high-protein, low-CHO diets promote weight loss, but rapid weight loss occurs largely because of water loss, not loss of fat. When CHO intake is inadequate to meet the body's energy requirements, protein is broken down and used for energy, resulting in the excretion of large amounts of water in order to rid the body of the nitrogenous wastes. The weight that is temporarily lost is regained when fluid balance is restored.
- Protein is a status food. Protein intake, namely the intake of meat, increases as income increases. Conversely, low meat intakes are associated with low socio-economic status.
- Meat intake is essential if the body is to get enough protein. Because the average American diet contains considerably more protein than the RDA, most Americans could completely eliminate meat, fish, and poultry from their diets and still meet their RDA for protein. In fact, studies show that even though lacto-ovo and strict vegetarians eat less protein than meat-eaters, they still eat more than the RDA. *Nutrients* are essential; *particular foods*, including meats, are not.

Table 2-10
The Percentage of Fat Calories in Selected Meat, Poultry, Milk, Cheese, and Eggs

Product (3 ounces, cooked, unless noted otherwise)	Calories from Fat (%)	Total Calories
BEEF		
Processed lunch meat, lean roast beef (2 oz)	39	70
Processed lunch meat, lean corned beef (2 oz)	37	80
Processed lunch meat, lean pastrami (2 oz)	37	80
Liver, braised	27	137
Eye of round, roasted, ⅛-in trim	40	171
Top round, broiled, ⅛-in trim	39	185
Tip round, roasted, ⅛-in trim	49	195
Meat loaf	53	197
Bottom round, braised, ⅛-in trim	53	230
Top sirloin, broiled, ⅛-in trim	54	222
Ground beef, extra lean, broiled medium	58	217
Corned beef, cured, brisket, cooked, ¼-in trim	68	213
Ground beef, lean, broiled medium	61	231
Bologna (about 2 slices)	83	170
Frankfurter, cured (about 1 frank, 5 in. long, ⅞ in around; 8 per 1-lb package)	81	173
Salami, cooked (3 oz is about 4 slices, 4 in around, ⅛ in thick)	71	216
Chuck, arm pot roast, braised, ⅛-in trim	63	277
Ground beef, regular, broiled medium	64	246
LAMB (ALL CUTS ARE TRIMMED TO 1/8 IN FAT EXCEPT GROUND LAMB)		
Leg, shank, roasted	47	186
Loin, broiled	63	255
Ground lamb, broiled	63	240
Shoulder, arm, braised	61	289
Rib, roasted	73	292
PORK (FRESH UNLESS NOTED OTHERWISE) (ALL CUTS ARE TRIMMED TO 1/4 IN FAT)		
Ham, cured, boneless, extra lean, roasted	34	123
Loin, tenderloin, roasted	31	147
Ham, cured, boneless, regular, roasted	46	151
Italian sausage, cooked (about ⅔ link; links packed 4 per lb)	72	177
Loin, center rib, rib chop, bone-in, broiled	53	223
Bratwurst, cooked (about ⅔ link; links packed 4 per 12-oz pkg)	78	164
Loin, sirloin (sirloin roasts), bone-in, roasted	55	222
Liver sausage, liverwurst (about 3¼ slices; slice is 2½ in diameter, ¼ in thick)	79	178
Knockwurst	82	261
Chitterlings, simmered	85	258
Bacon, cooked (broiled, pan fried, or roasted) (about 9 slices)	77	314
Spareribs, braised	69	338
Salami, dry or hard (3 oz is about 8½ slices; slice is 3⅛ in diameter, 1/16 in thick)	75	345

(continued)

Table 2-10 *(Continued)*
The Percentage of Fat Calories in Selected Meat, Poultry, Milk, Cheese, and Eggs

Product (3 ounces, cooked, unless noted otherwise)	Calories from Fat (%)	Total Calories
VEAL (ALL CUTS ARE TRIMMED TO 1/4 IN FAT)		
Shoulder, arm, roasted	40	156
Sirloin, roasted	47	171
Loin (chops), roasted	51	184
Rib roast, lean and fat, roasted	55	194
CHICKEN		
Processed lunch meat, lean chicken breast (2 oz)	25	59
Chicken, roasting, light meat without skin, roasted	24	130
Breast, without skin (3 oz is about 1/2)	20	140
Chicken roll, light meat, about 2 slices or 2 oz	42	87
Drumstick, without skin (3 oz is about 2)	30	146
Breast with skin (3 oz is about 1/2)	35	168
Chicken hot dog, about 1	68	142
Thigh, with skin (3 oz is about 1 1/2)	56	210
Wing, with skin (3 oz is about 2 1/2 wings)	60	247
TURKEY		
Breast, without skin	5	115
Ground turkey, breast meat only, cooked	20	130
Processed lunch meat, lean turkey breast (2 oz)	28	61
Breast, with skin	19	130
Wing, without skin	19	139
Processed lunch meat, lean turkey ham (2 oz)	43	75
Leg, without skin	21	135
Turkey roll, light meat, about 2 slices or 2 oz	44	81
Leg, with skin	29	145
Wing, with skin	43	176
Ground turkey, meat and skin, cooked	50	200
MILK (1 CUP UNLESS NOTED OTHERWISE)		
Skim milk	4	86
Buttermilk	20	99
Low-fat milk, 1% fat	22	102
Low-fat milk, 2% fat	34	121
Whole milk, 3.3% fat	48	150
YOGURT AND SOUR CREAM (1 CUP UNLESS OTHERWISE NOTED)		
Plain yogurt, nonfat	3	127
Yogurt, fruited, low fat	10	231
Plain yogurt, low-fat	21	144
Sour cream, imitation, 2 tbsp	85	35
Sour cream, 2 tbsp	87	52

(continued)

Table 2-10 (Continued)
The Percentage of Fat Calories in Selected Meat, Poultry, Milk, Cheese, and Eggs

Product (3 ounces, cooked, unless noted otherwise)	Calories from Fat (%)	Total Calories
CHEESE (1 OZ UNLESS NOTED OTHERWISE)		
Cottage cheese, low fat (1%), ½ c	13	82
Romano, grated, 1 tbsp	63	19
Parmesan, grated, 1 tbsp	59	23
Reduced fat and low-sodium cheese—American, cheddar, colby, monterey jack, muenster, or provolone	54	71
Mozzarella, part-skim	55	72
Reduced fat cheese—American, cheddar, colby, monterey jack, muenster, provolone, or string cheese	55	79
Ricotta, part-skim (¼ cup)	52	86
Cottage cheese, creamed, ½ c	38	117
Mozzarella	69	80
American processed cheese spread, pasteurized	66	82
Feta	72	75
Neufchatel	81	74
Camembert	73	85
American processed cheese food, pasteurized	68	93
Swiss	65	107
Monterey jack	73	106
Roquefort	75	105
American processed cheese, pasteurized	75	106
Colby	73	112
Cheddar	74	114
Cream cheese, 2 tbsp	90	101
EGGS AND EGG SUBSTITUTES		
Egg white	0	17
Egg substitute, frozen, ¼ c	63	96
Whole egg, large	60	75
Egg yolk	78	59

Source: NIH, NHLBI (1994). Step by Step Eating to Lower Your High Blood Cholesterol. NIH Publication No. 94-2920.

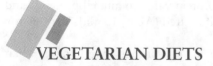

VEGETARIAN DIETS

A growing number of Americans consider themselves vegetarians. In addition to various religious, political, and economic reasons for becoming vegetarian, people are abstaining from meat because of health concerns. In fact, vegetarian diets come closer to the *Dietary Guidelines for Americans* than the typical average American diet.

Types of Vegetarian Diets

Vegetarianism is loosely defined as the abstinence from animal products. Pure vegetarians, or **vegans**, eat only plants; because of this, proper diet planning is essential to ensure adequate intakes of calories, vitamin B_{12}, vitamin D, iron, and calcium. Contrary to popular belief, protein requirements are rather easily met by vegans. As with the general population, average protein intake among vegans is well above the RDA.

Most vegetarians in the United States are classified as either **lacto- or lacto-ovo vegetarians**, whose diets include milk products or milk products and eggs, respectively. Their diets are not likely to be deficient in any nutrients. Many Americans consider themselves vegetarians simply because they avoid eating red meat.

An extreme type of vegetarian diet that was devised during the 1960s by the writer George Ohsawa was called the Zen-macrobiotic diet. In a series of 10 steps, the diet advances from meat-containing meals to a highly restrictive intake that consists mainly of brown rice, which supposedly is the ultimate food. The "higher" diets are dangerous and have caused severe cases of malnutrition and even death.

Potential Health Benefits

Compared with nonvegetarians, vegetarians have a lower mortality from coronary artery disease, and lower rates of hypertension and non–insulin-dependent diabetes mellitus. In some studies, reduced intake of meat and animal protein has been associated with decreased colon cancer, and research suggests that vegetarians are at decreased risk for breast cancer. Vegetarians, especially vegans, have body weights that are closer to desirable weight than do nonvegetarians (ADA, 1993a). However, vegetarians are not assured of either a low-fat or a healthful diet, for their diets can be high in fat if whole milk, whole milk cheeses, eggs, oils and other fats, nuts, seeds, and high-fat desserts are used extensively.

Nutritional Considerations

If the diet is varied and calorically adequate, plant sources of protein alone can provide adequate supplies of essential and nonessential amino acids; special attention to combining complementary proteins is unnecessary (ADA, 1993a). Soy protein has been shown to be nutritionally equivalent in protein value to animal proteins, and can serve as the sole source of protein intake, if desired (ADA, 1993a). Various soy products appear in the display, Soy Facts.

Although most vegetarian diets tend to provide less protein than nonvegetarian diets, most meet or exceed the RDA for protein. Lower intakes of protein may help improve calcium retention. Vegetable proteins have the advantage of being lower in fat and saturated fat, and are cholesterol-free. They also provide fiber, unlike animal proteins, which are devoid of fiber.

Vegetarians in the United States are not at greater risk for iron deficiency than nonvegetarians; not only is their intake of iron adequate, but adequate amounts of vitamin C (an iron absorption enhancer) are also consumed.

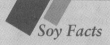

Soy Facts

DRY SOYBEANS

Dry soybeans are members of the legume family. To shorten their cooking time, dry soybeans should be soaked in water at room temperature for 6 to 8 hours or overnight. After draining and rinsing, the beans can be cooked in fresh water. Seasonings like onion, garlic, and bay leaf may be added.

GREEN VEGETABLE SOYBEANS

Green vegetable soybeans are similar in size and color to green peas and have a firm, crisp texture. They may be eaten as a side dish or snack, or combined with other ingredients in salads and soups.

TOFU

Tofu, also known as soybean curd, is a soft, cheeselike food that is made by curdling fresh hot soymilk with a coagulant. The curds are then pressed into a solid block. Although bland-tasting alone, tofu acts like a sponge to soak up flavors added to it. It can be crumbled into soup, blended with cocoa for chocolate pie filling, or added in chunks to casseroles. In American grocery stores, the three types of tofu that are sold are firm, soft, and silken. Tofu is rich in protein, a good source of B vitamins and iron, and low in sodium. Although 50% of the calories are from fat, that translates into only 6 g per 4-oz serving. It is low in saturated fat, cholesterol-free, and the softer the tofu, the lower the fat.

TEMPEH

Tempeh, a traditional Indonesian food, is a chunky cake of fermented soybeans with a smoky, nutty, or mushroomlike taste and a chewy consistency. It can be grilled, chunked, and added to casseroles and soups, or steamed, grated, and mixed with mayonnaise for a sandwich filling. It provides fiber, calcium, B vitamins, and iron.

MISO

Miso is a rich, salty condiment used extensively in Japanese cooking. It is made from soybeans and sometimes a grain, salt, and a mold culture that is aged for 1 to 3 years, although newer techniques speed processing time. Variations in ingredients and processing time account for different types of miso that vary greatly in flavor, texture, color, and aroma. Miso can be used to flavor soups, sauces, dressings, marinades, and pates. It is high in sodium.

SOYMILK

Soymilk is made from whole soybeans and can be purchased plain, or flavored with chocolate, vanilla, carob, or almond. Soymilk can be used by people with lactose intolerance and cow's milk allergies. It provides high-quality protein, B vitamins, and iron; lower fat varieties are available.

SOY PROTEIN ISOLATES

Soy protein isolates are a refined soy product of 90% protein used by food manufacturers to improve texture and taste. Soy protein isolates may be found in infant formulas, enteral formulas, and health food supplements, as well as breads and baked goods, breakfast cereals, pasta, snacks, desserts, soups, and sauces.

MEAT ANALOGS

Meat analogs are nonmeat foods made from soy protein and other ingredients to simulate various kinds of meat. They can be flavored to taste like beef, pork, chicken, and tunafish and can be made into imitation hot dogs, deli meats, and burgers. Although they are intended to be used in place of meat, they don't necessarily have the taste or texture of meat.

TEXTURED SOY PROTEIN

Textured soy protein, also known as TSP or TVP (textured vegetable protein), is made from soy flour that is compressed until the protein fibers change in structure. It is used as an extender in many food products and is sold to home cooks in dry, granular form. When rehydrated, TSP has a texture that is similar to that of ground beef. It also comes in chunks that resemble stew meat when rehydrated.

Vegetarians who include milk or eggs in their diet are not likely to be deficient in vitamin B_{12}, which is found only in animal products. Pure vegans should include a reliable source of B_{12} in their diets; spirulina, seaweed, tempeh, and other fermented foods are not considered "reliable" because as much as 80% to 94% of the vitamin B_{12} in these sources may be in inactive analogs (ADA, 1993a). "Reliable" sources include supplements and fortified foods such as some breakfast cereals, soy beverages, some brands of nutritional yeast, and other products.

Although certain substances in plants inhibit calcium absorption, the effect does not appear significant within the context of a total diet. Calcium deficiency in vegetarians is rare; they tend to absorb and retain more calcium than nonvegetarians (animal proteins have a calciuric effect).

Nutritional Adequacy

Obviously, the more foods that are restricted, the greater the chance that the diet will be nutritionally inadequate. However, with careful planning, all types of vegetarian diets, including vegan diets, can be nutritionally adequate for almost all healthy adults, infants, children, and adolescents; however, pure vegans should consume a reliable source of vitamin B_{12} and should have a reliable source of vitamin D (ADA, 1993a). Calcium, iron, and zinc intakes are usually adequate if adequate calories are consumed and the diet is varied. Table 2-11 lists good sources of minerals and vitamins that may be limited in vegan diets. Suggested food groups and serving sizes for vegetarians appears in Table 2-12. Suggested daily intakes for lacto-ovo vegetarians and total vegetarian diets at three different calorie levels appear in Tables 2-13 and 2-14, respectively.

Table 2-11
Good Sources of Nutrients That May Be Limited in Vegetarian Diets

Nutrient	Sources
MINERALS	
Calcium	Dark green, leafy vegetables ("greens"), broccoli, brussels sprouts, okra, legumes, rutabaga, almonds, filberts, calcium-fortified soybean milk, and tofu curdled with calcium salts
Iron	Dark green, leafy vegetables, whole grain and enriched grains, dried fruit, winter squash, sweet peas, dried peas and beans, lentils, iron that leaches into foods cooked in uncoated cast-iron pots
Zinc	Whole grain breads and cereals, dried yeast, dry beans, and nuts
VITAMINS	
Riboflavin	Whole grains, enriched breads, fortified cereals, dark green, leafy vegetables, broccoli, nuts, mushrooms, and avocado
Vitamin B_{12}	Fortified soybean milk, dietary supplements, yeast grown on B_{12}-enriched media, and meat analogs
Vitamin D	Sunlight, fortified soybean milk, and dietary supplements

Table 2-12
Food Groups and Serving Sizes for Vegetarian Diets

Food Group	Daily Servings	Serving Size
Breads, grains, cereals (50% whole grain)	6–11	1 slice bread 1 oz ready-to-eat cereal (¾ to 1 cup) ½ cup cooked cereal, rice, or pasta 6-in tortilla 1 small roll, or muffin ½ bagel or English muffin
Legumes	1–2	½ cup cooked dry beans, lentils, peas, limas, etc. ½ cup tofu, soy products, or meat analogs
Vegetables, dark green and green leafy vegetables*	3–5	½ cup cooked vegetable 1 cup raw, leafy vegetables or salad ¾ cup vegetable juice
Fruits	2–4	1 medium apple, banana, or orange ½ cup chopped, cooked, or canned fruit ¼ cup dried fruit ¾ cup fruit juice
Nuts and seeds	1–2	1 oz almonds, walnuts, seeds, etc. (¼ to ⅓ cup) 2 tbsp peanut butter, almond butter, tahini
Milk, yogurt, and/or cheese	2–3	1 cup low-fat (or nonfat) milk or yogurt 1.5 oz low-fat cheese ½ cup part-skim ricotta
Milk alternatives (soymilk) and tofu*		1 cup milk fortified with calcium and vitamin D and B$_{12}$ alternatives 1 cup tofu
Eggs	½	≤3 egg yolks/wk (may be deleted)
Fats, oil		1 tsp oil, margarine, or mayonnaise 2 tsp salad dressing ⅛ avocado 5 olives
Sugar		1 tsp sugar, jam, jelly, honey, syrup, etc.

 * The total vegetarian meal plan must include at least two servings of calcium-rich food items daily such as: 240 mL (1 cup) milk alternative fortified with calcium, Vitamin D, and Vitamin B$_{12}$; 168 g (1 cup) firm tofu; 186 g (1 cup) cooked broccoli; and 186 g (1 cup) cooked greens (*eg*, collards, dandelion, kale, mustard).
 Source: Haddad, E. (1994). Development of a vegetarian food guide. Am J Clin Nutr, 59(suppl), 12485–14545.

Well-planned vegan diets can be adequate for pregnant and lactating women, with special attention to vitamin B$_{12}$ and vitamin D. Like nonvegetarians, pregnant vegans are generally advised to take supplemental iron and folic acid.

Dietary Recommendations for Vegetarians

In addition to use of the suggested food guide and serving sizes for vegetarians as a general guide for meal planning (Haddad, 1994), the following recommendations are appropriate:

Table 2-13
Suggested Dietary Patterns for Lacto-ovovegetarian Diets at Three Energy Levels[1]

	Pattern A (1600 kcal)	Pattern B (2200 kcal)	Pattern C (2800 kcal)
	Servings/day		
Bread, grains, cereals[2]	6	9	11
Legumes, plant proteins	1	2	3
Vegetables	3	4	5
Fruits	2	3	4
Nuts, seeds	1	1	1
Milk, yogurt, cheese	2–3[3]	2–3[3]	2–3[3]
Eggs	1/2	1/2	1/2
Added fats and oils[4]	2	4	6
Added sugar[5]	3	6	9
Approximate composition			
Protein (g)	70	88	103
Fat (g)	50	62	74
Energy as fat (%)	28	25	24
Saturated fat (g)	16	18	20
Energy as saturated fat (%)	9	7	6

[1] Energy levels if low-fat or nonfat dairy and low-fat bakery food items are selected.
[2] At least half of the servings from whole grain breads and cereals.
[3] Three servings for women who are pregnant or breast-feeding, for teenagers, and for young adults aged ≤24 y.
[4] Fat added to food during food preparation or used as spreads and dressings.
[5] Sugar and other caloric sweeteners (*eg,* syrup, honey) added to food and bakery items during food preparation and used in drinks, beverages, and desserts.
Source: Haddad, E. (1994). Development of a vegetarian food guide. Am J Clin Nutr, 59(suppl), 12485–14545.

Eat a variety of foods, and be sure to consume adequate calories.

Choose whole grain or unrefined grain products whenever possible, or use fortified or enriched cereal products.

Avoid "empty calorie" foods (ie, sweets and fats) that provide few nutrients other than calories.

Eat a variety of fruits and vegetables, especially those high in vitamin C.

If milk and milk products are consumed, choose low-fat or nonfat varieties.

Limit egg yolks to 3 to 4 per week.

Be aware of the potential nutrient deficiencies in a pure vegan diet. Be sure to include a reliable source of vitamin B_{12}. If exposure to sunlight is limited, a vitamin D supplement may be indicated.

Vegetarian infants, like nonvegetarian infants, who are solely breast-fed beyond 4 to 6 months of age should receive supplements of iron and vitamin D, if sunlight exposure is limited.

Table 2-14
Suggested Dietary Patterns for Total Vegetarian Diets at Three Energy Levels[1]

	Pattern D (1600 kcal)	Pattern E (2200 kcal)	Pattern F (2800 kcal)
Bread, grains, cereals[2]	8	10	12
Legumes, plant proteins	1	2	3
Vegetables	2	3	4
Dark-green leafy vegetables	2	2	2
Fruits	2	4	6
Nuts, seeds	1	1	1
Fortified soy drinks and tofu[3]	2–3[4]	2–3[4]	2–3[4]
Added fats and oils[5]	2	4	6
Added sugar[6]	3	6	9
Approximate composition			
Protein (g)	60	76	95
Fat (g)	46	58	78
Energy as fat (%)	26	24	25
Saturated fat (g)	8	10	12
Energy as saturated fat (%)	5	4	4

[1] Energy levels if low-fat or nonfat dairy and low-fat bakery food items are selected.
[2] At least half of the servings from whole-grain breads and cereals.
[3] Milk alternatives fortified with calcium, Vitamin D, and Vitamin B_{12}, and multivitamin and mineral supplements and other supplements.
[4] Three servings for women who are pregnant or breast-feeding, for teenagers, and for young adults aged ≤24 y.
[5] Fat added to food during food preparation or used as spreads and dressings.
[6] Sugar and other caloric sweeteners (*eg,* syrup, honey) added to food and bakery items during food preparation and used in drinks, beverages, and desserts.
Source: Haddad, E. (1994). Development of a vegetarian food guide. Am J Clin Nutr, 59(suppl), 12485–14545.

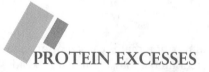

PROTEIN EXCESSES

Infants have a limited capacity to tolerate protein; their immature kidneys are unable to concentrate the urine sufficiently to excrete large quantities of nitrogenous wastes that result from a high protein intake (see Chapter 11). However, protein intakes that are two to three times higher than the RDA appear to be harmless to healthy adults.

Diets that are high in protein, particularly animal protein, however, may not be optimal. If animal protein foods are consumed at the expense of adequate quantities of fruits, vegetables, and grain products, then the intake of fiber and certain vitamins and minerals may be inadequate. Diets that are high in animal protein also tend to be high in saturated fat and cholesterol; thus, eating a high–animal protein diet may increase risk for the development of atherosclerosis.

According to some studies, a high protein intake increases the excretion of calcium, which may accelerate bone loss, increase the risk of calcium renal stones, and increase the risk of osteoporosis (see Chapter 20). Long-term high protein consumption may also damage the kidneys. According to animal studies, age-related decline in kidney function can be avoided by consumption of a low-protein diet; less nitrogenous waste means less work for the kidneys. Researchers believe the same may be true for people.

Lastly, diets that are high in animal protein generally are expensive.

PROTEIN DEFICIENCY

With the exception of the elderly, hospitalized patients, fad dieters, and people of low socioeconomic status, protein deficiency is rare in the United States and other affluent nations. However, in the developing countries, protein-calorie malnutrition (PCM) is a major health concern (see Food for Thought, Plant Biotechnology).

Protein-calorie malnutrition is estimated to cause 50% of infant deaths in developing countries; infants and children are more susceptible to nutritional deficiencies because they have high nutritional requirements relative to their weight. Kwashiorkor and marasmus are the most severe forms of PCM. Children who display symptoms of both diseases are said to have marasmic kwashiorkor, a less severe form of PCM.

Experts have questioned whether kwashiorkor and marasmus are actually two different problems, because the diets implicated in each are not significantly different. They hypothesize that marasmus may be a normal adaptive response to starvation, and that kwashiorkor occurs when the body cannot adapt to starvation because of a superimposed illness or infection. Such maladaptation may be responsible for the clinical and biochemical differences between kwashiorkor and marasmus.

Kwashiorkor

Kwashiorkor is a syndrome of severe protein malnutrition that is caused by an inadequate intake of good-quality protein; total protein intake may or may not be adequate. Starchy foods usually provide a marginal intake of calories.

In African dialect, kwashiorkor literally means "the disease of the deposed baby when the next one is born," which is an accurate description because it occurs most commonly after children are weaned because another child is born.

Kwashiorkor is most often seen between the ages of 1 and 4 years in areas where economic, social, and cultural factors combine to prevent an adequate protein intake, such as in 19 of the 21 countries in the Americas, India, most Middle and Far Eastern countries, and all the countries and territories of Africa south of the Sahara. In the United States, kwashiorkor most often occurs secondary to malabsorption disorders, cancer and cancer therapies, certain kidney diseases, hypermetabolic illnesses, and iatrogenic causes.

Signs and symptoms that may indicate kwashiorkor include edema and bloating related to low serum albumin; low weight, which may not be apparent because of

FOOD for THOUGHT

Plant Biotechnology: Food for Tomorrow

The earth's population is expected to double by the year 2033, with an estimated eleven thousand people born every hour (ADA and Monsanto, 1995). To meet the increased demand for food, plant biotechnology is coming to the forefront as a method to improve the quality, nutritional value, and variety of food available, as well as to increase the efficiency of food production and processing (ADA, 1993).

Biotechnology, also known as genetic engineering, recombinant DNA technology, or genetic modification, is the application of living organisms to develop new products. It can be used to develop modified plants with desired traits (plant hybridization), or to develop entirely new plant varieties with selected desirable traits. Biotechnology is also being used to develop herbicide-tolerant plants, so that farmers can use herbicides without risk of harming crops. Researchers are also working to develop plants that are resistant to certain types of plant viruses and insects, thus maximizing crop yield. Lastly, biotechnology can improve the quality and quantity of plant crops.

You may already be eating genetically engineered products. Biotechno tomatoes, known as Flavr Savrs™, are engineered to soften more slowly after harvest; thus they can remain on the vine longer to allow time for their natural flavor to develop (International Food Information Council, 1994). Approximately two thirds of U.S. manufactured cheese is made with a genetically engineered enzyme called chymosin, which is an exact replica of the animal enzyme rennin traditionally used to coagulate milk. Thus, instead of scraping the stomach linings of slaughtered calves for rennin, manufacturers can buy biotechno enzymes (Schardt, 1994).

In the future, biotechnology may lead to:

More tomatoes, peppers, and tropical fruits that ripen at controlled rates, thus allowing crops to be shipped long distances without spoiling

Potatoes and tomatoes with higher solid content, offering decreased processing costs because less energy is needed to extract water when producing products made from them

Corn and soybeans with higher essential amino acid content, to be used for food and animal feed

Coffee that is naturally decaffeinated

Plants with altered fatty acid contents, so that more healthful oils can be produced

The FDA is consulted during the plant development process to consider food composition and safety issues. Should the nutrition or composition of a new plant variety be substantially different from the original, the FDA requires a product approval process.

edema; retarded growth and maturation; mental apathy; muscular wasting; depigmentation of hair and skin; and scaly, flaky skin.

Without adequate and timely nutritional intervention, protein depletion can lead to fatty infiltration of the liver and increased susceptibility to infection. Diarrhea and malabsorption develop because of the decrease in both the number of intestinal cells and the quantity of digestive enzymes secreted. Numerous nutrient deficiencies develop secondary to malabsorption, and also because the synthesis of transport proteins for the bloodstream is limited. For example, a severe vitamin A deficiency leading to permanent blindness can occur when the protein that is required to move vitamin A through the blood is unavailable. Other complications of protein depletion include growth failure severe enough to cause permanent damage to physical and mental development and a high mortality rate, usually before 5 years of age.

Marasmus

Marasmus is a condition of chronic protein and calorie undernutrition that varies in severity. It occurs most often in 6- to 18-month-old infants whose parents are poor, uneducated, or mentally or emotionally disturbed. In addition to suffering from total food deprivation, the infant is usually lacking in emotional and physical care. Marasmus may also occur secondary to tuberculosis, malabsorption disorders, chronic infections, anorexia nervosa, and alcoholism. Isolated or hospitalized elderly patients are also at risk for PCM.

Marasmus may produce the following signs and symptoms: muscle wasting and loss of subcutaneous fat, leading to an emaciated appearance; physical and mental growth impairment; apathy; and lowered body temperature. Severe growth failure and diarrhea are common complications.

TREATMENT AND PREVENTION OF KWASHIORKOR AND MARASMUS

Of primary importance in the initial treatment of both kwashiorkor and marasmus is adequate replacement of both fluid and potassium. Diuresis is expected about 7 days after the treatment of kwashiorkor begins. Clinical symptoms may disappear within 4 to 6 weeks with intake of a diet that is adequate in high-quality protein, calories, and all other required nutrients; an increase to 30% above the RDA in both protein and calories is recommended. Vitamin supplements are generally indicated but should not be taken during the first 2 weeks of treatment.

Prevention of kwashiorkor and marasmus is far more effective than treatment, especially if the child is returned to the same environment and conditions after nutritional rehabilitation is completed. Prevention of both kwashiorkor and marasmus requires that broad, sweeping actions be taken, such as the following:

Resolve socioeconomic and psychological problems
Increase education in agriculture, nutrition, and health: Breast-feeding should be
  encouraged for the first 6 months of life; thereafter, a nutritionally adequate
  diet should be initiated and continued
Implement effective policies to improve nutrition and health care
Achieve a balance between population and food supply
Provide food aid to victims of manmade and natural disasters
Control infectious diseases

KEY CONCEPTS

- Protein is a component of every living cell. Except for bile and urine, every tissue and fluid in the body contains some protein.
- Amino acids, which are composed of carbon, hydrogen, oxygen, and nitrogen atoms, are the building blocks of protein. There are 22 known amino acids; 9 are

considered essential because they cannot be made by the body. The remaining amino acids are no less important, but are considered nonessential because they can be made by the body.

- The function of protein in the diet is to furnish adequate amounts and proportions of amino acids so that body proteins can be synthesized. Protein also helps regulate fluid balance, transports many substances through the blood, and can be oxidized to produce energy.

- Dietary protein is found in milk, meat, vegetables, and grains. Generally, animal sources of protein are considered complete proteins because they provide all the essential amino acids in adequate amounts and proportions to support protein synthesis. Plant sources of protein are considered incomplete because they are deficient in one or more essential amino acids.

- The small intestine is the principal site of protein digestion; amino acids and some dipeptides are absorbed through the portal bloodstream.

- Protein anabolism (buildup) and catabolism (breakdown) occur simultaneously and continuously within every cell. The net effect of othese reactions determines whether a person is in a neutral, positive, or negative nitrogen balance.

- The RDA for protein for adults is 0.8 g/kg. Most experts recommend protein contribute 10% to 20% of total calorie intake. Most Americans consume almost double their RDA for protein.

- Diets high in protein may also be high in fat. Excessive protein intake may also promote urinary calcium excretion and thus contribute to bone loss and calcium renal stones.

- Pure vegans eat no animal products. Most American vegetarians are lacto- or lacto-ove vegetarians, whose diets include milk products or millk products and eggs, respectively.

- Vegetarian diets tend to be closer to the Dietary Guidelines for Americans than the typical American diet. Most vegetarian diets meet or exceed the RDA for protein and are nutritionally adequate for almost all healthy adults, infants, children, and adolescents. However, pure vegans should consume a reliable source of vitamin B_{12} and vitamin D.

- Protein deficiency is rare in the United States. The elderly, hospitalized patients, fad dieters, and people of low socioeconomic status are at greatest risk for protein deficiency. In developing countries, protein–calorie malnutrition is a major health concern.

REFERENCES

American Dietetic Association (1993a). Position of the American Dietetic Association: Vegetarian diets. J Am Diet Assoc 93(11), 1317–1319.

American Dietetic Association (1993b). Position of The American Dietetic Association: Biotechnology and the future of food. J Am Diet Assoc, 93(2), 189–192.

American Dietetic Association and Monsanto (1995). Plant Biotechnology. Harvesting Solutions for Tomorrow's World. St. Louis: Monsanto.

Centers for Disease Control and Prevention (1994). Energy and Macronutrient intakes of persons ages 2 months and over in the United States: Third National Health and Nutrition Examination Survey, Phase 1, 1988–1991. Advance Data, No 255.

Haddad, E. (1994). Development of a vegetarian food guide. Am J Clin Nutr, 59(suppl), 1248S–1454S.

International Food Information Council (1994). Biotech tomato rolls to market. Food Insight. July/August, 5.

National Research Council: Recommended Dietary Allowances. 10th ed. Washington, DC: National Academy Press, 1989.

Schardt, D. (1994). Diving into the gene pool. Nutrition Action Health Letter, 21(6), 8–9.

United States Department of Agriculture (1992). The Food Guide Pyramid. Home and Garden Bulletin No. 252.

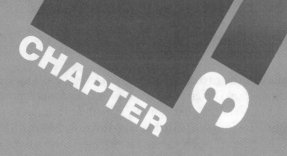

CHAPTER 3

Lipids

Chapter Outline

Key Terms

Brown fat
Diglycerides
Essential fatty acids
Fats
Fatty acids
Glycerol
Hydrogenation

Invisible fats
Lipids
Long-chain fatty acids
Medium-chain fatty acids
Monoglycerides
Monounsaturated fatty acids
Omega-6 fatty acids

Omega-3 fatty acids
Phospholipids
Polyunsaturated fatty acids
Short-chain fatty acids
Triglycerides
Unsaturated fatty acids
Visible fats

*L*ipids, commonly referred to as **fats**, are a group of organic compounds that are insoluble in water but soluble in alcohol, ether, chloroform, and other fat solvents. Of the three major classes of lipids in the diet, triglycerides ("fats and oils") represent 95% of the total fat intake; the remaining 5% comes from phospholipids (eg, lecithin) and sterols (eg, cholesterol).

SOURCES OF FAT

In some foods (eg, butter, margarine, and oils), fat provides 100% of the total calories. In other foods, such as meat, eggs, dairy products, desserts, and sweets, the percentage of calories from fat varies.

According to the exchange lists developed by the American Diabetes Association and the American Dietetic Association, fat is found mostly in the Meat and Fat groups (Table 3-1). Fats that can be easily identified, such as butter, oils, and the fat around meat, are known as **visible fats. Invisible fats** are hidden in foods that do not appear to be "fatty," such as the fat marbled throughout meat, and the fat in egg yolks, whole milk and whole milk products, nuts, desserts, and baked goods. Some items within the milk and bread groups also contain fat or "invisible" fat, as do many items in the "Other Carbohydrates" list, such as sweets, snacks, and desserts. Table 3-2 lists the fat content of selected sweets and snacks. Unless they are prepared with added fat, the fruit and vegetable groups are virtually fat free, with the exception of avocados, olives, and coconuts.

FUNCTIONS OF FAT

Because they supply 9 cal/g, fats and oils are the most concentrated source of energy in the diet, providing more than twice the fuel value of CHO and protein. With the exception of the central nervous system and erythrocytes, which normally rely solely

Table 3-1
Sources of Fat Based on the American Diabetic Association/American Dietetic Association Exchange Lists

Group	Serving Size	CHO (g)	Protein (g)	Fat (g)	Calories
EXCHANGE LISTS CONTAINING FAT					
Meat					
Very lean	1 oz	0	7	0–1	35
Lean	1 oz	0	7	3	55
Medium-fat	1 oz	0	7	5	75
High-fat	1 oz	0	7	8	100
Fat	Varies	0	0	5	45
EXCHANGE LISTS THAT MAY CONTAIN FAT, DEPENDING ON THE SELECTION					
Milk					
Skim	1 cup	12	8	0–3	90
Low-fat	1 cup	12	8	5	120
Whole	1 cup	12	8	8	150
Other carbohydrates	Varies	15	—	0–10	Varies
EXCHANGE LISTS CONTAINING NO FAT (IF PREPARED WITHOUT ADDED FAT)					
Starch		15	3	1 g or less	80
Bread	1 slice				
Cereal, cooked	½ cup				
Most ready-to-eat unsweetened cereal, dry	¾ cup				
Starchy vegetable, pasta	½ cup				
Rice	⅓ cup				
Vegetable	½ cup cooked or 1 cup raw	5	2	0	25
Fruit	Varies	15	0	0	60

Table 3-2
Fat Content of Selected "Sweets" and "Snacks"

Food	Serving Size	Total Calories	g Fat	% Calories From Fat
DESSERTS				
Cake doughnut, plain	1	198	10.8	49
Apple pie	1/8 of 9" pie	297	13.8	42
Chocolate cake with chocolate frosting	1/8 of 18-oz cake	235	10.5	40
Yellow cake with chocolate frosting	1/8 of 18-oz cake	242	11.2	42
Pound cake	1/10 of 10.75-oz cake	117	6.0	46
Cheesecake	1/6 of 17-oz cake	256	18	63
CANDY				
Chocolate fudge	1-oz piece	108	2.4	20
Milk chocolate bar	1 oz	145	8.7	54
COOKIES				
Oatmeal cookie	1 (2/3 oz)	81	3.3	37
Chocolate chip cookie	1 (2 1/4" around)	48	2.3	43
Chocolate brownie	1 2" square	139	6.6	43
FROZEN DESSERTS				
Vanilla ice cream, regular	1/2 cup	132	7.3	50
French vanilla soft ice cream	1/2 cup	185	11.2	54
Vanilla ice cream, rich (16% fat)	1/2 cup	178	12	61
Chocolate premium ice cream	1/2 cup	216	15.3	64
SNACKS				
Popcorn popped with oil	2 1/2 cups	142	8.0	51
Corn chips	1 oz	153	9.5	56
Tortilla chips, nacho flavor	1 oz	141	7.3	47
Potato chips	1 oz	152	9.8	58

Source: National Institutes of Health, National Heart, Lung, Blood Institute (1994). Step by Step. Eating to Lower Your High Blood Cholesterol. NIH Publication No. 94-2920.

on glucose for energy, all body cells can directly oxidize fatty acids to produce energy. However, because fat metabolism is more complicated than CHO metabolism, CHO is generally the preferred fuel.

Linoleic acid and linolenic acid are **essential fatty acids (EFA)** because they cannot be synthesized by the body and must therefore be supplied in the diet. Because linoleic acid is a precursor of arachidonic acid, arachidonic acid becomes an EFA when linoleic acid intake is deficient. Essential fatty acids play a role in the metabolism of cholesterol and, by some unknown mechanism, help lower serum cholesterol levels. Essential fatty acids also help maintain the function and integrity of capillaries and cell membranes. They are precursors of prostaglandins, a group of hormonelike substances with various metabolic functions, and of phospholipids, the structural lipids found in cell membranes and myelin sheaths (the insulating covers around nerves that speed the transmission of nerve impulses).

Fat improves the palatability and flavor of food and influences its texture. It delays gastric emptying time—fat may remain in the stomach for 3.5 to 4 hours after a meal, providing a feeling of fullness (satiety) and delaying the return of hunger. In addition, the presence of fat in the duodenum stimulates the release of a hormone in the stomach that inhibits hunger contractions. The absorption of the fat-soluble vitamins A, D, E, and K through the intestinal mucosa depends on fat.

Like phospholipids, cholesterol is a major component of cell membranes and myelin. Cholesterol has other essential metabolic functions, including being the precursor of steroid hormones and bile (see section on Other Lipids).

Fat, in the form of triglycerides, that is not used as an immediate energy source or needed for other functions is stored in adipose tissue. White fat and brown fat are the two forms of adipose tissue. **White fat,** the most abundant type of fat in the body, normally accounts for 15% to 25% of total body weight. It is deposited under the skin, in the abdominal cavity, and to a lesser extent in intramuscular tissue. Its functions are to provide energy in time of need, to insulate and protect the body against cold environmental temperatures, and to support internal organs such as the kidneys and heart, protecting them against mechanical injury. **Brown fat** is much less abundant—the largest quantity of brown fat is found in the body during infancy, and the amount then decreases with age. Less than 1% of an adult's body weight is attributable to brown fat. It is located only in certain areas in the body, mostly around the neck and chest. Its primary function is thermogenesis—that is, generating heat to protect against the cold. Brown fat, or the lack of it, has been theorized to play a role in the development of obesity (see Chapter 13).

COMPOSITION AND STRUCTURE OF FAT

Fats are made of the elements carbon, hydrogen, and oxygen in the form of one glycerol molecule with one, two, or three fatty acids attached. Although fats contain the same elements as CHO, they have proportionately less oxygen and more hydrogen and carbon atoms; because of this, they are higher in calories.

Glycerol

Glycerol is an alcohol made of a three–carbon atom stem with alcohol groups attached to each; all glycerol molecules are the same. After fat is broken down through the process of digestion into fatty acids and glycerol, the glycerol molecule is absorbed directly into the portal vein.

$$
\begin{array}{c}
\text{H} \\
| \\
\text{H}-\text{C}-\text{OH} \\
\text{H}-\text{C}-\text{OH} \\
\text{H}-\text{C}-\text{OH} \\
| \\
\text{H}
\end{array}
$$

Fatty Acids

Fatty acids are composed of a straight chain of carbon atoms with hydrogen atoms attached and an acid group at one end. Most fatty acids have an even number of carbon atoms ranging from 2 to 24. Two variables that determine the physical properties of fatty acids are the length of the carbon chain and the degree of saturation.

CARBON CHAIN LENGTH

Based on the length of the carbon chain, fatty acids may be classified as **short-chain fatty acids,** which contain 2 to 4 carbon atoms, **medium-chain fatty acids,** which contain 6 to 12 carbon atoms, or **long-chain fatty acids,** which contain 14 or more carbon atoms (Table 3-3). Most food fats contain predominantly long-chain fatty acids.

Table 3-3
Some Naturally Occurring Saturated and Unsaturated Fatty Acids

Fatty Acids	Number of Carbon Atoms	Food Sources
SATURATED FATTY ACIDS		
Short-chain		
Butyric acid	4	Butter
Medium-chain		
Caproic acid	6	Butter
Caprylic acid	8	Butter, coconut oil
Capric acid	10	Butter, coconut oil, and palm oil
Lauric acid	12	Butter, coconut oil
Long-chain		
Myristic acid	14	Butter, coconut oil
Palmitic acid	16	Beef, pork, lamb, and most vegetable oils
Stearic acid	18	Beef, pork, lamb, and most vegetable oils
Arachidic acid	20	Peanut oil, lard
MONOSATURATED FATTY ACIDS (1 DOUBLE BOND)		
Long-chain		
Palmitoleic acid	16	Butter, seed oils
Oleic acid	18	Meats, olive oil, and most other fats and oils
POLYUNSATURATED FATTY ACIDS		
Long-chain		
Linoleic acid	18 (2 double bonds)	Corn, cottonseed, soybean, sunflower, and safflower oils; poultry, walnuts
Linolenic acid	18 (3 double bonds)	Soybean oil, other vegetable oils, and egg yolk
Arachidonic acid	20 (4 double bonds)	Very little in foods

DEGREE OF SATURATION

The degree of saturation refers to the number of double bonds between carbon atoms. If all of the carbon atoms in a fatty acid are "saturated" with all the hydrogen atoms they can hold, no double bonds can exist. Such fatty acids are classified as **saturated**. All short- and medium-chain fatty acids are saturated; long-chain fatty acids may be either saturated or unsaturated. The major saturated fatty acids are palmitic acid and stearic acid.

```
    H  H  H  H  H  H  H  H  H  H  H  H  H  H  H  O
    |  |  |  |  |  |  |  |  |  |  |  |  |  |  |  ||
H – C– C– C– C– C– C– C– C– C– C– C– C– C– C– C– C– O – H   (palmitic acid)
    |  |  |  |  |  |  |  |  |  |  |  |  |  |  |
    H  H  H  H  H  H  H  H  H  H  H  H  H  H  H
```

Unsaturated fatty acids have one or more double bonds between carbon atoms. The carbon atoms are not saturated with hydrogen atoms, and thus double bonds form between carbon atoms to satisfy nature's law that each carbon atom have 4 bonds connecting it to the other atoms. **Monounsaturated fatty acids** contain only one double bond between carbon atoms. The most prevalent monounsaturated fatty acid in the diet is oleic acid.

```
    H  H  H  H  H  H  H  H  H  H  H  H  H  H  H  H  O
    |  |  |  |  |  |  |  |        |  |  |  |  |  |  ||
H – C– C– C– C– C– C– C– C– C= C– C– C– C– C– C– C– C– O – H   (oleic acid)
    |  |  |  |  |  |  |  |        |  |  |  |  |  |
    H  H  H  H  H  H  H  H        H  H  H  H  H  H
```

Polyunsaturated fatty acids (PUFA) have two or more double bonds between carbon atoms. In **omega-6 PUFA**, the first double bond occurs six carbon atoms from the methyl carbon. Linoleic acid, an omega-6 fatty acid, is one of the PUFA most commonly found in both plants and foods.

```
    H  H  H  H  H  H  H  H  H  H  H  H  H  H  H  H  O
    |  |  |  |  |  |  |  |  |  |  |  |  |  |  |  |  ||
H – C– C– C– C– C– C= C– C– C= C– C– C– C– C– C– C– C– O – H   (linoleic acid)
    |  |  |  |  |        |        |  |  |  |  |  |
    H  H  H  H  H        H        H  H  H  H  H  H
```

Omega-3 PUFA have their first double bond three carbon atoms from the methyl carbon. The most abundant omega-3 fatty acids are linolenic acid, which is found in plants, and the "fish oils," eicosapentaenoic acid (EPA) and docosahexaenoic acid (DHA).

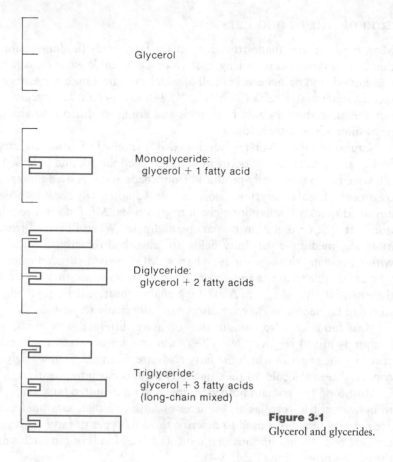

Glycerol

Monoglyceride:
glycerol + 1 fatty acid

Diglyceride:
glycerol + 2 fatty acids

Triglyceride:
glycerol + 3 fatty acids
(long-chain mixed)

Figure 3-1
Glycerol and glycerides.

FOOD FATS: TRIGLYCERIDES

Glycerol molecules that are bound with only one fatty acid are known as **monoglycerides** (Fig. 3-1). When two fatty acids are attached to a glycerol molecule, the result is a **diglyceride**. Both monoglycerides and diglycerides, which represent a very small percentage of the lipids in the diet, function as emulsifiers to keep fat particles dispersed and suspended in solution. For this reason, they often are used as food additives.

Triglycerides, which have three fatty acids attached to a glycerol molecule, make up about 95% of the lipids in food. Just as amino acids can be arranged in limitless combinations to form different proteins, fatty acids can attach to glycerol molecules in various ratios and patterns to form a large variety of triglycerides within a single food fat. The types and amounts of fatty acids in triglycerides determine their nature; in turn, the composition of triglycerides influences the characteristics of food fats. For instance, butter tastes and acts differently than corn oil, which tastes and acts differently than lard.

Composition of Most Food Fats

Most food fats are made from long-chain fatty acids (ie, long-chain triglycerides) that have a typical carbon length of 16 or 18; notable exceptions include milk fat, coconut oil, and palm kernel oil, all of which contain a high percentage of short- and medium-chain fatty acids (Shils et al, 1994). Long-chain fatty acids are less soluble in water than shorter-chain fatty acids and are more difficult to absorb than short- or medium-chain fatty acids.

Natural medium-chain triglycerides (MCT) consist of saturated fatty acids with 6 to 12 carbon atoms; they occur in milk fat, coconut oil, and palm kernel oil. MCT oil, which is commercially produced from coconut oil, is used therapeutically in the treatment of malabsorption disorders (see Chapter 16) because it is digested and absorbed quickly. Unlike long-chain triglycerides, MCT do not require emulsification with bile or digestion by pancreatic lipase. When liberated from the glycerol molecule, medium-chain fatty acids are absorbed directly into the portal system without moving through the lymphatics. MCT provide needed calories to patients who are unable to digest and absorb dietary fat; however, they are unpalatable, lack the essential fatty acids (EFA are long-chain, unsaturated fatty acids), and are not stored in fat deposits. They are also financially costly to provide.

Most food fats also contain two or more different fatty acids, and hence are known as mixed triglycerides. The characteristics of mixed triglycerides are influenced by the order in which the fatty acids are arranged. Simple triglycerides, which contain three molecules of the same fatty acid, occur infrequently.

Most food fats contain both saturated and unsaturated fatty acids. When applied to individual triglycerides and sources of fat in the diet, *saturated* and *unsaturated* are not absolute terms used to describe the only types of fatty acids present; rather, they are relative descriptions that indicate which kinds of fatty acids are included in the largest proportion (Table 3-4).

UNSATURATED FATS

Generally, food fats that are high in polyunsaturated fatty acids tend to be soft or liquid at room temperature and have low melting points—the more double bonds in a fatty acid, the lower the melting point. Poultry fat, for instance, is softer than beef fat because it has a higher percentage of unsaturated fatty acids. All vegetable oils, with the exception of coconut, palm kernel, and palm, are high in unsaturated fats (see Table 3-4). Although they are foods from animal sources, chicken and fresh-water fish are also high in unsaturated fat.

Polyunsaturated fats, especially the EFA, are susceptible to rancidity when exposed to light and oxygen over a prolonged period of time. The chemical change that occurs results in an offensive change in taste and smell and the loss of vitamins A and E. The two major antioxidants that are added to fats (ie, BHA and BHT) extend shelf life and protect vitamins A and E. Minimizing storage time and avoiding high temperatures also protect fats against rancidity.

Table 3-4
The Percentage of Polyunsaturated, Monounsaturated, and Saturated Fatty Acids in Selected Fats and Oils

	% Polyunsaturated Fatty Acids	% Monounsaturated Fatty Acids	% Saturated Fatty Acids
"UNSATURATED" OILS			
Safflower	75	15	10
Sunflower	60–70	24	12
Corn	55	25	13
Soybean	58	23	15
Cottonseed	51	18	30
Cashew nut	35	30	24
Walnut	70	15	10
"MONOUNSATURATED" FATS AND OILS			
Olive oil	10	71	17
Stick margarine	29	48	18
Canola oil	32	53	7
Soft tub margarine	31	47	18
Peanut oil	33	49	13
Chicken, turkey, egg	21	42	30
"SATURATED" FATS AND OILS			
Coconut oil	2	6	88
Palm kernel oil	2	11	81
Butter	3	26	65
Palm oil	10	38	52
Beef fat	2	42	53
Lard (pig)	10	46	42

Source: Shils, M., Olson, J., and Shike, M. (1994). Modern Nutrition in Health and Disease. 8th ed. Philadelphia: Lea & Febiger; and Proctor & Gamble (1993). Compare the Dietary Fats.

SATURATED FATS

Food fats that are high in saturated fatty acids tend to be solid at room temperature and have high melting points. With the exception of those found in poultry and freshwater fish, all animal fats are high in saturated fats (see Table 3-4). The only saturated vegetable fats are coconut, palm kernel, and palm oils.

HYDROGENATED FATS

Hydrogenated fats are unsaturated vegetable oils (usually corn, soybean, cottonseed, safflower, peanut, or olive) that have hydrogen atoms added to some of the double bonds to make the fat more saturated—the more hydrogen atoms added, the more saturated and harder the resulting product. The degree of hydrogenation varies according to the desired use of the fat in foods; most are slightly or partially hydrogenated. Oils may be slightly hydrogenated to improve stability yet still remain in their liquid form. Semisolid forms of margarine and shortening are made with a higher degree of hydrogenation. Hydrogenated products are less likely to oxidize and become rancid because they are chemically more stable. Therefore, they have a longer shelf-life. However, they bear little resemblance to the original oil.

Unfortunately, hydrogenated fats have a lower unsaturated fatty acid content than is found in the original oil; unsaturated fats may help lower serum cholesterol, thereby helping to reduce the risk of atherosclerosis. Also, some of the unsaturated fatty acids that remain are structurally different from the original molecule: Some double bonds in the *cis*-position, which occur naturally in nature, are converted to the *trans*-position (Fig. 3-2). Unfortunately, *trans*-polyunsaturated fatty acids do not perform essential fatty acid functions, nor are they made by the body or naturally abundant in foods. Although they are assumed to be safe, their effect on metabolism and health is unknown.

OTHER LIPIDS

The other 5% of lipids in the diet are phospholipids (lecithin is the most common) and sterols, including cholesterol. Lipoproteins are compound lipids that serve to transport lipids and cholesterol through the blood.

Phospholipids

Phospholipids are a group of compound lipids that are similar to triglycerides in that they contain a glycerol molecule and two fatty acids. However, in place of the third fatty acid, phospholipids have a phosphate group to which is attached a molecule of choline or a similar compound containing nitrogen atoms. Phospholipids are found

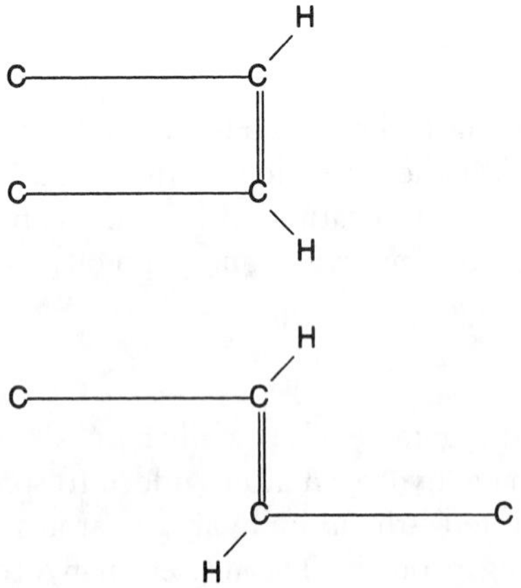

Cis-fatty acid configuration: both hydrogen atoms are on the same side of the double bond.

Trans-fatty acid: the hydrogen atoms are on opposite sides of the double bond.

Figure 3-2
Cis- and *trans*-fatty acid configurations.

naturally in almost all foods, and because they are soluble in both water and fat, they are used extensively by the food industry as emulsifiers.

Lecithin is the best-known phospholipid. Numerous claims that lecithin should be supplemented in the diet because it is an essential nutrient are untrue. Although lecithin does have important roles in maintaining the body, it is not required in the diet because the body synthesizes it. Also, lecithin that is consumed in the diet is not absorbed intact and transported throughout the body to perform super-functions. Instead, lecithin is broken down by enzymes in the intestinal tract, and its individual components are absorbed and sent to the liver to be used as needed.

Phospholipids serve as a structural component of cell membranes and are able to transport water-soluble and fat-soluble substances across membranes. Phospholipids are precursors of prostaglandins, a group of fatty-acid derivatives with hormonelike actions that perform the following functions: 1) help regulate blood pressure; 2) assist with nerve impulse transmission; 3) regulate gastric secretions and muscular contractions of the gastrointestinal tract; 4) stimulate uterine contractions; 5) induce labor and abortions; and 6) inhibit lipid catabolism.

Cholesterol

Cholesterol is a member of the sterol family, which includes bile acids, sex hormones, the adrenocortical hormones, and vitamin D. Although cholesterol performs vital functions in the body, it is not essential in the diet because it is synthesized primarily in the liver from glucose or saturated fatty acids. In fact, every day the body manufactures more than twice the amount of cholesterol contained in the average American diet.

Cholesterol is found only in animal products and is most abundant in organ meats and egg yolks (Table 3-5). Like other lipids, cholesterol is transported through the blood contained in lipoproteins.

Cholesterol is an essential constituent of all cell membranes and is especially abundant in brain and nerve cells. About 80% of metabolized cholesterol is used to synthesize bile acids; the cholesterol in bile acids is recycled. A high-fiber diet enhances the excretion of bile acids and, therefore, reduces cholesterol in the body. Cholesterol is a precursor of the steroid hormones and vitamin D: cholesterol in the skin + ultraviolet light = the formation of vitamin D.

There has been much debate about the role of dietary cholesterol in the development of atherosclerosis, a condition characterized by the formation of fatty plaques (containing mostly cholesterol) along the inside of arteries. A high serum cholesterol level is one of many risk factors associated with atherosclerosis, and diet influences serum cholesterol levels. Because most of the cholesterol that is circulating in the bloodstream is made by the liver from saturated fats, a high intake of saturated fat has a greater impact on serum cholesterol levels than a high intake of cholesterol. To help lower serum cholesterol levels, researchers recommend reducing total fat and saturated fat intake, replacing some saturated fat intake with PUFA and monounsaturated fats, and limiting dietary intake of cholesterol. See Chapter 17 for more on diet and heart disease.

Table 3-5
Cholesterol Content of Selected Foods

	Cholesterol (mg)			Cholesterol (mg)
BEEF (3 OZ COOKED)			**FISH (3 OZ COOKED)**	
Liver	331		Haddock	63
Sirloin, lean only	77		Cod	47
Chuck, pot roast, lean only	86		Salmon, sockeye	74
Salami, cooked	51		Lobster, northern	61
			Shrimp	167
LAMB (3½ OZ COOKED)			Scallops	47
Loin chop, lean	85		Blue crab	85
Arm chop, lean only	103		Oyster	89
			Squid, fried	221
PORK (3½ OZ COOKED)			**MILK (8 OUNCES)**	
Liver	302		Skim	4
Chitterlings	122		Buttermilk	9
Ham, cured	50		1% Fat	10
Knockwurst	48		2% Fat	18
			Whole	33
VEAL (3½ OZ COOKED)			**CHEESE**	
Ground veal, broiled	87		Mozzarella, 1 oz, part skim	16
Loin, chop, lean only	87		Swiss, 1 oz	26
			Cheddar, 1 oz	30
POULTRY (3½ OZ COOKED)			Cream cheese, 2 tbsp	32
Turkey, breast with skin	77		**EGGS***	
Turkey, breast without skin	71		White only	0
Turkey, leg without skin	101		Whole egg	213
Chicken, light meat without skin	64		Yolk	213
Duck, flesh only	76		Egg substitute, frozen, ¼ cup	1
Goose, flesh only	82		**FROZEN DESSERTS (½ CUP)**	
Turkey bologna, 2 oz	54		Sherbet	5
Chicken frankfurter, 1	55		Ice milk, hard	9
Venison, roasted	95		Ice cream, French vanilla, soft	78
			Ice cream, vanilla, rich (16% fat)	45
FATS (1 TABLESPOON)			Ice cream, chocolate, premium (23% fat)	98
Lard	12			
Butter	28			

Source: NIH, NHLBI (1994). Step by Step. Eating to Lower Your High Blood Cholesterol. NIH Publication No. 94-2920.

Lipoproteins

Lipoproteins are compound lipids that contain both protein and various types and amounts of lipids. They are made mostly in the liver and are used to transport water-insoluble lipids through the blood. Elevated levels of certain kinds of lipoproteins (hyperlipoproteinemias) represent a risk factor for the development of atherosclerosis (see Chapter 17). The following are classifications of lipoproteins based on density:

- Chylomicrons: composed mainly of triglycerides encased in a protein and phospholipid coating. Chylomicrons form for the purpose of transporting absorbed triglycerides from the intestines to the liver. High serum chylomicron levels do not increase the risk of atherosclerosis.
- Very-low-density lipoproteins (VLDL): contain primarily triglycerides with some protein and cholesterol. VLDL transport endogenous triglycerides from the liver to the tissues. High serum VLDL levels may increase the risk of atherosclerosis.
- Low-density lipoproteins (LDL): composed largely of cholesterol. LDL function to transport cholesterol from the liver to the tissues. High serum LDL levels greatly increase the risk of atherosclerosis. Diets that are high in saturated fat are associated with elevations in LDL cholesterol.
- High-density lipoproteins (HDL): contain primarily protein, with small amounts of triglycerides and cholesterol. HDL transport cholesterol from the tissues to the liver to be metabolized. High serum HDL levels are protective against the development of atherosclerosis.

HOW THE BODY HANDLES FAT

Digestion

A minimal amount of chemical digestion of fat occurs in the stomach through the action of a gastric lipase that breaks down short-chain triglycerides (found in butter) into fatty acids and glycerol (Fig. 3-3).

Through a series of events, fat in the duodenum stimulates the gallbladder to contract and release bile, which is not an enzyme but an emulsifier. Bile is continually produced in the liver and concentrated and stored in the gallbladder. Bile contains

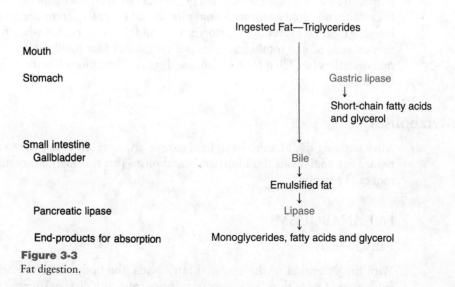

Figure 3-3
Fat digestion.

bile salts, cholesterol, phospholipids, bilirubin, and electrolytes. As an emulsifier, bile breaks down fat globules into smaller particles to increase the surface area on which pancreatic lipase can work.

Pancreatic lipase is the most important and powerful lipase, or fat-digesting enzyme. It splits off one fatty acid at a time from triglyceride molecules. Because removal of fatty acids is an increasingly difficult task, only one third to one half of the total fat is actually broken down completely to fatty acids and glycerol.

The end-products of triglyceride digestion are fatty acids, glycerol, and monoglycerides.

Absorption

Short- and medium-chain free fatty acids, glycerol, and medium-chain triglycerides are absorbed directly through the mucosal cells into the portal vein and are transported to the liver.

Monoglycerides and long-chain fatty acids, which are insoluble in water but dissolve in micelles, are formed from bile salts. Micelles then transport the monoglycerides and long-chain fatty acids to the mucosal cells of the villi, where they diffuse into the cells. The released bile salts return to the intestine, where most are reabsorbed in the terminal ileum, transported back to the liver, and recycled (enterohepatic circulation).

Within the mucosal cells of the small intestine, intestinal lipase breaks down monoglycerides into fatty acids and glycerol; the fatty acids and glycerol are then reformed into triglycerides. The reformed triglycerides, along with other lipids, such as cholesterol and phospholipids, become encased in protein to form chylomicrons.

Chylomicrons enter the bloodstream via the lymph system and the thoracic duct. Their destination is the liver by way of the hepatic artery.

About 95% of consumed fat is absorbed, mostly in the duodenum and jejunum. Normally, 4 to 5 g of fat is excreted in the feces daily. Inadequate bile output, a high-fiber diet, and rapid gastrointestinal motility all decrease fat absorption and thereby increase fecal fat excretion. Steatorrhea, a condition that occurs when fecal fat excretion exceeds 6% of total fat intake, is a symptom of fat maldigestion or malabsorption disorders (see Chapter 16; also, see display, Conditions Requiring Alterations in Fat Intake).

Metabolism

After entering the bloodstream, lipids are transported to either the liver or adipose tissue. Fat anabolism (buildup) and catabolism (breakdown) are regulated by hormones (Table 3-6).

FAT ANABOLISM

Fatty Acid Synthesis

With the exception of the essential fatty acids, the body can synthesize fatty acids from acetyl Co-A; thus, an excess of calories from any dietary source can be used. A

Conditions Requiring Alterations in Fat Intake

LOW-FAT DIETS ARE USED FOR

Chronic pancreatitis

Cystic fibrosis

Other malabsorption syndromes

Possibly for gallbladder disease

Obesity, as part of an overall reduction in calorie intake

MODIFIED FAT DIETS (SUCH AS LOW CHOLESTEROL, LOW SATURATED FAT, INCREASED UNSATURATED FAT DIETS) MAY BE USED

To treat hyperlipoproteinemias

As a preventive measure against coronary heart disease

As part of a diabetic diet as prevention against long-term complications resulting from altered fat metabolism

A HIGH-FAT DIET MAY BE USED

To induce ketosis in patients with epilepsy or other seizure disorders

group of enzymes known as fatty acid synthetases catalyze the series of reactions that take place predominantly in the liver.

Triglyceride Synthesis

The liver can synthesize triglycerides from an excess intake of CHO or protein through the process of lipogenesis. Through a complex series of steps, glucose is converted to glycerol and fatty acids, which may then be synthesized into triglycerides for storage in adipose tissue, or converted to lipoproteins, phospholipids, or cholesterol as needed. Ketogenic amino acids that remain after protein requirements are met can be converted to and stored as fat.

FAT CATABOLISM

If the body is to use stored fat for energy, lipases within the cell must first split the triglycerides into their component parts—a glycerol molecule and fatty acids.

Table 3-6
Hormones Affecting Fat Metabolism

Hormone	Effect on Fat Metabolism
ACTH (adrenocorticotropic hormone)	Increases fat mobilization
Epinephrine	Increases the rate of fat mobilization
Glucagon	Increases fat mobilization; decreases fat synthesis
Glucocorticoids	Increases the rate of fat mobilization
Growth hormone	Stimulates the release of free fatty acids from adipose tissue
Insulin	Stimulates fat synthesis
Thyroxine	Increases the rate of fat mobilization

The glycerol molecule is then converted to glucose (gluconeogenesis) and is either metabolized for energy or converted to glycogen or fat.

Through a complex series of reactions, fatty acids are catabolized by the liver (β oxidation) to two-carbon fragments. These fragments, known as acetyl coenzyme A (Co-A), can be oxidized for energy.

During normal fat metabolism, which requires oxygen and a compound generated by glucose (CHO) metabolism, small quantities of ketone bodies are formed (ketogenesis) and used for energy. However, when fat catabolism is excessive, such as when CHO intake is inadequate (or unavailable to meet the body's energy needs as in the case of uncontrolled diabetes), ketones accumulate in the bloodstream, leading to the condition known as ketosis. Normal fat catabolism cannot proceed if the supply of oxygen is inadequate, as occurs during overly strenuous exercise or with respiratory disease.

FAT ALLOWANCES, RECOMMENDATIONS, AND CONSUMPTION TRENDS

Saturated fatty acids, monounsaturated fatty acids, and cholesterol can be synthesized in the body. Therefore, no dietary requirement exists. Linoleic acid, which is known as *the* EFA because it alone can alleviate symptoms of EFA deficiency, should supply 1% to 2% of the total calorie intake in adults, or a minimum daily intake of 3 to 6 g (see display, How Much is a Gram?) This requirement is easily met in the typical American diet; safflower, sunflower, corn, cottonseed, and soybean oils are excellent sources of EFA. It is estimated that even in a totally fat-free diet, as little as one teaspoon of corn oil would supply enough linoleic acid to meet EFA requirements. For infants consuming 100 cal/kg of body weight/day, the EFA requirement is approximately 0.2 g/kg.

Although only 3 to 6 g of fat per day may truly be required, additional fat may be included in the diet to fulfill energy (calorie) requirements. However, because the body can get calories from other sources (eg, carbohydrates), a fat requirement to meet calorie needs has not been established.

The Fourth Edition of *Dietary Guidelines for Americans* (USDA/USDHHS, 1995) recommends that Americans choose a diet low in fat, saturated fat, and cholesterol. The suggestions for implementing these recommendations appear in the display, Suggestions for a Diet Low in Fat, saturated fat, and cholesterol and also in the display, Very Lean and Lean Meats (for more information on this, see also Chapter 8). According to *The Surgeon General's Report on Nutrition and Health* (PHS/USDHHS, 1988), a reduction in total fat intake, especially saturated fat, is emerging as the priority for dietary change in American diets. Research indicates that diets that are high in fat, saturated fat, and cholesterol increase the risk of obesity, heart disease, and certain cancers (see below). Indeed, the National Cholesterol Education Program (NCEP) recommends that all adult Americans limit fat intake to 30% of total calories or less, and saturated fat to 8% to 10% of total calories (NCEP, 1993). In addition, the American Cancer Society advises people to consume 30% or fewer total calories from fat (American Cancer Society, 1993) and the American Heart

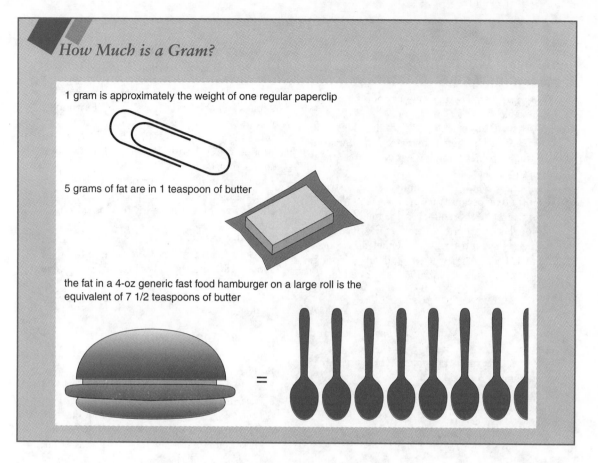

How Much is a Gram?

1 gram is approximately the weight of one regular paperclip

5 grams of fat are in 1 teaspoon of butter

the fat in a 4-oz generic fast food hamburger on a large roll is the equivalent of 7 1/2 teaspoons of butter

=

Association urges Americans to choose diets with less than 30% of calories from fat (AHA, 1991).

According to advance data of the Third National Health and Nutrition Examination Survey (NHANES), 34% of total calories in the average American diet come from fat, down from 36% of calories in the years 1976–1980 (CDC, 1994). Although this sounds like progress has been made toward lowering total fat intake, further research reveals that the average fat intake during these years remained the same; the percentage of fat calories dropped only because total calorie intake increased (Liebman, 1994).

NHANES data also indicate that we consume 12% of total calories from saturated fat (compared to the recommendation for less than 10%), 12.5% from monounsaturated fat (up to 15% is recommended), and 7% from polyunsaturated fat (less than 10% is recommended).

Although some progress is being made toward reducing and modifying fat intake, more change is needed. To achieve the necessary changes in fat intake, Americans must become more knowledgeable about their total fat allowance based on individual calorie requirements (see display, Figuring Fat) and must learn how to read labels to evaluate the fat content of foods (see display, Fat Label Facts). Although fat

Suggestions for a Diet Low in Fat, Saturated Fat, and Cholesterol

FATS AND OILS

- Use fats and oils sparingly in cooking and at the table.
- Use small amounts of salad dressings and spreads such as butter, margarine, and mayonnaise. Consider using low-fat or fat-free dressings for salads.
- Choose vegetable oils and soft margarines most often, because they are lower in saturated fat than solid shortenings and animal fats, even though their caloric content is the same.
- Check the Nutrition Facts Label to see how much fat and saturated fat are in a serving; choose foods lower in fat and saturated fat.

GRAIN PRODUCTS, VEGETABLES, AND FRUITS

- Choose low-fat sauces with pasta, rice, and potatoes.
- Use as little fat as possible to cook vegetables and grain products.
- Season with herbs, spices, lemon juice, and fat-free or low-fat salad dressings.

MEAT, POULTRY, FISH, EGGS, BEANS, AND NUTS

- Choose two to three servings of lean fish, poultry, meats, or other protein-rich foods, such as beans, daily. Use meats labeled "lean" or "extra lean." Trim fat from meat; take skin off poultry. (Three ounces of cooked lean beef or chicken without skin—a piece the size of a deck of cards—provides about 6 grams of fat; a piece of chicken with skin or untrimmed meat of that size may have as much as twice this amount of fat.) Most beans and bean products are almost fat-free and are a good source of protein and fiber.
- Limit intake of high-fat processed meats such as sausages, salami, and other cold cuts; choose lower fat varieties by reading the Nutrition Facts Label.
- Limit the intake of organ meats (three ounces of cooked chicken liver have about 540 mg of cholesterol); use egg yolks in moderation (one egg yolk has about 215 mg of cholesterol). Egg whites contain no cholesterol and can be used freely.

MILK AND MILK PRODUCTS

- Choose skim or low-fat milk, fat-free or low-fat yogurt, and low-fat cheese.
- Have two to three low-fat servings daily. Add extra calcium to your diet without added fat by choosing fat-free yogurt and low-fat milk more often. (One cup of skim milk has almost no fat, 1 cup of 1% milk has 2.5 grams of fat, 1 cup of 2% milk has 5 grams [one teaspoon] of fat, and 1 cup of whole milk has 8 grams of fat.) If you do not consume foods from this group, eat other calcium-rich foods.

(Source: USDA, USDHHS, 1995)

intake should be less than 30% of total calories, foods providing more than 30% are not necessarily contraindicated as long as they are balanced with low-fat foods so that overall intake approximates 30%.

Although the main sources of fat in the American diet continue to be fats and oils and meat (Fig. 3-4), choices within each category have changed in recent years (ADA, 1991). Since the 1950's, margarine consumption has surpassed that of butter and shortening intake has exceeded that of lard (see display, Margarine and Spreads). Beef consumption has dropped and poultry intake has increased. Reduced-fat and fat-free foods made with fat replacements are becoming increasingly popular as Americans try to lower their fat intake (see Food for Thought: Fake Fats).

Very Lean and Lean Meats

Item	Very Lean 0–1 g fat/oz (unless otherwise specified)	Lean 3 g fat/oz (unless otherwise specified)
Poultry	Chicken or turkey (white meat, no skin); cornish hen (no skin)	Chicken, turkey (dark meat, no skin); chicken white meat (with skin); domestic duck or goose (well-drained of fat, no skin)
Fish	Fresh or frozen cod, flounder, haddock, halibut, trout; tuna, fresh or canned in water	Herring (uncreamed or smoked); oysters (6 med); salmon (fresh or canned), catfish; sardines (canned) (2 med); tuna (canned in oil, drained)
Shellfish	Clams, crab, lobster, scallops, shrimp, imitation shellfish	None
Game	Duck or pheasant (no skin); venison; buffalo; ostrich	Goose (no skin); rabbit
Cheese	**Cheese with 1 gram or less fat per ounce:** Nonfat or low-fat cottage cheese (¼ c) Fat-free cheese	4.5%-fat cottage cheese (¼ c); grated parmesan (2 tbsp); cheeses with 3 grams or less fat per ounce
Other	Processed sandwich meats with 1 gram or less fat per ounce, such as deli thin, shaved meats, chipped beef, turkey ham; egg whites (2); egg substitutes, plain (¼ cup); hot dogs with 1 gram or less fat per ounce; kidney (high in cholesterol); sausage with 1 gram or less fat per ounce; dried beans, peas, lentils (cooked)	Hot dogs with 3 grams or less fat per ounce (1½ oz); processed sandwich meat with 3 grams or less fat per ounce, such as turkey pastrami or kielbasa); liver, heart (high in cholesterol)
Pork	None	Lean pork, such as fresh ham; canned, cured, or boiled ham; Canadian bacon; tenderloin, center loin chop
Lamb	None	Roast, chop, leg
Veal	None	Lean chop, roast
Beef	None	USDA Select or Choice grades of lean beef trimmed of fat, such as round, sirloin, and flank steak; tenderloin; roast (rib, chuck, rump); steak (T-bone, porterhouse, cubed), ground round

Source: ADA Exchange Lists.

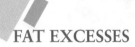

Figuring Fat

To determine total daily fat allowance:

1. Multiply total number of calories in the diet by 30% (0.30) to determine the desired maximum number of calories from fat:

$$\begin{array}{r} 1800 \text{ calories} \\ \times\ 0.30 \\ \hline 540 \text{ calories from fat} \end{array}$$

2. Divide the total number of fat calories by 9 calories/g to determine the total grams of fat recommended per day:

540 fat calories

divided by 9 calories/g = 60 g fat

FAT EXCESSES

An "excess of fat" is hard to define because actual fat requirements are so small. Most nutrition and health experts agree that Americans consume too much fat, which increases our risk for the following:

- Obesity. True, obesity can result from eating more calories than the body needs regardless of the source. However, because fats are a concentrated source of energy, eating 50 extra grams of fat (50 g × 9 cal/g = 450 calories) causes weight gain to occur more quickly than with 50 extra grams of either CHO or protein (50 g × 4 cal/g = 200 extra calories). High-fat diets are high in calories, and extremely low-fat diets tend to be unpalatable and lack satiety, that is, they leave you feeling hungry shortly after eating. An acceptable solution is moderate fat intake (ie, 30% of calories), which eliminates excess calories but not palatability and satiety.
- Coronary heart disease. Heart disease is not a foregone conclusion for *individuals* who eat a diet rich in fat, saturated fat, and cholesterol. However, epi-

Fat Label Facts

FAT

Fat free: Less than 0.5 g of fat per serving

Saturated fat free: Less than 0.5 g per serving and the level of *trans*-fatty acids does not exceed 1% of total fat

Low fat: 3 g or less per serving, and if the serving is 30 g or less or 2 tablespoons or less, per 50 g of the food

Low saturated fat: 1 g or less per serving and not more than 15% of calories from saturated fatty acids

Reduced or less fat: At least 25% less per serving than reference food

Reduced or less saturated fat: At least 25% less per serving than reference food

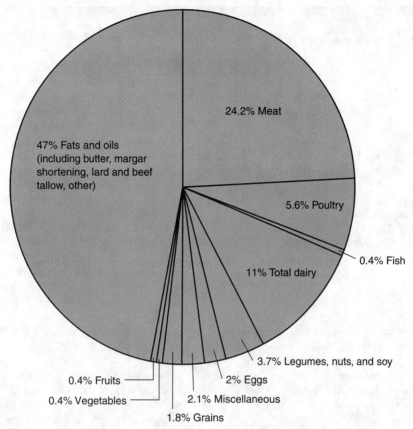

24.2% Meat

47% Fats and oils
(including butter, margar
shortening, lard and beef
tallow, other)

5.6% Poultry

0.4% Fish

11% Total dairy

3.7% Legumes, nuts, and soy

0.4% Fruits

2% Eggs

0.4% Vegetables

2.1% Miscellaneous

1.8% Grains

Figure 3-4
Fat contributed from major food groups to the U.S. food supply, 1990.

demiologic, animal, and clinical studies show that *population groups* who consume diets rich in fat have elevated serum cholesterol and lipoprotein levels, which are major risk factors in the development of atherosclerosis and coronary heart disease. The American Heart Association, in an effort to help prevent heart and vascular diseases, recommends that adults limit their intake of total fat to less than 30% of total calories, and limit saturated fat consumption to 10% or less of total calories (AHA, 1991).

• Certain types of cancer. Although the role of diet in the development of cancer is far from clear, the American Cancer Society estimates that 30% to 35% of all cases of cancer are diet-related. Based on numerous epidemiologic and animal studies, it appears that high-fat diets increase the risk of colon cancer and possibly other cancers. Although fat itself probably does not cause cancer, it seems to promote its development. In view of this, the Committee on Diet, Nutrition, and Cancer of the National Research Council/National Academy of Sciences recommends that Americans limit total fat intake to 30% of calories to reduce cancer risk. Interestingly, polyunsaturated fats seem just as likely to

Margarines and Spreads

The food industry has given the health-conscious American public a variety of choices to help decrease fat intake, especially in the butter aisle. To make the best choice, consider the product's physical form and intended use.

BUTTER

Standards set by the USDA and the FDA require butter to contain at least 80% fat by weight and to be fortified with vitamin A. Butter must be made from cream and milk; salt and/or coloring is optional. Butter is an all-purpose fat; however, it provides 11 g of fat (mostly saturated fat), 100 calories, and 28 mg of cholesterol per tablespoon.

MARGARINE

Like butter, products called margarine are required to contain at least 80% fat by weight and be fortified with vitamin A. Margarine must contain vegetable oil, water, and/or milk; salt, other vitamins, food coloring, emulsifying agents, and preservatives are optional. Margarine, available in stick and tub varieties, is also an all-purpose fat, but provides 11 g of fat and 100 calories per tablespoon.

SPREADS

A spread is classified as any butter or margarine that is less than 80% fat by weight. The percentage of fat by weight, which must appear on the label, ranges from 0% to 79%; generally, the softer the spread, the lower the fat content. Some or all of the fat may be replaced with water, gums, gelatins, or various starches; air is whipped into some. They come in sticks, tubs, liquids, and sprays. Unsalted and fat-free varieties are available. All are suitable for tabletop use; those with 50% fat or more may be used for sauteing, pan frying, and griddling. Spreads are generally not suitable for baking.

BLENDS

Blends are made from vegetable oil, milk fat, and other dairy ingredients used to provide a buttery taste. Their fat content can be reduced or be up to 80%. All blends are appropriate for tabletop use; they may or may not be suitable for cooking and baking, depending on the actual fat content.

BUDS

Butter-flavored buds, although made with a small amount of dehydrated butter, are considered "fat-free" and "cholesterol-free." They are intended to be sprinkled on hot, moist foods, like steaming vegetables, potatoes, and pasta. Mixed with water, they can be used to make butter-flavored sauces. They are not suitable for other uses.

(Source: Morgan, K, ed. (1995). Margarines and spreads: Definitions and uses. Nutrition Update. Winter 1995.)

promote cancer as saturated fats, and cholesterol appears to contribute no added risk (NRC, 1989).

FAT DEFICIENCY

Inadequate total fat intake is not likely to occur, because the body can synthesize fats from other sources. Moreover, the average American diet contains an abundance of fat. When an inadequate consumption of fat does occur, specifically resulting from an inadequate intake of calories, it is most likely related to one or more of the following problems:

FOOD *for* THOUGHT

Fake Fats

The market for artificial fats is booming, as Americans are caught between not wanting to give up the taste of their favorite high-fat foods, yet realizing the importance of reducing their fat intake. Fat substitutes, which are used to replace fat to varying degrees, simulate the texture, appearance, and taste of full-fat foods while reducing fat calories. As such, they have the potential to help Americans "have their cake and eat it too." Artificial fats may be classified as carbohydrate based, protein based, and fat based.

Carbohydrate-based artificial fats are used as thickeners, bulking agents, moisturizers, and stabilizers in lower fat and fat-free frozen desserts, cheeses, baked goods, salad dressings, sauces, gravies, processed meats, sour cream, yogurt, and pudding. Because they do not melt, they cannot be used for frying. They provide 1 to 4 cal/g, depending on how well they are digested.

Dextrins
    bland, nonsweet CHO made from starch
    gel-forming capacity simulates the texture and
        mouth feel of fat
    caloric content varies with the concentration
        used

Maltodextrin
    derived from cornstarch, potato starch, or
        tapioca starch
    can replace up to 100% of the fat in foods like
        margarine, frozen desserts, salad dressings,
        cereals, and snacks

Polydextrose
    a nonsweet starch polymer
    used as a bulking agent to replace some of the
        volume that is lost when fat and/or sugar are
        removed from a food
    most passes through the body unabsorbed;
        does not interfere with the absorption of vit-
        amins, minerals, or amino acids

Cellulose
    made from purified wood pulp
    forms a colloidal gel; can be used to replace up

to 100% of the fat in products such as salad
        dressings, sauces, and frozen desserts
    noncaloric

Gums
    provide creamy mouth feel when water
        replaces fat in foods, and help stabilize
        emulsions like pourable salad dressings and
        low-fat spoonable dressings
    are not digested, except by colonic bacteria;
        caloric value is negligible

Protein-based fat replacements may be made from whey protein concentrate, egg white, or soy and corn proteins; Simpless (The Nutrasweet Company, Deerfield, IL) is the most noted. They have the "mouth feel" of fat (ie, they feel creamy to the tongue), help retain moisture, and help stabilize emulsions in sauces, spreads, and salad dressings. Protein-based fat replacements can be used in cheese, butter, mayonnaise, salad dressings, frozen dairy desserts, sour cream, and baked goods. Because protein is not an effective conductor of heat, protein-based fat replacements cannot be used for frying, but they can be used in many high-temperature situations (ADA, 1991). Like carbohydrate-based artificial fats, they cannot be used for deep frying. They provide between 1 and 4 cal/g, depending on the degree of hydration.

Fat-based ingredients have the same physical properties as fats, such as taste, texture, and mouth feel. They are actual fats that are modified to provide fewer calories and less available fat to foods; some are structurally modified to provide no calories or fat.

Caprenin
    a reduced-calorie fat because it is only partially
        absorbed
    functional properties are similar to cocoa but-
        ter; it is intended to replace cocoa butter in
        soft candy and candy coatings

Olestra (brand name is Olean by Procter and
    Gamble, Cincinnati, OH

(continued)

formed from sucrose (but is not sweet) and long-chain fatty acids

resembles fat in appearance, taste, texture, and function

is suitable for frying, cooking, and baking, but approved for use only in salty-type snack foods like potato chips and crackers

is calorie free because it is not absorbed

manufacturers of foods made with Olestra are required to add vitamins A, D, E, and K because heavy use of Olestra impairs the absorption of the fat-soluble vitamins

DDM, EPG, and TATCA are other fat-based fat replacements currently under development.

- Disease- or drug-induced anorexia (eg, cancer and cancer therapies)
- Anorexia nervosa (the psychological disorder of self-imposed starvation)
- Altered digestion and absorption, associated with pancreatic insufficiency, celiac sprue, lactose intolerance, and other malabsorption syndromes

An EFA deficiency is rare but may develop in adults who are taking prolonged EFA-free parenteral feedings or in infants who are consuming EFA-deficient formulas. Essential fatty acid–deficient infants may exhibit inadequate growth rates and decreased resistance to infection, possibly resulting from an inadequate production of prostaglandins.

Possible signs and symptoms of an inadequate fat intake include a thin, emaciated appearance related to the loss of subcutaneous adipose tissue; sensitivity to cold; dry, dull hair; constipation (fat in the intestine acts as a lubricant); secondary deficiencies of the fat-soluble vitamins; and secondary protein malnutrition.

KEY CONCEPTS

- Ninety-five percent of lipids consumed in the diet are triglycerides, which are composed of one glyceride molecule and 3 fatty acids. Most fatty acids in foods are long chain, containing 16 or 18 carbon atoms. Phospholipids and sterols are the other 2 types of dietary lipids.
- All of the calories in pure fats and oils (eg, butter, margarine, olive oil) are from fat; the percentage of calories from fat varies in meat, milk, dairy products, sweets, and snacks. Most fruits and vegetables are fat free.
- Per equivalent amounts, fat provides more than twice the calories as either carbohydrates or protein. Fatty acids can be oxidized for energy by all body cells, with the exception of the central nervous system and erythrocytes, which normally rely exclusively on glucose for energy.
- Because they perform vital functions and cannot be synthesized in the body, linoleic acid and linolenic acid are essential fatty acids; arachidonic acid becomes an essential fatty acid when linoleic acid intake is deficient. Because all other fats can be synthesized in the body, no dietary requirement has been established.

- Saturation refers to the hydrogen atoms attached to the carbon atoms in the fatty acid chain. Saturated fatty acids do not have any double bonds between carbon atoms; thus each carbon is "saturated" with hydrogen. Unsaturated fats have one (mono) or more (poly) double bonds between carbon atoms. When used to describe food fats, these terms are relative descriptions of the type of fat present in the largest amount; all foods contain a mixture of saturated, monounsaturated, and polyunsaturated fatty acids.

- Because saturated fats tend to raise serum cholesterol, a risk factor for the development of coronary heart disease, experts recommend Americans limit their intake of saturated fat to less than 10% of total calories. Saturated fats are found mostly in animal sources, and also predominate in coconut, palm, and palm kernel oil.

- Cholesterol, a component of all cell membranes, is used to synthesize bile acids and is a precursor of vitamin D and the steroid hormones. Because the body makes cholesterol, it does not need to be consumed in the diet. It appears that dietary cholesterol has less of an impact on serum cholesterol than does saturated fat intake.

- Short-chain and medium-chain fatty acids, glycerol, and medium-chain triglycerides are absorbed into the portal vein, mostly in the duodenum and jejunum. Because they are insoluble in water (blood), triglycerides, cholesterol, and phospholipids are absorbed into the lymph system, not the portal vein.

REFERENCES

American Cancer Society (1993). Nutrition, Common Sense, and Cancer. American Cancer Society.

American Diabetes Association, American Dietetic Association (1995). Exchange Lists for Meal Planning. Chicago: American Diabetes Association.

American Dietetic Association (1991). Position paper of the American Dietetic Association: Fat replacements. JADA, 91(10), 1285–1288.

American Heart Association (1991). An Eating Plan for Healthy Americans. Dallas: American Heart Association.

CDC (1994). Advance data. Energy and macronutrient intakes of persons ages 2 months and over in the United States: Third National Health and Nutrition Examination Survey, Phase 1, 1988–91. DHHS Publication No. (PHS) 95-1250.

International Food Information Council (1995). Uses and nutritional impact of fat reduction ingredients. IFIC Review, November 1995.

International Food Information Council (1995). Sorting out the facts about fat. IFIC Review, January 1995.

International Food Information Council (1995). Fats and fat replacers. Food Insight, September/October, 1, 4–5.

Liebman, B. (1994). Confusing fat. Nutrition Action Health Letter, 21(4), 4.

National Cholesterol Education Program (1993). Second Report of the Expert Panel on Detection, Evaluation, and Treatment of High Blood Cholesterol in Adults. NIH Publication No. 93-3095.

National Research Council (1989). Recommended Dietary Allowances. 10th ed. Washington, DC: National Academy Press.

Public Health Service, United States Department of Health and Human Services (1988). The Surgeon General's Report on Nutrition and Health: Summary and Recommendations. DHHS (PHS) Publication No. 88-50211. Washington, DC: Government Printing Office.

Shils, M., Olson, J., and Shike, M. (1994). Modern Nutrition in Health and Disease. 8th ed. Philadelphia: Lea & Febiger.

United States Department of Agriculture, and United States Department of Health and Human Services (1995). Nutrition and Your Health: Dietary Guidelines for Americans. 4th ed. Home and Garden Bulletin No. 232.

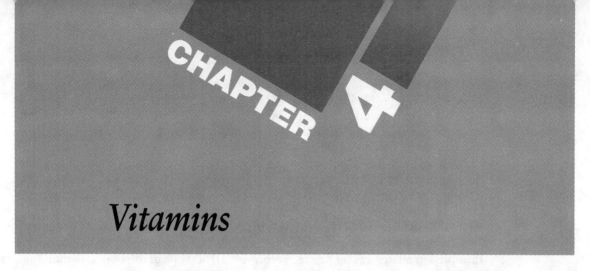

CHAPTER 4

Vitamins

Chapter Outline

Key Terms

Antioxidants   Hypervitaminosis   Provitamins
Antivitaminosis   Megadose   Vitamins
Antivitamins   Organic substances
Free radicals   Phytochemicals

CHARACTERISTICS OF VITAMINS AS A GROUP

Vitamins are chemical compounds made of the elements carbon, hydrogen, oxygen, and sometimes nitrogen or other elements. The presence of carbon classifies vitamins as **organic substances**, which can be converted to other forms and are susceptible to oxidation and destruction. Vitamins are soluble in either water or fat. Solubility influences their absorption, movement through the blood, storage, and excretion.

The body needs vitamins in very small amounts to help regulate body processes, such as the synthesis of numerous body compounds like bones, skin, nerves, brain, and blood. Vitamins do not provide energy (calories) but are required for the metabolism of energy-providing nutrients (CHO, protein, and fat). Most vitamins function by combining with a protein (apoenzyme) to form a coenzyme that promotes the action of enzymes. Without vitamins, thousands of chemical reactions cannot occur, and health and life are seriously threatened.

Most vitamins cannot be synthesized by the body; others are produced in inadequate amounts (see Appendices 2 and 3). Therefore, vitamins are an essential part of a healthy diet. The body can make vitamin D, vitamin A, and niacin *if* the proper precursors are available. Microorganisms in the gastrointestinal (GI) tract can synthesize vitamin K and vitamin B_{12} but not in sufficient amounts to meet the body's needs.

Vitamins are present in foods only in very small amounts; vitamins usually are measured in milligrams (mg), which represent 1/1000 of a gram, or micrograms (µg), 1/1000 of a milligram (Fig. 4-1).

INDIVIDUAL VITAMINS

Individual vitamins vary greatly in the way their elements are arranged, so that each is a distinct chemical individual. Each vitamin has one or more specific functions and cannot be converted to or substituted for another. Individual vitamins may exist in several different active forms; different forms perform different functions.

DEFINITIONS

Provitamins

Provitamins (or vitamin precursors) are vitamin-related compounds that can be converted to active vitamins in the body under proper conditions. Examples include tryptophan (an amino acid), which can be converted to niacin; carotene, which can be converted to vitamin A; and cholesterol, which can be converted to vitamin D.

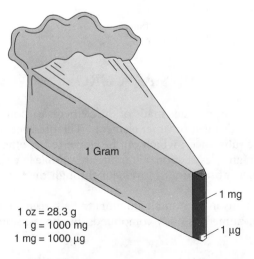

1 Gram

1 mg

1 oz = 28.3 g
1 g = 1000 mg
1 mg = 1000 µg

1 µg

Figure 4-1
Comparative units of measure.

Antivitamins

Antivitamins (vitamin antagonists or antimetabolites) are substances that block the synthesis or metabolism of a vitamin. Some drugs, like methotrexate (a folic acid antagonist), antibiotics (because they interfere with vitamin K synthesis), and dicumarol (an antagonist of vitamin K), are common antivitamins.

Avitaminosis

Avitaminosis means literally "without vitamins." When followed by the letter of a vitamin, avitaminosis means that that particular vitamin is deficient (eg, avitaminosis A).

Hypervitaminosis

When followed by the letter of a vitamin, **hypervitaminosis** means that an excess of that particular vitamin has accumulated in the body to toxic levels. Examples include hypervitaminosis A and hypervitaminosis D.

Megadose

A **megadose** is an amount at least 10 times greater than the RDA. Vitamins in megadoses have pharmacologic strength and act more like drugs than nutrients.

VITAMIN SOURCES

Although the American Diabetic Association and American Dietetic Association exchange lists are useful for identifying the sources and amounts of CHO, protein, and fat contained in the diet, the exchange lists do not indicate sources of vitamins and minerals. Likewise, dietary recommendations made by leading health organizations focus mostly on avoiding excesses of nutrients (sugar, protein, fats, and cholesterol), rather than on obtaining adequate amounts of vitamins and minerals. Despite the emphasis on avoiding too much, a "balanced diet" (ie, the food-group approach to meal planning) is still important to ensure nutritional adequacy.

The USDA's Food Guide Pyramid (see Chapter 8) divides foods into five major groups. Although the Pyramid is nonspecific with regard to quantities of *nutrients* that must be consumed, daily amounts of foods are recommended from each group. It is assumed that the vitamin and mineral content of the diet will be adequate if appropriate amounts of a variety of foods from each food group are chosen.

However, a person may eat the recommended number of servings from each of the food groups and still not have an adequate vitamin intake, if food selections are not varied. Because not all foods within a group are nutritionally equivalent (eg, pork is rich in thiamine but other meats are not), actual vitamin intake varies considerably depending on actual food choices. Also, vitamin retention in foods, especially of water-soluble vitamins, depends on proper handling, storage, and preparation. The theoretical vitamin content of a food that is listed in a food composition table may greatly exceed the amount of vitamin actually provided after that food has been prepared for consumption. And lastly, people with individual needs that are higher than normal because of metabolic disorders, inadequate absorption, the use of certain medications, substance abuse, or genetic background may require additional vitamins, which may be obtained through either dietary intake or use of vitamin supplements.

VITAMIN DEFICIENCIES

Before the 1940s, vitamin deficiencies were prevalent in the United States and throughout the world. As a result of an abundant food supply, selected fortification of certain foods, and better methods of determining and improving the nutrient content of foods, vitamin deficiency diseases have virtually been eliminated in developed countries. However, many researchers are questioning whether prevention of deficiencies should be the sole criterion in determining daily requirements; perhaps larger doses of certain vitamins, specifically those known as antioxidants, offer protection against chronic health problems like heart disease and certain cancers (see display, Antioxidants). Certainly, an exciting area of nutrition research focuses on phytochemicals—substances in fruits and vegetables that could be the vitamins of tomorrow (see Food for Thought: Phytochemicals).

Antioxidants

Free radicals are highly unstable, highly reactive molecule fragments that are produced continuously in cells as a byproduct of normal metabolism, as when oxygen is burned, and also by other means, such as by smoking tobacco. Because they have an unpaired electron, free radicals quickly react with other compounds to gain an electron, causing a chain reaction that generates even more free radicals. For instance, free radicals that are formed within cells can attack weak bonds in cell membranes or DNA in their search for an electron; in doing so, the oxidized molecule (the molecule that lost an electron) is impaired structurally and functionally, the free radicals become new stable molecules, and other free radicals are formed. Damage caused by free radicals is believed to contribute to aging and various health problems. Polyunsaturated fatty acids in the cell membrane are particularly vulnerable to the effects of free radicals.

Antioxidants are substances that can reduce (donate electrons to) another substance (ie, free radicals); by reducing the other substance, antioxidants themselves become oxidized and thus are destroyed. In the body, naturally occurring antioxidants and antioxidant vitamins (vitamins C and E and beta-carotene) sacrifice themselves to protect body cells from free radical damage.

Because free radicals have such a short lifetime, it is difficult to measure their role in the cause of disease. Yet, researchers speculate that damage to cell membranes or DNA that is caused by free radicals influences the process and may be implicated in the development of certain cancers, atherosclerotic heart disease, and cataracts. Conversely, antioxidants may prevent or forestall disease caused by free radical damage. However, health officials believe it is premature to recommend dietary supplements containing antioxidants because it may be that other substances in fruits and vegetables, like phytochemicals, are what protects us from disease.

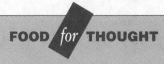

Phytochemicals

Over the past 20 years, researchers have consistently found that people who eat the most fruits and vegetables have lower rates of most cancers, especially epithelial cancers of the lung, bladder, cervix, mouth, larynx, throat, esophagus, stomach, pancreas, colon, and rectum. Although some vegetables appear to be better at guarding against certain cancers (eg, for lung cancer, carrots and green leafy vegetables seem most protective), fruits and vegetables, in general, are credited with the lower risk.

True, fruits and vegetables provide vitamins, minerals, and fiber that may also protect us against disease, but it is their hundreds or maybe thousands of **phytochemicals**, naturally occurring "plant" chemicals that may alter human metabolism to protect us from cancer, that are so intriguing (ADA, 1995). In laboratory and animal studies, phytochemicals appear to be potent anticarcinogens; however, that doesn't mean they work the same way in people. All fruits and vegetables have them in varying combinations and concentrations—tomatoes are estimated to have 10,000 phytochemicals. They are also found in grains, legumes, seeds, soy, and green tea. While no one can say that phytochemicals prevent cancer, the American Dietetic Association recognizes that phytochemicals may have a beneficial role in health as part of a varied diet

(ADA, 1995). And everyone agrees that eating more fruits and vegetables is a good idea. Raw or cooked, canned, frozen, juiced, or peeled, the more the better. Today's phytochemicals may be tomorrow's vitamins. . . .

Limonene in citrus fruits increases the production of enzymes that may destroy potential carcinogens

Allyl sulfides that are found in garlic, onions, leeks, and chives influence the production of an enzyme that may promote carcinogen excretion. Other allium compounds may impair tumor cell reproduction

Dithiolthiones in broccoli may trigger enzymes that block carcinogens from damaging a cell's DNA

Ellagic acid in grapes scavenges carcinogens and may prevent them from altering DNA

Isothiocyanates in cruciferous vegetables (bok choy, broccoli, brussels sprouts, cabbage, cauliflower, collards, kale, rutabaga) promote the formation of an enzyme that may block carcinogens from damaging a cell's DNA

P-*Coumaric acid and chlorogenic acid* found in tomatoes, green peppers, pineapples, strawberries, and carrots block the formation of nitrosamines.

Although severe vitamin deficiencies occur rarely in the United States, food consumption surveys indicate that very few people consume 100% of the RDA for all nutrients. However, because RDA are intended to exceed the needs of most healthy people, the vast majority of Americans consume at least their average need (77% of the RDA) of all 14 nutrients for which data are available (ADA, 1994). The vitamins most likely to be consumed at suboptimal levels are vitamin A, vitamin C, and folic acid (ADA, 1994). Those most likely to consume inadequate nutrients are adolescent girls, people on limited incomes, pregnant and lactating women, and the elderly. Smokers, alcoholics, and chronic users of certain medications; people who are chronically ill; and people with psychological disturbances are also at risk.

Although the actual biochemical and clinical findings vary, depending on which vitamin is deficient, the progression of the deficiency is the same for all vitamins (Fig. 4-2).

VITAMIN SUPPLEMENTS

It is estimated that Americans spend $3.7 billion a year on dietary supplements (Slesinski et al, 1995). Although estimates vary, 25% to 35% of American adults take a vitamin and/or mineral supplement daily; 9% of people polled consumed more than one type of supplement daily (Slesinski et al, 1995). Generally, supplement use is most common in the western United States and among whites, women, the elderly, people with higher incomes, those with higher education, nonsmokers (especially former smokers), and those who do not drink alcohol heavily (ADA, 1996).

Healthy adults who consume a variety of properly prepared foods from each of the food groups rarely require vitamin supplements. In the National Research Council's report entitled *Diet and Health*, eating a variety of foods, not consuming supplements, was recommended as the desirable way for the general public to obtain adequate amounts of nutrients (NRC, 1989). It is virtually unheard of to overdose on vitamins and minerals from food, and it may be that there are hundreds or thousands of other chemicals in foods (especially in fruits and vegetables) that are necessary for optimal health that haven't yet been identified. However, a supplement may be indicated when intake is marginal or unbalanced, or lacks variety. Examples include vitamin B_{12} for vegans, folic acid for women of childbearing age, vitamin D for those with limited milk intake and sunlight exposure; calcium for those with lactose intolerance or milk allergy; and a multivitamin and mineral supplement for people on very-low-calorie diets (ADA, 1996). Other population groups who may benefit from the use of supplements include people with increased vitamin requirements who may not be able to consume adequate amounts of vitamins through diet alone, such as pregnant and lactating women, people with malabsorption disorders or certain other chronic diseases, and people who use specific medications that interfere with the absorption or metabolism of vitamins. Severe physical stress, such as major surgery, second- and third-degree burns, large bone fractures, and multiple injuries, increases the need for vitamin C and certain other nutrients. Despite advertising

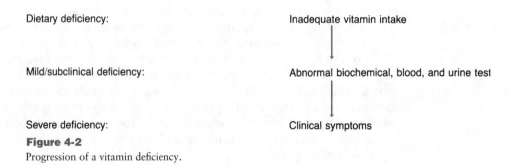

Figure 4-2

Progression of a vitamin deficiency.

claims, it has never been determined what, if any, effect psychological stress has on vitamin requirements.

People who need vitamin supplements should take them. People who do not need them are wasting their money and risk health problems if they take vitamins in excess of the RDA, especially high doses of single nutrients. Many people self-prescribe vitamins based on widespread beliefs that the typical American diet is deficient in vitamins; that taking supplements will provide energy, increase endurance, and combat stress; and that vitamin supplements can prevent or cure a wide variety of ills like cancer, colds, and arthritis. Many vitamin users are convinced that supplements help them cope better during times of stress or worry, and that supplements can make up for a "bad" diet.

Certainly, food is the best and safest source of nutrients. But those who choose to take unprescribed supplements should take a balanced multivitamin instead of only one or two vitamins, because vitamins work best together and when they are in balanced proportions. Too much of one vitamin can mask a deficiency of another. For instance, folic acid can reverse anemia caused by B_{12} deficiency but not the neurologic symptoms, which may remain undiagnosed and can cause permanent damage. In addition, people who are deficient usually need more than one vitamin because singular vitamin deficiencies, especially of the B complex vitamins, are rare (see display, Supplements: Buying Basics).

FAT-SOLUBLE VITAMINS

Vitamins A, D, E, and K are the four fat-soluble vitamins. A summary of the fat-soluble vitamins is outlined in Table 4-1.

Group Characteristics

As a group, fat-soluble vitamins have the following characteristics:

- They are absorbed into the lymphatic system with fat. Fat-soluble vitamin deficiencies can occur secondary to any condition that interferes with fat absorption, such as malabsorption syndromes, and pancreatic and biliary diseases.
- They must be attached to protein carriers to be transported through the blood, because fat is not soluble in water (blood).
- They are not excreted when consumed in excess of need; rather, they are stored primarily in the liver and adipose tissue.
- They can be toxic when consumed in large doses over a prolonged period of time, particularly vitamin A and vitamin D.
- Fat-soluble vitamin deficiency symptoms are slow to develop.
- Because of the body's storage reserve, they do not have to be consumed every day.
- They are fairly stable when subjected to heat, that is, they are not easily destroyed by cooking.

Supplements: Buying Basics

COMPOSITION

For an all-purpose, insurance-type supplement, stick to ones that provide only 100% of the Daily Value (the old USRDA) for the 12 vitamins and 8 minerals for which there are established Daily Values. It's easy to find multivitamin supplements; multivitamins with multiminerals at 100% Daily Value are more scarce.

If you go the megavitamin route, keep in mind that, with few exceptions, manufacturers are free to add or leave out whatever nutrients they choose. What they put in is often based on economics, not health. For instance, because biotin is expensive, only small amounts, if any, are found in supplements. Conversely, most of the other Bs are cheap, so they are often used abundantly. Buyer beware:

- The nutrient content on some brands is listed as a "serving," but you need to take 2 or 3 "servings" a day
- Taking more than 100% of the RDA for vitamins like thiamine, riboflavin, or niacin is usually not harmful, but it doesn't offer any advantage
- Taking more than 100% of the RDA for vitamins A, D, and B_6 is potentially harmful
- Average vitamin C intake exceeds the RDA even without supplements. Studies show that bioflavinoids do not appear to promote the absorption of vitamin C, despite label claims to the contrary, and despite costing 3 to 4 times more than vitamin C without bioflavinoids (Johnson and Luo, 1994).
- Dietary deficiencies of biotin and pantothenic acid are practically unheard of . . . why take more?
- Studies on vitamin E and its role in reducing the risks of heart disease, cancer, and cataracts use doses of 100 to 400 IU or more daily—more than the amount any diet or most multivitamins supply. To get that much, separate supplements are needed.
- Recent studies showed that people taking large doses of beta-carotene (20 mg or 33,333 IU) actually had a higher incidence of lung cancer and that their risk of heart disease may actually have been increased also; this despite observational studies that show populations who eat large amounts of fruits and vegetables, especially those rich in carotenes, have a lower risk of most cancers (Liebman, 1994). It may be that other carotenes or other substances in fruits and vegetables are protective, and that taking large doses of only one kind of beta-carotene may interfere with the absorption, transport, or utilization of the anticancer substance. Until more is known, it is best to get beta-carotene from fruits and vegetables, and avoid it in supplements.
- The average diet provides enough iodine, manganese, boron, molybdenum, and chloride (minerals)
- The average diet supplies more than the RDA for phosphorus; taking more can weaken bones
- Men and postmenopausal women are at low risk for iron deficiency and do not need to exceed their RDA of 10 mg. Unless it is medically indicated, premenopausal women should not exceed the Daily Value of 18 mg.

(continued)

Vitamin A

Vitamin A was recognized in 1913 as the first identified fat-soluble vitamin. Although it is relatively stable, vitamin A is destroyed gradually by continued exposure to air, light, and heat.

Pre-formed vitamin A exists as a group of compounds commonly known as retinoids. These include retinol, retinaldehyde, and retinoic acid. Vitamin A activity

Supplements: Buying Basics (Continued)

- Nickel, silicon, and boron are essential for animals, but because a human deficiency has not been identified, it is impossible to say whether humans need these trace elements
- Cadmium, lead, lithium, tin, and vanadium may remotely be needed by humans in minute amounts, amounts easily met through intake of food, water, and air.

NATURAL IS NOT NATURALLY BETTER

Marketing tactics that promote vitamins as "natural" and "organic" are open to interpretation. In fact, "natural" often means synthetic mixed with plant extracts. Regardless of whether a vitamin is synthetically prepared in a laboratory or extracted from natural food sources, the chemical structure is the same. For instance, the body cannot distinguish between inexpensive synthetic vitamin C and vitamin C from rosehips that costs twice as much. The only exception appears to be vitamin E: Natural vitamin E appears to be slightly better absorbed than the synthetic variety. To find natural vitamin E, ignore "natural" on the label and look for "*d*-alpha tocopherol" on the ingredient list, not "*dl*-alpha tocopherol."

THEY'VE GOT TO DISINTEGRATE

According to the Dietary Supplement Health and Education Act of 1994, supplements must meet appropriate specifications for quality, including tablet or capsule disintegration. Voluntary standards for disintegration and dissolution are in the *U.S. Pharmacopeia*. But, if you want to be sure the supplement will disintegrate, choose a chewable variety—either adult or children's. However, many chewables are low in minerals.

HIGHER COST DOESN'T NECESSARILY MEAN HIGHER QUALITY

Vitamin supplements do not necessarily follow the dictum of "you get what you pay for." Because large retail chains like K-Mart and Wal-mart are high-volume customers, they can demand, and get, their own top quality "store brand" supplements from vitamin manufacturers; their cost is usually significantly less than that of brand name varieties, yet the quality and content are similar.

Many high-priced supplements contain optional ingredients that aren't essential, like inositol, bioflavinoids, and herbs. Why buy what you don't need?

FRESHNESS COUNTS

Freshness should be a consideration, because over time, supplements can decompose or become too hard to dissolve. Prolonged storage, especially under hot, humid conditions like those in a bathroom, causes vitamins to lose their potency. Unfortunately, the FDA does not require expiration dates on vitamin supplements, so look for one that's dated, preferably at least a few months ahead.

Source: Liebman, B., and Schardt, D. (1995). Vitamin Smarts. Nutrition Action Health Letter, 22(9), 1, 6–10.

differs among retinoids. Preformed vitamin A is found only in animal sources such as any kind of liver (beef, veal, pork, lamb, chicken, and turkey), butter, cream, and egg yolk. Significant amounts of vitamin A are supplied by foods fortified with vitamin A, such as milk, dairy products, and breakfast cereals. Fish oils are rich in vitamin A but are not generally consumed as foods.

The precursors of vitamin A are carotenes or carotenoids, the yellow pigment in yellow fruits and yellow and dark green vegetables (the green pigment, chlorophyll,

Table 4-1
Summary of Fat-Soluble Vitamins

Vitamin	Functions	Deficiency Signs and Symptoms
VITAMIN A Vitamin precursor: carotene Vitamin: retinol **Adult RDA** Men: 1000 µg RE* Women: 800 µg RE Pregnancy: 800 µg RE Lactation: 1300 µg RE	The formation of visual purple, which enables the eye to adapt to dim light Normal growth and development of bones and teeth The formation and maintenance of mucosal epithelium to maintain healthy functioning of skin and membranes, hair, gums, and various glands Important role in immune function	Night blindness, or the slow recovery of vision after flashes of bright light at night Bone growth ceases; bone shape changes; enamel-forming cells in the teeth malfunction; teeth crack and tend to decay. Skin becomes dry, scaly, rough, and cracked; keratinization or hyperkeratosis develops; mucous membrane cells flatten and harden: Eyes become dry (xerosis); irreversible drying and hardening of the cornea can result in blindness. Decreased saliva secretion → difficulty chewing, swallowing → anorexia Decreased mucous secretion of the stomach and intestines → impaired digestion and absorption → diarrhea, increased excretion of nutrients Susceptibility to respiratory, urinary tract, and vaginal infections increases.

Food Sources
Preformed retinol is found in liver, fish liver oils, whole + fortified milk and dairy products, fortified margarine, and fortified breakfast cereals. Carotenes are found in dark-green and yellow vegetables, such as sweet potatoes, winter squash, carrots, broccoli, spinach, "greens," peaches, apricots, and cantaloupe

Vitamin	Functions	Deficiency Signs and Symptoms
VITAMIN D Vitamin precursors: ergosterol, 7-dehydro-cholesterol Vitamins: D$_2$ (ergocholecalciferol), D$_3$ (cholecalciferol) **Adult RDA** 19–24-year olds: 10 µg After age 24: 5 µg Pregnancy or lactation: 10 µg	Helps maintain optimal serum levels of calcium and phosphorus for normal bone mineralization by stimulating the intestinal absorption of calcium Mobilizing calcium and phosphorus from the bone Stimulating reabsorption of calcium by the kidney Increasing reabsorption of phosphorus by the kidney	Rickets (in infants and children) Retarded bone growth Bone malformations (bowed legs) Enlargement of ends of long bones (knock-knees) Deformities of the ribs (bowed, with beads or knobs) Delayed closing of the fontanel → rapid enlargement of the head Decreased serum calcium and/or phosphorus Malformed teeth; decayed teeth Protrusion of the abdomen related to relaxation of the abdominal muscles Increased secretion of parathyroid hormone Osteomalacia (in adults) Softening of the bones → deformities, pain, and easy fracture Decreased serum calcium and/or phosphorus, increased alkaline phosphatase Involuntary muscle twitching and spasms

(continued)

Table 4-1 (Continued)
Summary of Fat-Soluble Vitamins

Vitamin	Functions	Deficiency Signs and Symptoms

Food Sources
Fortified milk, margarine, and breakfast cereals; small amounts are found in butter, egg yolk, liver, salmon, sardines, and tuna fish

VITAMIN E

Tocopherol (alpha, beta, and gamma tocopherol)	Acts as an antioxidant to protect vitamin A and PUFA from being destroyed	Increased RBC hemolysis
Adult RDA	Protects cell membranes	In infants, anemia, edema, and skin lesions
Men: 10 mg α-TE†		
Women: 8 mg α-TE		
Pregnancy: 10 mg-TE		
Lactation: 12 mg α-TE		

Food Sources
Vegetable oils, wheat germ, leafy vegetables, soybeans, corn, peanuts, pecans, walnuts, and margarine and salad dressings made with vegetable oils

VITAMIN K

Vitamin K_1 (phylloquinone)	Essential for the formation of 5 proteins necessary for normal blood clotting	Delayed blood clotting $\rightarrow$ hemorrhage
Vitamin K_2 (menaquinone)		Hemorrhagic disease of the newborn
Adult RDA		
Men: 80 µg		
Women: 65 µg		
Pregnancy or lactation: 65 µg		

Food Sources
K_1: Green leafy vegetables, cabbage, cauliflower, spinach, cheese, egg yolk, and liver.
K_2: Synthesized by GI flora

* RE = retinol equivalents. 1 retinol equivalent = 1 µg retinol or 6 µg β-carotene
† α = tocopherol equivalents. 1 mg d = α tocopherol = 1 α-TE

masks the presence of carotenes in green vegetables). Although there are some 500 naturally occurring carotenoids in plants and some animal fats, only 50 are precursors of vitamin A. Beta carotene is the most common of these. Because not all carotenes can be converted into vitamin A, the color intensity of a fruit or vegetable is not a reliable indicator of provitamin A content. Excellent sources include sweet potatoes, winter squash, carrots, broccoli, spinach, green leafy vegetables, peaches, apricots, and cantaloupe. The RDA for vitamin A is measured in retinol equivalents.

FUNCTIONS

Vitamin A is best known for its role in night vision, the normal growth of bones and teeth, and the formation and maintenance of mucosal epithelium for the normal function of skin, hair, gums, various glands, and mucous membranes. The role of vitamin A is less well understood in reproduction, cell membrane stability, the synthesis of corticosterone (a hormone produced by the adrenal glands), the output of thyroxine (the hormone secreted by the thyroid gland), the development of the nervous system, red blood cell (RBC) production, and immune system functioning.

CLINICAL APPLICATIONS

Vitamin A Deficiency

Even if the diet is devoid of vitamin A, it may take several years for a vitamin A deficiency to become apparent because the body is capable of storing large amounts of vitamin A and deficiency symptoms do not appear until body stores are exhausted. Vitamin A deficiency is often associated with protein-calorie malnutrition.

Vitamin A deficiency may be caused by an inadequate intake (primary deficiency) or may occur secondary to malabsorption disorders, pancreatic and biliary diseases, disorders that interfere with vitamin A storage, or conditions that prevent the conversion of carotenes to vitamin A.

Severe vitamin A deficiency occurs rarely in the United States, although mild vitamin A deficiency may be seen among low socioeconomic groups. In many developing nations, vitamin A deficiency is the major cause of blindness.

Clinical Findings

Vitamin A deficiency may produce the following clinical findings:

Night blindness or changes in the eyes, such as dryness, wrinkling, keratinization, ulceration, or softening and perforation of the cornea may occur.
Skin may appear dry, scaly, or bumpy.
Diarrhea may develop, and susceptibility to respiratory infections increases.
Teeth may appear cracked or decayed.
Fatigue and other symptoms of anemia may develop.

Treatment

Acute vitamin A deficiency is treated with large doses of oral supplements; the more severe the symptoms, the longer the response time to vitamin A therapy.

Vitamin A Toxicity

The occurrence of vitamin A toxicity is not likely to result from problems with diet alone; toxicity is usually associated with megadoses of vitamin A supplements. Toxicity can develop in adults who have sustained daily intakes exceeding 15,000 µg. Short of consuming liver or fish liver oils daily, this dose cannot be achieved from foods alone. Children can develop toxic reactions to vitamin A at lower doses. Individual tolerance to vitamin A varies considerably. However, toxicity occurs only from excessive intakes of pre-formed vitamin A, not from the vitamin A precursor carotene, which is not converted to vitamin A quickly enough to cause a toxicity. Instead, carotene is stored in adipose tissue and may accumulate under the skin to the extent that it causes the skin color to turn yellowish orange, a harmless condition known as hypercarotenemia.

Manifestations of vitamin A toxicity include anorexia, abnormal skin pigmentation, nausea, vomiting, abdominal pain, diarrhea, weight loss, irritability, fatigue, ascites and portal hypertension, brittle nails, loss of hair, dry skin, bone pain and fragility, hydrocephalus and vomiting (in infants and children), and spleen enlargement. Extensive liver damage may occur. Symptoms can be reversed if toxicity is detected early and vitamin supplementation is stopped, although complete recovery may take several weeks. Permanent damage can result if prompt action is not taken.

Pharmacologic Uses of Vitamin A

Large doses of vitamin A may be used pharmacologically to treat vitamin A deficiency; they also may be used to treat severe, resistant forms of acne. By some unknown mechanism, the drug Accutane (a retinoid, 13-*cis*-retinoic acid, or isotretinoin; Roche Laboratories, Nutley, NJ) can cause a complete and prolonged remission of acne. Although vitamin A toxicity may develop depending on the dose and duration of treatment, Accutane appears to be safer and more effective than other forms of vitamin A that were used in the past (eg, retinol). Because large doses of vitamin A can cause spontaneous abortion and fetal abnormalities, Accutane should not be used by women who are or may be pregnant.

Vitamin A has also been used experimentally to block the conversion of precancerous cells to cancerous cells. Studies have shown that the incidence of epithelial cancers, particularly lung, larynx, esophagus, and bladder cancers, is higher among people whose diets are low in vitamin A, particularly beta-carotene. Vitamin A does not seem to prevent the initiation of cancer but may prevent or retard tumor development, possibly through its ability to enhance the immune system (Baumgartner, 1994). Another possible mechanism is its role as an antioxidant. Research has also shown that animals injected with known carcinogens developed significantly fewer tumors when given doses of 13-*cis*-retinoic acid. This compound and other synthetic retinoids appear to be more effective and less toxic than natural vitamin A, at least in test animals. However, studies have shown an increase in the incidence of lung cancer among people taking large doses of supplemental beta-carotene (Liebman, 1994). For now, researchers recommend eating lots of fruits and vegetables rich in beta-carotene, which poses no harm, and avoiding beta-carotene supplements (see Supplements: Buying Basics).

Nutrient/Drug Interactions

Supplements of vitamin A may:

- Enhance hepatotoxicity of alcohol (if hypervitaminosis A exists)
- Increase the risk of vitamin A toxicity from the drug isotretinoin (13-*cis*-retinoic acid/Accutane)
- Enhance intracranial hypertension induced by tetracycline

Drugs that affect absorption of vitamin A are as follows:

- Cholestyramine: decreases vitamin A and carotene absorption
- Clofibrate: decreases carotene absorption
- Colchicine: decreases carotene absorption

- Mineral oils: decrease vitamin A absorption
- Oral contraceptives: increase plasma vitamin A levels

Vitamin D (Calciferol)

Vitamin D was discovered in 1918 and isolated in 1930. It is very stable and is resistant to heat, aging, and storage.

7-Dehydrocholesterol, a precursor of vitamin D that is found in some animal sources, is converted to cholecalciferol (vitamin D_3) in the skin by ultraviolet light. D_2 (ergocalciferol) is the other major form of vitamin D. Its precursor is ergosterol, which is a plant sterol that is converted to vitamin D_2 when exposed to ultraviolet light. Ergocalciferol is produced commercially for use in vitamin supplements.

Both vitamin D_2 and vitamin D_3 must be converted to the active form of vitamin D. The liver converts vitamin D_3 to a more potent form of vitamin D (25-hydroxycholecalciferol), which the kidneys convert to calcitriol, the most potent and active form of vitamin D. Because calcitriol can be synthesized in the kidney and stimulates functional activity elsewhere in the body, vitamin D is considered by some to be a hormone, not a vitamin.

There are few food sources of vitamin D in the diet, except for liver, fish liver oils, and eggs. Fortified foods are the major source of vitamin D in the average American diet. Fortunately, the body can synthesize all the vitamin D it needs if enough sunlight is available. However, the amount of vitamin D that is synthesized in the skin depends on the area of skin exposed, the length of exposure, and the character of the skin. For instance, light skin synthesizes vitamin D more readily than dark skin, and aging reduces an 80-year-old's synthesizing ability to about half that of a 20-year-old.

Because the body is capable of synthesizing vitamin D, a dietary source is unnecessary if exposure to sunlight is regular and under optimal conditions. However, because few people meet those conditions, a dietary source of vitamin D is considered essential (see Table 4-1). Some studies have found that average daily consumption of vitamin D is below the RDA, and that because of a decreased ability to produce vitamin D that occurs with aging, the RDA may be set too low for certain age or sex groups.

FUNCTIONS

Because of its role in calcium and phosphorus metabolism, vitamin D is essential for normal growth and development (see Table 4-1).

CLINICAL APPLICATIONS

Vitamin D Deficiency

A deficiency of vitamin D results in rickets in children and osteomalacia in adults. Children at high risk for rickets are those who have malabsorption syndromes, are born prematurely, or are given vitamin D–deficient formulas or are breast-fed by vegan mothers, as well as those who have received anticonvulsant therapy for a long time. The fortification of foods with vitamin D has almost eliminated rickets in the United States, although it continues to be a problem in underdeveloped countries.

Clinical osteomalacia occurs rarely in the United States but may be observed in women who have had chronically low intakes of vitamin D and multiple pregnancies. Also at risk are house-bound or institutionalized elderly people, because aging impairs the ability to synthesize vitamin D, and exposure to sunlight is limited. Pure vegans are at risk because they exclude milk and dairy products, which are fortified with vitamin D, from their diet. Secondary vitamin D deficiency can develop in people with liver or kidney diseases, because the conversion of previtamins to the active form of vitamin D is impaired, or from fat malabsorption syndromes that interfere with vitamin D absorption.

Vitamin D deficiency may also occur when exposure to sunlight is limited, such as in northern climates. Unfortunately, ultraviolet light cannot penetrate atmospheric pollution, fog, smoke, glass, or clothing; even dark pigment in the skin limits the synthesis of vitamin D.

Clinical Findings

Children with rickets may be observed to have the following:

Profuse sweating and restlessness, which may be the first sign of rickets
Tetany and convulsions
Growth retardation
Skeletal deformities, such as bowed legs or knock-knees; enlarged, malformed skull; beading on the ribs and pigeon chest; curvature of the spine; enlarged wrists and ankles
Delayed tooth eruption; defective enamel

In adults, signs and symptoms of osteomalacia may include the following:

Softening of the bones, leading to bone deformities, especially of the limbs, chest, and pelvis
Muscular weakness and back pain
Development of a waddling gait

Treatment

Symptoms of rickets and osteomalacia are reversible with therapeutic doses of vitamin D daily; calcium supplements may also be prescribed, and exposure to the sun is encouraged. Intramuscular injection may be necessary in adults with malabsorption.

Vitamin D Toxicity

Vitamin D may be the most toxic fat-soluble vitamin. Although vitamin D toxicity generally occurs when large doses are consumed over time, toxic levels for some groups may be as low as five times the RDA. Individual tolerance varies significantly; however, young children are especially vulnerable to toxicity. An excess of vitamin D produces hypercalcemia, which causes excessive calcification of the bones and soft tissues, formation of kidney stones, and the potential for permanent kidney damage and irreversible cardiovascular damage. Symptoms include nausea, vomiting, headache, weakness, weight loss, constipation, polyuria, and polydipsia. Children may also experience mental and physical growth retardation, and failure to thrive. Drowsiness and coma may develop in severe cases.

Toxicity is treated by discontinuing the vitamin supplement, correcting fluid and electrolyte imbalances, reducing calcium intake, and administering a loop diuretic to increase renal calcium excretion. Glucocorticoid therapy may be used to lower serum calcium levels.

Pharmacologic Uses of Vitamin D

Vitamin D preparations may be used to treat hypocalcemic diseases such as vitamin D–dependent rickets, renal osteodystrophy, postoperative tetany, idiopathic tetany, and hypoparathyroidism. In healthy people, vitamin D in excess of the RDA offers no known benefit and introduces the possibility of toxicity; therefore, intakes greater than the RDA are not recommended.

Nutrient/Drug Interactions

Supplements of vitamin D may precipitate cardiac arrhythmias in patients receiving digoxin who have vitamin D–induced hypercalcemia.

Drugs that affect vitamin D are as follows:

- Adrenal corticosteroids: antivitamin D activity inhibits intestinal absorption of calcium
- Anticonvulsants: increase inactivation of vitamin D
- Barbiturates: increase inactivation of vitamin D
- Cholestyramine: decreases intestinal absorption of vitamin D
- Mineral oil: prolonged use causes vitamin D malabsorption
- Thiazide diuretics: may potentiate vitamin D–induced hypercalcemia in hypoparathyroid patients
- Isoniazid (antituberulosis): interferes with vitamin D metabolism; long-term use of isoniazid may necessitate the use of vitamin D supplements

Vitamin E

Vitamin E was discovered in 1922 and first synthesized in 1937. Processing, storage, and preparation techniques may result in large losses of vitamin E in foods.

Compounds with vitamin E activity are known as tocopherols. Alpha-tocopherol is the most active form of vitamin E and the most abundant in food. Vitamin E is found in plant fat and is especially abundant in vegetable oils, products made with vegetable oils (like margarine and shortening), wheat germ, nuts, and to a lesser extent, green leafy vegetables. Animal fats are poor sources of vitamin E. The actual vitamin E content of the diet varies considerably depending on the type and amount of fat consumed. The RDA for vitamin E is expressed as tocopherol equivalents.

FUNCTIONS

Although the mechanism by which it functions is not fully understood, vitamin E is the primary antioxidant in the body, and it protects biologic membranes from oxidative damage by trapping free radicals. Studies show that tobacco smokers need to consume more than the RDA for vitamin E in order to meet their physiologic needs, because vitamin E is used to reduce free radicals that are formed from smoking tobacco (Giraud et al, 1995).

The need for vitamin E increases as the intake of PUFA increases; fortunately, both are found in the same foods. Because cell membranes, especially RBC membranes, are rich in PUFA, vitamin E helps maintain cell membrane integrity and protects RBC against hemolysis.

CLINICAL APPLICATIONS

Vitamin E Deficiency

Premature and very-low-birth-weight infants are at risk for vitamin E deficiency because they are born with low body reserves, their intestinal absorption is impaired, and accelerated growth rates increase vitamin E demand. Feeding these infants commercial formulas with high concentrations of PUFA and iron, which destroys vitamin E, compounds the problem.

The only other population group likely to develop vitamin E deficiency are people with chronic fat malabsorption related to celiac disease, cystic fibrosis, or pancreatic disorders. Vitamin E deficiency related to poor intake is not likely to occur.

Clinical Findings

In infants, symptoms of hemolytic anemia, edema, and skin lesions may develop. In adults, neurologic symptoms appear, but not until malabsorption has persisted for 5 to 10 years.

Treatment

Infants may be given formula with added vitamin E, vitamin E drops, or, when severe deficiency develops, injections of vitamin E. Adults may be given supplements of vitamin E or a multivitamin containing vitamin E.

Vitamin E Toxicity

Compared to vitamin A and vitamin D, vitamin E appears to be relatively nontoxic. Although individual tolerance varies, it appears that oral doses in adults of up to 100 to 800 mg/day are harmless and useless (NRC, 1989). Diarrhea, cramps, blurred vision, headaches, and dizziness may occur with higher doses. Megadoses of vitamin E can also interfere with vitamin A metabolism and normal blood clotting, and may increase the risk of hemorrhagic stroke.

Pharmacologic Uses of Vitamin E

The only established pharmacologic use of vitamin E is to treat or prevent vitamin E deficiency. Numerous beliefs about the uses of vitamin E are unfounded. These include claims that it can be used to treat infertility, diabetes, ulcers, skin disorders, burns, shortness of breath, and muscular dystrophy, as well as increase physical performance and sexual potency, protect against air pollution, reverse gray hair and wrinkles, and slow the aging process.

However, the use of vitamin E in premature infants to reduce the toxic effects of oxygen therapy on lung parenchyma and the retina is being investigated. Also, because of its role as an antioxidant, studies are under way to determine if vitamin E can slow or prevent heart disease, cancer, and cataracts (see display, Antioxidants).

Nutrient/Drug Interactions

Vitamin E may enhance anticoagulant response to warfarin and can reduce the efficacy of oral iron supplements. Mineral oil can cause vitamin E malabsorption.

Vitamin K

Vitamin K was recognized as the antihemorrhagic factor in 1935. It is resistant to heat and air but is destroyed by light, strong acids and alkalis, and oxidizing agents. The body is able to store small amounts of vitamin K in the liver, heart, skin, muscles, and kidney.

Vitamin K occurs naturally in two forms: phylloquinone, which is found in dark green leafy vegetables and members of the cabbage family; and menaquinones, which are synthesized in the intestinal tract by bacteria. Animals provide both forms of vitamin K. The RDA for vitamin K was established for the first time in 1989.

FUNCTIONS

Vitamin K is essential for the synthesis of prothrombin and at least five other proteins that are required for normal blood clotting.

CLINICAL APPLICATIONS

Vitamin K Deficiency

Because intestinal bacteria and a balanced diet provide ample amounts of vitamin K, a deficiency is not likely to occur in a healthy person. However, research indicates that intestinal synthesis is not sufficient to meet total vitamin K needs, and alterations in clotting factors result when dietary intake of vitamin K is restricted. Unlike other fat-soluble vitamins, stores of vitamin K are quickly depleted if intake is deficient (Harris, 1995).

Newborns are prone to vitamin K deficiency because they have sterile GI tracts; thus, lack of bacteria results in absence of vitamin K synthesis. Newborns are exposed to intestinal bacteria when they pass down the birth canal; however, it takes 1 to 2 days for the bacteria to become established in the GI tract. In addition, newborns may not have an immediate dietary source of vitamin K; initial feedings are often delayed for a number of hours, and breast milk is a poor source of vitamin K. Because of this, a single parenteral dose of vitamin K is usually given prophylactically at birth.

A secondary deficiency may result from impaired intestinal synthesis related to prolonged use of antibiotics or vitamin K antagonists (see Nutrient/Drug Interactions), or from impaired vitamin K absorption related to chronic fat malabsorption, or chronic biliary obstruction. People who are taking long-term total parenteral nutrition are also at risk.

Clinical Findings

Signs of hemorrhaging may be observed. These are related to delayed blood clotting.

Treatment

Vitamin K deficiency in adults is treated with either oral or intramuscular administration of vitamin K.

Vitamin K Toxicity

Excessive doses of vitamin K that are taken over long periods of time have failed to produce toxic symptoms. However, menadione may cause hemolytic anemia and hyperbilirubinemia in the newborn.

Pharmacologic Uses of Vitamin K

Vitamin K is used pharmacologically to treat coagulation disorders related to impaired vitamin K synthesis or absorption, and prophylactically to treat hemorrhagic disease of the newborn. Vitamin K also is given for oral anticoagulant–induced prothrombin deficiency.

Nutrient/Drug Interactions

Vitamin K in liquid food supplements may inhibit the hypoprothrombic effect of warfarin. Drugs that affect vitamin K are as follows:

- Coumarin and indanedione anticoagulants: interfere with hepatic synthesis of vitamin K–dependent clotting factors. Although it is not necessary for clients who are taking anticoagulants to avoid foods that contain vitamin K (with the exception of kale and significant amounts of parsley), they should try to maintain a consistent vitamin K intake so that appropriate coagulation status can be maintained (Harris, 1995).
- Cholestyramine: decreases vitamin K absorption
- Mineral oil: decreases vitamin K absorption
- Salicylates: antagonize vitamin K
- Tetracyclines: decrease intestinal synthesis of vitamin K

WATER-SOLUBLE VITAMINS

The water-soluble vitamins include vitamin C and the B-complex vitamins (all of which perform one or more functions in the body and must be supplied in the diet), as well as pantothenic acid and biotin. Recommended dietary allowances have been established for vitamin C and six B vitamins: thiamine, riboflavin, niacin, vitamin B_6, folate, and vitamin B_{12}. Estimated safe and adequate intakes have been established for pantothenic acid and biotin. Table 4-2 is a summary of the water-soluble vitamins.

Group Characteristics

As a group, water-soluble vitamins have the following characteristics:

They are absorbed through the intestinal wall directly into the bloodstream, where they travel freely and without the aid of protein carriers.

Water-soluble vitamins are filtered through the kidneys and excreted in the urine when consumed in excess of need.

Although some tissues are able to hold limited amounts, water-soluble vitamins are generally considered nontoxic. However, that belief has come under scrutiny since 1983, when neurologic abnormalities were reported in people who were taking megadoses of vitamin B_6.

Table 4-2
Summary of Water-Soluble Vitamins

Vitamin	Functions	Deficiency Signs and Symptoms
VITAMIN C (ASCORBIC ACID)		
Adult RDA Men and women: 60 mg Pregnancy: 70 mg Lactation: 95 mg	Acts as an antioxidant Formation of collagen Enhances intestinal absorption of iron Converts folate to its active form Involved in the metabolism of certain amino acids	Bleeding gums, pinpoint hemorrhages under the skin Scurvy, characterized by Hemorrhaging Muscle degeneration Skin changes Delayed wound healing: reopening of old wounds Softening of the bones → malformations, pain, easy fractures Soft, loose teeth Anemia Increased susceptibility to infection Hysteria and depression

Food Sources
Guava, broccoli, brussels sprouts, green peppers, strawberries, "greens," citrus fruits, potatoes, tomatoes, and cabbage

THIAMINE (VITAMIN B₁)		
Adult RDA Men: 1.2–1.5 mg Women: 1.0–1.1 mg Pregnancy: 1.5 mg Lactation: 1.6 mg	Energy metabolism, especially the metabolism of CHO Normal nervous system functioning	Beriberi Mental confusion Fatigue Peripheral paralysis Muscle weakness and wasting Painful calf muscles Anorexia Edema Enlarged heart Sudden death from heart failure

(continued)

Table 4-2 (Continued)
Summary of Water-Soluble Vitamins

Vitamin	Functions	Deficiency Signs and Symptoms

Food Sources
Pork, liver, organ meats, whole grain and enriched grains, nuts, legumes, potatoes, eggs, and milk

RIBOFLAVIN (VITAMIN B₂)

Adult RDA
Men: 1.4–1.7 mg
Women: 1.2–1.3 mg
Pregnancy: 1.6 mg
Lactation: 1.8 mg
	CHO, protein, and fat metabolism
	Other metabolic roles
		Ariboflavinosis
		  Dermatitis
		  Cheilosis
		  Glossitis
		  Photophobia
		  Reddening of the cornea

Food Sources
Milk and dairy products, organ meats, eggs, enriched grains, and green leafy vegetables

NIACIN

Adult RDA
Men: 15–19 mg NE
Women: 13–15 mg NE
Pregnancy: 17 mg NE
Lactation: 20 mg NE
	CHO, protein, and fat metabolism	Pellagra: 4 (Ds)
		  Dermatitis (bilateral and symmetrical)
		    and glossitis
		  Diarrhea
		  Dementia, irritability, mental confusion
		    → psychosis
		  Death, if untreated

Food Sources
Kidney, liver, poultry, lean meat, fish, yeast, peanut butter, enriched and whole grains, dried peas and beans, and nuts

VITAMIN B₆ (PYRIDOXINE)

Adult RDA
Men: 2.0 mg
Women: 1.6 mg
Pregnancy: 2.2 mg
Lactation: 2.1 mg
	Amino acid metabolism
	Blood formation
	Maintenance of nervous tissue
	Conversion of tryptophan to niacin
		Dermatitis, cheilosis, glossitis, abnormal
		  brain wave pattern, convulsions, and
		  anemia

Food Sources
Chicken, fish, peanuts, oats, yeast, wheat germ, pork, organ meats, egg yolk, whole grain cereals, corn, potatoes, and bananas

FOLATE

Adult RDA Men: 200 µg Women: 180 µg Pregnancy: 400 µg Lactation: 280 µg	Amino acid metabolism DNA and RNA synthesis; proliferation of cells Blood formation	Glossitis, diarrhea, macrocytic anemia

Food Sources
Enriched cereals, green leafy vegetables, asparagus, broccoli, liver, organ meats, milk, eggs, yeast, wheat germ, and dried peas and beans

VITAMIN B₁₂ (COBALAMIN)

Adult RDA
Men and Women: 2 µg
Pregnancy: 2.2 µg
	RNA and DNA synthesis
	Blood formation
	Maintenance of nervous tissue
		GI changes: glossitis, anorexia, indigestion,
		  recurring diarrhea or constipation, and
		  weight loss

(continued)

Table 4-2 *(Continued)*
Summary of Water-Soluble Vitamins

Vitamin	Functions	Deficiency Signs and Symptoms
VITAMIN B₁₂ (COBALAMIN) (continued)		

Vitamin	Functions	Deficiency Signs and Symptoms
VITAMIN B$_{12}$ (COBALAMIN) (continued)		
Adult RDA (continued) Lactation: 2.6 µg	CHO, protein, and fat metabolism Folate metabolism	Macrocytic anemia → pallor, dyspnea, weakness, fatigue, and palpitations Neurologic changes: paresthesia of the hands and feet, decreased sense of position, poor muscle coordination, poor memory, irritability, depression, paranoia, delirium, and hallucinations
Food Sources Liver, kidney, fresh shrimp and oysters, meats, milk, eggs, and cheese		
PANTOTHENIC ACID		
Adult RDA Men and women: safe and adequate intake 4 mg to 7 mg	CHO, protein, and fat metabolism	Not observed in humans
Food Sources Animal tissues, whole grain cereals, legumes, milk, vegetables, fruit		
BIOTIN		
Adult RDA Men and women: safe and adequate intake 30 µg to 100 µg	Fat and CHO metabolism Glycogen formation	Observed only under experimental conditions
Food Sources Liver, organ meats, egg yolk, milk, and yeast Synthesized by GI flora.		

Because tissue reserves of water-soluble vitamins are minimal, deficiency symptoms often develop rapidly when intake is inadequate.

Water-soluble vitamins should be supplied in the diet daily.

Vitamin C (Ascorbic Acid)

Vitamin C was not isolated in its pure form until 1932. Although the association between intake of citrus fruits and the prevention of scurvy has long been known, it was not until the 20th century that vitamin C was discovered to be the anti-scurvy ingredient. Vitamin C is labile, that is, it is easily destroyed by heat, air, alkalis, drying, and aging.

Active vitamin C exists in two forms: ascorbic acid and dehydroascorbic acid. The richest sources of vitamin C are citrus fruits, green and red peppers, collard greens, broccoli, spinach, tomatoes, and strawberries. Although potatoes and root vegetables are low in vitamin C, they contribute substantial amounts of vitamin C to the diet because they are eaten in large quantities. Ascorbic acid is often added to processed foods for its antioxidant properties.

The RDA for vitamin C is listed in Table 4-2. However, there is considerable controversy over how much vitamin C is needed for optimal health. Even among different nations, recommended allowances vary, from 30 mg/day in Canada to 60 mg/day in the United States and 75 mg/day in Germany. The vitamin C requirement does increase in response to fever, chronic illness, infection, burns, multiple wounds, and smoking; the National Research Council recommends that regular cigarette smokers consume at least 100 mg of vitamin C daily. Although many people habitually take 1000 mg or more of vitamin C without toxic side effects, the long-term risks of such large doses are not known. Routine use of megadoses is not recommended.

In the absence of continuous intake, vitamin C is poorly retained in the body. Vitamin C that is consumed in excess of need is excreted in the urine.

FUNCTIONS

Vitamin C has many important functions in the body, although the mechanism by which it works is not clearly understood. Vitamin C is needed for the formation of collagen, the most abundant protein in fibrous tissue such as connective tissue, cartilage, bone matrix, tooth dentin, skin, and tendon. The integrity of this "intracellular cement" is important for maintaining capillary strength, promoting wound healing, and resisting infection.

Vitamin C also acts as an antioxidant to protect vitamin A, vitamin E, PUFA, and iron from destruction. It is involved in many metabolic reactions, including the promotion of iron absorption, the conversion of folacin to its active form, the formation of some neurotransmitters, the synthesis of thyroxine, the metabolism of amino acids, and the absorption of calcium and its deposition and withdrawal from teeth.

CLINICAL APPLICATIONS

Vitamin C Deficiency

According to advance data of the Third National Health and Nutrition Examination Survey, Phase 1, 1988–1991, vitamin C intake exceeds the RDA for all sex and age groups (CDC, 1994). Groups most at risk for vitamin C deficiency are alcoholics, people who do not eat fruits and vegetables, people with increased vitamin C requirements, and people of low socioeconomic status.

Clinical Findings

When the body's supply of vitamin C is exhausted and intake is inadequate, symptoms of scurvy appear. Defects in collagen synthesis are evidenced by swollen, inflamed gums that bleed easily and pinpoint hemorrhages under the skin that are related to capillary fragility. Hemorrhaging worsens as the disease progresses. Softening of the ends of the long bones can lead to painful malformations and fractures, and ankle and wrist joints may appear swollen. Wound healing is delayed and previous wounds may reopen. Secondary infections are more likely to occur. Changes in skin and teeth may become apparent. In addition, psychological symptoms of hysteria and depression may develop. Internal hemorrhage may lead to heart failure and sudden death.

Treatment

Scurvy can be cured as quickly as 5 days after moderate doses of vitamin C are administered (100 mg).

Vitamin C Toxicity

Although large doses of vitamin C generally are considered nontoxic, it is possible that megadoses may cause undesirable side effects such as nausea, abdominal cramps, and diarrhea; also, iron absorption may become excessive. Large doses of vitamin C also can cause a false-positive test for glucose in the urine. An increase in oxalic acid excretion (excess vitamin C may be excreted as vitamin C or oxalic acid, a waste product of vitamin C metabolism) theoretically increases the risk for oxalate renal stone formation. Certain population groups, including some black Americans, Sephardic Jews, and Orientals, may develop hemolytic anemia because they lack an enzyme that normally protects against the effects of large amounts of vitamin C and other strong reducing agents. Because the body becomes conditioned to catabolizing and excreting large amounts of vitamin C, rebound scurvy may develop during the time between cessation of megadoses and restoration of normal vitamin C metabolism.

Pharmacologic Uses of Vitamin C

The only proven effective therapeutic use of vitamin C is to prevent or treat scurvy. In large doses, vitamin C may have pharmacologic or druglike effects. For instance, vitamin C may be used as adjunctive therapy to promote wound healing, as in the treatment of severe burns and multiple or serious pressure ulcers, and during postoperative periods. Vitamin C is the most frequently supplemented nutrient in the United States, with reported estimates of regular vitamin C use ranging from 8% of the general population to 44% of elderly women (Johnson and Luo, 1994).

Vitamin C and the Common Cold, a book written by Nobel Prize winner Linus Pauling in 1970, claims that taking 1 g of vitamin C daily can reduce the incidence of colds by 45% and that during a cold, doses of 500 to 1000 mg of vitamin C every hour alleviates symptoms (Pauling, 1970). However, most studies conclude that megadoses of vitamin C do not prevent colds, and although large amounts of vitamin C may lessen the duration and severity of colds, the benefit is so small that supplements are not recommended.

Researchers are also investigating the role of vitamin C in cancer prevention. Studies indicate that foods that are high in vitamin C may protect against certain kinds of cancer, such as cancer of the stomach and esophagus. However, it has not been determined whether vitamin C alone, or vitamin C together with some other components in those foods, is to be credited for the reduced risk. It is known that vitamin C may help prevent cancer by blocking the conversion of nitrites and amines (both present in food) to nitrosamines, which are potent animal carcinogens.

Although vitamin C may reduce the risk of cancer from nitrosamines, that is not the same as saying vitamin C prevents cancer. Most experts agree that the recommendation to take megadoses of vitamin C to prevent cancer is premature and unsupported by current evidence. However, the American Cancer Society does recommend that Americans choose foods rich in vitamin C to reduce their risk of cancer (American Cancer Society, 1993).

In some hypercholesterolemic people, large doses of vitamin C have lowered serum cholesterol levels; however, these results have not been confirmed by others.

Although vitamin C has been shown to relieve infertility caused by nonspecific sperm agglutination, the men who were successfully treated tended to be deficient in vitamin C. Evidence that vitamin C cures infertility in well-nourished people is lacking.

Nutrient/Drug Interactions

Supplements of vitamin C may

- Interfere with the absorption of fluphenazine, an antipsychotic agent.
- Decrease prothrombin time in clients receiving oral anticoagulants.
- Increase the excretion of acidic drugs (salicylates, barbiturates) and increase the excretion of basic drugs (quinidine, atropine, amphetamines, tricyclic antidepressants, phenothiazines).
- Increase the risk of crystalluria with sulfonamides.
- Enhance absorption of oral iron supplements.

Drugs that affect vitamin C are as follows:

- Adrenal corticosteroids: increase urinary excretion of vitamin C
- Barbiturates: increase urinary excretion of vitamin C
- Indomethacin: decreases plasma and platelet ascorbic acid levels
- Levodopa: increases the need for vitamin C
- Oral contraceptives: decrease serum, leukocyte, and platelet levels of vitamin C
- Phenacetin: increases urinary excretion of vitamin C
- Salicylates: increase urinary excretion of vitamin C
- Sulfonamides: increase urinary excretion of vitamin C

Thiamine (Vitamin B_1)

Thiamine was discovered in 1921 and synthesized in 1936. Thiamine is lost during cooking, especially when cooking is prolonged or at high temperatures. Alkalis also destroy thiamine.

Rich sources of thiamine include unrefined and enriched grains, pork, organ meats, legumes, seeds, and nuts. Enriched and fortified grains and cereals contribute substantial amounts of thiamine to the diet.

Thiamine requirements are based on the calorie content of the diet—a high-CHO diet increases the need for thiamine. The heart and brain are the tissues that store, or become saturated with, thiamine when intake exceeds requirement; thiamine that remains after tissues are saturated is excreted in the urine.

FUNCTIONS

Thiamine is an important component in the coenzyme thiamine pyrophosphate (TPP), which is involved in converting CHO (glucose) to energy. Thiamine is also necessary for protein and fat metabolism and for normal nervous system functioning.

CLINICAL APPLICATIONS

Thiamine Deficiency

Significant thiamine depletion can develop within 3 weeks on a diet devoid of thiamine. In the United States, thiamine deficiency is most commonly related to alcohol abuse, which alters thiamine intake, absorption, and metabolism. Other high-risk groups include renal patients undergoing long-term dialysis, patients receiving long-term parenteral nutrition, people with chronic fever, and the relatively few people with thiamine-responsive inborn errors of metabolism.

Severe thiamine deficiency, known as *beriberi*, is rare in the United States, although subclinical deficiencies may be seen. Throughout history, countries in the Orient, which rely heavily on milled rice (refining rice removes much of the thiamine content) and foods with antithiamine activity, have had a high incidence of beriberi. However, food enrichment programs have virtually eradicated beriberi in Japan and the Philippines.

Clinical Findings

Beriberi, which translates literally to "I can't, I can't," is an accurate description of the weakening disease that primarily affects the nervous and cardiovascular systems. Adult beriberi produces symptoms of anorexia, fatigue, nausea, vomiting, irritability, mental confusion, muscular weakness, peripheral paralysis, emotional instability, depression, and general lethargy.

Beriberi may be classified as "mixed," which is characterized by neuritis and heart failure, "dry," in which polyneuritis is the major finding, or "wet," which is identified by edema and heart failure. Without treatment, most patients die from sudden heart failure.

Infantile beriberi is common in breast-fed infants living in underdeveloped countries. Symptoms include restlessness, pallor, inability to sleep, edema, diarrhea, muscle wasting, and breathing difficulties. Death caused by acute heart failure may occur 1 to 2 days after the onset of symptoms.

Treatment

Large oral doses of thiamine or a thiamine derivative are administered. Wet beriberi responds within a few hours after treatment is initiated if the nervous system is not badly damaged; recovery from dry beriberi is slower. Infantile beriberi is treated by giving thiamine both to the lactating mother and to the infant. Because thiamine deficiency rarely occurs alone, a B-complex multivitamin preparation frequently is given.

Thiamine Toxicity

Thiamine that is consumed orally produces no known toxic effects; large parenteral doses may produce evidence of toxicity.

Pharmacologic Uses of Thiamine

The only pharmacologic use of thiamine is to treat thiamine deficiency, which is most commonly associated with alcoholism.

Nutrient/Drug Interactions

Supplements of thiamine can enhance the response to peripherally acting muscle relaxants.

Drugs that affect thiamine are as follows:

- Antacids: destroy thiamine
- Barbiturates: decrease thiamine absorption
- Diuretics, mercurial: increase urinary excretion of thiamine

Riboflavin (Vitamin B$_2$)

Riboflavin was discovered in 1932 and synthesized in 1935. Although it is resistant to heat, acid, and oxidation, riboflavin is quickly destroyed by light.

Riboflavin is widely distributed in foods but only in small amounts. Good sources include milk and dairy products, followed by meats, poultry, and fish. Enriched and fortified grains and cereals contribute large amounts of riboflavin to the diet.

The RDA listed for riboflavin is a recommended minimum daily intake. Actual riboflavin requirements are based on calorie intake: As calorie intake increases, the amount of riboflavin needed also increases. Because only small amounts of riboflavin are "stored" in the liver and kidney, a daily intake is necessary. However, riboflavin that is consumed in excess of need is excreted in the urine; protein-wasting conditions increase riboflavin excretion.

FUNCTIONS

Riboflavin is part of the coenzymes FAD (flavin adenine dinucleotide) and FMN (flavin mononucleotide), which have vital metabolic roles in energy metabolism, DNA and protein synthesis, and gluconeogenesis. Riboflavin is also involved in the activation of vitamin B$_6$, the conversion of folacin to its coenzyme, the synthesis of corticosteroids, the production of RBC, and the activity of thyroid enzymes.

CLINICAL APPLICATIONS

Riboflavin Deficiency

Riboflavin deficiency is uncommon in the United States. However, people with marginal calorie intakes, such as adolescent women, alcoholics, and the elderly, are at risk for riboflavin deficiency, as are people with malabsorption syndromes and those using certain drugs (see Nutrient/Drug Interactions).

Clinical Findings

Signs of riboflavin deficiency may not appear for several months on a riboflavin-deficient diet. Early symptoms include oral lesions, dermatitis, normocytic anemia, and scrotal and vulval skin changes.

Cheilosis (fissuring of the lips), angular stomatitis (cracks in the skin at the corners of the mouth), a purplish swollen tongue, and reddening of the cornea are characteristics of a severe riboflavin deficiency (ariboflavinosis).

Treatment

Riboflavin deficiency is treated with large oral doses of riboflavin or B-complex vitamins; severe deficiency may require parenteral administration. Lesions may heal within a few days or weeks.

Riboflavin Toxicity

Riboflavin produces no known toxic effects.

Pharmacologic Uses of Riboflavin

Riboflavin is used pharmacologically only to treat riboflavin deficiency.

Nutrient/Drug Interactions

Drugs that affect riboflavin are as follows:

- Amitriptyline: interferes with riboflavin metabolism
- Chloramphenicol: may increase the need for riboflavin
- Chlorpromazine: may interfere with riboflavin metabolism
- Imipramine: may interfere with riboflavin metabolism
- Probenecid: increases urinary excretion of riboflavin

Niacin or Nicotinic Acid

Although it has been known since 1867, niacin was not recognized as a vitamin until 1936. Niacin is relatively stable to heat, oxidation, light, acid, and alkalis; therefore, little is lost through food preparation, cooking, or storage. However, bioavailability of niacin may be low in some foods.

Lean meats, kidney, liver, poultry, fish, yeasts, and peanut butter are excellent sources of niacin. Enriched and whole grain products, dried peas and beans, and nuts contain lesser amounts of niacin.

The body is able to synthesize niacin from its precursor tryptophan, an amino acid that is abundant in milk, eggs, and other foods rich in protein. At least 1% of total protein intake is in the form of tryptophan, and 60 mg of tryptophan is needed to synthesize 1 mg of niacin (ie, 60 g of protein = 0.6 g [or 600 mg] tryptophan, which may be converted to 10 mg of niacin).

The RDA for niacin represents the minimum total milligrams of niacin equivalents that are required daily; as with riboflavin, actual need is based on total calorie intake: Increased calorie intake increases niacin requirements. "Niacin equivalents" is the total amount of niacin available in the diet from preformed niacin and the precursor tryptophan. Little niacin accumulates in the body, and amounts that are consumed in excess of need are excreted in the urine.

FUNCTIONS

As part of the coenzymes NAD (nicotinamide adenine dinucleotide) and NADP (nicotinamide adenine dinucleotide phosphate), niacin (nicotinamide is its active form) is required by all living cells for oxidation and the release of energy from CHO, protein, and fat. NAD also plays a role in glycogenesis. Reduced NADP is required for the synthesis of fatty acids, cholesterol, and steroid hormones.

CLINICAL APPLICATIONS

Niacin Deficiency

A severe deficiency of niacin leads to pellagra, which literally means "rough skin." In the United States, pellagra is uncommon and most often associated with alcohol abuse or clinical stresses. Pellagra is widespread in areas that rely on corn as a staple, such as parts of Africa and Asia, and it occurred frequently in the southern United States before grain products were enriched.

Clinical Findings

The symptoms of niacin deficiency are similar to those of a deficiency of riboflavin. Early symptoms include anorexia, apathy, weakness, indigestion, and skin lesions. Classic symptoms of pellagra are the "four Ds":

- Dermatitis, which occurs bilaterally and symmetrically—especially on skin exposed to the sun; the tongue also becomes smooth, sore, and "beefy"
- Diarrhea
- Dementia; also irritability, depression, confusion, psychosis, and tremors
- Death, if untreated

Treatment

Niacin deficiency may be treated with niacin and/or tryptophan. However, because a deficiency of niacin rarely occurs alone, treatment is most effective when other B-complex vitamins are also administered, especially thiamine and riboflavin.

Severe pellagra may be treated with oral doses of 150 to 600 mg of nicotinic acid or nicotinamide several times daily (nicotinamide is preferred because it produces fewer side effects). Response may begin within the first 24 hours of treatment and may be complete within a few weeks; some mental disturbances may be permanent if their onset is related to chronic malnutrition.

Niacin Toxicity

Large doses of nicotinic acid may produce flushing and itching. Daily doses of 3 to 9 g of nicotinic acid decrease serum lipids and impede mobilization of fatty acids from adipose during exercise. Other reported side effects include nausea, vomiting, diarrhea, hypotension, tachycardia, fainting, hypoglycemia, and liver damage.

Pharmacologic Uses of Niacin

Niacin is used pharmacologically to treat niacin deficiency and pellagra. Total daily doses of nicotinic acid may be used as adjunctive therapy to lower serum cholesterol in people who do not respond adequately to diet and weight loss. Initially, 1500 mg to 3000 mg may be taken in three divided doses after meals; the dose may be increased to 6000 mg/day (Skidmore-Roth, 1995). However, it is not clear whether nicotinic acid has a positive, negative, or neutral effect on morbidity or mortality that is related to atherosclerosis or coronary heart disease. Adverse reactions include nausea, vomiting, abdominal pain, diarrhea, GI disorders, generalized flushing, sensation of warmth, and dry, itchy, tingling skin.

Although "orthomolecular therapists" use megadoses of niacin alone or in combination with large doses of other vitamins and minerals, enzymes, hormones, diets, and electroconvulsant therapy to treat schizophrenia, its efficacy and safety are unproven.

Nutrient/Drug Interactions

Large doses of niacin can potentiate the vasodilating effect of sympathomimetic blocking–type antihypertensive drugs and may cause postural hypotension.

Niacin can reduce the effectiveness of oral hypoglycemic agents by elevating blood glucose levels.

The drug that affects niacin is as follows:

- Isoniazid: causes pyridoxine depletion; pyridoxine is necessary for the conversion of tryptophan to niacin

Vitamin B_6

Vitamin B_6 was identified in 1934 and isolated in 1939. Food processing can cause considerable losses of vitamin B_6.

Vitamin B_6, sometimes referred to as pyridoxine, is actually a group of three active compounds: pyridoxine, pyridoxal, and pyridoxamine. Chicken, fish, kidney, liver, pork, and eggs are rich sources of vitamin B_6. Whole-wheat products, peanuts, walnuts, oats, and unmilled rice are also good sources.

The vitamin B_6 requirement is related directly to protein intake: As protein intake increases, so does the need for vitamin B_6. Very little vitamin B_6 is stored in the body. The most recent edition of the RDA lowered the recommendations for vitamin B_6 because metabolic maintenance is observed with lower intakes than were previously suggested. Approximately 40 drugs are known to affect vitamin B_6 metabolism or bioavailability (see Nutrient/Drug Interactions).

FUNCTIONS

As part of the coenzyme pyridoxal phosphate (PLP) or pyridoxamine phosphate, vitamin B_6 is involved in more than 60 biochemical reactions, especially in protein and amino acid metabolism. Vitamin B_6 is also important for the synthesis and conversion of tryptophan to niacin, the synthesis of gamma-aminobutyric acid (GABA, a compound that inhibits neurotransmitters in the brain), the formation of heme for hemoglobin, the metabolism of fatty acids, the synthesis of myelin sheaths, and the maintenance of cellular immunity.

CLINICAL APPLICATIONS

Vitamin B_6 Deficiency

Because vitamin B_6 is so widespread in foods and the daily requirement is small, a dietary deficiency of vitamin B_6 is uncommon. When a dietary deficiency does develop, it most often occurs in people with multiple B vitamin deficiencies.

A primary deficiency of vitamin B_6 occurs in people with an inborn error of vitamin B_6 metabolism, which prevents the synthesis of GABA. Infants who are born with the disorder become mentally retarded and develop uncontrollable convulsions unless they are treated early in the neonatal period with large daily doses of vitamin B_6.

A secondary deficiency may result from malabsorption syndromes, alcohol abuse, or certain drug therapies.

Clinical Findings

Deficiency symptoms include depression, nausea, vomiting, irritability, drowsiness, dermatitis, weight loss, increased susceptibility to infection, cheilosis, glossitis, anemia, abnormal brain wave pattern, and convulsions. A high protein intake increases the severity and speeds the onset of vitamin B_6 deficiency symptoms.

Treatment

Deficiency is treated with oral doses of vitamin B_6; parenteral injections are used if oral intake is contraindicated or absorption is impaired. Patients with vitamin B_6 dependency syndromes require large doses for life.

Vitamin B_6 Toxicity

Although acute toxicity occurs infrequently, high doses of vitamin B_6 (ie, gram quantities) used for months or years have been blamed for neurologic problems, such as difficulty in walking, numbness of the feet and hands, clumsiness, and nerve degeneration. Damage is not permanent, and symptoms improve gradually when the vitamin is discontinued.

Pharmacologic Uses of Vitamin B_6

In pharmacologic doses, vitamin B_6 is used to treat vitamin B_6 deficiency related to poor intake or malabsorption, or secondary to drug therapy or inborn errors of metabolism.

Vitamin B_6 has also been used experimentally in doses of 10 to 15 mg to relieve malaise and depression in women who use oral contraceptives, and to alleviate symptoms of premenstrual syndrome, even though its efficacy has not been proven in controlled, double-blind studies. Vitamin B_6 has also been used with some success to relieve nausea and vomiting during pregnancy and after radiation therapy.

New research has found that victims of sickle cell anemia have low plasma levels of B_6. When given 50 mg of the vitamin twice a day for 2 months, the sickest patient had much shorter, much less severe crises. Further studies must be conducted to determine the relationship between sickle cell disease and vitamin B_6. By happenstance, during this study, it was discovered that all healthy "controls" (participants without sickle cell anemia) who had low vitamin B_6 levels also had bronchial asthma. An earlier study that was done with asthmatic children found that 200-mg supplements of vitamin B_6 given for 1 month decreased asthmatic symptoms. Like sickle cell, this is an area for future investigation.

Nutrient/Drug Interactions

Supplements of vitamin B_6 may

- Reverse the antiparkinsonism of the drug levodopa.
- Reduce phenytoin levels.
- Correct drug-induced peripheral neuropathy caused by hydralazine, isoniazid, and penicillamine.

Drugs that affect vitamin B_6 are as follows:

- Adrenal corticosteroids: increase the need for vitamin B_6
- Alcohol: promotes B_6 destruction and excretion
- Chloramphenicol: may increase the need for vitamin B_6
- Cycloserine: decreases serum vitamin B_6
- Diuretics: increase urinary excretion of vitamin B_6
- Hydralazine: inactivates vitamin B_6 and increases its urinary excretion
- Isoniazid: increases urinary excretion of vitamin B_6; causes vitamin B_6 depletion
- Levodopa: vitamin B_6 antagonist; depletes vitamin B_6
- Oral contraceptives (estrogen-containing): increase vitamin B_6 requirement
- Penicillamine: inhibits pyroxidal-dependent enzymes

Folic Acid (Folate, Folacin)

Folate was synthesized in 1946. Unfortunately, up to 50% of folate in foods may be lost during preparation, processing, and storage.

Folate is widespread in the diet. Excellent sources of folate include enriched cereals, green leafy vegetables, asparagus, broccoli, liver, organ meats, milk, eggs, yeast, wheat germ, and dried peas and beans; beef, potatoes, whole grain cereals, nuts, bananas, cantaloupe, lemons, and strawberries are also good sources.

In its most recent edition, the RDA for folate was lowered by one-half the previous recommendation because adult diets providing only 200 µg adequately maintained folate status and liver stores. Folate requirements increase in response to pregnancy, lactation, alcohol abuse, malabsorption syndromes, certain medications, and other stresses.

FUNCTIONS

The conversion of folate to the coenzyme tetrahydrofolic acid may depend on an adequate supply of vitamin B_{12}. As a coenzyme, folate plays a role in the synthesis of RNA (ribonucleic acid) and DNA (deoxyribonucleic acid) and is therefore necessary for the proliferation of cells and the transmission of inherited characteristics. It is because of its role in cellular proliferation that folic acid is thought to protect against neural tube defects in newborns (see Chapter 10). Other functions of folic acid include the formation and maturation of RBC and white blood cells, and the synthesis of enzymes. Through its role in amino acid metabolism, some researchers believe adequate folic acid intake may help prevent cardiovascular disease: It appears that folic acid deficiency leads to the accumulation of the amino acid homocysteine in the blood, which may damage arteries and set the stage for the development of atherosclerosis.

CLINICAL APPLICATIONS

Folate Deficiency

Folate deficiency is widespread in all parts of the world. In developing nations, folate deficiency commonly is caused by parasitic infections; the incidence of folate deficiency that is related to inadequate intake alone is difficult to estimate.

Americans who are most at risk for folate deficiency are alcoholics because of poor folate intakes, impaired folate absorption, and altered folate metabolism. At risk for deficiency related to poor intake are the elderly, minorities, fad dieters, and the poor. Because the relationship between inadequate folic acid intake and neural tube defects is so strong, the CDC recommends that women of childbearing age consume 400 micrograms/day; both mean and medium intakes of folic acid by women have been found to be below this level (CDC, 1994). The March of Dimes urges all women who are capable of becoming pregnant to eat a balanced diet AND take a daily multivitamin that contains folic acid. Because growth increases folate requirements, infants, adolescents, and pregnant women may have difficulty consuming adequate amounts. Lastly, risk is increased when absorption is altered, which may occur secondary to certain medications (see Nutrient/Drug Interactions), malabsorption syndromes, and general effects of aging. Absorption can be improved by eating a rich source of vitamin C with folate-containing foods. Policymakers are currently debating whether to require folic acid fortification of cereal grains, and if so, to what level.

Clinical Findings

Folate deficiency results in macrocytic or megaloblastic anemia, which is characterized by large, immature RBC; anemia leads to fatigue, weakness, and pallor.

Other symptoms that may be observed include diarrhea, weight loss, and glossitis.

Treatment

Large oral doses result in rapid improvement of most symptoms; however, anemia is gradually reversed.

Folic Acid Toxicity

Folic acid produces no known toxic effects, although large doses may interfere with anticonvulsant therapy and precipitate convulsions in epileptics controlled by phenytoin. Large parenteral doses of folic acid given to animals can produce kidney damage and hypertrophy.

Pharmacologic Uses of Folic Acid

Pharmacologic doses of folic acid are used to treat megaloblastic anemia related to inadequate folic acid intake, impaired absorption, altered requirements, or altered metabolism. Folic acid may be used prophylactically during pregnancy to prevent anemia.

Nutrient/Drug Interactions

Supplements of folic acid may

- Alter response to the drug methotrexate.
- Decrease the anticonvulsant action of the drug phenytoin.

Drugs that affect folic acid are as follows:

- Adrenal corticosteroids: increase the need for folic acid
- Alcohol: decreases folic acid absorption
- *p*-Aminosalicylic acid: decreases folic acid absorption
- Anticonvulsants: may decrease serum folate levels
- Azathioprine: acts as a folic acid antagonist
- Barbiturates: increase the need for folic acid
- Chloramphenicol: can antagonize response to folic acid
- Cycloserine: may decrease serum folate
- Isoniazid: may decrease serum folate
- Methotrexate: acts as a folic acid antagonist
- Nitrofurantoin: decreases serum folate
- Oral contraceptives: may impair folic acid metabolism and produce folate depletion
- Pyrimethamine: decreases serum folate
- Salicylates: decrease serum folate in patients with rheumatoid arthritis
- Sulfasalazine (salicylazosulfapyridine): decreases folic acid absorption
- Triamterene: acts as a folic acid antagonist
- Trimethadione: may lower serum folate levels when used on a long-term basis
- Trimethoprim: may decrease folic acid absorption

Vitamin B_{12} (Cobalamin)

Vitamin B_{12} was discovered in 1948 and synthesized in 1974. It is stable during normal cooking.

Vitamin B_{12} is found only in animal products and is especially abundant in kidney, liver, fresh shrimp and oysters, milk, eggs, fish, cheese, and muscle meats. Although GI flora synthesize small amounts of vitamin B_{12}, it is not absorbed because it is synthesized beyond the terminal ileum.

Vitamin B_{12} equilibrium can be maintained over a wide range of intakes. Excess vitamin B_{12} is stored in the liver in amounts that are sufficient to last 5 to 6 years or longer. The actual RDA for vitamin B_{12} is set high enough to maintain stores at substantial levels in view of the increasing evidence that vitamin B_{12} absorption appears to decrease in the elderly.

FUNCTIONS

Vitamin B_{12} is essential for the normal function of all cells, especially those of the GI tract, bone marrow, and the nervous system. Vitamin B_{12} plays a role in the synthesis of RNA and DNA and is therefore required for growth and RBC maturation. Myelin formation, and CHO, protein, fat, and folic acid metabolism are additional functions of vitamin B_{12}.

CLINICAL APPLICATIONS

Vitamin B_{12} Deficiency

Vitamin B_{12} deficiency may develop from impaired absorption related to aging; many elderly lack sufficient gastric acid and pepsin to liberate vitamin B_{12} from food. Other causes include iron deficiency, hypothyroidism, malabsorption syndromes, intestinal infestations, and intestinal resections that bypass the ileum. Impaired absorption accounts for more than 95% of the cases of vitamin B_{12} deficiency in the United States.

The absorption of vitamin B_{12} from the lower ileum requires the presence of intrinsic factor (IF), a glycoprotein that is secreted in the stomach. Conditions that alter IF secretion, such as gastric surgery or gastric cancer, lead to vitamin B_{12} malabsorption and a megaloblastic anemia called *pernicious anemia* (see Chapter 17).

A dietary deficiency of vitamin B_{12} is generally rare, except among the elderly and pure vegetarians who consume no animal products and who do not supplement their diet. Even then, symptoms may not develop for 5 to 10 years.

Clinical Findings

Symptoms related to anemia that may be observed include pallor, dyspnea, weakness, and fatigue. Gastrointestinal changes may become apparent, including glossitis, anorexia, indigestion, recurring diarrhea or constipation, and weight loss.

Observe for neurologic changes, including paresthesia of the hands and feet, decreased sense of position, poor muscle coordination, poor memory, irritability, depression, paranoia, delirium, and hallucinations.

Treatment

Vitamin B_{12} deficiency that is caused by an inadequate intake can be reversed with oral vitamin B_{12} supplements, as can deficiency in the elderly that is related to decreased gastric acid and pepsin. When vitamin B_{12} deficiency is related to impaired absorption, intramuscular injections are necessary.

Correct diagnosis and early treatment are necessary to prevent irreversible nervous system damage. Folic acid supplements will relieve vitamin B_{12} deficiency symptoms of anemia and GI changes, but they do not halt the progressive nervous system damage that only vitamin B_{12} can treat.

Vitamin B_{12} Toxicity

Large oral doses of vitamin B_{12} produce no known toxic effects, nor do they offer any benefit.

Pharmacologic Uses of Vitamin B_{12}

Pharmacologic doses of vitamin B_{12} are used only to treat vitamin B_{12} deficiency.

No evidence exists to support claims that vitamin B_{12} relieves infectious hepatitis, multiple sclerosis, poor appetite, poor growth, aging, or fatigue.

Nutrient/Drug Interactions

Drugs that affect vitamin B_{12} are as follows:

- Alcohol: decreases vitamin B_{12} absorption
- *p*-Aminosalicylic acid: decreases vitamin B_{12} absorption; causes a depletion in serum levels
- Anticonvulsants: may decrease serum levels of vitamin B_{12}
- Barbiturates: decrease serum vitamin B_{12} levels
- Chloramphenicol: may increase the need for vitamin B_{12}
- Cholestyramine: may decrease absorption of vitamin B_{12}; decreases serum levels
- Clofibrate: decreases vitamin B_{12} absorption
- Colchicine: decreases vitamin B_{12} absorption; decreases serum levels
- Cycloserine: may decrease serum vitamin B_{12} levels
- Metformin: decreases vitamin B_{12} absorption; decreases serum levels
- Methotrexate: decreases vitamin B_{12} absorption; decreases serum levels
- Neomycin: decreases vitamin B_{12} absorption; decreases serum levels
- Oral contraceptives: may alter tissue distribution of vitamin B_{12}
- Phenformin: decreases vitamin B_{12} absorption
- Phenobarbital: decreases serum and cerebrospinal fluid levels of vitamin B_{12}
- Potassium chloride: decreases vitamin B_{12} absorption
- Pyrimethamine: decreases serum levels of vitamin B_{12}
- Sodium nitroprusside: depletes plasma vitamin B_{12} by increasing urinary vitamin B_{12} excretion

Pantothenic Acid

Pantothenic acid was discovered in 1933 and synthesized in 1940. It is stable in moist heat, but destroyed by dry heat, acid, alkalis, and certain salts.

Pantothenic acid is found to some degree in all plants and animals. The richest sources of pantothenic acid are animal tissues, whole-grain cereals, and legumes; milk, vegetables, and fruit are also good sources. Pantothenic acid may be synthesized by GI flora.

An RDA has not been established for pantothenic acid because of a lack of conclusive evidence regarding dietary requirements. An estimated safe and adequate daily intake of 4 to 7 mg is probably adequate for adults, most of whom consume 5 to 10 mg/day. Pantothenic acid that is consumed in excess of need is excreted in the urine.

FUNCTIONS

As part of coenzyme A, pantothenic acid is important in the metabolism of CHO, protein, and fat; it is essential to most living things.

CLINICAL APPLICATIONS

Pantothenic Acid Deficiency

No cases of pantothenic acid deficiency from natural causes have been reported. Laboratory-induced pantothenic acid deficiency produces dermatitis, burning sensations of the feet, fatigue, insomnia, nausea, intestinal disturbances, irritability, depression, and increased susceptibility to infections.

Pantothenic Acid Toxicity

Pantothenic acid produces no known toxic effects, although large amounts may cause diarrhea.

Nutrient/Drug Interactions

Drugs that affect pantothenic acid are as follows:

- Mercaptopurine: may antagonize pantothenic acid
- Probenecid: decreases urinary excretion of pantothenic acid

Biotin

Biotin was discovered in 1935 and synthesized in 1942. It is resistant to heat, but is unstable to alkali and oxidation, and may be leached from food by water.

Biotin is widely distributed in nature. Biotin that is bound to protein is fat-soluble and found in animal tissues. The richest sources are liver, organ meats, egg yolk, milk, and yeast. Biotin that is found freely in nature is water soluble and occurs mostly in plants and plant products: legumes, nuts, soy flour, and cereals. Gastrointestinal flora synthesize significant amounts of biotin, but it is not known how much is available for absorption.

Although an RDA for biotin cannot be established on the basis of the information that is currently available, it is assumed that the average American diet contains amounts that are adequate to meet the needs of most healthy adults. The newest estimated safe and adequate daily dietary intake is lower than those that appeared in previous editions of the RDA.

FUNCTIONS

As a coenzyme, biotin plays a role in the metabolism of fats and CHO, the conversion of tryptophan to niacin, and the formation of glycogen, as well as in chemical reactions that add or remove carbon dioxide from other compounds.

CLINICAL APPLICATIONS

Biotin Deficiency

Biotin deficiency symptoms have been induced in humans only by adding the equivalent of 24 raw egg whites to a biotin-deficient diet. Avidin, a chemical in raw egg white, prevents the absorption of biotin from the intestinal tract and leads to a dry, scaly dermatitis, anorexia, nausea, vomiting, glossitis, pallor, and mental depression. A biotin deficiency may also result from long-term use of biotin-free total parenteral nutrition. Biotin supplements reverse most deficiency symptoms within 2 to 3 days; all symptoms are alleviated after 3 months of biotin therapy.

Biotin Toxicity

Biotin produces no known toxic effects.

Pharmacologic Uses of Biotin

None known.

Nutrient/Drug Interactions

None known.

KEY CONCEPTS

- Vitamins are organic compounds that are soluble in either water or fat; solubility determines how they are absorbed, transported through the blood, stored, and excreted.
- Vitamins do not provide energy (calories) but are needed for the metabolism of carbohydrates, protein, and fat. Most vitamins function by joining with specific proteins to form coenzymes, which promote the action of enzymes.
- Vitamins are needed by the body in small amounts (microgram or milligram measures). They are essential in the diet because they cannot be made by the body or are synthesized in inadequate amounts.
- The RDA for each vitamin is set at a level to prevent deficiency disease, plus a safety factor. Because it appears that higher doses of certain vitamins may offer additional health benefits, some experts are suggesting the focus of the RDA shift from disease avoidance to health promotion.
- Fortification and enrichment have virtually eliminated vitamin deficiencies in healthy Americans. It is assumed that if a variety of foods and the recommended number of servings from each of the Food Guide Pyramid groups are chosen, the vitamin content of the diet will be adequate.
- Groups at risk of vitamin deficiencies include people on very-low-calorie diets, finicky eaters, strict vegans, and the elderly.
- Because vitamins share similar food sources, when deficiencies do occur, they are often deficiencies of multiple vitamins, not just of one particular vitamin.
- Vitamins A, D, E, and K are the fat-soluble vitamins. Because they are stored in the liver and adipose tissue, they do not need to be consumed daily. Vitamins A and D can be toxic when consumed in large quantities over a long period of time.

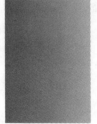

- Vitamin C and the B-complex vitamins are water-soluble vitamins. Although some tissues are able to hold limited amounts of certain water-soluble vitamins, they are generally not stored in the body, so a daily intake is necessary. Because they are not stored, they are considered nontoxic; however, adverse side effects can occur from taking megadoses of certain water-soluble vitamins over a prolonged period.
- Phytochemicals are plant chemicals that occur naturally in fruits and vegetables; it appears they may be protective against certain types of cancer.

REFERENCES

American Cancer Society (1993). Nutrition, Common Sense, and Cancer. Atlanta: American Cancer Society.

American Dietetic Association (1996). Position of The American Dietetic Association: Vitamin and mineral supplementation. J Am Diet Assoc, 96(1), 73–77.

American Dietetic Association (1995). Position of The American Dietetic Association: Phytochemicals and functional foods. J Am Diet Assoc, 95(4), 493–496.

American Dietetic Association (1994). Positions of The American Dietetic Association: Enrichment and fortification of foods and dietary supplements. J Am Diet Assoc, 94(6), 661–663.

Baumgartner, T. (1994). Antioxidants in modern nutrition. NewsLines, 3(3).

Centers for Disease Control and Prevention (1994). Advance Data. Dietary intake of vitamins, minerals, and fiber of persons ages 2 months and over in the United States: Third National Health and Nutrition Examination Survey, Phase 1, 1988–1991. DHHS Publication No. 95-1250.

Committee on Diet and Health, National Research Council (1989). Diet and Health. Implications for reducing chronic disease risk (executive summary). Washington, DC: National Academy Press.

Giraud, D., Martin, D., and Driskell, J. (1995). Plasma and dietary vitamin C and E levels of tobacco chewers, smokers, and nonusers. J Am Diet Assoc, 95(7), 798–800.

Harris, J. (1995). Interaction of dietary factors with oral anticoagulants: Review and applications. J Am Diet Assoc, 95(5), 580–584.

Johnson, C. and Luo, B. (1994). Comparison of the absorption and excretion of three commercially available sources of vitamin C. J Am Diet Assoc, 94(7), 779–781.

Liebman, B. (1995). Folic acid: For the young and heart. Nutrition Action Health Letter, 22(7), 1, 4–6.

Liebman, B. (1994). Antioxidants: Surprise, surprise. Nutrition Action Health Letter, 21(5), 4.

Liebman, B. and Schardt, D. (1995). Vitamin Smarts. Nutrition Action Health Letter, 22(9), 1, 6–10.

Malseed, R.T. (1990). Pharmacology Drug Therapy and Nursing Considerations. 3rd ed. Philadelphia: JB Lippincott.

National Research Council (1989). Recommended Dietary Allowances. 10th ed. Washington, DC: National Academy Press.

Pauling, L. (1970). Vitamin C and the Common Cold. San Francisco: WH Freeman.

Schardt, D. (1994). Phytochemicals: Plants against cancer. Nutrition Action Health Letter, 21(3), 1, 9–11.

Skidmore-Roth, L. (1995). Mosby's 1995 Nursing Drug Reference. St. Louis: Mosby–Year Book.

Slesinski, M., Subar, A., and Kahle L. (1995). Trends in use of vitamin and mineral supplements in the United States: The 1987 and 1992 National Health Interview Surveys. J Am Diet Assoc, 95(8), 921–923.

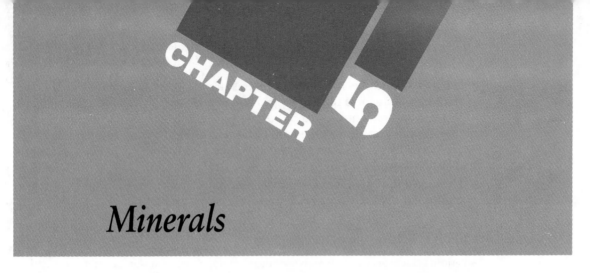

Minerals

Chapter Outline

Key Terms

Macrominerals   Minerals   Trace elements

GROUP CHARACTERISTICS

Unlike the energy nutrients and vitamins, **minerals** are *inorganic elements*; as such, minerals are not metabolized, that is, they are not broken down and rearranged in the body, nor are they destroyed during food preparation. However, some minerals in food may be lost through excessive soaking and cooking in water. Minerals are contained in the ash that remains after food has been digested.

Although only about 4% of the body's total weight comprises minerals, they are found in all body fluids and tissues, either in the form of salts (eg, sodium chloride) or combined with organic compounds (eg, iron in hemoglobin). In their ionic form, minerals are water soluble. Minerals function as structural components in the body and serve to regulate body processes (Table 5-1).

Although they have several common group characteristics, there are distinct differences between individual minerals. For instance, some minerals are excreted in the urine, whereas others are excreted in the feces. Minerals that are easily

Table 5-1
General Functions of Minerals

Mineral	Regulating Function	Structural Function
Calcium	Nerve cell transmissions Muscle contractions Blood clotting	Bones and teeth
Phosphorus	Acid–base balance	Bones and teeth Soft tissues
Magnesium	Nerve cell transmission Muscle contractions	Bones and teeth
Fluorine		Bones and teeth
Sulfur	Vitamin, enzyme, and hormonal activity	Skin Hair Nails Soft tissues
Iron		Blood (hemoglobin) Soft tissues
Potassium	Fluid balance	Soft tissues
Sodium ⎱ Chlorine ⎰	Acid–base balance Fluid balance	
Zinc ⎫ Manganese ⎪ Cobalt ⎪ Copper ⎬ Chromium ⎪ Iodine ⎪ Selenium ⎭	Vitamin, enzyme, and hormonal activity	

excreted do not accumulate to toxic levels in the body; others are stored and can produce symptoms of toxicity when consumed in excess of need. Toxicities are not likely to occur from eating a balanced diet; rather, they are most often related to excessive use of mineral supplements, environmental or industrial exposure, human errors in commercial food processing, or alterations in metabolism (eg, a genetic defect in iron absorption causes hemosiderosis, an excessive accumulation of iron in the liver).

Three minerals that are discussed in this chapter, calcium, phosphorus, and magnesium, are classified as **macrominerals** because they are found in the body in amounts greater than 5 g and are needed by the body in relatively large amounts (100 mg/day or more). Nine minerals that are discussed in this chapter are considered **trace elements**, or microminerals, because they are found in the body in amounts less than 5 g and are needed in only very small amounts (15 mg/day or less). Other elements, such as cobalt, nickel, and vanadium, may prove essential to human nutrition in the future. At present, their functions and requirements have not been established (see Food for Thought: Other Trace Elements—Future RDA Candidates?).

FOOD *for* **THOUGHT**

Other Trace Elements—Future RDA Candidates?

Although definitive evidence is lacking, future research may reveal that other trace elements are essential for human nutrition. Unfortunately, evidence is difficult to obtain, and quantifying human need is even more formidable. And, as in the case of all trace elements, the potential for toxicity exists.

ARSENIC, NICKEL, SILICON, AND BORON

Although "poison," "plastic," or cleaning solutions may come to mind, these trace elements are recognized as essential nutrients for animals. However, a deficiency in humans has not been identified, and therefore it is impossible to estimate human requirement.

CADMIUM, LEAD, LITHIUM, TIN, AND VANADIUM

They sound like pollutants, and in some cases they are. Yet it is remotely possible that humans need them in minute amounts, amounts easily met by levels naturally occurring in food, water, and air.

COBALT

Cobalt is an essential component of vitamin B_{12}; however, there is no evidence that cobalt intake is limiting in the diet, and no RDA is necessary.

MAINTENANCE OF MINERAL BALANCE IN THE BODY

The body has several mechanisms by which it maintains mineral balance, or homeostasis, depending on the mineral involved. Some minerals can be released from storage and redistributed as needed, which is what happens when calcium is released from the bones to restore normal serum calcium levels. The body can also compensate for low or high levels of some minerals by increasing or decreasing the amount of mineral absorbed. For example, the normal absorption rate of iron from a mixed diet is only 10%, but the rate may increase to up to 50% during iron deficiency. Finally, the excretion rate of some minerals can be adjusted as needed, as in the case of sodium. Virtually all the sodium consumed in the diet is absorbed, and the only way the body can get rid of it is by excreting it in the urine. Hence, for healthy individuals, the higher the sodium intake, the greater the urinary sodium excretion.

Mineral balance is significantly influenced by mineral-mineral interactions and by mineral interactions with other dietary components. For instance, high intakes of zinc impair copper absorption; iron absorption is enhanced by vitamin C and impaired by tannins in tea. Thus, mineral status should be viewed as a function of the total diet, not just from the standpoint of how much of each particular mineral is consumed. Much has yet to be learned about mineral interactions and "nutritional adequacy" as it applies not only to avoiding deficiencies, but to promoting optimal health. Like the RDA for vitamins, future recommendations may focus on optimal nutrient levels to protect against chronic disease.

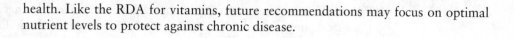

MACROMINERALS

Calcium, phosphorus, and magnesium are macrominerals. A summary of each appears in Table 5-2. Although sodium, potassium, and chlorine are also macrominerals, they function primarily as electrolytes and are discussed in Chapter 6.

Calcium

Calcium is the most abundant mineral in the body, making up about half of the body's total mineral content. Almost all of the body's calcium (99%) is combined with phosphorus, magnesium, and other elements to give rigidity and structure to bones and teeth. As a large, dynamic reservoir of calcium, bones continually take up

Table 5-2
Summary of Macrominerals

Mineral and Sources	RDA	Estimated Average Adult Intake in the U.S.	Functions
CALCIUM			
Milk and dairy products Green leafy vegetables Whole grains Nuts Legumes	18–24 yo: 1200 mg 25 and older: 800 mg	Males: 976 mg Females: 744	Bone and teeth formation and maintenance Blood clotting Nerve transmission Muscle function Cell membrane permeability
PHOSPHORUS			
Meat Poultry Fish Eggs Legumes Milk and dairy products Soft drinks	18–24 yo: 1200 mg 25 and older: 800 mg	1000–1700 mg	Bone and teeth formation and maintenance Acid–base balance Energy metabolism Cell membrane structure Regulation of hormone and coenzyme activity
MAGNESIUM			
Green leafy vegetables Nuts Legumes Whole grains Seafood	Men: 350 mg Women: 280 mg	238–321 mg	Bone formation Smooth muscle relaxation Protein synthesis CHO metabolism

and release calcium to keep serum calcium levels within a narrow range. The remaining 1% of calcium in the body is found in plasma and other body fluids. It plays important roles in blood clotting, nerve transmission, muscle contraction and relaxation, cell membrane permeability, and the activation of certain enzymes.

Milk and milk products are the richest sources of calcium in the diet, so much so that an inadequate intake of calcium is likely if dairy products are omitted from the diet. It is estimated that dairy products contribute more than 55% of calcium intake in the average American diet. Canned fish with bones may also be an excellent source of calcium. Although green leafy vegetables, whole grains, nuts, and legumes are good sources of calcium, fiber and other binding agents decrease the amount of calcium that is available for absorption. See Appendix 12 for the calcium content of selected foods.

ABSORPTION AND EXCRETION

Normally, only 30% to 40% of the calcium that is consumed in the average mixed diet is absorbed. The percentage of calcium absorbed is known to increase in response to body need, such as during pregnancy, lactation, growth, and recovery from bone fractures. Lactose, which is the CHO in milk and dairy products, and vitamin D both promote calcium absorption. At normal and below-normal intakes of protein, calcium absorption is enhanced; however, protein intakes in excess of the RDA do not offer any additional benefit. Phosphorus, in all forms except phytate phosphorus, has little if any negative effect on calcium absorption.

Calcium absorption is impaired because of reduced transit time when gastrointestinal (GI) motility is increased. Likewise, excessive fat intake and fat malabsorption syndromes cause calcium to precipitate into insoluble calcium soaps, which are excreted in the feces. Phytates and oxalates, chemicals found in whole wheat and green, leafy vegetables, respectively, also combine with calcium to prevent its absorption. Excessive intakes of certain fibers may impair calcium absorption, as can excessive intakes of magnesium or iron. Because of changes in the levels of circulating vitamin D metabolites, the efficiency of calcium absorption decreases with age. Calcium that is not absorbed is excreted in the feces.

The kidneys help maintain serum calcium levels by increasing urinary excretion when serum levels rise. Calcium excretion is also influenced by other factors. Studies using purified proteins showed that a high protein intake increases urinary calcium excretion. However, when red meat was used as the protein source, there was no effect on urinary calcium, nor on fecal calcium, calcium balance, or intestinal absorption. An increase in phosphorus intake decreases calcium excretion. Because many sources of protein are also high in phosphorus (milk, eggs, and meat), an increase in the intake of one of these sources is usually accompanied by an increase in the other. The net effect on calcium balance is negligible at recommended levels of calcium intake.

In the past, it was believed that high intakes of phosphorus combined with low calcium consumption led to secondary hyperparathyroidism and loss of calcium from the bones. However, studies on humans have failed to establish a negative effect of phosphorus intake on calcium balance when calcium intake is adequate.

MAINTENANCE OF SERUM CALCIUM LEVELS

Normal serum calcium = 4.5–5.3 mEq/liter or 9–11 mg/dl

Serum calcium levels, and the ratio of serum calcium to phosphorus, are held relatively constant at the expense of bone when dietary intake of calcium is inadequate. Through the action of hormones, the body can correct deviations in calcium levels by increasing the amount of calcium that is absorbed, by depositing or withdrawing calcium from the bones, or by increasing urinary excretion.

Low serum calcium levels are raised by *vitamin D*, which increases calcium absorption, mobilizes calcium from the bone, and, to a small extent, increases renal reabsorption of calcium. *Parathyroid hormone* also functions to raise serum calcium by increasing calcium absorption, mobilizing calcium from the bone, and increasing renal reabsorption of calcium. High serum calcium levels are corrected by *calcitonin*, which prevents further bone resorption. Altered serum calcium levels are not related to dietary intake, but rather are the result of hormonal abnormalities or may occur secondary to other clinical conditions. Hypocalcemia (low serum calcium levels) is caused by an inadequate secretion of parathyroid hormone related to idiopathic or surgically induced hypoparathyroidism (thyroidectomy, parathyroidectomy, or neck dissections). Tetany, a symptom of hypocalcemia, is characterized by severe, intermittent, tonic contractions of the extremities, muscular cramps, uncontrolled seizures, and possible convulsions. Tetany occurs when serum calcium levels fall in response to an increase in serum phosphorus levels, possibly due to an excessive phosphorus intake or a decrease in parathyroid hormone secretion.

Hypercalcemia (elevated serum calcium levels) can cause nausea, vomiting, anorexia, abdominal pain, constipation, polyuria, polydipsia, mental changes, calcium renal stones, and excessive calcification of the bones and soft tissues. Coma and death may result if it is not treated. Hypercalcemia may be caused by cancer, excessive combined intakes of vitamin D and calcium, hyperparathyroidism (increased secretion of parathyroid hormone), thyroid disorders, and hypophosphatemia.

Resorptive hypercalciuria is a condition that occurs during periods of prolonged immobility when an excessive amount of calcium is withdrawn from the bone and excreted in the urine, which increases the risk of calcium renal stones.

See Chapter 18 for more on alterations in calcium metabolism.

RECOMMENDED DIETARY ALLOWANCE AND AVERAGE INTAKE

The RDA for calcium is 800 mg/day for both women and men 25 years of age and older. The newest edition of the RDA raised the RDA for men and women 18 to 24 years of age to 1200 mg/day, in view of the evidence that peak bone mass is not attained before age 25, and that an apparent protective measure against osteoporosis later in life is to maximize genetically programmed peak bone mass by consuming an adequate calcium intake during early adulthood.

Because the body has the ability to adapt during times of inadequate calcium intake, and because evidence of inadequate intake is slow to develop, there is considerable controversy regarding how much calcium is actually needed to maintain calcium balance. Some studies have shown that at intakes of 800 mg/day, a substantial percentage of ambulatory people are in negative calcium balance. Increasing calcium intake to 1200 mg caused a significant increase in calcium balance; however, intakes of 2000 mg and higher did not offer any real improvement in calcium balance. Because 800 mg does not appear adequate to maintain calcium balance, and because calcium losses increase with aging, many researchers believe that the RDA should be higher, especially for women. In fact, The National Institutes of Health Consensus Development Panel on Optimal Calcium intake recommends higher calcium intakes than the current RDA: 1500 mg calcium/day for postmenopausal women who are not on estrogen replacement therapy and everyone over 65 years old; 1200 to 1500 mg/day for females 11 to 24 years of age, and pregnant or lactating women; and 1000 mg/day for both men and women 25 to 49 years of age and postmenopausal women 50 to 64 years of age who are on estrogen replacement therapy (IFIC, 1994).

According to advance data from the Third National Health and Nutrition Examination Survey, Phase 1, 1988–1991, both mean and median calcium intakes are lower than the RDA for almost all female racial and ethnic groups over 12 years of age, and thus they are much lower than National Institutes of Health recommendations (CDC, 1994). The mean calcium intake of all females was 744 mg compared to the mean calcium intake for males of all ages of 976 mg (CDC, 1994).

CLINICAL APPLICATIONS

Calcium Deficiency

Calcium deficiency may be related to an inadequate calcium intake or may occur secondary to malabsorption syndromes, vitamin D deficiency, or endocrine disorders. A long-standing deficiency of calcium, which causes loss of calcium from the bones in order to maintain serum calcium levels, can result in osteoporosis, a prevalent condition among middle-aged and elderly women that is characterized by a negative calcium balance and a loss of total bone mass. Although all people lose bone with age, the rate of bone loss appears to be accelerated by a calcium deficiency (see Chapter 20 for more on osteoporosis).

Calcium Excess

Although intakes of up to 2500 mg/day have not produced adverse effects in healthy people, high calcium intakes may cause constipation and increase the risk of calcium urinary stones in men with hypercalciuria. In addition, absorption of iron, zinc, and other minerals may be inhibited, and the potential for hypercalciuria, hypercalcemia, and renal function deterioration exists.

Future Directions

Some studies have shown that high calcium intakes protect against high blood pressure; other studies have failed to establish a relationship. Another area of future research is the role played by calcium in the prevention of colon cancer that is promoted by fat and bile acids.

Nutrient/Drug Interactions

When taken together, calcium decreases the absorption of tetracycline, phenytoin, and iron salts and may antagonize the action of calcium channel–blocking drugs.

Drugs that affect calcium are as follows:

- Acetazolamide: increases urinary calcium excretion
- Adrenal corticosteroids: decrease calcium absorption
- Anticonvulsants: may decrease serum levels of vitamin D and calcium
- Capreomycin: decreases serum calcium
- Cholestyramine: decreases calcium absorption with long-term use; decreases serum calcium; increases urinary calcium excretion
- Cycloserine: may decrease calcium absorption
- Dactinomycin: decreases calcium absorption
- Digitalis glycosides: may increase urinary calcium excretion
- Ethacrynic acid: increases urinary calcium excretion
- Furosemide: increases urinary calcium excretion; decreases serum calcium in hypercalcemia
- Glutethimide: may alter calcium need; long-term use may cause osteomalacia
- Lithium: increases urinary calcium excretion, decreases calcium uptake by bone
- Mercurial diuretics: increase urinary calcium excretion
- Neomycin: decreases calcium absorption
- Petrolatum, liquid: decreases calcium absorption
- Phenolphthalein: decreases vitamin D and calcium absorption
- Probenecid: increases urinary calcium excretion
- Spironolactone: increases urinary calcium excretion
- Tetracyclines: decrease absorption of calcium
- Thiazide diuretics: single dose increases calcium excretion; long-term use tends to decrease calcium excretion and increase serum calcium
- Triamterene: may increase urinary calcium excretion
- Viomycin: can cause hypocalcemia; causes excessive urinary excretion of calcium, which persists after the drug is discontinued

Phosphorus

Next to calcium, phosphorus is the second most abundant mineral in the body. Approximately 85% of the body's phosphorus is found in bones; along with calcium, it is essential for their formation and maintenance. The rest of the body's phosphorus is metabolically active and is found in every body cell. It performs numerous functions, such as regulating acid–base balance, metabolizing energy, providing structure to cell membranes, serving as an essential component of nucleic acids, regulating the activity of hormones and coenzymes, aiding in the absorption and transportation of fats, and facilitating the absorption of glucose.

Almost all foods contain phosphorus. Foods that are rich in protein (meat, poultry, fish, eggs, legumes, and nuts) and calcium (milk and milk products) are also high in phosphorus. In the average adult American diet, soft drinks and processed foods supply a significant amount of phosphorus. Grains, eggs, nuts, and legumes are also good sources. See Appendix 12 for the phosphorus content of selected foods.

ABSORPTION, EXCRETION, AND MAINTENANCE

Normally, about 50% to 70% of the phosphorus in the adult diet is absorbed. Like calcium, the absorption of phosphorus is enhanced by the presence of vitamin D and is regulated by parathyroid hormone. The major route of phosphorus excretion is the urine.

Normal serum inorganic phosphorus is maintained at 2.5 to 4.8 mg/dl. Hyperphosphatemia (high serum phosphorus level), which may be related to renal insufficiency or hypoparathyroidism, is characterized by symptoms of hypocalcemic tetany. Hypophosphatemia (low serum phosphorus levels) may occur as a result of administering long-term, phosphorus-free total parenteral nutrition, or it may result from excessive use of phosphate-binding antacids, malabsorption syndromes, vitamin D deficiency leading to rickets or osteomalacia, hyperparathyroidism, treatment of diabetic acidosis, or alcoholism. Clinical findings include anorexia, weakness, circumoral paresthesia, and hyperventilation.

RECOMMENDED DIETARY ALLOWANCE AND AVERAGE INTAKE

With the exception of young infants, who need less phosphorus in relation to calcium, the RDA for phosphorus equals the RDA for calcium for all age and sex groups. The typical adult American diet supplies 1000 to 1700 mg/day (CDC, 1994), well above the RDA of 800 mg, and those figures may even be underestimated by 15% to 20% because of the prevalence of phosphorus-containing additives in the diet.

CLINICAL APPLICATIONS

Phosphorus Deficiency

Because phosphorus is pervasive in the diet, a dietary deficiency is rare. However, premature infants who are fed only breast milk may develop hypophosphatemic rickets resulting from a low phosphorus intake during a period when need is increased because of rapid bone mineralization.

Phosphorus deficiency may be induced in people who are receiving long-term aluminum hydroxide (antacid) therapy, because aluminum hydroxide binds with phosphorus, making it unavailable for absorption. Weakness, anorexia, malaise, and pain characterize the loss of bone.

Phosphorus Excess

In animals, an excessive phosphorus intake has been shown to lower serum calcium levels and to cause secondary hyperparathyroidism and loss of bone. In humans, lowered serum calcium levels have been the only result. An intake of phosphorus that is excessive enough to cause adverse effects is not likely to occur in normal diets.

Nutrient/Drug Interactions

Drugs that affect phosphorus are as follows:

- Aluminum hydroxide: decreases phosphorus absorption; may cause hypophosphatemia if used frequently and on a long-term basis
- Magnesium hydroxide: may decrease phosphorus absorption
- Petrolatum, liquid: decreases phosphorus absorption

Magnesium

Of the 20 to 28 g of magnesium in the adult body, approximately 60% is deposited in the bone with calcium and phosphorus. The rest of the body's magnesium is distributed in various soft tissues, muscles, and body fluids. Magnesium plays a role in smooth muscle relaxation, sodium and potassium metabolism, protein synthesis, CHO metabolism, cellular growth and reproduction, and hormonal activity. Serum magnesium concentration is held constant in healthy individuals by poorly understood homeostatic mechanisms and does not appear to be controlled by hormones.

Magnesium is abundant in the diet, especially in green, leafy vegetables as a component of chlorophyll (green pigment). Other sources include whole grains, nuts, legumes, seafood, cocoa, and chocolate.

ABSORPTION AND EXCRETION

Average magnesium absorption occurs at a rate of 40% to 60% of intake. An inverse relationship exists between magnesium intake and absorption—as intake increases, absorption decreases. In animal studies, the absorption of calcium and magnesium is competitive and mutually exclusive. The higher the intake of calcium, the lower the absorption of magnesium. However, studies with humans have not shown magnesium absorption or balance to be altered by calcium intakes of up to 2000 mg/day. Factors that decrease the absorption of magnesium include phytates and oxalates, and the presence of fat. Because the kidneys efficiently conserve magnesium, urinary excretion is very low.

RECOMMENDED DIETARY ALLOWANCE AND AVERAGE INTAKE

It is reported that the mean male intake of magnesium is 321 mg per day and the mean female intake is 238 mg (CDC, 1994), figures that fall below the current RDA of 350 mg and 280 mg for men and women, respectively. Magnesium intake has declined in the United States over the last few decades, a possible result of milling of whole grains, which removes many micronutrients that are not replaced (Mertz, 1994). However, there is no evidence that magnesium deficiency is common among healthy American adults.

Factors that may increase the need for magnesium include diets high in calcium, protein, vitamin D, or alcohol, as well as psychological or physical stress, including athletic training.

CLINICAL APPLICATIONS

Magnesium Deficiency

A dietary deficiency of magnesium has not been reported in people who consume a normal mixed diet (NRC, 1989). However, magnesium deficiency may occur secondary to malabsorption syndromes, renal dysfunction, and general malnutrition and alcoholism; it may also result from iatrogenic causes such as nasogastric suctioning and parenteral or enteral feedings that are deficient in magnesium, or it may be a side effect of certain medications.

Hypomagnesemia (low serum magnesium level of less than 1.8 mg/dl) is uncommon because of the supply of magnesium that is available on the surface of bones, coupled with the kidneys' ability to conserve magnesium. However, hypomagnesemia may occur secondary to numerous clinical conditions, including GI disorders such as malabsorption, vomiting, and diarrhea, or as a side effect of certain medications (see Nutrient/Drug Interactions); it may also be associated with alcoholism, kwashiorkor, hyperthyroidism and parathyroid disorders, diabetic acidosis, the administration of magnesium-free parenteral fluids after surgery, postsurgical stress, renal disease, and rickets in patients who are receiving massive doses of vitamin D.

Signs and symptoms of hypomagnesemia include increased neuromuscular and central nervous system irritability, which progresses to loss of muscular control, tremors, disorientation, tetany, positive Trousseau's signs, positive Chvostek's signs, and convulsions.

Magnesium Excess

Large oral intakes of magnesium appear to be safe when renal function is normal. However, hypermagnesemia (high serum magnesium level greater than 3.0 mg/dl) may occur in people with impaired renal function who take therapeutic doses of magnesium. Central nervous system depression, coma, and hypotension may result.

Nutrient/Drug Interactions

When they are taken together, magnesium decreases the absorption of tetracycline. Drugs that affect magnesium are as follows:

- Alcohol: increases urinary excretion of magnesium
- Amphotericin B: decreases serum magnesium
- Capreomycin: decreases serum magnesium
- Cycloserine: may decrease magnesium absorption
- Digitalis glycosides: may increase urinary excretion of magnesium
- Ethacrynic acid: increases urinary excretion of magnesium; can cause hypomagnesemia
- Furosemide: increases urinary excretion of magnesium
- Gentamicin: increases urinary excretion of magnesium
- Lithium: increases plasma magnesium
- Mercurial diuretics: increase urinary excretion of magnesium; may induce magnesium depletion

- Phenobarbital: decreases serum magnesium levels
- Phenytoin: decreases serum magnesium levels
- Probenecid: increases urinary excretion of magnesium
- Spironolactone: increases urinary excretion of magnesium
- Tetracyclines: may decrease magnesium absorption, but result is not clinically significant
- Thiazides: increase urinary excretion of magnesium; can cause magnesium depletion
- Viomycin: can cause hypomagnesemia; excessive urinary excretion of magnesium persists after the drug is discontinued

TRACE ELEMENTS

Iron, iodine, and zinc are the best-known trace elements. Iron has always been listed in the RDA tables; iodine first appeared in 1968, and zinc was added in 1974. Selenium was upgraded to RDA status for the first time in 1989. A summary of trace elements with defined RDA appears in Table 5-3.

In 1980, estimated safe and adequate daily intakes for copper, manganese, fluoride, chromium, and molybdenum were listed separately from the RDA table (Table 5-4). Research shows that arsenic, nickel, silicon, and boron are essential in animals; however, human requirement has not been proven. Lead and mercury are toxic, nonessential trace elements (see Food for Thought: Other Trace Elements—Future RDA Candidates?).

Table 5-3
Summary of Essential Trace Elements with Defined RDAs

Trace Element	RDA	Estimated Average Adult Intake in the United States	Major Sources	Function	Signs of Deficiency	Signs of Toxicity
Iron (Fe)	Men: 10 mg Women: 15 mg	Men: >13 mg Women: 10–13 mg	Liver, lean meat, dried beans, fortified cereals	Oxygen transport via hemoglobin and myoglobin; constituent of enzyme systems	Depletion of iron stores, anemia (microcytic, hypochromic), pallor, decreased work capacity	Hemochromatosis, hemosiderosis Acute poisoning → GI cramping, nausea, vomiting, possible shock, convulsions, and coma
Iodine (I)	150 μg	170 μg–250 μg	Iodized salt, seafood, milk, eggs, bread	Constituent of thyroid hormones that regulate BMR	Goiter (not a problem in the United States)	Acnelike skin lesions, "iodine goiter"

(continued)

Table 5-3 *(Continued)*
Summary of Essential Trace Elements with Defined RDAs

Trace Element	RDA	Estimated Average Adult Intake in the United States	Major Sources	Function	Signs of Deficiency	Signs of Toxicity
Zinc (Zn)	Men: 15 mg Women: 12 mg	8 mg to 16 mg	Meat, oysters, seafood, milk, egg yolks, legumes, whole grains	Tissue growth, development, and healing; sexual maturation and reproduction; constituent of many enzymes in energy and nucleic acid metabolism	Impaired growth, sexual maturation, and immune system functioning; skin lesions; acrodermatitis enteropathica; decreased sense of taste and smell	Excess use of supplements may cause anorexia, vomiting, nausea, diarrhea, muscle pain, lethargy, drowsiness, and bleeding gastric ulcers; may also interfere with copper metabolism and decrease serum levels of high-density lipoproteins (HDL, the "good" form of cholesterol)
Selenium (Se)	Men: 70 µg Women: 55 µg	108 µg	Seafood, kidney, liver, meat, some grains	Protects against oxygen damage and heavy metals; constituent of an enzyme that acts as an antioxidant	Usually occurs in combination with protein-energy malnutrition or other nutrient deficiency; may produce cardiomyopathy	Loss of hair, brittle fingernails, and fatigue

Group Characteristics

Because trace elements are required in such infinitesimal amounts, measuring their presence in both food and the body is difficult. With the exception of iron, manganese, and copper, food composition tables generally do not provide data on trace elements. Compounding the problem of not knowing how much of trace elements are provided in the diet is the variable of bioavailability. The metabolism of individual trace elements is strongly influenced by other dietary factors, so that absorption and utilization of an element can vary depending on the source of the nutrient and the presence of other food components that are consumed at the same time. Assessing dietary intake of trace elements is extremely difficult.

In the body, reliable and valid indicators of trace element status (eg, measuring serum levels, conducting balance studies, determining enzyme activity) are not

Table 5-4
Summary of Trace Elements With Estimated Safe and Adequate Daily Dietary Intakes

Newer Trace Element	Adult Estimated Safe and Adequate Daily Intakes	Average Estimated Intake in the United States	Major Sources	Function	Signs of Deficiency	Signs of Toxicity
Copper (Cu)	1.5 mg– 3.0 mg	1 mg	Organ meats, seafood, nuts, seeds	Integrity of heart and large arteries; bone and blood formation; antioxidant	Anemia, altered bone formation, impairment of cardio-vascular system, hypercholes-terolemia	None known
Manganese (Mn)	2.0 mg– 5 mg	2.2 mg–2.7 mg	Whole grains and cereals, fruits, vegetables	Constituent of enzymes in mucopoly-saccharide metabolism and in fat synthesis; also needed for growth, reproduc-tion, and blood clotting	Deficiency in humans is unknown	Dietary excess unlikely
Fluoride (Fl)	1.5 mg to 4 mg	0.9 mg–1.7 mg	Fluoridated water, tea, bottled water, infant formulas	Structure of enamel of teeth; promotes enamel re-mineraliza-tion through-out life; role in bone for-mation and integrity	Dental caries; may in-crease the risk of osteoporosis	2 mg/day to 8 mg/day may cause mottling of the teeth; doses of 20 mg to 80 mg may induce bone changes years later
Chromium (Cr)	50 µg– 200 µg	25 µg–33 µg	Brewers yeast, whole grains, liver, kidney	Cofactor for insulin	Insulin resis-tance; impaired glucose tol-erance; low serum chro-mium is cor-related with coronary heart dis-ease in humans.	Dietary toxicity unlikely; occu-pational expo-sure to chromium dusts corre-lated to increase in bronchial cancer

(continued)

Table 5-4 (Continued)
Summary of Trace Elements With Estimated Safe and Adequate Daily Dietary Intakes

Newer Trace Element	Adult Estimated Safe and Adequate Daily Intakes	Average Estimated Intake in the United States	Major Sources	Function	Signs of Deficiency	Signs of Toxicity
Molybdenum (Mo)	75 µg– 250 µg	76 µg–109 µg	Milk, beans, breads, cereals	Component of enzymes and flavo- protein, and therefore important for normal body metabolism	Sulfur amino acid toxicity; decreased production of uric acid (dietary deficiency unlikely)	Interferes with copper metabolism

available for all microminerals; therefore, assessing trace element status is not always possible.

It appears that each trace element has its own curve or range of safe and adequate intakes over which the body can maintain homeostasis. The margin of safety may be narrower for some minerals than others. Extremely excessive or deficient intakes of any element have the potential to cause death. Somewhere in between optimal function and obvious alteration in function lies a gray area of marginal deficiency or marginal toxicity—an area that generates much controversy and interest. People who consume an adequate diet derive no further benefit from using supplements, and because a delicate balance exists among minerals, a large intake of one element may induce a deficiency of another. However, people with marginally deficient intakes may experience improved health through the judicious use of supplements.

Trace element deficiencies may be related more to geographic location than to "bad" eating habits. Because plants, and ultimately animals and humans, depend on

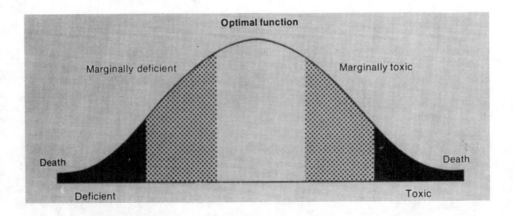

the soil for trace elements, some mineral deficiencies (eg, goiter) are related to living in areas with soil that is poor in minerals (eg, the "goiter belt" area around the Great Lakes). Thus, foods that have been evaluated for their trace element content may not represent the actual amount of a trace element a person consumes, depending on where the food was harvested.

Iron

Of the 3 to 5 g of iron in the body, approximately 67% is in the heme portion of hemoglobin, and 27% is stored as ferritin in the liver, bone marrow, and spleen. The remaining iron is found in transferrin (the transport carrier of iron) in myoglobin, and in enzyme systems that are active in energy metabolism.

Iron in the diet exists in two forms: heme iron, which constitutes about half of the iron in animal sources such as meat, fish, and poultry; and nonheme iron, which comprises the remaining half of the iron found in animal sources and all of the iron found in plants such as grains, vegetables, legumes, and nuts. Although heme iron is much better absorbed, nonheme iron accounts for a larger percentage of total iron intake. Table 17-8 lists heme and nonheme sources of iron.

ABSORPTION AND EXCRETION

Although the average rate of iron absorption is about 10% of the total consumed, the rate varies significantly during times of need. When iron requirements are increased, such as during growth, pregnancy, and iron deficiency, as much as 50% of the iron consumed may be absorbed, and iron absorption becomes more efficient for both forms of iron.

Heme and nonheme iron are absorbed by different mechanisms. Heme iron generally is absorbed at a rate of about 15% to 35% of the amount consumed; the rate is influenced by body need. Nonheme iron is less well absorbed, with a rate of only 3% to 8% of that consumed. In addition to need, its absorption rate is influenced by the presence of absorption enhancers and inhibitors. Factors that increase the absorption of nonheme iron include vitamin C, when consumed at the same meal; certain animal proteins, such as meat, fish, and poultry; alcohol; and gastric acidity, which increases iron solubility. Nonheme iron absorption decreases in the presence of tea, coffee, and binding agents like bran, phosphates, oxalates, phytates, phosvitin, and EDTA (a metal-sequestering food additive). Alkalinity (eg, from the use of antacids), diarrhea, and steatorrhea are also associated with decreased iron absorption.

Iron absorption from supplements and enriched and fortified foods also varies with the particular form of iron used. Ferrous sulfate, lactate, fumarate, succinate, glycine sulfate, and glutamate are well absorbed; ferrous citrate, tartrate, and pyrophosphate are poorly absorbed (see Chapter 17 for more on iron).

Because the body maintains iron balance primarily by adjusting the rate of absorption, little or no iron is excreted in the urine. Even iron that is contained in hemoglobin and other body substances is recycled as the cells are replaced. However, a small amount of iron is lost daily through the skin, hair, feces, nails, sweat, and GI cells. Menstrual blood loss accounts for additional lost iron.

RECOMMENDED DIETARY ALLOWANCE AND AVERAGE INTAKE

To compensate for an average absorption rate of 10% and the daily (and monthly) iron losses, the RDA for iron is set at 10 mg/day for men and postmenopausal women and 15 mg/day for women of childbearing age. The previous RDA for women of childbearing age was 18 mg/day; that figure is still used as the Daily Value on food labels. Adult men typically consume more iron than women and exceed the RDA for all adolescent and adult age groups (CDC, 1994). The mean iron intake among all adult female age groups was below the RDA.

Iron requirements increase during periods of growth (infancy, adolescence, pregnancy) and in response to heavy or chronic blood loss related to menstruation, surgery, injury, childbirth, GI bleeding, and aspirin abuse. Iron needs may also increase secondary to the use of medications that alter iron absorption (see Nutrient/Drug Interactions).

CLINICAL APPLICATIONS

Iron Deficiency

Iron may be the most frequently deficient nutrient in the United States, especially among infants, adolescents, menstruating women, and pregnant women. Daily supplements of 30 to 60 mg are often prescribed for pregnant women. Because menstruating women, infants, and adolescents may not eat enough iron to meet their needs, iron supplements may be indicated (see Chapter 17 for more on iron deficiency).

Iron Toxicity

Iron toxicity is uncommon, because the body normally decreases the rate of iron absorption when its iron status is adequate. However, a rare genetic defect in iron metabolism, known as hemochromatosis, causes iron to accumulate in excessive amounts, which can eventually saturate the body's tissues, especially the skin, liver, and pancreas, and end in multiple-system organ failure.

Because alcohol enhances iron absorption, alcoholics and even people with a history of alcoholism absorb iron at rates much higher than average. One report found iron absorption rates as high as 50% among alcoholics who had abstained from alcohol for 4 weeks before the study, a rate similar to that noted in hemochromatosis. The result may be toxic overload.

In the absence of genetic defects or alcohol abuse, excessive iron storage from diet alone is unlikely. However, taking iron supplements or vitamin pills with iron is a leading cause of accidental poisoning in young children, who have a much lower tolerance for iron loads than adults. Signs and symptoms of acute iron poisoning include GI cramping and pain, vomiting, and nausea, which may lead to shock, convulsions, and coma.

Nutrient/Drug Interactions

When they are taken together, iron may decrease the absorption of tetracycline.
Drugs that affect iron are as follows:

- Alcohol: increases absorption of ferric iron
- Antacids (carbonate): decrease iron absorption
- Chloramphenicol: increases serum iron, total iron-binding capacity
- Cholestyramine: can decrease iron absorption; decreases iron reserves (high dose in animal studies)
- Clofibrate: decreases iron absorption
- Dactinomycin: decreases iron absorption
- Indomethacin: may cause anemia
- Neomycin: decreases iron absorption
- Oral contraceptives: may increase serum levels of iron
- Salicylates: may cause iron-deficiency anemia with long-term use or overuse

Iodine

The average adult body has 20 to 50 mg of iodine, which is found in muscles, the thyroid gland, skin, skeleton, endocrine tissues, the central nervous system, and the bloodstream. It is an essential component of thyroxine (T_4) and triiodothyronine (T_3), the thyroid hormones responsible for regulating basal metabolic rate.

The major source of iodine in the American diet is iodized salt, even though about half of the salt sold in the United States is not iodized. Because iodine is abundant in ocean water, seafood is an excellent source of iodine. Plants that are grown in iodine-rich soil, which includes most areas of the United States except the Rocky Mountain states and the Great Lakes areas, are also good sources of iodine. Although it is a naturally poor source of iodine, milk now provides a significant amount of iodine in the diet because of both the iodized salt licks that are given to cows and the use of iodine chemicals to sanitize and disinfect udders, milking machines, and milk tanks. Iodates that are used as bread dough conditioners also contribute to iodine intake.

ABSORPTION AND EXCRETION

Dietary iodine is rapidly and almost completely absorbed from the small intestine in the form of iodides. Approximately two thirds of the amount absorbed is excreted in the urine; the small amount of iodine found in the feces comes from bile.

RECOMMENDED DIETARY ALLOWANCE AND AVERAGE INTAKE

The RDA for both men and women is set at 150 µg/day, which includes a measure of safety for the as-yet unquantified effect of goitrogens (thyroid antagonists found in members of the cabbage family) on iodine requirements. The average iodine intake is estimated at 250 µg for men and 170 µg for women, excluding the intake from iodized salt. This figure represents a gradual decline in iodine intake over the last decade, which is most probably a result of reduction in the use of the iodine-containing red dye erythrosine (FD&C Red No. 3) in ready-to-eat cereals. Still, it is recommended that no new sources of iodine be added to the U.S. food supply (NRC, 1989).

CLINICAL APPLICATIONS

Iodine Deficiency

A deficiency of iodine leads to a decrease in the production of thyroid hormones. Over time, the thyroid hypertrophies, or develops endemic goiter. Severe and prolonged iodine deficiency may result in hypothyroidism, an endocrine disorder that affects the uptake of iodine by the thyroid gland (see Chapter 18).

Before the introduction of iodized salt, goiter was prevalent in the United States. Now, the problem of goiter occurs only in developing countries.

Iodine Toxicity

Most people are unaffected by excess iodine; for those who are affected, the amount of iodine that is required to cause adverse effects is highly individualized. Iodine toxicity may manifest itself as thyroiditis (inflammation of the thyroid gland), goiter, hypothyroidism (inhibited synthesis of the thyroid hormone), hyperthyroidism, or sensitivity reactions (ie, allergic and anaphylactic responses); acute responses may occur with large doses (cardiovascular collapse, convulsions, asthma attacks). Intake of large amounts of iodine can be fatal.

Nutrient/Drug Interactions

None known.

Zinc

Although zinc is present in the body in only a small quantity (about 2 g), it is found in many tissues, including the eye, bones, skin, hair, muscles, pancreas, liver, kidney, and male reproductive organs. It is a component of DNA, RNA, insulin, and numerous enzyme systems that function in tissue growth, maintenance, and healing; the metabolism of CHO, protein, fat, and nucleic acids; sexual maturation and reproduction; the senses of taste and smell; and the development of immune reactions.

Generally, animal products are good sources of zinc, especially meats, oysters and other seafood, milk, and egg yolks. Legumes and whole grains are good sources of zinc but are less well absorbed.

ABSORPTION AND EXCRETION

On the average, only 15% to 35% of ingested zinc is absorbed; however, people with low zinc status absorb zinc more efficiently than people with good status, and small doses of zinc are absorbed more efficiently than large doses. The bioavailability of zinc varies significantly depending on the source. Whereas fiber and phytates interfere with zinc availability, the effect may be negligible in the average U.S. diet. Protein, phosphorus, and iron may have greater impact on zinc status, but results from studies are inconsistent and contradictory.

Zinc homeostasis is strongly regulated, and its excretion, primarily through the feces, is directly proportional to zinc status. Fecal excretion includes unabsorbed dietary zinc and zinc from enteropancreatic circulation. Small amounts of zinc are excreted in bile; under normal conditions, there is no urinary excretion of zinc.

RECOMMENDED DIETARY ALLOWANCE AND AVERAGE INTAKE

For the first time, sex-specific recommendations were made for zinc in the 10th edition of the RDA. Research shows that men need more zinc than women, as reflected in the RDA, which recommends 15 mg/day for men and 12 mg/day for women.

Zinc intake is related to total calorie intake: As calorie content increases, zinc content increases. The mean zinc intake among adult males ranges from 10.72 to 15.96 mg. Among adult females, mean intake ranges from 7.82 to 9.67 mg (CDC, 1994). It is estimated that men consume 90% or more of the RDA for zinc and women select diets that provide less than 81% of the RDA for zinc. The difference in zinc intake between men and women appears to be related solely to calorie intake, not to the zinc density of foods chosen.

CLINICAL APPLICATIONS

Zinc Deficiency

Although average zinc intake among Americans may be marginal, mild to marginal zinc deficiency states may not be apparent because clinical deficiency symptoms are not observed (Shils et al, 1994). Vegetarians who consume a high-fiber diet, as well as children, adolescents, and pregnant women, may be especially at risk for zinc deficiency. Zinc deficiency can also occur secondary to malabsorption syndromes because zinc absorption is decreased while excretion is increased. Sickle cell anemia, long-term use of total parenteral nutrition, and a rare inborn error of metabolism that interferes with zinc absorption also can lead to zinc deficiency.

Growth retardation, hypogonadism, mild anemia, hypogeusia (decreased taste acuity), delayed wound healing, alopecia, and a dermatitis called acrodermatitis enteropathica characterize zinc deficiency. Symptoms are dramatically reversed with zinc supplements.

Zinc Toxicity

Muscle incoordination, GI irritation, vomiting, diarrhea, dizziness, drowsiness, lethargy, renal failure, and anemia may be caused by large supplemental doses of zinc. Zinc toxicity may also impair copper metabolism and decrease serum HDL (high-density lipoproteins, the "good" cholesterol).

Nutrient/Drug Interactions

When they are taken together, zinc may decrease the absorption of tetracycline. Drugs that affect zinc are as follows:

- Adrenal corticosteroids: increase urinary zinc excretion
- Alcohol: increases urinary zinc excretion

- Chlorthalidone: increases urinary zinc excretion
- Dimercaprol: binds zinc; alters taste acuity
- Mercaptopurine: may cause zinc deficiency
- Methotrexate: may cause zinc deficiency
- Oral contraceptives: high estrogen preparations increase erythrocyte zinc levels
- Penicillamine: binds zinc; increases urinary zinc excretion; decreases taste acuity
- Tetracyclines: may decrease zinc absorption, although not to a clinically significant extent
- Thiazide diuretics: increase urinary zinc excretion

Selenium

Selenium is a component of the enzyme glutathione peroxidase, which acts as an antioxidant. As such, selenium has a close metabolic relationship with vitamin E, the body's primary antioxidant. Selenium deficiency has been postulated to be a predisposing condition to a disorder of cardiomyopathy known as Keshan disease. Other functions of selenium are being explored.

Good sources of selenium include seafoods, kidney, liver, and other meats. The selenium content of grains and seeds depends on the selenium content of the soil in which they are grown. Grains, vegetables, and meat raised in South Dakota, Wyoming, New Mexico, and Utah are high in selenium; the selenium content of the soil in the southern states and on both coasts of the United States is considerably lower.

RECOMMENDED DIETARY ALLOWANCE AND AVERAGE INTAKE

The RDA for selenium was established for the first time in 1989. Based on studies of Chinese men, the RDA has been set at 70 μg for men and 55 μg for women. Previously, the estimated safe and adequate daily intake was 50 to 200 μg: Average daily adult intake in the United States is 108 μg.

CLINICAL APPLICATIONS

Selenium Deficiency

In animals, simultaneous deficiencies of vitamin E and selenium cause many diseases that can be prevented or cured by supplements of either nutrient alone (NRC, 1989). Muscular discomfort or weakness that develops in humans who are receiving long-term total parenteral nutrition that is devoid of selenium responds to selenium supplementation. Cardiomyopathy may also develop.

Selenium Toxicity

It is not known exactly how much selenium is toxic. The residents of one particular county in China developed toxicity after consuming 50,000 μg per day. Symptoms included itchy scalp, dry brittle hair, cracked fingernails, mottled teeth, and blistering lesions over the limbs. Some people had nervous system alterations, such as numbness, convulsions, paralysis, and even death. In the United States, people who took an improperly manufactured supplement that contained 27.3 mg of selenium per tablet developed nausea, abdominal pain, diarrhea, nail and hair changes, peripheral neuropathy, fatigue, and irritability (NRC, 1989). The margin of error between the present RDA and toxicity dose appears to be at least 500 µg.

Future Directions

Both laboratory and epidemiologic studies suggest that selenium may be protective against cancer. However, the evidence is not complete, and other contradictory studies have shown that large doses of vitamin C and selenium actually increase tumor growth. Because the long-term safety of selenium supplements and the possible interactions with other nutrients are not known, researchers refuse to endorse the use of supplements.

Nutrient/Drug Interactions

None known.

"NEWER" TRACE ELEMENTS

Five other trace elements—copper, manganese, fluorine, chromium, and molybdenum—are considered essential for human nutrition. However, because not enough is known to firmly establish their RDA, they have been assigned estimated safe and adequate daily dietary intake ranges (see Table 5-4).

KEY CONCEPTS

- Because minerals are inorganic substances, they cannot be broken down and rearranged in the body like organic nutrients (carbohydrates, protein, fat, and vitamins).
- Mineral toxicities are not likely to occur from diet alone; rather, they are most often related to excessive use of mineral supplements, environmental exposure, or from alterations in metabolism.
- Calcium, phosphorus, and magnesium are considered to be macrominerals because they are needed in relatively large amounts (more than 100 mg/day) and are found in the body in quantities greater than 5 g.
- Trace elements are needed in very small amounts (less than 15 mg/day) and are found in the body in amounts less than 5 g.
- Depending on the mineral involved, the body can maintain mineral balance by altering the rate of absorption, altering the rate of excretion, or releasing minerals from storage when needed.
- The absorption of many minerals is influenced by mineral–mineral interactions; thus too much of one mineral may promote a deficiency of another.

REFERENCES

American Dietetic Association (1994). Positions of The American Dietetic Association: Enrichment and fortification of foods and dietary supplements. J Am Diet Assoc, 94(6), 661–663.

American Dietetic Association (1994). Position of The American Dietetic Association: The impact of fluoride on dental health. J Am Diet Assoc, 94(12), 1428–1431.

Centers for Disease Control and Prevention (1994). Advance data. Dietary intake of vitamins, minerals, and fiber of persons ages 2 months and over in the United States: Third National Health and Nutrition Examination Survey, Phase 1, 1988–1991. DHHS Publication No. (PHS) 95-1250.

International Food Information Council (1994). Calcium: Make no bones about it. Food Insight, Sept/Oct, 1, 4.

McBean, L., Forgac, T., and Finn, S. (1994). Osteoporosis: Visions for care and prevention—A conference report. J Am Diet Assoc, 94(6), 668–671.

Mertz, W. (1994). A balanced approach to nutrition for health: The need for biologically essential minerals and vitamins. J Am Diet Assoc, 94(11), 1259–1262.

Mertz, W. (1993). Essential trace metals: New definitions based on new paradigms. Nutrition Reviews, 51, 287–295.

National Research Council (1989). Recommended Dietary Allowances. 10th ed. Washington, DC: National Academy Press.

Shils, M., Olson, J., and Shike, M. (1994). Modern Nutrition in Health and Disease. 8th ed. Philadelphia: Lea & Febiger.

Fluid and Electrolytes

Chapter Outline

Key Terms

Acids
Acidosis
Alkalosis
Anions
Blood hydrostatic pressure
Blood osmotic pressure
Buffers

Cations
Electrolytes
Extracellular fluid
Hyperkalemia
Hypernatremia
Hypervolemia
Hypokalemia

Hyponatremia
Hypovolemia
Intracellular fluid
Oncotic pressure
Pseudohyperkalemia

Body fluids are composed of water and electrolytes. Water is more vital to life than food because it is required for numerous functions, cannot be stored in the body, and is excreted daily. It is estimated that adults of normal weight can live about 70 days without food, but in a moderate climate, they die within 10 days without water.

Electrolytes are chemical compounds that dissociate into charged ions when dissolved in water. Together, water and electrolytes regulate the body's fluid balance and acid–base balance. The three major electrolytes are sodium, potassium, and chloride.

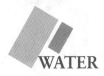

WATER

Water is absorbed rapidly into the blood and lymph by diffusion; it passes easily between body compartments, primarily by osmosis, depending on the concentration of electrolytes.

As the major constituent of every body cell, water accounts for 50% to 60% of adult body weight. Muscle and visceral cells have the highest concentration of water; skeletal cells are low in water, and fat is practically water free. Therefore, the higher the muscle mass, the greater the proportion of body water.

About two thirds of the body's water is within the cells (**intracellular fluid** or ICF); the rest of the body's fluid is called **extracellular** fluid (ECF) and includes plasma fluid, interstitial fluid, and all other body fluids such as lymph, cerebrospinal fluid, and gastrointestinal (GI)-tract fluids. Total body water and ECF decrease with age; ICF increases with an increase in body mass.

Water is involved in virtually every body function. Approximately 7 to 9 liters of water are secreted into the GI tract daily to aid in digestion and absorption. With the exception of 100 ml of water that is lost in the feces, almost all of the water contained in these secretions (saliva, gastric secretions, bile, pancreatic secretions, and intestinal mucosal secretions) is reabsorbed in the ileum and colon.

Water is the medium for all chemical reactions and a participant in many. Water is a solvent that dissolves many solutes, and as a component of blood, it helps transport nutrients to, and carry wastes away from, cells. By evaporating from the skin, water helps to regulate body temperature. Water also acts as a lubricant along mucous membranes and between moving parts.

Water Balance

A state of water balance exists when the total fluid volume in the body is adequate and appropriately distributed among the body compartments. Normally, water intake equals water output to maintain water balance (Fig. 6-1).

WATER INTAKE

For most healthy people, thirst is a reliable indicator of the body's need for water: A decrease in the ECF volume or an increase in the osmotic pressure of the blood stimulates the sensation of thirst by way of thirst receptors in the hypothalamus. However, thirst may not be a reliable indicator of need during illness, and among infants and the elderly. Intense, sustained physical activity may also inactivate normal thirst mechanisms.

Most of the water that is consumed in the average American diet does not come from water, but from other beverages (see Food for Thought: Better Bottled). Mean intake of water is estimated at 2.8 cups; the total amount of other beverages con-

Water Intake		Water Output	
Fluids	500 ml-1700 ml	Urine	600 ml-1600 ml
Water in food	800 ml-1000 ml	Water in feces	50 ml-200 ml
Metabolic water	200 ml-300 ml	Water in expired air	
		and perspiration	850 ml-1200 ml
	Total=1500 ml-3000 ml		Total=1500 ml-3000 ml

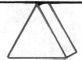

Figure 6-1
Water balance: Intake vs. output.

sumed (milk, coffee, tea, and soft drinks) is approximately 4.5 cups/day (NRC, 1989). Many solid foods provide water; fruits and vegetables are the best sources (Table 6-1). Another source of water is metabolic water, which is produced from the oxidation of food. Every 100 g of CHO, protein, and fat that is oxidized yields 55, 41, and 107 g of water, respectively.

When oral intake is contraindicated, fluid can be given intravenously in the form of glucose solutions, blood, plasma, or protein hydrolysate mixtures. Water may also be administered rectally in the form of isotonic saline solutions, or it may be given subcutaneously.

WATER OUTPUT

Measurable water loss (sensible) occurs through the urine and feces. Water that is lost through expired air and perspiration is continuous, largely unnoticeable, and unmeasurable (insensible). Generally, about 350 ml of water is lost daily through expired air. The amount of water that is lost through perspiration varies with activity and climate: As the amount of water excreted through perspiration increases, the volume of urine decreases.

Urine

By far the largest output of water is through the urine. The amount of urine excreted daily varies with the amount of water consumed in the diet; normal adult urine output ranges from 600 to 1600 ml/day; the minimum or obligatory urine output that is needed to excrete nitrogenous and other wastes is about 600 ml.

When water intake is inadequate, the kidneys, under the influence of antidiuretic hormone (ADH), compensate by concentrating the urine to conserve water. Kidney diseases have a profound impact on water balance.

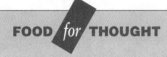

FOOD *for* THOUGHT

Better Bottled

The average American drinks 8 gallons of bottled water each year. Taste and safety are the most common reasons why Americans choose bottled over tap water. However, despite the fact that bottled water can cost 300 to 1200 times more per gallon than tap water, 25% of bottled water is nothing more than tap water. And it is possible that bottled water could contain harmful levels of contaminants that are not allowed in tap water. Without standard definitions for terms like "ground water" and "spring water," the consumer was left in the dark, and possibly in danger.

But all that changed when new FDA regulations took effect mid-1996. Bottled water is now required to meet the same safety standards set by the EPA for municipal water, except that the standard for lead is even more strict. Standard definitions for the terms "artesian water," "ground water," "mineral water," "purified water," "sparkling bottled water," "spring water," "sterile water," and "well water" have helped eliminate consumer confusion. Any bottled water that comes from a municipal water supply must now clearly state so on the label, in lettering as large as the brand's name. And labels now have to disclose any nutrients that are contained in significant amounts, so that the buyer will know how much sodium, calcium, or iron he or she is getting.

Feces

Normally, only a small amount of water (50 to 200 ml) is excreted daily in the feces. Conditions that interfere with intestinal reabsorption of water (eg, diarrhea and malabsorption syndromes) greatly increase water excretion and seriously affect the body's water balance.

Table 6-1
Approximate Percentage of Water in Selected Foods

Food	% Water
Vegetables	70–95
Fruit	75–90
Whole milk	87
Eggs	75
Ice cream	60
Meats	40–75
White bread	36
Butter	15
Gelatin	13
All-purpose flour	12
Dried beans	11
Dry cereals	5
White sugar	0.5

Recommended Dietary Allowance

The requirement for water is highly variable and impossible to determine because actual need varies in response to other factors. The amount of water required is that needed to replace insensible losses, which vary considerably, and maintain a normal solute load, which can vary with diet and other factors. For practical purposes, adults need 1 ml/cal of energy expenditure, under average conditions of energy expenditure and environmental exposure (NRC, 1989). Because the risk of water intoxication is minimal, 1.5 ml/cal is often recommended to compensate for any variations in activity level, perspiration, and solute load. The recommendation for infants is 1.5 ml/cal of energy expenditure because they have proportionately higher needs, are unable to express thirst, and have limited ability to concentrate the urine.

Clinical Applications

NORMAL FLUID BALANCE

The volume of water in the body and how it is distributed among body compartments are determined largely by the concentration of solutes in solution, namely sodium and potassium. Sodium in the ECF draws water from the ICF (water follows salt); potassium inside the cell attracts water from the ECF. Water moves easily and reversibly between the ECF and the ICF from areas of low-solute concentration to areas of high-solute concentration to equalize the solute concentration on both sides of the semipermeable membrane (Fig. 6-2). For instance, a slight increase in the sodium concentration of the ECF causes water to move from the ICF to the ECF to equalize the solute concentration in both compartments.

The movement of water between body compartments is directed by the dynamic interplay of two opposing forces: hydrostatic pressure (a pushing force) and osmotic pressure (a pulling force). The net effect of these forces determines the direction of water's movement. **Blood hydrostatic pressure**, the blood pressure (push) at the capillary level, is related to the pressure created each time the heart contracts. It seeks to push fluid from the blood vessel to the interstitium. **Blood osmotic pressure** tries to pull water across cell membranes into the blood. It is directly proportional to the total number of dissolved particles in solution. **Oncotic pressure**, the pressure at the capillary membrane caused by dissolved protein in the plasma and interstitial fluid, contributes to osmotic pressure. Protein acts to prevent plasma fluid in the blood vessels from leaking into the interstitial fluid. However, changes in the concentration of water, water and solutes, or serum protein influence the movement of fluid.

Interstitial fluid hydrostatic pressure, the push exerted by interstitial fluid against tissues and cells, tries to move fluid into the blood. **Interstitial fluid osmotic pressure** is the pull of water from the blood vessel to the interstitium that is exerted by proteins in the interstitial fluid.

FLUID VOLUME DEFICIT

Fluid volume deficit, also known as **hypovolemia**, occurs when water output exceeds water intake, and may result from water deprivation, injection of hypertonic solu-

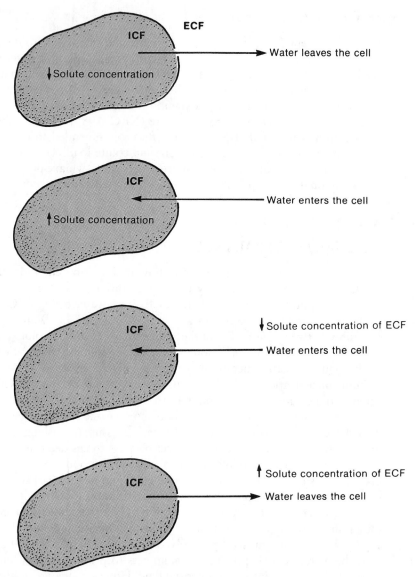

Figure 6-2
The movement of water across cell membranes.

tions, a reduction in the total quantity of electrolytes, or excessive fluid loss. Conditions that increase fluid losses include fever; profuse perspiration caused by intense physical activity, especially during hot environmental temperatures accompanied by high humidity; and a variety of clinical conditions such as diarrhea, vomiting, fistulas, excessive urination (eg, uncontrolled diabetes), hemorrhage, and severe burns. The use of drainage tubes also contributes to increased fluid losses.

Symptoms vary in intensity according to the degree of depletion. Intense thirst; dry mucous membranes; weak and rapid pulse; orthostatic hypotension; lowered body temperature; vomiting; confusion; and oliguria may occur. Hematocrit is usually elevated, as is BUN. Urine becomes concentrated, and specific gravity is usually increased. As the fluid volume deficit worsens, stupor, hypotension, and coma are common. Hypovolemia is life-threatening when more than 10% of body weight is lost.

When fluid volume deficit is mild, oral fluids that contain electrolytes may adequately restore fluid volume. Severe cases of fluid volume deficit may be treated with IV administration of an isotonic electrolyte solution, such as lactated Ringer's solution or isotonic saline solution (0.9% NaCl). Intake and output are closely monitored (see display, Fluid Equivalents).

FLUID VOLUME EXCESS

Fluid volume excess is also known as **hypervolemia**. Fluid intoxication resulting from excessive water intake is rarely observed in healthy adults. Fluid volume excess, however, can occur secondary to impaired fluid output or altered sodium balance, as in the case of renal failure, congestive heart failure, excessive sodium intake, corticosteroid therapy, cirrhosis, or Cushing's syndrome. In addition, excessive oral or parenteral infusion of fluid over a short period of time can cause hypervolemia.

Symptoms, which vary in intensity with the degree of fluid volume excess, may include peripheral edema, rapid weight gain, bounding pulse, distended neck veins, moist crackles in the lung, polyuria, and dilute urine if renal function is not impaired. Severe fluid volume excess can lead to ascites and pulmonary edema.

If fluid volume excess is mild, oral and IV fluid and electrolytes may be withheld until fluid balance is restored. Diuretics and a sodium-restricted diet may be required for moderate to severe cases. More intense medical therapy is indicated if ascites or pulmonary edema develops.

ELECTROLYTES

By definition, electrolytes carry electrical charges when they are dissolved in solution. **Cations**, such as sodium and potassium, are positively charged ions; **anions**, like chloride, are negatively charged ions. In an electrolyte solution, the total number of cations is equal to the total number of anions.

Fluid Equivalents

1 oz = 30 cc	4 oz = 120 cc
2 oz = 60 cc	8 oz = 240 cc

Within the body, the concentration of electrolyte ions or number of electrical charges in a liter of solution is expressed in milliequivalents per liter (mEq/liter). The concentration of electrolytes is maintained within a narrow range in both the ECF and ICF. Normally, serum contains about 150 mEq of cations/liter and 150 mEq of anions/liter, for a total serum osmolarity of about 300 mEq/liter. A summary of the requirements, sources, and functions of the electrolytes sodium, potassium, and chloride appears in Table 6-2.

EXAMPLE

$$\text{Milliequivalents} = \frac{\text{milligrams}}{\text{atomic weight}}$$

$$\frac{2000 \text{ mg of sodium}}{23 \text{ (atomic weight of sodium)}} = 86.96 \text{ mEq of sodium}$$

$$\frac{2000 \text{ mg of potassium}}{39 \text{ (atomic weight of potassium)}} = 51.3 \text{ mEq of potassium}$$

Sodium

Approximately 30% of the 120 mg of sodium in the body is located on the surface of the bone crystals; it is available for use in maintaining serum sodium levels if hyponatremia develops. The rest of the body's sodium is in the ECF, mostly in plasma and in nerve and muscle tissue. As the major extracellular cation, sodium largely determines plasma osmolality, which is a measure of serum concentration. It regulates cell permeability and the movement of fluid, electrolytes, glucose, insulin,

Table 6-2
Summary of Sodium, Potassium, and Chloride

Electrolyte	Adult Estimated Minimum Requirement	Sources	Functions
Sodium	500 mg	Sodium chloride, processed foods like canned soups, meats, vegetables, pickled foods, snack items, convenience foods, soft water, milk, meats	Fluid balance, acid–base balance, maintain muscle irritability, regulates cell membrane permeability and nerve impulse transmission
Potassium	2000 mg	Fruits and vegetables, legumes, whole grains, milk, meats	Fluid balance, acid–base balance, nerve impulse transmission, catalyst for many metabolic reactions, involved in skeletal and cardiac muscle activity
Chloride	750 mg	Sodium chloride, same sources as sodium	Fluid balance, acid–base balance,

and amino acids. Sodium functions to maintain fluid balance, maintain acid–base balance, maintain muscular irritability, and regulate nerve impulse transmission.

Sodium makes up 39% of salt, or sodium chloride, by weight. Because salt is used extensively in food processing and manufacturing, it is estimated that processed foods account for 75% of the total amount of sodium consumed. Canned meats and soups, condiments, pickled foods, foods prepared in brine solutions, and traditional snack items are high in added sodium. Naturally occurring sources of sodium, like milk, meats, eggs, carrots, beets, spinach, celery, artichokes, and asparagus, provide only about 10% of the sodium consumed. Salt added during cooking and at the table provides 15% of total sodium (see Chapter 17 for high- and low-sodium foods).

ABSORPTION AND EXCRETION

About 95% of ingested sodium is absorbed, with the remaining 5% excreted in the feces. Sodium that is absorbed in excess of need is excreted by the kidneys. The hormone aldosterone acts to increase the reabsorption of sodium when blood volume, cardiac output, or extracellular sodium is low, or when extracellular potassium is high.

Normally, the amount of sodium ingested equals the amount of sodium excreted. When a salty meal is consumed, thirst is stimulated so that the transitory increase in sodium in the body can be diluted to normal concentration. With the increase in both sodium and fluid in the body, kidneys excrete more sodium and fluid to normalize blood volume. When sodium and fluid are both depleted, as in the case of profuse sweating, vomiting, or diarrhea, and only water is taken in, hyponatremia develops and water intoxication results. Symptoms of muscle weakness, apathy, nausea, and anorexia are alleviated with correction of fluid and electrolyte imbalance.

RECOMMENDATIONS AND AVERAGE INTAKE

The minimum amount of sodium that is needed by a healthy adult to replace obligatory losses and to provide for growth is probably only 115 mg/day. To compensate for wide variations in physical activity and climatic exposure, 500 mg has been set as the estimated minimum requirement for healthy adults. The Daily Value for sodium, which appears on the Nutrition Facts label, is set at 2400 mg, which is approximately 1 teaspoon of salt (see display, Sodium Math Facts). Definitions of

Sodium Math Facts

1 tsp. salt weighs 6000 mg

Because 39% of salt is sodium, 6000 mg × .39 is approximately 2300 mg sodium in each teaspoon of salt

sodium claims that appear on labels are provided in the display, Sodium label definitions.

The Fourth Edition of the *Dietary Guidelines for Americans* suggests that Americans choose a diet that is moderate in salt and sodium because average intake greatly exceeds actual need (USDA/USDHHS, 1995). Suggestions for consuming less salt and sodium appear in the display, To Consume Less Salt and Sodium. A reduction in sodium intake is urged because *population* studies show that a high sodium intake is associated with higher blood pressure; however, because blood pressure is influenced by numerous variables, it is not possible to predict which *individuals* may lower blood pressure by limiting sodium intake. Because there is no risk from lowering sodium intake and the potential advantage is great, even people with normal blood pressure are urged to reduce sodium intake to help protect against hypertension and cardiovascular diseases in the future.

Calculating average sodium intake is extremely difficult, especially because "average" can vary considerably from day to day, depending on the amount of processed foods consumed. Also, the discretionary use of salt, which tends to be highly variable and can be considerable in amount, is practically impossible to estimate from dietary surveys. According to advance data from the third National Health and Nutrition Examination Survey, mean sodium intake for adult males ranges from 2861 to 4659 mg; a mean intake of 2248 to 3002 mg is cited for adult women. These figures include naturally occurring sodium, sodium used in food processing, and a calculated amount of sodium used in food preparation. They do not include sodium that is consumed from salt added at the table (CDC, 1994).

CLINICAL APPLICATIONS

Normal serum sodium equals 135 to 145 mEq/L.

Sodium Deficiency

Hyponatremia occurs when serum sodium falls below 135 mEq/L, or when the ratio of sodium to water falls, because of either excessive sodium loss or excessive fluid retention. Excessive sodium loss may be caused by severe vomiting or profuse sweating in high temperatures; cystic fibrosis; hypothyroidism; adrenal insufficiency (Addison's disease); use of thiazide diuretics; sodium-wasting renal disorders; and

---

Sodium Label Definitions

Sodium free: less than 5 mg per serving

Low sodium: 140 mg or less per serving and, if the serving is 30 g or less or 2 tablespoons or less, per 50 g of the food

Very low sodium: 35 mg or less per serving and, if the serving is 30 g or less or 2 tablespoons or less, per 50 g of the food

Reduced or less sodium: at least 25% less per serving than reference food

To Consume Less Salt and Sodium

- Read the Nutrition Facts Label to determine the amount of sodium in the foods you purchase. The sodium content of processed foods—such as cereals, breads, soups, and salad dressings—often varies widely.

- Choose foods that are lower in sodium and ask your grocer or supermarket to offer more low-sodium foods. Request less salt in your meals when eating out or traveling.

- If you salt foods in cooking or at the table, add small amounts. Learn to use spices and herbs, rather than salt, to enhance the flavor of food.

- When planning meals, consider that fresh and most plain frozen vegetables are low in sodium.

- When selecting canned foods, select those prepared with reduced or no sodium.

- Remember that fresh fish, poultry, and meat are lower in sodium than most canned and processed ones.

- Choose foods that are lower in sodium content. Many frozen dinners, packaged mixes, canned soups, and salad dressings contain a considerable amount of sodium. Remember that condiments such as soy and many other sauces, pickles, and olives are high in sodium. Ketchup and mustard, when eaten in large amounts, can also contribute significant amounts of sodium to the diet. Choose lower-sodium varieties.

- Choose fresh fruits and vegetables as a lower-sodium alternative to salted snack foods.

(Source: USDA, USDHHS, 1995)

excessive diuresis or excessive salt restriction. Excessive fluid retention, as can be seen in congestive heart failure (CHF) and the syndrome of inappropriate antidiuretic hormone (SIADH), causes hyponatremia by dilution. Clinical findings include anorexia, nausea, vomiting, abdominal cramping, headache, and fatigue. Clients who are also dehydrated may experience dizziness, hypotension, and tachycardia; clients who have fluid overload present with edema and elevated blood pressure (Bove, 1996). Worsening hyponatremia can lead to headaches, lethargy, restlessness, irritability, disorientation, confusion, and possibly seizures, stroke, coma, and death.

As with other electrolyte imbalances, treatment begins with identifying and correcting the underlying problem. For mild hyponatremia, oral sodium in the form of salty foods, salty broth, or salt tablets may be given; oral fluid may be restricted. IV administration of a hypertonic solution may be necessary when sodium levels are lower than 110 mEq/L; although this level is rare, it is life-threatening and requires aggressive intervention. Because a rapid rise in serum sodium can damage cells, serum levels should not increase by more than 2 mEq/L per hour (Bove, 1996).

Sodium Excess

Hypernatremia, which is characterized by a serum sodium greater than 148 mEq/L, is an excess of sodium compared to water. It is not likely to occur simply from eating too much sodium: Most people can tolerate a wide range of sodium intakes because the kidneys are able to compensate by excreting more or less sodium in the urine. When hypernatremia does occur, it is most likely related to excessive fluid losses, such as those caused by profuse diarrhea, high fever, and thermal injuries; or, it may be due to inadequate fluid intake, Cushing's syndrome, or diabetes insipidus. Excessive parenteral administration of sodium may also cause hypernatremia.

Signs and symptoms of hypernatremia include fatigue, muscle weakness, restlessness, flushed appearance, and low-grade fever. Confusion, disorientation, lethargy, and seizures may develop. Severe hypernatremia can lead to coma.

The treatment of hypernatremia includes correcting the underlying disorder and diluting serum sodium with water, which can be achieved by providing oral intake or by using IV administration of a hypotonic solution, such as 0.45% sodium chloride, or a sodium-free solution, like 5% dextrose. Dietary sodium may be limited. Treatment should proceed slowly to avoid rapid fluid shifts (Bove, 1996).

Nutrient/Drug Interactions

Drugs that affect sodium are as follows:

- Castor oil: inhibits sodium absorption
- Captopril: may cause hyponatremia
- Colchicine: decreases sodium absorption
- Corticosteroids: cause sodium retention
- Diuretics: increase sodium excretion
- Levodopa: increases urinary sodium excretion
- Neomycin: decreases sodium absorption
- Probenecid: increases urinary excretion of sodium

Potassium

Most of the body's approximately 270 mg of potassium is located inside the cells as the major ICF cation; the remainder is in the ECF, where it serves to maintain fluid balance, maintain acid–base balance, transmit nerve impulses, catalyze metabolic reactions in the body, aid in CHO metabolism and protein synthesis, and control skeletal muscle contractility.

Potassium is widespread in the diet and is especially abundant in unprocessed foods, fruits, many vegetables, and fresh meats. Many salt substitutes contain significant amounts of potassium in place of sodium, which may convey both potential health risks and benefits (see display, Sodium and Potassium Content of Salt Substitutes).

ABSORPTION AND EXCRETION

Potassium is absorbed readily from the small intestine at an efficiency rate of approximately 90%; up to 15% of potassium is excreted through the feces (Perez, 1995b). As with sodium, an excessive intake of potassium does not lead to an increase in serum concentration, because of the action of hormones. Aldosterone increases the urinary excretion of potassium when serum levels rise. Unfortunately, the kidneys cannot conserve potassium as efficiently as sodium, and urinary losses may be 200 to 400 mg/day, even when the body is potassium depleted.

Sodium and Potassium Content of Salt Substitutes

Salt Substitute	mg Na	mg K
	(per teaspoon)	
Morton Lite salt	1100	1500
Morton salt substitute	0	2800
Morton seasoned salt substitute	0	2100
No salt salt alternative	5	2500
No salt salt alternative, seasoned	2	1330
Nu-Salt	0	1
Adolph's Salt substitute	<0.5	2580
Adolph's Seasoned Salt	trace	1750
Mrs. Dash, Original	4	38
Mrs. Dash, Extra Spicy	4	38
Lite, Lite, Lite Papa Dash	360	trace
Papa Dash Salt Lover's Blend	960	trace

RECOMMENDATIONS AND AVERAGE INTAKE

In the 10th Edition of the RDA, an estimated minimum requirement for potassium for healthy adults was set at 2000 mg/day (NRC, 1989). Previously, a daily intake of 1875 to 5625 mg/day for adults was recommended as safe and adequate.

There is no dietary guideline that specifically addresses potassium intake. However, discussion around the guideline to choose a diet that is moderate in salt and sodium includes the advice to consume more fruits and vegetables to increase potassium intake, because potassium may help reduce blood pressure. Foods that provide potassium appear in the display, Some Good Sources of Potassium.

Some Good Sources of Potassium*

- Vegetables and fruits in general, especially potatoes and sweet potatoes
  spinach, swiss chard, broccoli, winter squashes, and parsnips
  dates, bananas, cantaloupes, mangoes, plantains, dried apricots, raisins, prunes, orange juice, and grapefruit juice
  dry beans, peas, lentils

- Milk and yogurt are good sources of potassium and have less sodium than cheese; cheese has much less potassium and usually has added salt.

*Does not include complete list of examples.
(Source: USDA, USDHHS, 1995)

Potassium intake varies widely, depending on actual food selections. Diets that are high in fruits and vegetables may provide as much as 8 to 11 g/day. According to advance data from the Third National Health and Nutrition Examination Survey, mean potassium intake ranges from 2595 to 3451 mg for adult men, and from 2221 to 2547 mg for adult women (CDC, 1994).

CLINICAL APPLICATIONS

Normal serum potassium equals 3.5 to 5.0 mEq/L.

Potassium Deficiency

Hypokalemia develops when serum potassium falls below 3.5 mEq/L. It may occur from prolonged malnutrition and loss of protein tissue; prolonged GI loss related to vomiting, diarrhea, or gastric suctioning; kidney disease; diabetic ketoacidosis; and the use of potassium-wasting diuretics. In addition, volume depletion, which stimulates aldosterone secretion, promotes sodium and water conservation and potassium excretion. Hypokalemia can also be caused by alkalosis: As the body attempts to correct alkalemia by moving hydrogen ions out of cells into the bloodstream, potassium moves from the serum into the cells, resulting in a drop in serum potassium. Because insulin causes potassium to move into skeletal muscle and liver cells, clients who are on continuous insulin infusion or total parenteral nutrition (TPN) (high-glucose solution causes hypersecretion of insulin) may develop hypokalemia.

Because hypokalemia decreases the contractility of smooth, skeletal, and cardiac muscle, clients may complain of leg and generalized body cramps (Perez, 1995b). Other signs and symptoms are weakness, lethargy, anorexia, nausea, confusion, drowsiness, decreased gastric motility, and paralytic ileus. Glucose intolerance may develop. Severe hypokalemia can result in cardiac dysrhythmias, which may be fatal. Symptoms usually do not appear until serum potassium falls below 3.0 mEq/L, although clients taking digoxin may experience cardiac arrhythmias with even mild hypokalemia (Perez, 1995a).

Clients with severe or life-threatening hypokalemia are treated with IV potassium in the clinical setting. Mild hypokalemia is treated with routine potassium supplementation; the oral route is preferred over IV administration because it is slower and thereby allows the kidneys time to help conserve potassium. Oral potassium supplements, which are available in pill and powder form, can cause GI upset and ulcers. To minimize side effects, they should be taken with food or juice.

Potassium Excess

Hyperkalemia is characterized by a serum potassium level greater than 5.0 mEq/L. Clients with renal failure, who are unable to adequately excrete potassium, are at risk, as are clients with severe tissue damage, which causes potassium to leak from damaged cells into the bloodstream. Another cause of hyperkalemia is acidosis: The body tries to raise serum pH by moving hydrogen ions from the bloodstream into cells, with potassium moving in the opposite direction. Because aldosterone promotes potassium excretion, clients with aldosterone deficiency (ie, Addison's Disease) are prone to hyperkalemia. Hyperkalemia is also related to high blood glucose, which draws both water and potassium from the cells into the ECF. Other possible causes of hyperkalemia include excessive potassium supplementation, a too-rapid infusion of intravenous potassium, dehydration, and the use of ACE inhibitors. A false high potassium level, known as **pseudohyperkalemia**, can occur when blood cells in the sample break open and release potassium. This results from trauma that occurs during specimen collection or handling (Perez, 1995b).

Signs and symptoms of hyperkalemia include irritability, anxiety, listlessness, mental confusion, slurred speech, nausea, cramping, diarrhea, GI hyperactivity, muscular weakness, numbness of the extremities, hypotension, and cardiac arrhythmia. Potassium levels near 8 mEq/liter can cause paresthesia and ascending paralysis, which can progress to respiratory arrest. Sometimes the first sign of hyperkalemia is cardiac arrest (Perez, 1995b).

Treatment of hyperkalemia begins with discontinuing potassium replacement or supplementation, if appropriate. Calcium may be given intravenously if serum potassium exceeds 6.5 mEq/liter. This intervention does not lower serum potassium levels but does increase the cellular threshold potential of the heart, thus decreasing the likelihood of arrhythmias. Sodium bicarbonate or insulin may be given to move potassium out of the serum and into the cells. Increased fecal potassium excretion is achieved through the use of a cation exchange resin (eg, sodium polystyrene sulfonate) in sorbitol, which absorbs potassium in exchange for sodium in the large intestine, while sorbitol stimulates diarrhea and potassium excretion. Potassium-wasting diuretics (ie, loop and thiazide-type) may be used to promote urinary losses. Hemodialysis may be necessary for renal failure patients with life-threatening hyperkalemia.

Nutrient/Drug Interactions

Supplements of potassium may

- Cause hyperkalemia when used concurrently with potassium-sparing diuretics
- Cause hyperkalemia when used concurrently with salt substitutes that contain potassium

Increased serum potassium decreases both the toxicity and the effectiveness of digitalis drugs.

Drugs that affect potassium are as follows:

- Adrenal corticosteroids: increase urinary potassium excretion
- *p*-Aminosalicylic acid: can cause hypokalemia
- Amphotericin B: increases urinary potassium excretion
- Capreomycin: decreases serum potassium
- Captopril: causes potassium retention, leading to hyperkalemia
- Colchicine: decreases potassium absorption
- Diuretics (except spironolactone, triamterene): increase urinary excretion of potassium; may cause hypokalemia
- Gentamicin: increases urinary potassium excretion
- Levodopa: increases urinary excretion of potassium

- Neomycin: decreases potassium absorption
- Penicillin: can cause hypokalemia, renal potassium wasting
- Phenolphthalein: causes hypokalemia in laxative abusers
- Probenecid: increases urinary excretion of potassium
- Salicylates: increase urinary excretion of potassium
- Viomycin: can cause hypokalemia; excessive urinary excretion of potassium persists after drug is discontinued

Chloride

Chloride is the primary inorganic anion in the ECF; a relatively large amount is found as an essential component of hydrochloric acid (HCl) in the stomach. It also plays a role in maintaining acid–base balance, and in promoting the exchange of oxygen and carbon dioxide from hemoglobin in red blood cells. Its concentration in most cells is low.

Almost all the chloride in the diet comes from salt (sodium chloride); therefore, rich sources of sodium are also rich sources of chloride.

ABSORPTION AND EXCRETION

Chloride is almost completely absorbed in the small intestine; the kidneys excrete chloride that is absorbed in excess of need. Diarrhea and vomiting increase chloride losses.

RECOMMENDATIONS AND AVERAGE INTAKE

An RDA for chloride has not been established. Because both the sources of chloride and its normal losses from the body correspond to those of sodium, the estimated minimum requirements that are listed for all age and sex groups except infants are equal to those of sodium on a milliequivalent basis. For healthy adults, the estimated minimum requirement of 750 mg/day is easily exceeded because of the amount of salt consumed in the average American diet. It is estimated that added salt provides approximately 6000 mg of chloride daily (NRC, 1989).

CLINICAL APPLICATIONS

Normal serum chloride is 95 to 106 mEq/L.

Chloride Deficiency

Because sodium and chloride travel together, hypochloremia (serum chloride less than 95 mEq/liter) often occurs during hyponatremia. Prolonged vomiting, diarrhea, dehydration, chronic respiratory acidosis, gastric suctioning, the long-term use of certain diuretics (thiazides), fistula and tube drainage, cystic fibrosis, and excessive perspiration may lead to hypochloremia. Clinical findings include muscle spasms, twitching, and tetany, in addition to symptoms of hyponatremia. Depressed respirations and hypoventilation can progress to respiratory arrest (Bove, 1996).

Hypochloremia that is accompanied by hyponatremia is treated by limiting fluid intake and replacing lost electrolytes. Hypochloremia that occurs without hyponatremia may be treated with ammonium or potassium chloride rather than sodium chloride to avoid hypernatremia.

Chloride Excess

The only known cause of hyperchloremia (serum chloride greater than 106 mEq/L), which usually occurs with hypernatremia, is water-deficiency dehydration. Signs and symptoms are similar to those of hypernatremia, only they are more severe. Treatment for hyperchloremia is the same as for hypernatremia.

Nutrient/Drug Interactions

Drug that affects chloride:

* Probenecid: increases urinary excretion of chloride

ACID–BASE BALANCE

Acids are substances that donate hydrogen ions (H+) to neutralize bases; bases are H+ acceptors that neutralize acids. Acid–base balance refers to maintenance of the body's concentration of H+. Most of the body's hydrogen ion concentration is produced through the metabolism of food: The oxidation of CHO, protein, and fat for energy yields carbon dioxide and water, which combine to form carbonic acid, the most abundant acid in the body.

pH

The degree of acidity of a solution, or the concentration of hydrogen ions, is expressed in terms of pH, which ranges from 0 to 14. Normal blood pH is maintained between 7.35 and 7.45; other body fluids vary in pH from 1.2 to 8.6 (Fig. 6-3). A pH of 7 indicates that the solution is neutral, that is, it contains an equal number of hydrogen and hydroxide ions.

A pH lower than 7 indicates that the solution is acidic; the lower the number, the more acidic the solution. Acidic solutions have more hydrogen ions than hydroxide ions. Alkaline solutions have a pH greater than 7; the higher the number, the more alkaline the solution and the fewer the number of hydrogen ions.

Buffer systems, respirations, and the kidneys help regulate normal pH.

Buffer Systems

Buffers are substances that prevent drastic changes in pH by accepting or donating hydrogen ions to neutralize acids or bases. Most of the body's buffer systems are composed of a weak acid and a weak base, which can weaken strong acids and bases within a fraction of a second. There are three major buffer systems in the body.

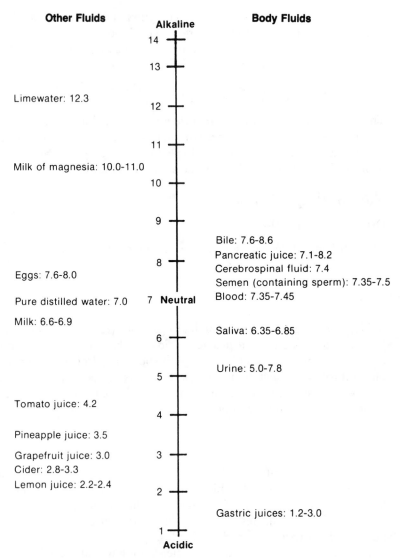

Figure 6-3
The pH of various body fluids and other fluids.

The carbonic acid–bicarbonate system functions to regulate the pH of blood. Carbonic acid (a weak acid) buffers strong bases like sodium hydroxide, and sodium bicarbonate (a weak base) buffers strong acids like hydrochloric acid.

The phosphate buffer system acts to regulate the pH of red blood cells and the kidney tubular fluids. Dihydrogen phosphate (a weak acid) buffers strong bases like sodium hydroxide, and monohydrogen phosphate (a weak base) buffers strong acids like hydrochloric acid.

The pH of body cells and plasma is regulated by the protein system. Amino acids are amphoteric—that is, they can act as either acids or bases because they have at least one carboxyl group that acts like an acid to buffer bases, and at least one amine group that acts like a base to buffer acids.

Respirations

The pH of body fluids can be changed within a matter of minutes by adjusting the rate of breathing. Carbonic acid, the most abundant acid produced by metabolic activity, is converted to carbon dioxide and is exhaled through the lungs. Changes in the carbon dioxide content of the blood can cause a change in the rate of breathing; likewise, a change in the rate of breathing causes a change in blood pH. For instance, a decrease in blood CO_2 causes an increase in pH. As a compensatory mechanism, breathing rate slows to retain CO_2 and lower pH. Conversely, an increase in blood CO_2 that is followed by a decrease in pH stimulates an increase in breathing rate so that CO_2 exhalation is increased and pH is ultimately increased.

The Kidneys

Although it may take as long as several hours to a few days, the kidneys are the most potent regulators of pH because of their ability to excrete hydrogen ions in the form of ammonium ions, weak acids, and small quantities of free hydrogen ions. The kidneys also regulate the excretion of electrolytes and bicarbonate. A decrease in the pH of body fluids (becomes more acidic) causes the kidneys to excrete more hydrogen ions. When the pH of body fluids increases (becomes more alkaline), the kidneys excrete more bicarbonate and retain hydrogen ions to lower pH.

ACID–BASE IMBALANCE

Acidosis

Acidosis is a condition that occurs when the hydrogen ion concentration of the blood increases, resulting in a pH of 7.35 to 6.8. Respiratory acidosis is caused by a decrease in respirations, which leads to an increase in the CO_2 content of the blood. Emphysema, pulmonary edema, pneumonia, and asphyxia can cause respiratory acidosis. Metabolic acidosis is caused by an increase in metabolic acids, like ketones or lactic acid, accompanied by a decrease in bicarbonate. It may be caused by diarrhea, lactic acidosis, uremia, diabetic ketoacidosis, shock, or starvation. Renal tubular disorders that cause an increase in the excretion of bicarbonate ions can also lead to metabolic acidosis.

Signs and symptoms of metabolic acidosis include anorexia, nausea, vomiting, headache, lethargy, drowsiness, abdominal pain, and weakness. Acute respiratory acidosis can cause behavioral changes, tremors, muscle twitching, headache, weakness, and paralysis. Acidosis depresses the central nervous system (CNS), which may result in confusion, coma, and death.

Treatment involves correcting the underlying disorder and replenishing fluid and electrolytes, as appropriate. Bicarbonate may be given for metabolic acidosis.

Alkalosis

Alkalosis, which is characterized by a pH of 7.45 to 7.8, occurs when the hydrogen ion concentration of the blood is abnormally low and bicarbonate is high. Respiratory alkalosis is caused by hyperventilation, which decreases the concentration of CO_2 in the blood. Salicylate poisoning, acute anxiety, fevers, infections, and high altitudes can cause respiratory alkalosis. Metabolic alkalosis occurs when the hydrogen ion concentration decreases in response to an increase in bicarbonate. Vomiting, which causes the loss of hydrogen ions in hydrochloric acid, as well as potassium depletion and the excessive use of alkaline drugs can cause metabolic alkalosis.

Nervousness, muscle spasms, and convulsions may develop as the nerves of both the CNS and the peripheral nervous system become overexcited and conduct impulses in the absence of stimulation. Other symptoms include anorexia, nausea, vomiting, sweating, and dry mouth.

Treatment of metabolic alkalosis involves correcting the underlying disorder. Potassium may be given if hypokalemia exists; clients with fluid volume deficit may be given sodium chloride. Treatment of respiratory alkalosis is aimed at correcting hyperventilation.

ACID AND BASE FORMERS

Because minerals are not broken down during metabolism, they leave an acid or alkaline ash in the body depending on their chemical composition. Calcium, sodium, potassium, and magnesium are bases; foods that contain large amounts of these cations are said to be alkaline-forming or alkaline-producing (see Ch. 19 display, Acid-Forming, Base-Forming, and Neutral Foods). Foods that contain predominantly chloride, sulfur, and phosphorus are acid-formers (see Ch. 19 display, Acid-Forming, Base-Forming, and Neutral Foods). Because they contain no minerals and, therefore, do not leave an ash, pure fats and pure CHO are considered neutral foods.

Even if the diet contains predominantly acid-forming or alkaline-forming foods, the pH of the blood is maintained by renal excretion of electrolytes. For instance, the higher the intake of sodium or potassium, the higher the quantity of these electrolytes in the urine. Although it is possible to treat renal stones by manipulating the diet to alter urinary pH, drug therapy is a much more effective and consistent method of treatment (see Chapter 19)

KEY CONCEPTS

- Because it is involved in almost every body function, is not stored, and is excreted daily, water is more vital to life than food.
- Under normal conditions, water intake equals water output to maintain water balance. In most healthy people, thirst is a reliable indicator of need.
- The body's need for water is influenced by many variables; to account for individual differences, 1.5 cc/cal is often recommended.

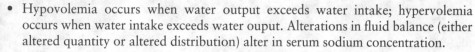

- Hypovolemia occurs when water output exceeds water intake; hypervolemia occurs when water intake exceeds water ouput. Alterations in fluid balance (either altered quantity or altered distribution) alter in serum sodium concentration.

- Electrolytes carry electrical charges when they are dissolved in solution. Cations, like sodium and potassium, are positively charged ions; anions, like chloride, are negatively charged.

- As much as 75% of the sodium consumed in the average American diet is from processed food. Americans are urged to reduce their intake of sodium because of its potential role in the development of hypertension.

- Normally, an intake greater than need of either sodium or potassium does not lead to a high serum level; rather, the excess is excreted in the urine.

- Potassium is widespread in the diet. Most people consume more than is required, but this is not deleterious.

- Normal pH is maintained through the action of buffer systems, respirations, and the kidneys.

REFERENCES

Bove, L. (1996). Restoring electrolyte balance. Sodium and chloride. RN, 59(1), 25–28.

Centers for Disease Control and Prevention (1994). Advance data. Dietary intake of vitamins, minerals, and fiber of persons ages 2 months and over in the United States: Third National Health and Nutrition Examination Survey, Phase 1, 1989–1991. DHHS Publication No. (PHS) 95-1250.

Cirolia, B. (1996). Understanding edema. Nursing 95, 26(2), 66–70.

National Research Council (1989). Recommended Dietary Allowances. 10th ed. Washington, DC: National Academy Press.

Perez, A. (1995a). Restoring electrolyte balance. Hypokalemia. RN, 58(12), 33–35.

Perez, A. (1995b). Electrolytes. Restoring the balance. Hyperkalemia. RN, 58(11), 32–36.

Public Health Service, United States Department of Health and Human Services (1988). The Surgeon General's Report on Nutrition and Health: Summary and Recommendations. DHHS (PHS) Publication No. 88-50211. Washington, DC: Government Printing Office.

Scherer, J. and Timby, B. (1995). Introductory Medical-Surgical Nursing. 6th ed. Philadelphia: JB Lippincott Company.

United States Department of Agriculture, United States Department of Health and Human Services (1995). Nutrition and Your Health: Dietary Guidelines for Americans. 4th ed. Home and Garden Bulletin No. 232.

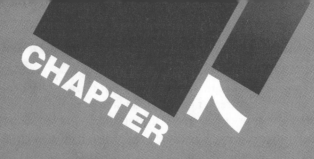

CHAPTER 7

Digestion, Absorption, and Metabolism

Chapter Outline

Key Terms

Acetyl molecules/acetyl
  Co-A
ATP/adenosine triphos-
  phate
Anabolism
Beta oxidation
Brush border
Catabolism
Chyme

Deamination
Electron transport chain
Gluconeogenesis
Glycogenesis
Glycogenolysis
Glycolysis
Ketogenesis
Ketone bodies
Lipogenesis

Microvilli
Oxidation
Pyruvate
TCA (tricarboxylic acid)
  cycle
Transamination
Villi

All foods are composed of water and solid matter, which includes carbohydrates, protein, fat, vitamins, and minerals. The varying proportions and combinations of these components are what determines a food's nutritional value and physical characteristics. Despite the differences in how foods may taste, smell, feel, and appear, their complex molecules are all reduced to common, basic units before being absorbed.

Digestion is the process by which the body breaks down complex molecules of carbohydrates, protein, and fat, into smaller, simpler units that can be absorbed. The physical breakdown and mixing of food that occurs through chewing and involuntary muscular activity along the GI tract is known as mechanical digestion. Chemical digestion occurs as food is mixed with secretions from the mouth, stomach, small intestine, liver, and pancreas. **Hydrolysis** is an example of chemical digestion that uses water to split large water-soluble molecules into smaller ones that can be used by the cells.

Absorption is the process by which nutrients pass through the GI mucosa into the blood (water-soluble nutrients) or lymph (fat-soluble nutrients). The small intestine is the primary site of absorption for the end-products of carbohydrate, protein, and fat digestion, and for most vitamins, minerals, and drugs. Electrolytes and more water are absorbed primarily from the colon. Alcohol is absorbed through the stomach and small intestine. Normally, 95% of ingested CHO, protein, and fat is absorbed.

The actual movement of substances across the mucosal membrane occurs through either passive diffusion (movement of a substance from an area of high concentration to one of lower concentration) or active transport (energy-dependent movement from an area of low concentration to one of higher concentration). Osmosis, the passage of water through a semipermeable membrane to equalize the osmotic pressure exerted by ions in solution, is the process by which water is absorbed.

The entire process of digestion and absorption generally takes 24 hours. Although motility is affected by numerous variables, including actual food and fluid intake, activity and muscle tone, emotional factors, certain drug therapies, and GI integrity, it is controlled primarily by the action of nerves and hormones.

Metabolism is a broad term that is defined as the sum total of all chemical reactions that occur in living cells. Energy metabolism involves the changes that occur as body cells extract and use energy from nutrients. It is a continuous process of two opposite actions: *anabolism*, the building up or synthesizing of new substances, and *catabolism*, the breaking down of substances into smaller units.

THE DIGESTIVE SYSTEM

The digestive system is composed of a continuous musculomembranous tubular structure called the gastrointestinal tract (alimentary canal) that begins at the mouth and ends at the anus (Fig. 7-1). The structure of the GI wall is consistent along the tube's entire length; the structure of the small intestine is depicted in Figure 7-2. Arbitrarily, the mouth, esophagus, stomach, duodenum, and jejunum are known as the upper GI tract; the ileum, large intestine (cecum, colon, and rectum), and anus make up the lower GI tract. The salivary glands, liver, pancreas, and gallbladder are accessory organs.

Mechanical Digestion

Mechanical digestion occurs as muscles of the GI tract contract and relax to push and mix the GI contents. The GI tract's muscular layer is composed of longitudinal (long) muscles on the outside surface and circular muscles that surround the tube

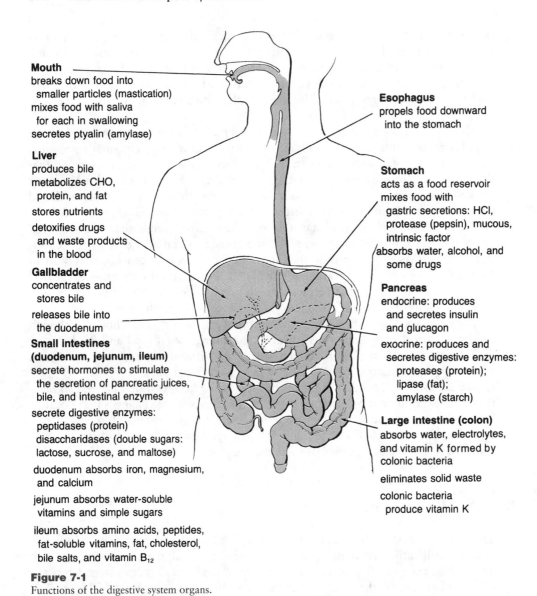

Mouth
breaks down food into
  smaller particles (mastication)
mixes food with saliva
  for each in swallowing
secretes ptyalin (amylase)

Liver
produces bile
metabolizes CHO,
  protein, and fat
stores nutrients
detoxifies drugs
  and waste products
  in the blood

Gallbladder
concentrates and
  stores bile
releases bile into
  the duodenum

**Small intestines
(duodenum, jejunum, ileum)**
secrete hormones to stimulate
  the secretion of pancreatic juices,
  bile, and intestinal enzymes

secrete digestive enzymes:
  peptidases (protein)
  disaccharidases (double sugars:
  lactose, sucrose, and maltose)

duodenum absorbs iron, magnesium,
  and calcium

jejunum absorbs water-soluble
  vitamins and simple sugars

ileum absorbs amino acids, peptides,
  fat-soluble vitamins, fat, cholesterol,
  bile salts, and vitamin B_{12}

Esophagus
propels food downward
  into the stomach

Stomach
acts as a food reservoir
mixes food with
  gastric secretions: HCl,
  protease (pepsin), mucous,
  intrinsic factor
absorbs water, alcohol, and
  some drugs

Pancreas
endocrine: produces
  and secretes insulin
  and glucagon

exocrine: produces and
  secretes digestive enzymes:
    proteases (protein);
    lipase (fat);
    amylase (starch)

Large intestine (colon)
absorbs water, electrolytes,
and vitamin K formed by
colonic bacteria

eliminates solid waste

colonic bacteria
  produce vitamin K

Figure 7-1
Functions of the digestive system organs.

(Fig. 7-3). Contraction of long muscles propels matter forward by a rhythmic, wave-like movement known as peristalsis. Peristaltic contractions occur continuously, regardless of whether food is present. Peristalsis is strongest in the esophagus, and weakest in the small intestine.

Circular muscles control the diameter of the tube by contracting and relaxing. Segmentation is a localized contraction in the small intestine that occurs as circular muscles periodically squeeze to constrict the diameter of the tube (Fig. 7-4). This

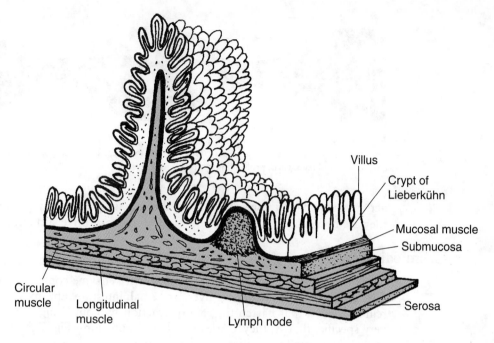

Figure 7-2
Diagram of the intestinal villi and columnar epithelial cells.

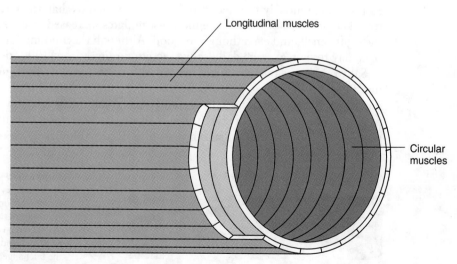

Figure 7-3
Longitudinal and circular muscles of GI wall.

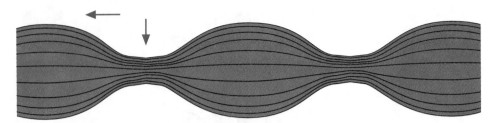

Figure 7-4
Segmentation of the small intestine. As circular muscles squeeze to constrict the diameter of the tube, chyme is forced backward, prolonging contact with digestive juices.

action forces the GI contents backward a few inches, thereby prolonging the time they are in contact with digestive juices and the absorptive surface.

Chemical Digestion

Chemical digestion occurs as food is mixed with enzyme-containing secretions from the mouth, stomach, pancreas, liver, and small intestine. Enzymes are complex protein molecules that hasten the rate of reaction without being consumed. They are very specific; that is, they work on only one substrate (Fig. 7-5). Because they are reused, only small quantities of enzymes are needed.

A large amount of fluid is pumped into the GI tract to facilitate digestion. Normal adults secrete about 6 to 10 liters of fluid into the GI tract daily, in addition to the 1 to 2 liters that are normally consumed. Usually, all but 10% is reabsorbed (Shils et al, 1994).

SALIVA

Saliva is continuously secreted into the mouth by glands that are under nervous control. The presence of food in the mouth stimulates increased saliva secretion, as can the sight, smell, and even thought of food. Although the amount varies considerably from day to day, average daily saliva secretion ranges from 1000 to 1500 ml.

Saliva moistens mucous membranes and food to promote chewing and swallowing. By dissolving food, saliva enhances the sense of taste and facilitates chemical digestion. It also contains salivary amylase (ptyalin), an enzyme that begins the process of breaking down starch into maltose. Because food is usually held in the mouth only briefly, limited starch digestion occurs. However, swallowed amylase

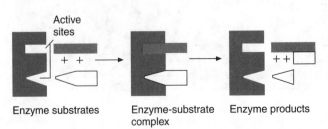

Active sites

Enzyme substrates   Enzyme-substrate complex   Enzyme products

Figure 7-5
Lock-and-key mechanism of enzyme action. Like keys, substrates fit in the active sites of the enzyme. Following the reaction, the products separate and the unchanged enzyme is available to catalyze production of additional products.

Table 7-1
Components of Saliva

Component	Function
Water (99.5%)	Dissolves food; provides medium for digestive reactions
Solutes (.5%):	
Amylase	Begins hydrolysis of starch into maltose
Lingual lipase	Has a limited role in beginning fat digestion
Chlorides	Activate salivary amylase
Bicarbonates and phosphates	Buffer chemicals; help keep saliva pH between 6.35 and 6.85
Urea and uric acid	Body wastes excreted by salivary glands
Mucin	Forms mucus when dissolved in water; mucus lubricates food to promote swallowing
Lysozyme	Destroys bacteria to protect mucous membrane from infection and teeth from decay

may continue to work for another 15 to 30 minutes in the stomach until it is inactivated by gastric acids. The components of saliva are listed in Table 7-1.

GASTRIC JUICE

Among other substances (Table 7-2), gastric juice contains hydrochloric acid, which is responsible for the very low stomach pH of about 2. The acid environment has many advantages, including activating gastric enzymes, killing most food bacteria, and promoting the absorption of calcium and iron.

Chemically, the primary function of the stomach is to begin breaking down protein into smaller peptide molecules through the action of the enzyme pepsin. Pepsin is first secreted in its inactive form pepsinogen; it is converted to pepsin in the presence of HCl. To help protect the stomach lining from being digested, activated pepsin stimulates the secretion of mucus, which coats and protects the mucosa.

PANCREATIC, LIVER, AND INTESTINAL SECRETIONS

The small intestine is the primary site of chemical digestion of all three energy nutrients (CHO, protein, fat) (Fig. 7-6).

Table 7-2
Components of Gastric Juice

Component	Function
Hydrochloric acid	Activates pepsin from pepsinogen; destroys most food bacteria; promotes calcium and iron absorption
Pepsinogen	Inactive form of pepsin; pepsin hydrolyzes proteins into polypeptides
Gastric lipase	Limited role; splits butterfat molecules found in milk
Mucus	Acts as a barrier to protect stomach wall from digestion
Intrinsic factor	Facilitates the absorption of vitamin B_{12}

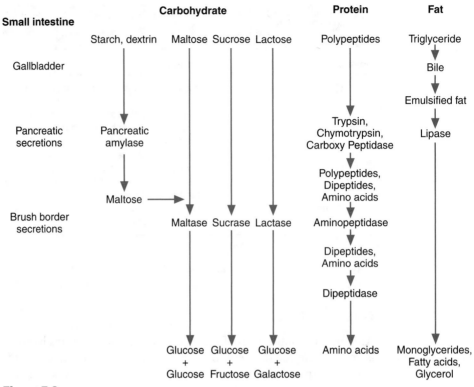

Figure 7-6
Chemical digestion within the small intestine.

Pancreatic secretions, which contain enzymes, bicarbonate, and electrolytes, are delivered into the duodenum through a duct. Pancreatic enzymes (amylases, proteases, and lipases) are responsible for the digestion of carbohydrates, protein, and fat, respectively. Sodium bicarbonate and fluid transform acidic chyme to a neutral or slightly alkaline semiliquid.

Bile, which is made in the liver and concentrated and stored in the gallbladder, passes through the common bile duct to reach the duodenum. Its secretion is stimulated by fat in the duodenum; bile is not an enzyme, but an emulsifier that promotes fat digestion by suspending fat particles in solution, thereby increasing the surface area on which lipases can work.

The lining of the small intestine has hundreds of folds covered with **villi**, which are fingerlike projections into the intestinal lumen (Fig. 7-7). Each villus is covered with a layer of epithelial cells that are coated with projections called **microvilli**; these microvilli greatly increase the surface area of the small intestine. The microvilli collectively form what is known as the **brush border**, which contains both digestive enzymes and cells that absorb nutrients.

Digestion and Absorption: Putting It All Together

Normally, food enters the GI tract by way of the mouth, also known as the oral or buccal cavity. The process of mechanical digestion begins in the mouth as the teeth

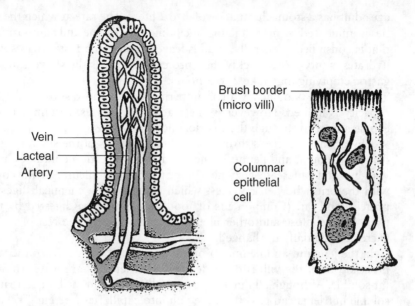

Brush border
(micro villi)

Vein

Lacteal

Artery

Columnar
epithelial
cell

Figure 7-7
Villi and microvilli.

and tongue work to reduce food to a soft, pliable mass. Swallowed food, called bolus, is directed into the esophagus (and away from the trachea) by closure of the epiglottis.

In the esophagus, food is aided downward by peristalsis and gravity. Very soft foods and liquids may reach the stomach in about 1 second; solid or semisolid food may take 4 to 8 seconds. No chemical digestion or absorption occurs in the esophagus.

At both ends of the esophagus, circular muscles called sphincters control the passage of food. The upper esophageal sphincter relaxes (opens) during swallowing to allow food to pass from the laryngopharnyx into the esophagus. The lower esophageal sphincter relaxes to allow food to pass from the esophagus into the stomach. Both sphincters contract (close) to prevent the backflow of food.

As food enters the upper portion of the stomach (cardia), gentle churning and mixing with gastric secretions transforms it into a semiliquid paste called **chyme**. Chyme may remain in the fundus for an hour or more, during which time muscular activity is slight, but salivary amylase can continue digesting starch. Vigorous churning occurs when chyme enters the body of the stomach. Chyme must pass through the pyloric sphincter to enter the duodenum, and it does so in very small amounts so as not to overwhelm the small intestine. As "gatekeeper" for the duodenum, the pyloric sphincter normally remains almost, but not quite, completely closed. Wavelike forward and backward "splashing" of GI contents helps force chyme through the sphincter, but some backflow does occur. This continued churning accounts for most of the mixing of the GI contents.

The position and size of the stomach change continuously: The stomach seemingly "shrinks" when empty, but stretches to accommodate a large meal. The average adult has a stomach capacity of 1 to 2 liters. The rate at which the stomach empties is influenced by many factors, including the volume and composition of the food that is consumed. Generally, liquids leave the stomach faster than solids do, carbohydrates empty more quickly than protein, and fat is the slowest mover. Complete gastric emptying may take 2 to 6 hours.

Because the stomach wall is impermeable to most substances, its absorptive capacity is limited. However, some water, electrolytes, certain drugs, and alcohol can be absorbed through the gastric mucosa.

Chyme then proceeds through the three portions of the small intestine: the duodenum, jejunum, and ileum. In the duodenum, digestion continues as chyme mixes with bile and pancreatic enzymes. In the jejunum and ileum, chyme comes in contact with the brush border enzymes, which complete the chemical digestion of CHO, protein, and fat. (Components of food that cannot be digested by the human GI tract, like cellulose and other fibers, continue through the rest of the tract and are excreted essentially unchanged.)

In the jejunum and ileum, absorbable nutrients enter cells of the villi. How they proceed out of the villi is dependent on whether they are water (blood)-soluble or fat-soluble. Although all nutrients eventually end up in the bloodstream, only water-soluble nutrients can pass from the villi into capillaries (see Fig. 7-7) and then enter portal circulation. This is the route taken by monosaccharides, amino acids, glycerol, water-soluble vitamins, minerals, short-chain fatty acids, and medium-chain fatty acids. Long-chain fatty acids, once inside the villi, are further digested into glycerol and fatty acids; then, they are recombined to form triglycerides. The re-formed triglycerides, along with vitamins A, D, E, and K, and cholesterol, leave the villi as chylomicrons by way of the lymphatic system, traveling into the thoracic duct, through the subclavian veins, to the liver.

Unabsorbed material exits the small intestine through the ileocecal valve and enters the large intestine, which is composed of the cecum, colon, rectum, and anal canal. Electrolytes and large amounts of water are absorbed in the colon. Colonic microflora synthesize significant amounts of vitamin K, and smaller amounts of vitamin B_{12}, biotin, thiamine, and riboflavin. The semisolid waste that remains after absorption is completed is made of water, food residues, microorganisms, digestive secretions, and mucus. Feces is held in the rectum by muscular action until the anal sphincter opens to allow voluntary evacuation. Figure 7-8 depicts the site of nutrient absorption.

ENERGY METABOLISM

Energy metabolism refers to how the body obtains and uses energy from the energy-yielding nutrients after they are absorbed—glucose from carbohydrate digestion, glycerol and fatty acids from fat digestion, and amino acids from protein digestion (Fig. 7-9). It is a continuous process that includes energy-using reactions that build (**anabolism**) and energy-producing reactions that break down (**catabolism**). Many enzymes and cofactors, which are derived from vitamins and minerals, are necessary for these reactions. The liver plays a central part in numerous metabolic reactions, some of which are listed in the display, Some Metabolic Functions of the Liver. In a healthy adult, the rate of catabolism equals the rate of anabolism.

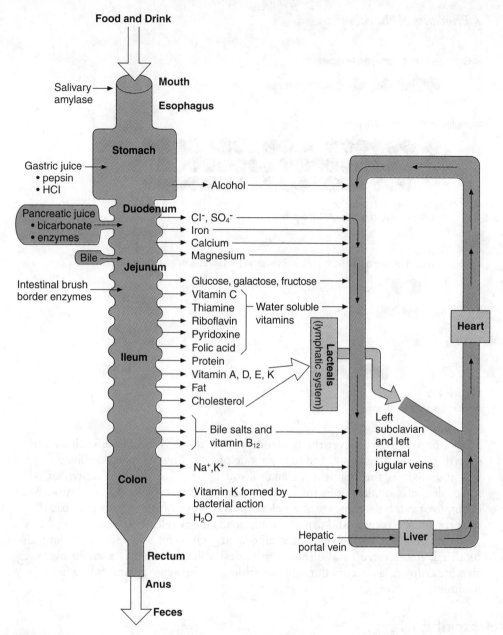

Figure 7-8
Sites of secretion and absorption in the gastrointestinal tract.

Anabolism is the building or synthesizing of more complex compounds from smaller molecules. It uses energy that is derived from catabolic reactions. Examples of anabolic reactions include glycogen synthesis from glucose, triglyceride synthesis from glycerol and fatty acids, and protein synthesis from amino acids. Anabolism occurs continuously in all people as cells or substances are replaced after normal wear and tear, and as excess nutrients are reassembled and stored for later use. Accelerated

a. Glucose from carbohydrate digestion

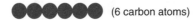 (6 carbon atoms)

b. Triglycerides from fat digestion

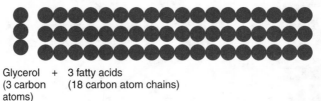

Glycerol   +   3 fatty acids
(3 carbon   (18 carbon atom chains)
atoms)

c. Three types of amino acids from protein digestion (with nitrogen already removed)

1. ●● (2 carbon atoms)

2. ●●● (3 carbon atoms)

3. (6 carbon atoms)

Figure 7-9
Basic units after digestion.

anabolism occurs whenever the demand for new tissue is increased, such as during growth periods, pregnancy, and the anabolic phase following injury or illness.

Catabolism is the opposite of anabolism: It refers to the breakdown of large molecules into smaller ones for the purpose of releasing energy. **Oxidation** is an example of catabolism in which an electron is removed from a molecule, usually in the presence of oxygen, and usually resulting in energy release. Glucose is the body's preferred fuel for oxidation, but amino acids, glycerol, and fatty acids are also oxidized. Accelerated catabolism is an undesirable state that is marked by excessive breakdown, as occurs during starvation and the acute period following injury or illness.

The Release of Energy

In order for cells to "work"—their roles include transporting ions, generating heat, synthesizing chemical compounds, and contracting muscles—they need energy. Their instant supply of energy is stored in a compound that is available in all cells and is known as **ATP (adenosine triphosphate)**. Chemically, ATP contains a purine (adenine), a sugar (ribose), and three phosphate molecules. When energy is needed, ATP is hydrolyzed, that is, a phosphate group is removed and energy is released, thereby forming the new lower-energy compound ADP (adenosine diphosphate). (An even lower-energy molecule is AMP [adenosine monophosphate], which forms when two phosphate groups are removed from ATP, or when one phosphate group

Some Metabolic Functions of the Liver

CARBOHYDRATE METABOLISM

Converts fructose and galactose to glucose

Makes, stores, and breaks down glycogen

Makes glucose from glycerol and some amino acids (gluconeogenesis)

FAT METABOLISM

Makes bile that emulsifies fat in the small intestine

Converts excess glucose, glycerol, fatty acids, and amino acids to triglycerides (lipogenesis)

Catabolizes triglycerides when needed (lipolysis)

Synthesizes and catabolizes phospholipids and cholesterol

Makes lipoproteins for the transport of fats through the blood

Makes ketone bodies (ketogenesis)

PROTEIN METABOLISM

Makes nonessential amino acids

Deaminates excess amino acids

Synthesizes urea from ammonia

Provides only site of albumin and fibrinogen synthesis. Makes other plasma proteins, such as heparin, prothrombin, and antibodies

OTHER

Stores fat-soluble vitamins, copper, and iron

Plays a role in the activation of vitamin D

Detoxifies alcohol, drugs, and poisons. Accumulates poisons that cannot be detoxified and excreted (eg, DDT)

Digests worn out red and white blood cells

is removed from ADP.) Of the energy that is released by these reactions, half or more is lost through heat; this is why metabolism raises temperature. If necessary (ie, to maintain body temperature), ATP can release all of its energy as heat. In muscle cells, creatine phosphate (CP) also provides a limited supply of immediate energy.

ATP is generated through the catabolism of all the energy-yielding nutrients. The **TCA cycle** (**tricarboxylic acid cycle**), or Krebs' cycle, is a complex series of aerobic (oxygen-requiring) reactions during which two-carbon compounds (**acetyl molecules**) are oxidized to produce energy and carbon dioxide. Acetyl molecules are formed directly through the breakdown of fatty acids and some amino acids, and indirectly from **pyruvate**, an intermediate that is formed during the breakdown of glucose, glycerol, and other amino acids. Thus, all energy-yielding nutrients enter the TCA cycle, although not all by the same route.

The final step in the release of energy is the **electron transport chain** (also known as oxidative phosphorylation), which is also dependent on oxygen. Through a complex series of oxidation and reduction reactions, energy that is produced by the TCA cycle is released and stored in ATP, where it is readily available for cellular use.

Glucose Catabolism

Absorbed monosaccharides, which are six carbon molecules, are transported to the liver, where fructose and galactose are converted to glucose. The complete oxidation of glucose, also known as cellular respiration, occurs in every cell in the body and is the body's major source of energy.

Glucose catabolism begins with the anaerobic process of **glycolysis** (glucose splitting), in which glucose is partially broken down into 2 molecules, each with 3 carbons. Glycolysis produces 2 molecules of ATP, about 8% of the total energy available from glucose (Berne and Levy, 1993). As illustrated in Figure 7-10, two pyruvate molecules (regardless of their original source) can be put back together to remake a glucose molecule, although the process isn't exactly reversible (other enzymes are needed). Glycolysis can provide the sole source of energy only briefly because the supply of glucose is limited, and because accumulated pyruvate is converted to lactate (lactic acid), which is ultimately deleterious. (See display, Food for Thought: Why Not to "Go for the Burn.")

If the cell needs more energy and oxygen is available, catabolism continues as a carbon splits off from pyruvate, leaving the two-carbon compound acetate. Notice in Figure 7-10 that this reaction is irreversible: Two-carbon compounds cannot be remade into glucose. The freed carbon atom joins with oxygen from water molecules to form carbon dioxide, which is released into the blood and eventually exhaled through the lungs. The acetate molecule combines with Co-A, an important enzyme in acetylation reactions, to become acetyl Co-A. Acetyl Co-A enters the TCA cycle where it is split into carbon dioxide and two more molecules of ATP.

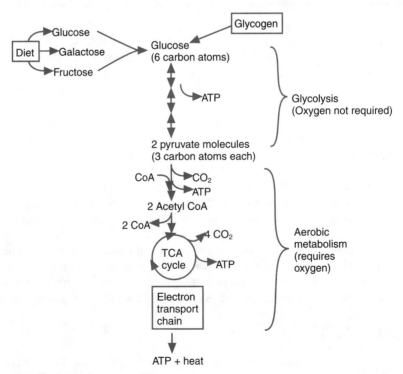

Figure 7-10
Complete oxidation of glucose.

FOOD for THOUGHT

Why Not to "Go for the Burn"

The energy metabolism discussed in this Chapter was primarily aerobic—that is, it is the means by which the body processes its fuel when adequate oxygen is available. However, sometimes oxygen isn't available, at least not quickly enough or in large enough supply, as in the case of intense or prolonged exercise. What happens then is anaerobic metabolism (glycolysis), the body's attempt to keep things moving when you can't "catch your breath."

Muscle cells' immediate fuel when activity begins is the energy trapped in ATP, of which every cell has a small supply. You'll remember that half or more of the energy released is lost as heat; thus exercise has an immediate warming effect. Muscle cells also utilize creatine phosphate, a high-energy compound, to augment the supply of ATP. Neither ATP nor creatine phosphate is dependent on the availability of oxygen. However, the supply of creatine phosphate is tiny, so if the activity lasts longer than 10 to 20 seconds, another source of fuel is needed.

Coming to the rescue is liver glycogen, which is broken down to release glucose into the blood. Muscle cells pick up this glucose and use it along with their own private supply of glycogen to generate energy through anaerobic glycolysis during the first 1 to 3 minutes of activity.

Which fuels are used next depends on the intensity and duration of the exercise. Low-intensity exercise, like leisurely walking, ballroom dancing, or any exercise that does not "take your breath away," is fueled aerobically, using about 90% fat, 10% glucose. Moderate exercise, like jogging, running, and swimming, is fueled with a mix of fat and carbohydrate, with the predominant fuel shifting during training toward fat to conserve glycogen. People exercising for weight control do so to lose fat, not glycogen, so this is a desirable use of fuel.

To extract all the available energy from glycogen and fat, adequate oxygen is required—oxygen that is obtained through deep regular breathing. During moderate aerobic exercise, a trained heart and circulatory system can adequately meet the muscles' demand for oxygen. However, when conditioning is less than optimal, or when activity is intense and/or prolonged, the heart and lungs cannot supply adequate oxygen quickly enough to maintain aerobic metabolism. When this occurs, muscles switch from using fat to only glucose, because it can be metabolized anaerobically, albeit incompletely. Fat can be broken down for energy only when oxygen is present; in fact, more oxygen is needed to catabolize fat than glucose.

In anaerobic metabolism, glucose is broken down into pyruvate, but pyruvate catabolism cannot continue. Instead, pyruvate accumulates, which stimulates the heart and lungs to work harder. If there is a break in the action, the increase in breathing (and therefore oxygen) will allow the body to switch back to aerobic metabolism and catabolize pyruvate through the TCA cycle (aerobically). Without adequate oxygen, the accumulated pyruvate is transformed into lactic acid, which accumulates until adequate oxygen becomes available. The body can quickly alternate between aerobic and anaerobic metabolism as the supply of oxygen changes.

The accumulation of lactic acid is deleterious: It is responsible for the burning-type pain in muscles, and can quickly lead to muscle exhaustion if it is not carried away by the blood. To avoid problems with lactic acid accumulation, rest periodically and breathe deeply. And, even more importantly, make a point of doing aerobic exercise regularly, for at least 20 to 30 minutes, three times per week. Regular aerobic exercise improves heart and lung capacity, which increases oxygen delivery to muscle cells. It also stimulates muscle cells to produce more structures within the cell in which aerobic metabolism takes place (mitochondria), thereby increasing the rate of energy synthesis.

Remember, if fat loss is what you're after, low-intensity, prolonged exercise is best. In general, the longer you exercise, the greater the proportion of fat used. But when you can't catch your breath, you're not burning fat. So avoid "the burn," and keep breathing!

Abbreviations: ATP, adenosine triphosphate; TCA, tricarboxylic acid

The final step in oxidation, and the one that produces most of the energy, is the electron transport chain. For every molecule of glucose that is completely oxidized, 36 molecules of ATP, 6 molecules of carbon dioxide, and 6 molecules of water are formed.

Glucose Anabolism

Most of the body's glucose is catabolized for energy. Glucose that remains after the body's energy needs are met can be used by liver and skeletal muscle cells to make glycogen, the storage form of glucose, through the process of **glycogenesis**. On average, the body can store about 1.1 pounds of glycogen (some in the liver, most in the skeletal muscle cells). Carbohydrate loading, a regime practiced by many long-distance athletes, can increase muscle glycogen storage as much as five times the normal amount. (Conversely, the breakdown of glycogen is **glycogenolysis**. Liver glycogen can be broken down to release glucose into the blood: This occurs between meals, when the body has used up the energy from the last meal. Muscle cells are able to break down glycogen for their own use, but cannot release glucose into the bloodstream.)

Glucose can be synthesized from pyruvate, the three-carbon molecule; thus, glycerol and certain amino acids that are converted to pyruvate can ultimately be converted to glucose if necessary, through the process known as **gluconeogenesis**.

Fat Catabolism

The basic units of fat digestion are fatty acids and glycerol, which are catabolized differently in the body (Fig. 7-11). Most naturally occurring fatty acids comprise an even number of carbon atoms in a chain, varying in length from 4 carbon atoms to 24 carbon atoms. Glycerol is a three-carbon compound to which one, two, or three fatty acids attach to form monoglycerides, diglycerides, or triglycerides, respectively. By weight, 5% of a typical fat molecule is glycerol; the remaining 95% is fatty acids.

With the exception of the central nervous system and red blood cells, all body cells can directly oxidize fatty acids to produce energy, thereby using the body's second choice of fuel. Through the process of **beta oxidation**, fatty acids are split, two carbon atoms at a time, into molecules of acetyl Co-A. For instance, the 18-carbon chain in the fatty acid linoleic acid is broken down into nine two-carbon molecules of acetyl Co-A. Those molecules can then enter the TCA cycle, followed by the electron transport chain. After undergoing complete oxidation, one 18-carbon fatty acid yields a net of 129 ATP molecules. It is important to note that because fatty acids are broken down into compounds containing two-carbon atoms, not three-carbon atoms, they cannot be re-formed into glucose.

Under normal conditions, the liver produces small quantities of **ketone bodies** (acetoacetic acid and acetone) through fatty acid metabolism by condensing two molecules of Co-A (**ketogenesis**). Ketones leave the liver, travel through the bloodstream, and diffuse into other body cells, where they are catabolized into Co-A, which enters the TCA cycle. A higher than normal level of ketones in the blood (ketosis) occurs during starvation and periods of extremely low carbohydrate intake as the body uses fatty acids instead of glucose for energy. Because ketones are mostly

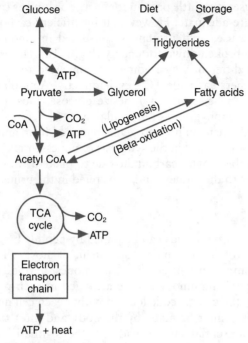

Figure 7-11
Fat metabolism.

acidic, ketosis can lead to acidosis, an undesirable condition of abnormally low blood pH.

The glycerol molecule of fat is easily converted to pyruvate, the three-carbon compound. From there it can be reassembled into glucose, or if energy is needed, pyruvate can be oxidized through the TCA cycle and electron transport chain.

Fat Anabolism

Glycerol and fatty acids that are not used for energy can be re-formed into triglycerides and stored in the liver and adipose tissue. When either carbohydrates or protein is consumed in excess of need, the excess is converted by liver cells into lipids through the process of **lipogenesis**. In people of normal weight, fat stores constitute 10% to 30% of total body weight. Unfortunately, the body has a virtually limitless capacity to store fat, and in very obese people, fat tissue can account for 80% of total weight (Berne and Levy, 1993).

Protein Catabolism

Amino acids are the basic units that remain after protein digestion is completed. Like glucose, glycerol, and fatty acids, they also have a carbon stem. Unique to amino acids is the nitrogen-containing amino group, which must be removed (**deaminated**) before amino acids can be used for energy.

Normally, the body uses very little protein for energy as long as carbohydrate and fat intake and storage are adequate. However, if insufficient carbohydrate and fat are available for energy use, or if protein is consumed in amounts greater than needed, amino acids are broken down for energy (Fig. 7-12). Different amino acids enter the TCA cycle in different ways: Some are converted to pyruvate, some to acetyl Co-A, and still others enter the TCA cycle directly. Amino acids that can be converted to pyruvate can be used to synthesize glucose; thus, protein can be a source of glucose when carbohydrate is not available.

Ammonia is produced when amino nitrogen is removed from amino acids. In the liver, some of this ammonia is used in the synthesis of nonessential amino acids. The remaining ammonia combines with carbon dioxide to make urea, which is released into the blood, circulates to the kidney, and is excreted in the urine.

Protein Anabolism

In almost every body cell, amino acids can be joined by peptide bonds to synthesize proteins. Not only are proteins a primary component of most cell structures, they are also the primary components of enzymes, hormones, antibodies, and clotting chemicals. The way in which amino acids are arranged in each particular type of protein is determined by the genetic code located within each cell nucleus.

Essential amino acids cannot be made by the body and must therefore be consumed in the diet. Nonessential amino acids can be synthesized by body cells

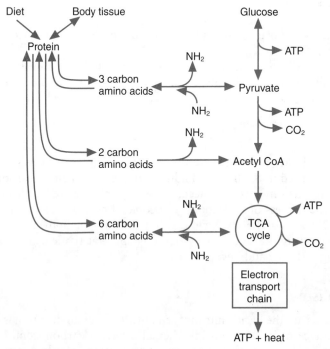

Figure 7-12
Protein metabolism.

through a process called **transamination,** wherein an amino group is transferred to a substance or acid of the TCA cycle (see Fig. 7-12). Protein synthesis occurs only when adequate amounts of the appropriate essential and nonessential amino acids are present in the cell.

ABSORPTIVE AND POSTABSORPTIVE STATES

At rest, a mixture of fuels is used to meet the body's energy needs, usually about 50% from carbohydrate, about 40% from fat, and about 5% to 10% from amino acids (Butterfield and Gates, 1994). The actual proportion of fuels that are used depends on the diet and the amount of time that has passed since the last meal was eaten.

The body alternates between two metabolic states: absorptive and postabsorptive (fasting). The absorptive state, which occurs for about 4 hours after each meal, is the period during which nutrients that have been absorbed into the bloodstream and lymphatic system are used for energy. If carbohydrate intake increases, as it typically does immediately after a meal, the proportion of energy that is obtained from glucose increases; if fat intake increases, an increase in fat usage does not seem to occur.

The postabsorptive (fasting) state occurs generally during late morning, late afternoon, and most of the evening, during which the body's energy needs are met by the breakdown of stored nutrients. During this time, the proportion of energy derived from fat increases as triglycerides are mobilized from stores. For people who eat three meals per day, the amount of time spent in each state is generally the same. Figure 7-13 depicts the anabolic and catabolic reactions summarized below.

Absorptive State

Carbohydrate digestion yields glucose, most of which enters the TCA cycle in body cells to produce energy (ATP). Glucose that remains after energy needs are met is converted to glycogen and stored in the liver and muscle cells. Glycogen storage is limited, though, so that any glucose that is left, in the form of excess pyruvate or acetyl molecules, is converted to fat (triglycerides) and stored.

Fat digestion yields glycerol and fatty acids. Glycerol is broken down into pyruvate, which can enter the TCA cycle to produce energy, can be synthesized into glucose, or can be used to synthesize fat. Fatty acids are broken down into acetyl molecules, which can enter the TCA cycle to produce energy. Excessive acetyl molecules are converted back to fatty acids, which combine with glycerol to form fat for storage.

Protein digestion yields amino acids, some of which are used to synthesize body proteins. If protein is eaten in excess of need, or if not enough carbohydrate and fat were consumed to meet energy needs, amino acids (stripped of their nitrogen) can enter the TCA cycle through several different pathways to be broken down into energy. If energy needs are met, deaminated amino acids can be converted, through the intermediates pyruvate and acetyl molecules, to fat for storage.

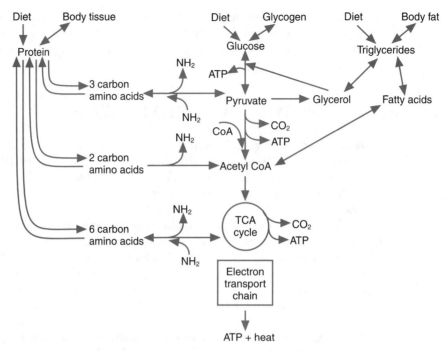

Figure 7-13
Summary of catabolic and anabolic reactions.

Postabsorptive State

Obviously, the body uses energy to perform physical activity through muscular action: The more physically active a person is, the more energy (calories) he or she requires. However, most people use less energy for voluntary activities than for involuntary activity. For instance, energy is used continuously to maintain normal body temperature and muscle tone, beat the heart, inflate the lungs, and propel the GI tract. The brain and central nervous system, which normally use only glucose for energy, account for about two thirds of the total glucose used each day. Before anything else, the body's top priority is to meet its energy needs.

In the postabsorptive state, when food is not available for energy, body stores are broken down. First, liver glycogen and fatty acids from fat storage are released into the bloodstream, where body cells use them in the TCA cycle to produce energy. When glycogen stores are exhausted, usually within 4 hours or so, low blood glucose signals hunger; eating returns the body to the absorptive state.

If eating does not occur, because of either voluntary or involuntary fasting, fat breakdown continues. In most body cells, fatty acids can be catabolized for energy. The exceptions are cells of the brain and nerves, which normally rely exclusively on glucose for energy. During the first few days of a fast, brain and nerve cells obtain about 10% of the glucose they need from glycerol, and the remaining 90% through the catabolism of body proteins, such as muscle and lean tissue. Although only certain amino acids can be converted to pyruvate and ultimately glucose, whole proteins must be broken down to make them available. The remaining amino acids from tissue breakdown that cannot be converted to glucose (ie, two-carbon molecules) are used for energy by other body cells. Breaking down body protein for energy is expensive; yet compared to the small amount of glucose that is available from glycerol in stored triglycerides, it is more efficient. If protein catabolism were to continue at this rate, death would occur within 3 weeks, regardless of the amount of stored fat a person may have.

Fortunately, the body adapts to starvation in an attempt to conserve body protein. Some brain cells are able to use ketone bodies, derived from fatty acid catabolism, for energy. Ketone production increases to meet demand, and after several weeks of fasting, about two thirds or more of the nervous system's energy requirements are supplied by ketones. Unfortunately, many brain cells are unable to convert to ketone use, so some body protein catabolism continues.

Another adaptive mechanism that occurs during prolonged fasting is a slowing of the metabolic rate (calories used for involuntary activities), which, when combined with a decrease in physical activity, results in a decrease in energy requirements. In long-term fasting, fatty acids supply about 90% of total energy requirements. If adequate fluids are consumed, a normal-weight person can survive up to 60 days before fat stores are exhausted. After that, protein catabolism quickly accelerates, and death follows.

KEY CONCEPTS

- Mechanical and chemical digestion breaks down complex molecules of carbohydrates, protein, and fat into smaller molecules that the body can absorb. Water, vitamins, minerals, and simple sugars do not undergo digestion before being absorbed.

- Enzymes are chemicals that facilitate reactions without being consumed. Most chemical digestion occurs in the small intestine through the action of enzymes produced by the brush border cells and the pancreas.

- Energy metabolism refers to how energy is extracted from carbohydrates, protein, and fat.

- In healthy adults, the rate of anabolism (tissue buildup) is equal to the rate of catabolism (tissue breakdown).

- ATP, generated through the catabolism of carbohydrates, protein, and fat, is a compound available to all cells that, when hydrolyzed, releases energy and heat.

- Glucose is the body's preferred fuel. Under normal conditions, red blood cells, the brain, and the nervous system rely solely on glucose for energy.

- Although they enter at different routes, carbohydrates, protein, and fat are all aerobically metabolized through the TCA cycle to produce ATP (energy). If more energy is required, oxidation continues through the electron transport chain, the process that yields the greatest amount of energy.

- Glucose that remains after energy needs are met can be converted to glycogen and fat.

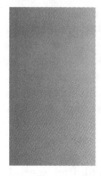

- Fat is the body's second-choice fuel. Excess fat that remains after energy needs are met is rearranged and stored as fat.
- Protein is used for energy only when it is consumed in excess of need, or if insufficient carbohydrate and fat are available. Ammonia is produced when the nitrogen group is removed from amino acids, a step that must occur before amino acids can enter the TCA cycle.
- During prolonged fasting, the brain and nervous system adapt to the shortage of glucose by using ketones that result from fat catabolism. However, body protein catabolism does continue (although at a slower rate) because not all cells are able to adapt to ketone use.

REFERENCES

Berne, R., Levy, M. (1993). Physiology. 3rd ed. St Louis: Mosby–Year Book, Inc.

Butterfield, G., Gates, J. (1994). Fueling Activity: Current Concepts. Topics in Nutrition and Food Safety, Fall 1994.

Shils, M., Olson, J., Shike, M. (1994). Modern Nutrition in Health and Disease. 8th ed. Philadelphia: Lea & Febiger.

Whitney, E, Cataldo, C., Rolfes, S. (1994). Understanding Normal and Clinical Nutrition. 3rd ed. St Paul: West Publishing Company.

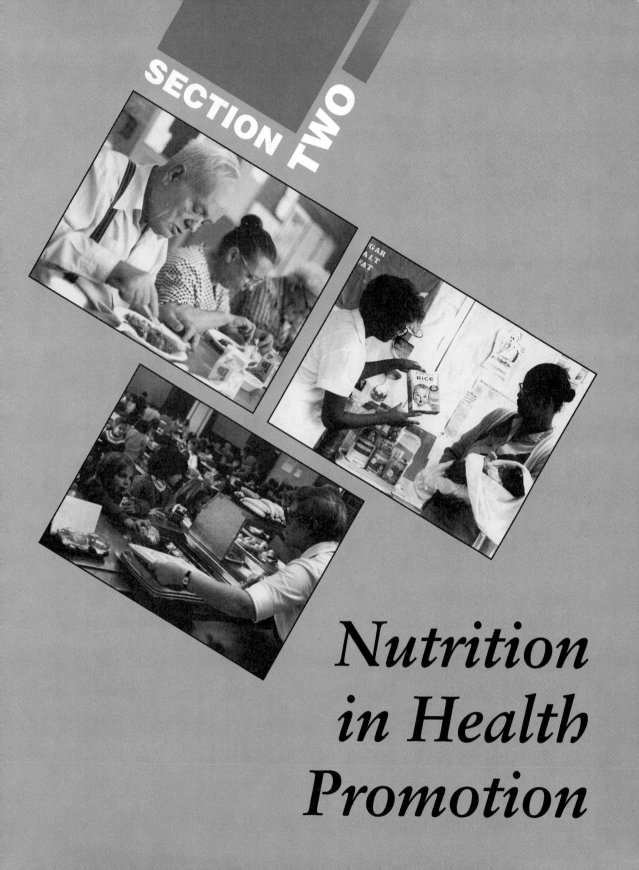

SECTION TWO

Nutrition in Health Promotion

CHAPTER 8

Planning an Adequate Diet: Nutritional, Cultural, and Safety Considerations

Chapter Outline

Key Terms

Daily Reference Values
  (DRVs)
Daily Value (DV)
Dietary Guidelines for
  Americans

Food Guide Pyramid
"Nutrition Facts"
Recommended Dietary
  Allowances

Reference Daily Intakes
  (RDIs)

*A*n adequate diet obviously provides a balanced intake of sufficient amounts of all nutrients that are required for growth and development and physical activity, as well as for maintenance or restoration of health. Exactly what constitutes an adequate diet, and for whom, is less obvious. Nutritional deficiency diseases now occur infrequently in the United States except among the poor, the elderly, alcoholics, fad dieters, and, ironically, hospitalized patients. In fact, public health concern has shifted away from undernutrition to overnutrition: Of the 10 leading causes of death in the United States today, 5 are associated with dietary excesses (Table 8-1). Alco-

Table 8-1
Leading Causes of Death Associated with Dietary Excesses

Disorder	Associated Dietary Excess
Heart diseases	Total fat, saturated fat, and cholesterol
Cancer (bowel and maybe breast)	Fat
Strokes	Sodium, calories
Diabetes (type II)	Calories
Atherosclerosis	Fat, saturated fat, cholesterol

hol plays a role in another three (chronic liver disease and cirrhosis, unintentional injuries, and suicide). Just how much of an impact diet actually has on these disorders is unknown, because diet is difficult to separate from genetic, behavioral, and environmental factors. However, it is certain that diet contributes to the development of these diseases and that dietary change can contribute to their prevention (USDHHS/PHS, 1988).

A "good" diet contains mostly "good" foods, but "good" can mean different things to different people. Nutritional guidelines are available from various governmental and health agencies to assist Americans in their efforts to choose a healthful diet. For instance, the Recommended Dietary Allowances can be used to plan a diet or to evaluate the nutritional adequacy of a diet. However, they deal with individual nutrients, not food groups, and are too complex for use by the general public. The *Dietary Guidelines for Americans* serves as the federal nutrition policy, outlining dietary suggestions for health promotion that are graphically illustrated in the Food Guide Pyramid (USDA/USDHHS, 1995). Nutrition labeling can assist consumers with food choices. For insight into Americans' attitudes, concerns, and behaviors about diet and health, see Food for Thought, Where We Stand.

Because eating supplies food for the body and the soul, diet planning is an art as well as a science. Although 84% of Americans in a recent poll indicated they are either concerned or very concerned that what they eat could have an effect on their future health (IFIC, 1994), nutritional considerations have a much lesser impact on most people's food choices than do personal food preferences and aversions, as influenced by culture, sociodemographic variables, and individual variables: Ignoring the significance of these individual variables can undermine diet planning (see Food for Thought). Other factors to consider while planning a diet include food quality, safety considerations, and economic feasibility.

NUTRITIONAL GUIDELINES

Recommended Dietary Allowances

The **Recommended Dietary Allowances (RDA)** were initially developed as a guide for planning and procuring food supplies for a wartime nutrition program in 1943.

FOOD *for* THOUGHT

Where We Stand

To get a better idea of what influences Americans' food choices, the Gallup Organization conducted a survey for the International Food Information Council (IFIC) and the American Dietetic Association. Seven hundred fifty-four adults over the age of 18 were interviewed by phone in December 1993. With that sample size, there is a 95% confidence level that the error attributable to sampling and other random effects could be plus or minus four percentage points.

On the plus side, the survey found:

- 94% agreed that balance, variety, and moderation are the keys to healthy eating
- 92% agreed that controlling portions or serving sizes is important to maintaining health
- 85% said that physical activity is very important to maintaining health
- 71% said they have made changes in their diet regarding fat
- 68% said they are likely to change their eating habits if advised to do so by a doctor
- 56% agreed that any food can be part of a total, healthy diet
- 48% are confident in their ability to choose a healthful diet

However:

- 75% said there are too many conflicting nutrition reports
- 75% said that the information about how to eat a healthy diet is too confusing, and 27% are very or somewhat confused about knowing how to choose a healthy diet
- 69% believe that foods should contain 30% or less calories from fat, misapplying the 30% guideline for total diet to individual foods
- only 30% said they are familiar with the Food Guide Pyramid
- the most common source for nutrition and food information is the media, with magazines the top choice at 34%; doctors were listed as the primary source of nutrition information by only 15%, and registered dietitians by only 5% of participants
- 68% said they are very or somewhat likely to change their food choices based on information from the media

So although Americans recognize the importance of nutrition for good health, misconceptions and confusion may be standing in the way of a healthful diet for many Americans.

Source: IFIC (1994). How are Americans making food choices? IFIC Review, October.

Today, they are used primarily by professionals both to plan and to evaluate the nutritional quality of diets, and to evaluate the adequacy of food supplies in meeting nutritional needs and the adequacy of government feeding programs (NRC, 1989). The RDA are useful in developing new food products, drawing up guidelines for nutrition labeling, and planning nutrition education programs. See display, Recommended Dietary Allowances.

In order to evaluate a person's intake according to the RDA, the nutritional composition of the diet must be calculated. This can be done using food composition references, either in computerized data bases or book form, which provide the average nutrient content for a given amount of food based on the chemical analysis of a number of samples (see Appendix 1). Food composition references are intended to

Recommended Dietary Allowances

Definition*	Comments
The levels of intake of essential nutrients that, on the basis of scientific knowledge, are judged by the Food and Nutrition Board to be adequate to meet the known nutritional needs of practically all healthy persons.	Recommended dietary allowances (RDA) have not been established for all the essential nutrients; therefore, a variety of foods should be consumed. RDA are revised periodically (about every 5 years) as more information becomes available. Does not guarantee to meet the needs of *all* healthy people: Some people consuming the RDA may not be meeting their individual needs for certain nutrients. The RDA are not appropriate for people who have acute or chronic illnesses, genetic disorders, or those using medications that alter nutritional requirements. The RDA also do not cover nutritional needs of low-birthweight infants.
RDA are recommendations for the average daily amounts of nutrients that population groups should consume over a period of time.	Designed for a reference population of Americans who live in a temperate climate and are moderately active. Separate categories have been established for age, sex, pregnancy, and lactation (Appendix 2). Estimated safe and adequate daily dietary intakes of additional selected vitamins and minerals supplement the 1980 edition of the RDA (Appendix 3). Estimated sodium, chloride, and potassium Minimum Requirements of Healthy Persons were added to the 1989 edition of the RDA. Because the body has adaptive mechanisms and the ability to store many nutrients, the RDA are more meaningful over a 5- to 8-day period than on any given day.
RDA should not be confused with requirements for a specific individual. Differences in the nutrient requirements of individuals are usually unknown. Therefore, RDA (except for energy) are estimated to exceed the requirements of most individuals and thereby to ensure that the needs of nearly all in the population are met. Intakes below the recommended allowance for a nutrient are not necessarily inadequate, but the risk of having an inadequate intake increases to the extent that intake is less than the levels recommended as safe.	The definition of requirement is the amount of a nutrient needed to prevent a deficiency; the definition of allowance is requirement plus a safety factor to account for individual variations. To accurately assess an individual's nutritional status and dietary adequacy, dietary factors, as well as anthropometric measurements, medical-socioeconomic data, biochemical findings, and clinical observations, should be evaluated (see Chap. 9).

* Data from National Research Council: Recommended Dietary Allowances, 10th ed. Washington, DC: National Academy Press, 1989.

be used as a standard reference for the nutritional value of foods consumed throughout the country on a year-round basis. Besides being used to calculate the nutrient intake of individuals or groups, food composition references also can aid in planning therapeutic diets with restricted or increased amounts of one or more nutrients, in developing food guides and nutrition education teaching materials, and in selecting nutritionally comparable alternatives among foods to control costs.

Although there are shortcomings inherent in using food composition tables to calculate nutrient intake that can then be compared to RDA values (see display, Food Composition Data Shortcomings), the RDA is still the only reference available that gives specific nutrient and calorie recommendations based on age and sex, and offers the advantage of providing close evaluation of actual intake. In addition, the RDA is revised periodically to reflect current data. The most recent edition of the RDA was published in 1989 and appears in Appendices 2, 3, and 4.

Unfortunately, the RDA are too complex for use by the general public and are established for healthy people only. Another disadvantage is that the RDA are appropriate for populations, but not necessarily for individuals. Ten percent of the population may be consuming a deficient diet even if they meet 100% of the RDA. Conversely, some people may habitually consume less than the RDA for some nutrients while still maintaining adequate intakes.

Because of the lack of research on the nutritional requirements of the elderly, the RDA for people 51 years of age and older has been extrapolated from studies on younger adults and may not be valid. In addition, there is no distinction made between the nutritional requirements of a 51-year-old and the requirements of a 90-year-old, although one can surmise that they may be different.

It may be necessary to exceed the RDA for some nutrients (eg, protein) in order to meet the RDA for others (eg, trace minerals such as iron and zinc), and the RDA do not take into consideration nutrient losses that are incurred during food storage and preparation.

Dietary Guidelines for Americans

Dietary Goals for the United States, the predecessor of the Dietary Guidelines, was published in 1977 by the Select Committee on Nutrition and Human Needs of the United States Senate. It recommended that Americans consume 30% of their total calories from fat, 12% from protein, and the remainder from carbohydrates, mostly

Food Composition Data Shortcomings

There may be wide variations in nutrient composition among different samples of the same food, related to the ripeness or maturity of the food, the portion of the food analyzed (eg, outer or inner leaves), the variety of a food, the length of time the food has been stored, the degree of processing and cooking used in preparation, the soil content where the food is grown, and the time of year the food is harvested.

Not all foods have been analyzed for their nutrient content (eg, food fads and convenience items).

Not all nutrients are listed in food composition tables (eg, trace elements like selenium).

Even if the nutrient composition of a food is known, the bioavailability of the nutrients in that food may be altered by other foods or nutrients that are consumed in a mixed diet (ie, orange juice can significantly increase the amount of iron absorbed from iron-fortified cereals).

in the form of starch and fiber. Because the goals generated a lot of controversy and criticism, the committee was disbanded and its responsibilities were delegated to the United States Department of Agriculture (USDA) and the United States Department of Health, Education, and Welfare (USDHEW), which later became the United States Department of Health and Human Services. Together these agencies published the first edition of *Dietary Guidelines for Americans* in 1980, which proved to be a less controversial, watered-down version of *Dietary Goals*. Public law now requires that the Guidelines be revised at least every 5 years.

The guidelines have evolved into the current (Fourth) edition, which was published in 1995. Their purpose is to provide guidance on diet and health to the general public by transforming current knowledge into prudent and practical recommendations that meet nutritional requirements, promote health, support active lives, and reduce the risk of chronic disease (USDA/USDHHS, 1995). They provide more "how to" advice than earlier editions, and negative suggestions ("avoid") have been replaced with positive ones ("choose a diet . . .").

The Guidelines stress the following points:

- Eating is one of life's greatest pleasures. Recognizing that food choices are influenced by culture, history, environment, and taste, in addition to energy and nutritional needs, the Guidelines emphasize variety, flexibility, and pleasure when choosing a healthful diet.
- Diet is important to health at all stages of life. The Guidelines provide advice for healthy Americans 2 years of age and older.
- Foods contain energy, nutrients, and other components that affect health. Focus is on the total diet, with avoidance of both deficiencies and excesses.
- Physical activity fosters a healthful diet.

The Guidelines are dietary suggestions to maintain health for the general population, not individuals. As such, they should be used as a starting point from which to develop an adequate diet for an individual (see display, Dietary Guidelines for Americans and Suggestions for Implementation).

The Food Guide Pyramid

The food group approach has long been used to teach basic principles of nutrition to the general public and to assist individuals in choosing balanced diets. Although they were simple and easy to use, traditional food group approaches (the Basic 4) were overly simplistic, generally only recommended minimum amounts of foods to consume, and did not address current concerns of overnutrition.

In 1992, a new generation of food guides was launched with the introduction of the USDA's **Food Guide Pyramid**, the official food guide for the United States and the only one recognized by federal agencies or departments (Achterberg et al, 1994). The pyramid is a complex graphic designed to illustrate the Dietary Guidelines for Americans, with an emphasis on variety, balance, and moderation (Fig. 8-1).

Unlike previous Basic 4 guidelines, the Food Guide Pyramid suggests *a range of daily servings* from each major food group, instead of *minimum* recommendations

(text continues on page 202)

Dietary Guidelines for Americans and Suggestions for Implementation

Guideline	Advice for Today	Suggestions for Implementation
Eat a variety of foods. *Rationale:* No single food supplies all 40-plus essential nutrients in amounts needed. Variety also helps reduce the risk of nutrient toxicity and accidental contamination.	Enjoy eating a variety of foods. Get the many nutrients your body needs by choosing among the varied foods you enjoy from these groups: grain products, vegetables, fruits, milk and milk products, protein-rich plant foods (beans, nuts), and protein-rich animal foods (lean meat, poultry, fish, and eggs). Remember to choose lean and low-fat foods and beverages most often. Many foods you eat contain servings from more than one food group. For example, soups and stews may contain meat, beans, noodles, and vegetables.	**Choose Foods from Each of Five Food Groups** The Food Guide Pyramid illustrates the importance of balance among food groups in a daily eating pattern. Most of the daily servings of food should be selected from the food groups that are the largest in the picture and closest to the base of the Pyramid. • Choose most of your foods from the grain products group (6–11 servings), the vegetable group (3–5 servings), and the fruit group (2–4 servings). • Eat moderate amounts of foods from the milk group (2–3 servings) and the meat and beans group (2–3 servings). • Choose sparingly foods that provide few nutrients and are high in fat and sugars. *Note:* A range of servings is given for each food group. The smaller number is for people who consume about 1600 calories a day, such as many sedentary women. The larger number is for those who consume about 2800 calories a day, such as active men.
Balance the food you eat with physical activity—maintain or improve your weight. *Rationale:* Excess weight increases the risk of numerous chronic diseases, such as hypertension, heart disease, and diabetes.	Try to maintain your body weight by balancing what you eat with physical activity. If you are sedentary, try to become more active. If you are already very active, try to continue the same level of activity as you age. More physical activity is better than less, and any is better than none. If your weight is not in the healthy range, try to reduce health risks through better eating and exercise habits. Take steps to keep your weight within the healthy range (neither too high nor too low).	**To Decrease Calorie Intake** • Eat a variety of foods that are low in calories and high in nutrients—check the Nutrition Facts Label. • Eat less fat and fewer high-fat foods. • Eat smaller portions and limit second helpings of foods high in fat and calories. • Eat more vegetables and fruits without fats and sugars added in preparation or at the table. *(continued)*

Dietary Guidelines for Americans and Suggestions
for Implementation (Continued)

Guideline	Advice for Today	Suggestions for Implementation
	Have children's heights and weights checked regularly by a health professional.	• Eat pasta, rice, breads, and cereals without fats and sugars added in preparation or at the table. • Eat less sugar and fewer sweets (like candy, cookies, cakes, soda). • Drink less or no alcohol.
Choose a diet with plenty of grain products, vegetables, and fruits. *Rationale:* Plant foods provide fiber, complex carbohydrates, vitamins, minerals, and other substances important for good health. They are also generally low in fat.	Eat more grain products (breads, cereals, pasta, and rice), vegetables, and fruits. Eat dry beans, lentils, and peas more often. Increase your fiber intake by eating more of a variety of whole grains, whole-grain products, dry beans, fiber-rich vegetables and fruits such as carrots, corn, peas, pears, and berries.	**For a Diet With Plenty of Grain Products, Vegetables, and Fruits, Eat Daily—** *6–11 servings of grain products (breads, cereals, pasta, and rice)* • Eat products made from a variety of whole grains, such as wheat, rice, oats, corn and barley. • Eat several servings of whole-grain breads and cereals daily. • Prepare and serve grain products with little or no fats and sugars. *3–5 servings of various vegetables and vegetable juices* • Choose dark green leafy and deep yellow vegetables often. • Eat dried beans, peas, and lentils often. • Eat starchy vegetables, such as potatoes and corn. • Prepare and serve vegetables with few or no fats. *2–4 servings of various fruits and fruit juices* • Choose citrus fruits or juices, melons, or berries regularly. • Eat fruits as desserts or snacks. • Drink fruit juices. • Prepare and serve fruits with little or no added sugars.
Choose a diet low in fat, saturated fat, and cholesterol. *Rationale:* High-fat diets increase the risk of obesity, heart disease, and certain types of cancer.	To reduce your intake of fat, saturated fat, and cholesterol, follow these recommendations, as illustrated in the Food Guide Pyramid, which apply to diets consumed over several days and not to single meals or foods. • Use fats and oils sparingly.	**For a Diet Low in Fat, Saturated Fat, and Cholesterol** *Fats and Oils* • Use fats and oils sparingly in cooking and at the table. • Use small amounts of salad dressings and spreads such as butter,

(continued)

Dietary Guidelines for Americans and Suggestions for Implementation (Continued)

Guideline	Advice for Today	Suggestions for Implementation
	• Use the Nutrition Facts Label to help you choose foods lower in fat, saturated fat, and cholesterol. • Eat plenty of grain products, vegetables, and fruits. • Choose low-fat milk products, lean meats, fish, poultry, beans, and peas to get essential nutrients without substantially increasing calorie and saturated fat intakes.	margarine, and mayonnaise. Consider using low-fat or fat-free dressings for salads. • Choose vegetable oils and soft margarines most often because they are lower in saturated fat than solid shortenings and animal fats, even though their caloric content is the same. • Check the Nutrition Facts Label to see how much fat and saturated fat are in a serving; choose foods lower in fat and saturated fat. *Grain Products, Vegetables, and Fruits* • Choose low-fat sauces with pasta, rice, and potatoes. • Use as little fat as possible to cook vegetables and grain products. • Season with herbs, spices, lemon juice, and fat-free or low-fat salad dressings. *Meat, Poultry, Fish, Eggs, Beans, and Nuts* • Choose two to three servings of lean fish, poultry, meats, or other protein-rich foods, such as beans, daily. Use meats labeled "lean" or "extra lean." Trim fat from meat; take skin off poultry. (Three ounces of cooked lean beef or chicken without skin—a piece the size of a deck of cards—provides about 6 grams of fat; a piece of chicken with skin or untrimmed meat of that size may have as much as twice this amount of fat.) Most beans and bean products are almost fat-free and are a good source of protein and fiber. • Limit intake of high-fat processed meats such as sausages, salami, and other cold cuts; choose lower fat varieties by reading the Nutrition Facts Label.

(continued)

Dietary Guidelines for Americans and Suggestions for Implementation *(Continued)*

Guideline	Advice for Today	Suggestions for Implementation
		• Limit the intake of organ meats (3 ounces of cooked chicken liver have about 540 mg of cholesterol); use egg yolks in moderation (one egg yolk has about 215 mg of cholesterol). Egg whites contain no cholesterol and can be used freely. *Milk and Milk Products* • Choose skim or low-fat milk, fat-free or low-fat yogurt, and low-fat cheese. • Have two to three low-fat servings daily. Add extra calcium to your diet without added fat by choosing fat-free yogurt and low-fat milk more often. [One cup of skim milk has almost no fat, 1 cup of 1% milk has 2.5 grams of fat, 1 cup of 2% milk has 5 grams (one teaspoon) of fat, and 1 cup of whole milk has 8 grams of fat.] If you do not consume foods from this group, eat other calcium-rich foods.
Choose a diet moderate in sugars. *Rationale:* Foods high in added sugar are often "empty calories." Both sugars and starches promote tooth decay.	Use sugars in moderation—sparingly if your calorie needs are low. Avoid excessive snacking, brush with a fluoride toothpaste, and floss your teeth regularly. Read the Nutrition Facts Label on foods you buy. The food label lists the content of total carbohydrate and sugars, as well as calories.	**For Healthier Teeth and Gums** • Eat fewer foods containing sugars and starches between meals. • Brush and floss teeth regularly. • Use a fluoride toothpaste. • Ask your dentist or doctor about the need for supplemental fluoride, especially for children.
Choose a diet that is moderate in salt and sodium. *Rationale:* A high salt intake is associated with higher blood pressure.	Fresh fruits and vegetables have very little sodium. The food groups in the Food Guide Pyramid include some foods that are high in sodium and other foods that have very little sodium, or that can be prepared in ways that add flavor without adding salt. Read the Nutrition Facts Label to compare and help identify foods lower in sodium within each group. Use herbs and spices to flavor food.	**To Consume Less Salt and Sodium—** • Read the Nutrition Facts Label to determine the amount of sodium in the foods you purchase. The sodium content of processed foods—such as cereals, breads, soups, and salad dressings—often varies widely. • Choose foods lower in sodium and ask your grocer or supermarket to

(continued)

Dietary Guidelines for Americans and Suggestions for Implementation *(Continued)*

Guideline	Advice for Today	Suggestions for Implementation
	Try to choose forms of foods that you frequently consume that are lower in sodium and salt.	offer more low-sodium foods. Request less salt in your meals when eating out or traveling. • If you salt foods in cooking or at the table, add small amounts. Learn to use spices and herbs, rather than salt, to enhance the flavor of food. • When planning meals, consider that fresh and most plain frozen vegetables are low in sodium. • When selecting canned foods, select those prepared with reduced or no sodium. • Remember that fresh fish, poultry, and meat are lower in sodium than most canned and processed ones. • Choose foods lower in sodium content. Many frozen dinners, packaged mixes, canned soups, and salad dressings contain a considerable amount of sodium. Remember that condiments such as soy and many other sauces, pickles, and olives are high in sodium. Ketchup and mustard, when eaten in large amounts, can also contribute significant amounts of sodium to the diet. Choose lower-sodium varieties. • Choose fresh fruits and vegetables as a lower-sodium alternative to salted snack foods.
If you drink alcoholic beverages, do so in moderation. *Rationale:* Current evidence suggests that moderate drinking is associated with a lower risk for coronary heart disease in some individuals. However, higher levels of alcohol intake raise the risk	If you drink alcoholic beverages, do so in moderation, with meals, and when consumption does not put you or others at risk.	**What Is Moderation?** Moderation is defined as no more than one drink per day for women and no more than two drinks per day for men. *Count as a drink—* • 12 ounces of regular beer (150 calories) • 5 ounces of wine (100 calories) • 1.5 ounces of 80-proof distilled spirits (100 calories)

(continued)

Dietary Guidelines for Americans and Suggestions for Implementation *(Continued)*

Guideline	Advice for Today	Suggestions for Implementation
for high blood pressure, stroke, heart disease, certain cancers, accidents, violence, suicides, birth defects, and overall mortality (deaths). Too much alcohol may cause cirrhosis of the liver, inflammation of the pancreas, and damage to the brain and heart.		**Who Should Not Drink?** Some people should not drink alcoholic beverages at all. These include: • Children and adolescents. • Individuals of any age who cannot restrict their drinking to moderate levels. This is a special concern for recovering alcoholics and people whose family members have alcohol problems. • Women who are trying to conceive or who are pregnant. Major birth defects, including fetal alcohol syndrome, have been attributed to heavy drinking by the mother while pregnant. While there is no conclusive evidence that an occasional drink is harmful to the fetus or to the pregnant woman, a safe level of alcohol intake during pregnancy has not been established. • Individuals who plan to drive or take part in activities that require attention or skill. Most people retain some alcohol in the blood up to 2–3 hours after a single drink. • Individuals using prescription and over-the-counter medications. Alcohol may alter the effectiveness or toxicity of medicines. Also, some medications may increase blood alcohol levels or increase the adverse effect of alcohol on the brain.

Source: USDA, USDHHS, 1995

(Table 8-2), thus addressing both undernutrition and overnutrition. More specific recommendations based on total calorie intake appear in the display, How Many Servings Do You Need Each Day? Other differences and teaching concepts and considerations appear in the display, Food Guide Pyramid Characteristics.

Nutrition Labeling

The Nutrition Labeling and Education Act of 1990 resulted in the most sweeping nutrition labeling reforms in American history, with the focus shifting away from avoiding nutrient deficiencies and toward avoiding nutrition-related chronic diseases

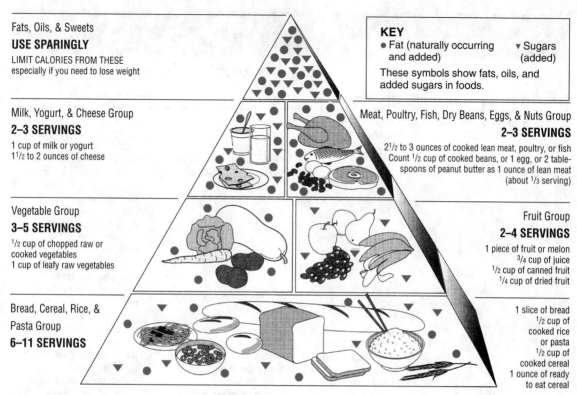

Figure 8-1
The Food Guide Pyramid (serving sizes depicted in boxes).

(Allen, 1995). The new law was fully implemented during 1994 and includes mandatory labeling, a new user-friendly nutrition label ("Nutrition Facts"), definitions of terms, the use of health claims, and changes in ingredient labeling.

MANDATORY LABELING

Nutrition information now appears on about 90% of processed food; exemptions are plain coffee and tea; some spices, flavorings, and other foods that contain no significant amounts of nutrients; ready-to-eat food prepared primarily on site, such as deli and bakery items; restaurant food; bulk food that is not resold; and food that is produced by small businesses. Manufacturers of foods in small packages are not required to list nutrition information on their labels unless they make a nutrition claim. Nutrition information is voluntary (point-of-purchase) for many raw foods, including frequently eaten raw fruits, vegetables, and fish, and major cuts of meat and poultry.

"NUTRITION FACTS"

"**Nutrition Facts**" is the name of the new label (Fig 8-2). Its format features a different set and sequence of nutrients that reflect current health concerns. As with the

Table 8-2
Guide to Daily Food Choices

Food Group	Nutritional Attributes	Suggested Daily Servings and Serving Sizes	Selection Tips
Bread, Cereal, Rice, and Pasta Group	Provide complex CHO, vitamins, minerals, and fiber	6–11 servings 1 serving is: 1 slice bread 1 oz ready-to-eat cereal ½ cup cooked cereal, rice, or pasta	For fiber, choose several servings a day of foods made from whole grains. Choose most often items made with little fat and sugar: bread, English muffins, rice, pasta. Avoid baked products high in fat and sugar: cakes, cookies, croissants, pastries. Limit fats and sugars used as toppings and spreads. When preparing package mixes, use only half the fat suggested, and if milk is called for, use low-fat.
Vegetable Group	Provide vitamins A, C, and folate; iron, magnesium, and fiber Naturally low in fat	3–5 servings 1 serving is: 1 cup raw leafy vegetables ½ cup other vegetables, cooked or chopped raw ¾ cup vegetable juice	Because different vegetables provide different nutrients, be sure to eat: • dark green leafy vegetables several times a week (broccoli, romaine lettuce, spinach) • deep yellow vegetables (carrots, sweet potatoes) • starchy vegetables (potatoes, corn, peas) • legumes several times a week (navy, pinto, and kidney beans) • other vegetables (lettuce, tomatoes, onions, green beans). Limit fat added to vegetables. Use low-fat salad dressing.
Fruit Group	Provide vitamins A and C and potassium Naturally low in fat and sodium	2–4 servings 1 serving is: 1 medium apple, banana, or orange ½ cup chopped, cooked, or canned fruit ¾ cup fruit juice	Choose fresh, frozen, canned or dried fruit and fruit juices. Eat whole fruits often. Eat fruits high in vitamin C regularly: citrus fruits, melons, berries. Choose 100% fruit juice instead of punches, ades, and drinks.

(continued)

Table 8-2 (Continued)
Guide to Daily Food Choices

Food Group	Nutritional Attributes	Suggested Daily Servings and Serving Sizes	Selection Tips
Meat, Poultry, Fish, Dry Beans, Eggs, and Nuts	Meat, fish, and poultry provide protein, B vitamins, iron, and zinc Dry beans, eggs, and nuts provide protein and most vitamins and minerals	2–3 servings, the equivalent of 5–7 ounces of cooked lean meat, poultry, or fish 1 serving is: 　2–3 ounces of cooked 　　lean meat, poultry, or fish For the other items in this group, 1 ounce of meat equals: 　½ cup cooked, dry beans 　1 egg 　2 tablespoons 　　peanut butter	Choose lean meat, poultry without skin, fish, and dried peas and beans often. They are lowest in fat. Use low-fat preparation techniques: Trim away visible fat, don't add fat during cooking. Limit egg yolks; use egg whites freely. Because nuts and seeds are high in fat, use them in moderation.
Milk, Yogurt, and Cheese Group	Provide protein, vitamins, calcium, and other minerals	2–3 servings 1 serving is (based on calcium content): 　1 cup milk or yogurt 　1½ ounces natural 　　cheese 　2 ounces process cheese	Choose skim milk and non-fat yogurt often; they are lowest in fat. Cottage cheese is lower in calcium than most cheeses; 1 cup cottage cheese = ½ cup milk. Limit high-fat cheese and ice cream. Choose "part skim" or low-fat cheeses and lower-fat milk desserts (ice milk, frozen yogurt)
Fats, Oils, and Sweets	Provide calories with little else nutritionally	Use sparingly	

Source: USDA (prepared by Human Nutrition Information Service), USDA's Food Guide Pyramid. Home and Garden Bulletin Number 249, Hyattsville, MD, 1992.

previous label, calories, total fat, total carbohydrate, protein, sodium, vitamins A and C, calcium, and iron must appear on the label. New items are calories from fat, saturated fat, cholesterol, sugars, and dietary fiber. Thiamine, riboflavin, and niacin are no longer required to be listed because deficiencies of these vitamins are no longer considered a public health concern. Voluntary items include calories from saturated fat, stearic acid (on meat and poultry products only), polyunsaturated fat, monounsaturated fat, potassium, soluble fiber, insoluble fiber, sugar alcohol, other carbohydrate, the percent of vitamin A present as beta-carotene, and amounts of other essential vitamins and minerals. If a food is fortified or enriched with any optional components, or if a health claim is made about any of them, the pertinent information then becomes mandatory.

How Many Servings Do You Need Each Day?

Calorie Level*	About 1,600	About 2,200	About 2,800
Bread group	6	9	11
Vegetable group	3	4	5
Fruit group	2	3	4
Milk group	2–3**	2–3**	2–3**
Meat group	2, for a total of 5 ounces	2, for a total of 6 ounces	3, for a total of 7 ounces

* These are the calorie levels if you choose low-fat, lean foods from the 5 major food groups and use foods from the fats, oils, and sweets group sparingly.
** Women who are pregnant or breast-feeding, teenagers, and young adults to age 24 need 3 servings.

"Nutrition Facts" have standardized serving sizes that are set by the FDA to allow consumers to make comparisons between similar items in a product line. The servings are also more representative of amounts that most people typically eat.

Nutrients are listed as the amount per serving and also as a percent "**Daily Value**," which is the new dietary reference designed to help consumers evaluate a food in the context of a total diet. Daily Values actually are composed of two sets of behind-the-scene standards: Daily Reference Values (DRV) and Reference Daily Intake (RDI). **Daily Reference Values** are the reference standards for fat, saturated fat, cholesterol, carbohydrate, protein, fiber, sodium, and potassium (see display, Daily Reference Values [DRVs]). DRV for energy-yielding nutrients are based on total calories consumed per day. For labeling purposes, a 2000-calorie diet is used as the standard; however, DRV for a 2500-calorie diet also appear on the label. DRV represent the maximum desirable amount.

Reference Daily Intake (RDI) replaces USRDA as the reference for essential vitamins and minerals, and in selected groups, protein. The standards that are used for RDI appear in the display, Reference Daily Intakes (RDI). They are derived from the 1968 Recommended Dietary Allowances.

DEFINITION OF TERMS

The terms "low," "free," "more," "reduced," "high," and "good source" have been defined for the first time (see display, Labeling Lingo). Any term that is used to describe the nutrient content of a food will be uniform on every product on which the term appears.

HEALTH CLAIMS

Health claims can be made about the relationship between certain nutrients or foods and the risk of a disease or health-related condition. The FDA allows such claims to appear on products it regulates if the product meets these three criteria:

Food Guide Pyramid Characteristics

Characteristics	Teaching Concepts and Considerations
Recommendations are for total diet, not minimum requirements to avoid deficiencies	Emphasize variety, proportion, and moderation Teach sequentially, beginning at the base of the pyramid and focusing on one group at a time Augment pyramid with Dietary Guidelines; sodium, weight control, and alcohol are not addressed in pyramid.
Foods are divided into five major food groups	Each group supplies some nutrients; no group supplies adequate amounts of all essential nutrients No one group is more important than any other Some food from each major group should be eaten every day The apex of the pyramid is another category (fats, oils, and sweets); it is not a major food group; therefore no foods are illustrated there. Items in the apex basically provide only calories; most are condiments like butter, jelly, honey. Foods like hot dogs and french fries do not belong in this group Many clients will not know how to classify mixed dishes like pizza, casseroles, and stew; mixed items should be analyzed according to their component parts
The food group names have changed from previous food group approaches	The names of the groups are longer and more cumbersome, but are intended to clarify the composition of each group The names are Bread, Cereal, Rice, and Pasta Group Milk, Yogurt, and Cheese Group Vegetable Group Meat, Poultry, Fish, Dried Beans, Fruit Group Eggs, and Nuts Group Children may not be familiar with all the terms (eg, pasta, poultry)
Fruit and vegetables are separated into two distinct groups	The Vegetable Group is placed to the left of the Fruit Group and occupies a bigger space than fruit, signifying more servings should be obtained from vegetables than fruit. A conscious effort should be made to emphasize that Vegetables and Fruit are separate groups; vegetables are rich in vitamins and minerals, whereas fruit contributes mostly vitamins
Each group has a different recommended number of daily servings, listed as a range	Some groups should be eaten in greater quantity than others Number of servings must be referenced with serving sizes to be meaningful Common misconceptions about the serving recommendations include • smaller people should eat the lower end of the range, larger people eat the higher end • dieters should eat the lower end of the range, people who want to gain weight should eat the upper end • it is appropriate to eat any amount within the range on any given day The term "sparingly" may not be understood by some
Serving sizes have changed for some foods and food groups	Serving sizes on the pyramid do not correspond to serving sizes on food labels; pyramid sizes are the recommended amounts, serving sizes on food labels represent the amount most Americans currently consume
Icons for fat and sugar have been added; circles represent added and naturally occurring fat; inverted triangles depict added, but not naturally occurring sugar	Icons may not be noticed by some consumers; others may think they are merely decorative The different concentration of icons in each group represents the relative amount of fat or sugar found in each group compared to another. Differences among individual selections within each group are not apparent on the pyramid, but need to be addressed (eg, the difference between skim milk and whole milk, the difference between a doughnut and a bagel)

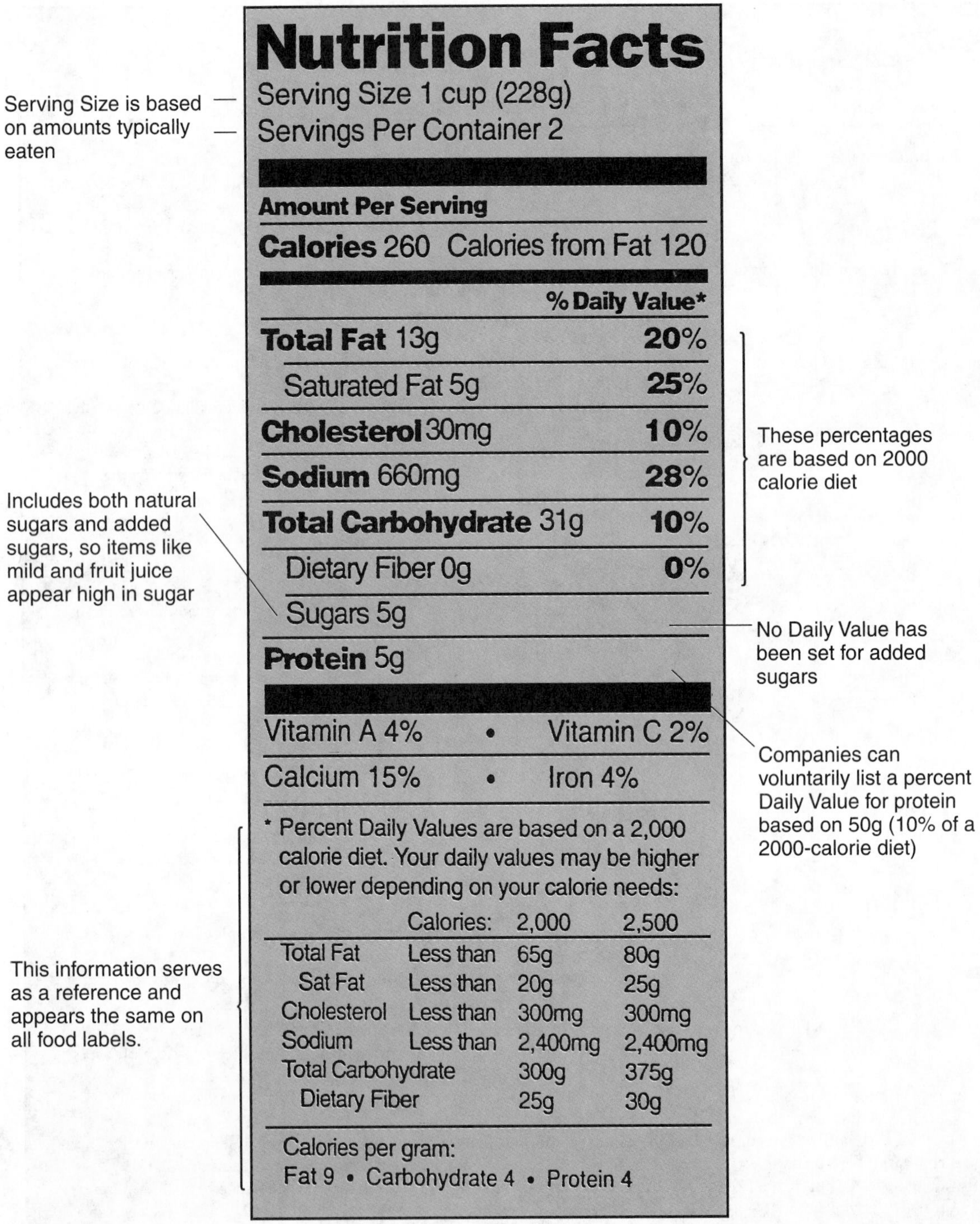

Serving Size is based on amounts typically eaten

Nutrition Facts
Serving Size 1 cup (228g)
Servings Per Container 2

Amount Per Serving

Calories 260   Calories from Fat 120

	% Daily Value*
Total Fat 13g	**20%**
Saturated Fat 5g	**25%**
Cholesterol 30mg	**10%**
Sodium 660mg	**28%**
Total Carbohydrate 31g	**10%**
Dietary Fiber 0g	**0%**
Sugars 5g	
Protein 5g	

Vitamin A 4%	•	Vitamin C 2%
Calcium 15%	•	Iron 4%

* Percent Daily Values are based on a 2,000 calorie diet. Your daily values may be higher or lower depending on your calorie needs:

	Calories:	2,000	2,500
Total Fat	Less than	65g	80g
Sat Fat	Less than	20g	25g
Cholesterol	Less than	300mg	300mg
Sodium	Less than	2,400mg	2,400mg
Total Carbohydrate		300g	375g
Dietary Fiber		25g	30g

Calories per gram:
Fat 9 • Carbohydrate 4 • Protein 4

Includes both natural sugars and added sugars, so items like mild and fruit juice appear high in sugar

These percentages are based on 2000 calorie diet

No Daily Value has been set for added sugars

Companies can voluntarily list a percent Daily Value for protein based on 50g (10% of a 2000-calorie diet)

This information serves as a reference and appears the same on all food labels.

Figure 8-2
Nutrition label format.

Daily Reference Values (DRV)*

Food Component	DRV	Standard Used
Fat	65 grams (g)	30% of total calories
Saturated fatty acids	20 g	10% of total calories
Cholesterol	300 milligrams (mg)	†
Total carbohydrate	300 g	60% of total calories
Fiber	25 g	11.5 g/1000 cal
Sodium	2400 mg	†
Potassium	3500 mg	†
Protein**	50 g	10% of total calories

*Based on 2000 calories a day for adults and children over 4 only

** DRV for protein does not apply to certain populations; Reference Daily Intake (RDI) for protein has been established for these groups: children 1 to 4 years: 16 g; infants under 1 year: 14 g; pregnant women: 60 g; nursing mothers: 65 g.

† Independent of total calorie intake

- The product does not exceed specific levels for total fat, saturated fat, cholesterol, and sodium. For instance, total fat may not exceed 13 g in a serving of food, 19.5 g in a serving of a main dish product, or 26 g of fat in a serving of a meal-type product. Standards have also been set for saturated fat, cholesterol, and sodium.
- It contains at least 10% of the Daily Value (before supplementation) for any one or all of the following: protein, dietary fiber, vitamin A, vitamin C, calcium, and iron.

Reference Daily Intakes (RDI)*

Nutrient	Amount	Nutrient	Amount
Vitamin A	5000 International Units (IU)	Folic acid	0.4 mg
Vitamin C	60 milligrams (mg)	Vitamin B_{12}	6 micrograms (µg)
Thiamine	1.5 mg	Phosphorus	1.0 g
Riboflavin	1.7 mg	Iodine	150 µg
Niacin	20 mg	Magnesium	400 mg
Calcium	1.0 gram (g)	Zinc	15 mg
Iron	18 mg	Copper	2 mg
Vitamin D	400 IU	Biotin	0.3 mg
Vitamin E	30 IU	Pantothenic acid	10 mg
Vitamin B_6	2.0 mg		

*Based on National Academy of Sciences' 1968 Recommended Dietary Allowances.

Labeling Lingo

Free
Contains virtually none of that nutrient
Can be used with calorie, sugar, sodium, salt, fat, saturated fat, and cholesterol

Low
Has a small enough amount of a nutrient that the product can be used frequently without concern about exceeding dietary recommendations
- Low sodium has no more than 140 mg sodium/serving
- Low calorie has no more than 40 calories/serving
- Low fat has no more than 3 g fat/serving
- Low saturated fat has no more than 1 g saturated fat/serving
- Low cholesterol has no more than 20 mg cholesterol/serving

Very low
Refers to sodium only; product has no more than 35 mg sodium/serving

Reduced or less
Has at least a 25% reduction in a nutrient compared to the regular product

Light or Lite
Has 1/3 fewer calories than a comparable product or 50% of the fat found in a comparable product

Good source
Has 10% to 19% of the Daily Value for a nutrient

High, Rich In, or Excellent Source
Has at least 20% of the Daily Value for a nutrient

More
Has at least 10% more of a desirable nutrient than does a comparable product

Lean
Refers to meat or poultry products with less than 10 g fat, less than 4 g saturated fat, and less than 95 mg cholesterol per standardized serving and per 100 g

Extra Lean
Refers to meat or poultry products with less than 5 g fat, less than 2 g saturated fat, and less than 95 mg cholesterol per standardized serving and per 100 g

- It meets the criteria listed in the display, Conditions for Allowable Health Claims.

INGREDIENT LABELING

All processed, packaged foods, including standardized foods that were previously exempt, must have all ingredients listed on their labels. For the first time, FDA-certified color additives must appear by name, and sources of protein hydrolysates must be listed. Foods that claim to be nondairy must state that the caseinate is a milk derivative, and beverages that claim to contain juices must declare the total percentage of juice on the information label.

PERSONAL CONSIDERATIONS

A person's food preferences, choices, and aversions are continuously shaped by evolving cultural, sociodemographic, and individual variables (Table 8-3). Before planning a diet, factors that influence food habits and their relative importance to

Conditions for Allowable Health Claims

To make a claim in this area	The product must
• Calcium and osteoporosis	Have at least 20% of the Daily Value for calcium
• Fat and cancer	Meet the requirement for "low fat"
• Saturated fat and cholesterol and risk of coronary heart disease	Meet requirements for "low saturated fat," "low fat," and "low cholesterol"
• Fiber-containing grain products, fruits, and vegetables and cancer	Contain grain products, fruits, or vegetables. It must also meet the requirement for "low fat" and be a "good source" of dietary fiber
• Fruits, vegetables, and grain products that contain fiber, and risk of coronary heart disease	Contain grain products, fruits, or vegetables. It must also meet the requirement for "low fat," "low saturated fat," and be a naturally "good source" of soluble fiber
• Fruits and vegetables and cancer	Be a fruit or vegetable, must meet the requirement for "low fat," and be a naturally "good source" of one or more of the following: vitamin A, vitamin C, dietary fiber
• Sodium and high blood pressure	Meet the requirement for "low sodium"

the person must be assessed. Positive aspects of an individual's food habits should be maintained and encouraged; dietary changes should be implemented prudently within the context of the person's normal diet.

Although they are not static, conservative traditional influences like culture, geographic region, and religion have a stabilizing effect on food habits. Even though these influences do not have an equal impact on all people within a group, generalizations can be made about characteristic food patterns and habits of the group.

Culture

Culture encompasses the total way of life of a particular population or community at a given time. It exerts an unconscious influence on its members, and has an inherent value system that defines what is desirable and what is undesirable. Because culture is transmitted from generation to generation, it is learned, not instinctive. Within any culture, individuals or groups of individuals participate differently, based on age, gender, social class, or income. In addition, culture is not a static influence, and although it resists change, culture may change at any given time to reflect ongoing changes in lifestyle, attitudes, technology, and environment.

As it pertains to the use of food, culture defines what is edible; which foods are appropriate for particular groups within the culture; how food is procured, distributed, handled, prepared, consumed, stored, and disposed; the meaning of food and eating; attitudes toward obesity and body size; and the relationship between diet and health. An unconscious food selection decision process appears in Figure 8-3.

As people of various ethnic backgrounds and nationalities have settled in the United States, different cultural food patterns have blended and adapted to Ameri-

Table 8-3
Variables Influencing Food Habits

Factors	Comment
CULTURAL VARIABLES	
Food value	Culture defines the value of a food, for instance what is a food (eg, cow) vs. what is a non-food (eg, dog). Culture also determines which foods signify prestige, prosperity, hospitality, and security. Failing to recognize a food's value can undermine health and nutrition counseling.
Beliefs	Represent an interpretation of food values as they relate to health, wellness, and weight, such as the belief that red wine "helps build blood" or that craving sweets during pregnancy means the baby will be a girl. Some cultures do not believe slimness is desirable; weight loss programs that lack cultural implicitness are likely to fail (Domel et al., 1992).
Customs/Rituals Symbolism	Customs are norms of behavior that are acquired as a member of a group; symbolism is the nonrational expression of the meaning of food. People feed on symbols as much as nutrients. Custom defines meal vs. snack, everyday vs. "company" foods, feminine vs. masculine foods, and holiday foods. Symbolically, food can be used to express love, reward or punish, display piety, express moral sentiments, demonstrate belongingness to a group, or proclaim the separateness of a group.
SOCIODEMOGRAPHIC VARIABLES	
Region	Region influences food availability and, like socioeconomic status and educational level, is a stronger predictor of dietary intake than race (Harland, et al., 1992).
Ethnicity	Ethnic differences in food choices may be independent of socioeconomic status and may be the result of cultural influences.
Age	Certain foods are associated with specific age groups: milk with infancy, peanut butter and jelly with childhood, hamburgers with adolescence, and tea and toast with the elderly.
Education	Educational level of the female head of household is positively related to total food expenditure, and often to dietary quality (Axelson, 1986). Educational level has been found to be inversely related to the use of convenience foods, directly related to the number of meals a household eats together, but not related to the number of meals eaten away from home (Axelson, 1986).
Income	Higher incomes do not necessarily mean better quality diets, but as personal income rises, the likelihood of an adequate diet increases. The intakes of dried peas and beans, rice, and eggs are inversely related to income.
Religion	Religion may assign a particular meaning to food or restrict its use (see section on Religion).
Gender	Physiology (eg, women are generally smaller and therefore need less food, so eat fewer calories) rather than culture may explain the differences in food consumption between men and women.
INDIVIDUAL VARIABLES	
Nutritional requirements	Although there is little variation in actual nutritional requirements among people, there is an infinite number of food and food combinations that can satisfy those requirements. Hunger is the least frequent reason for eating.
Health status	People often revert to childhood eating behaviors and food preferences when recovering from an illness (eg, they may request chicken noodle soup and ice cream because those foods are associated with recovery from childhood illnesses).
Taste physiology	Flavor is often irrelevant (eg, we don't have to taste a food to label it offensive or unacceptable because culture tells us what is fit to eat). For instance, you may like a food (cat) until you know what it is, disliking the *idea* of the food, rather than the actual food itself.

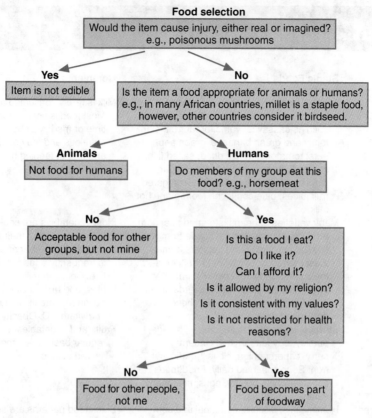

Figure 8-3
Food selection decision-making.

can culture. First-generation Americans usually adhere more closely to cultural food patterns than subsequent generations, and they may cling to traditional foods for the link they have with the past. Struggles to give up or keep ethnic food habits may continue for generations. Subsequent generations may follow cultural patterns only on holidays and at family gatherings, or they may give up ethnic foods but retain traditional methods of preparation. Even within a cultural group, food habits vary significantly among individuals and families. Table 8-4 outlines characteristics of certain ethnic diets.

Geographic Region

In addition to the sharing of cultural food patterns within the melting pot of the United States, advances in food technology and transportation have vastly increased the variety and availability of food across the country. Although "regional" foods are available anywhere, certain areas of the country are noted for certain foods:

- New England: Boston baked beans, clam chowder, lobster, and clam cakes

Table 8-4
Characteristics of Certain Ethnic Diets

Group and Place of Origin	Staple Foods	Comments
Hispanic Americans from Puerto Rico	Steamed white rice; many varieties of beans; wheat breads; starchy vegetables such as cassavas, yams, breadfruit, plantains, and green bananas; green peppers; tomatoes; garlic; dried, salted fish; salt pork, bacon; lard; olive oil; sugar; jams and jellies, sweet pastries; sugared fruit juices; cafe con lèche (coffee and hot milk)	Milk is rarely consumed as a beverage. Most food is cooked for long periods of time or fried. Malt beer is believed to be nutritious and may be given to children and breast-feeding mothers.
Hispanic Americans from Mexico, Central America	Many varieties of beans; steamed rice; corn products such as tortillas made from lime-soaked cornmeal; chili peppers; tomatoes; mangoes; prickly pear fruit; potatoes; meat and sausages; fish; poultry; eggs; milk cheeses; milk custards and bread puddings; lard; sweet chocolate and coffee drinks; cakes; pastries	Most vegetables are cooked so long that they lose most of their nutritional value. Diet is high in fiber and starch. Animal fat is frequently added during food preparation. Because milk, green leafy vegetables, and fruit intakes are low, diet may be inadequate in calcium, iron, vitamin A and vitamin C. Obesity is common.
Hispanic Americans from Cuba	Stews and casseroles flavored with sage, parsley, bay leaf, thyme, cinnamon, curry, capers, onion, cloves, garlic, saffron. Soup is served daily. Fried foods, especially fish, poultry, eggs; rice; many varieties of beans	Fruits and vegetables are not eaten on a regular basis. Main meal is usually served at lunch.
Southern black Americans from West Africa (many generations in United States)	Hominy grits; biscuits; cornmeal and corn bread; rice; legumes; potatoes; onions; tomatoes; hot peppers; green leafy vegetables cooked in fatback or salt pork; okra; sweet potatoes; squashes; corn; cabbage; melons; peaches; pecans; all parts of a pig; fresh meats and poultry; fish; thick stews; butter, shortening, and lard; sugar; bread puddings; pies and sweets	Black food patterns are similar to whites in same region. Northern blacks may be unfamiliar with "soul food." Frying is common; diet tends to be high in fat and salt, low in calcium. High rate of obesity.
Chinese Americans from China (diets vary sometimes with region)	Rice and rice gruel; wheat noodles; corn; green vegetables, especially from the cabbage family; squashes; cucumbers; eggplant; leafy vegetables; various shoots, including bamboo, mung, and soy; sweet potatoes; radishes; onions; peas and pods; mushrooms; roots; many local, seasonal vegetables; pickled vegetables; sea vegetables; plums; peaches; tangerines; kumquats and other citrus fruits; litchis; longans; mangoes; papayas; pomegranates; soybean products such as tofu (soybean curd), soy	Yin (feminine)-yang (masculine) concept of balancing intake; moderation is valued. Obesity is rare. Regional differences in food choices exist. Rice symbolizes life and fertility. Raw vegetables are rarely served. Diet is high in fiber and many nutrients, is low in fat, and may be low in protein.

(continued)

Table 8-4 (Continued)
Characteristics of Certain Ethnic Diets

Group and Place of Origin	Staple Foods	Comments
	sauces, bean noodles, and soy milk; tiny portions of meat, fish with bones, or poultry; seafood; soup or tea as beverage; sugar as seasoning	
Japanese Americans from Japan	Rice; vegetables; pickled vegetables; soy as miso (soup), tofu, bean paste, and soy sauce; fruits; salads; fish with bones; sugar as seasoning; sea vegetables; seafood; ginseng; green tea	Common preparation methods include broiling, steaming, boiling, and stir-frying. Meat portions are small. Milk is rarely used by adults. Diet is low in fat, rich in nutrients, high in sodium.
Vietnamese Americans from Vietnam	Rice, rice noodles; french bread and croissants with butter; hot peppers; curries of asparagus and potatoes; salads; tropical fruits and vegetables; lemons and limes; small portions of poultry; eggs; fish pâtés; nuoc nam (a strong, fermented fish sauce added to almost every cooked dish); sweets, candies, sweetened drinks; coffee; tea	Rice may be eaten at every meal. Fresh milk is not readily available; lactose intolerance is common. Little fat is used in preparation. Diet may be low in iron and calcium.
Native Americans (Indians)	*Southeast:* corn; cornmeal; coontie (flour from a palmlike plant); fried breads; swamp cabbage (now illegal to harvest); pumpkins; squashes; papayas; alligator, snake, wild hog, duck, fish, and shellfish. *Northeast:* blueberries; cranberries; beans; corn; pumpkins; fish; lobster; wild game; maple syrup. *Midwest:* bison; beans; corn; melons; squashes; tomatoes. *Southwest:* corn (many colors and varieties); beans; squash; pumpkins; chili peppers; melons; pinenuts; cactus. *Northwest:* salmon; caviar; other fish; otter; seal; whale; bear; elk; other game; wild fruits; acorns (and other wild nuts); wild greens.	Food has great religious and social significance. Corn is a status food for most tribes. Milk is used seldomly; calcium intake is usually low. Diets on some reservations are considered poor. High rate of obesity.

- Pennsylvania Dutch Country: shoofly pie, scrapple, and German-style sausage
- The South: grits, fried chicken, hot biscuits, greens, sweet potatoes, and corn bread
- Louisiana: French and Creole-style cooking
- Texas: chili con carne
- The Southwest: Mexican foods such as tortillas, tamales, enchiladas, and refried beans
- The Far West: citrus fruit, fresh produce, salads, and Oriental cooking
- The Midwest: dairy products and beef

Religion

Religion may assign a particular meaning to food or restrict its use, and religious affiliation may have a greater impact on food habits than nationality or culture (eg, Orthodox Jews follow kosher dietary laws regardless of their national origin).

- *Roman Catholics* do not eat meat on Ash Wednesday or Good Friday.
- *Muslims* cannot eat pork in any form. Alcohol is prohibited. Eating is a matter of worship.
- *Hindus* are vegetarians; beef is especially sacred.
- *Seventh Day Adventists* are lacto-ovovegetarians. Coffee, tea, and alcohol are prohibited. An interval of 5 to 6 hours between meals is recommended, with no snacking between meals.
- *Mormons (Church of Jesus Christ of the Latter-Day Saints)* do not use coffee, tea, alcohol, or tobacco.
- *Orthodox Jews* can eat only kosher meat and poultry that has been slaughtered according to ritual, soaked in water, salted, and washed. Shellfish and all pork products are prohibited. Milk and dairy products are used widely but cannot be consumed at the same meal as meat or poultry. Dairy products are not allowed within 6 hours after eating meat or poultry; meat and poultry cannot be eaten for 30 minutes after dairy products have been consumed. Separate utensils must be used for preparing and serving meat and dairy products.

Food preparation is prohibited on the Sabbath. Religious holidays are celebrated with certain foods. For example, only unleavened bread is eaten during Passover; a 24-hour fast is observed on Yom Kippur.

Because of the rigid dietary laws, Orthodox Jews rarely eat outside the home, with the exception of homes or restaurants with kosher kitchens.

- *Conservative Jews* may follow the Jewish dietary laws at home, but they take a more liberal attitude on social occasions.
- *Reform Jews* may not follow any religious dietary laws.

FOOD QUALITY AND SAFETY CONSIDERATIONS

Planning an adequate diet relates not only to nutritional adequacy and an individual's psychosocial and cultural needs, but also to food quality and safety concerns. Proper storage and preparation are vital to ensure that the vitamin and mineral content of a food is retained. Food-borne illness represents a threat when food is improperly handled or stored, and naturally occurring toxicants may be a much greater threat to health than manmade pesticides.

Retaining the Nutrient Content of Food

Even when it is carefully planned, there are no guarantees that a diet will provide optimal amounts of all nutrients, especially if the food that is eaten has been improperly stored or overly processed. Generally, food begins to lose its nutrients the moment that harvesting or processing begins, and the more that is done to a food before it is eaten, the greater the nutrient loss. Heat, light, air, soaking in water, mechanical injury, dry storage, and acidic or alkaline food processing ingredients can all hasten nutrient losses. Vitamins, minerals, and fiber are particularly vulnerable to the effects of food processing (see display, Retaining Nutrients in Food, for ways to minimize nutrient losses).

Retaining Nutrients in Food

FOOD PURCHASING

Don't buy produce that is damaged or wilted, or that has been improperly stored.

Whenever possible, buy frozen foods instead of canned foods. Canning procedures (blanching, sterilizing, and soaking) destroy nutrients.

Whenever possible, buy produce that was picked when fully ripe. It is higher in nutrients than produce picked when green.

FOOD STORAGE

Avoid storing foods for a long time.

Avoid exposing food to light, especially milk. As little as 2 hours of light can decrease the riboflavin content of milk by 20% to 80%. Keep milk cold and covered.

Refrigerate fruits and vegetables immediately to slow enzyme activity and retain nutrients; keep produce in the refrigerator crisper or in moisture-proof bags.

Avoid storing vegetables after they have been cut, because air can destroy nutrients (oxidation). Wrap cut produce tightly.

Store frozen foods at 0°F or below; even the nutrients in canned foods will be preserved better if stored below 65°F.

FOOD PREPARATION

Wash produce, but don't soak, to avoid leaching nutrients.

Use the dark outer leaves of salad plants whenever possible. They are higher in vitamins and iron than the light inner leaves.

Avoid peeling and paring vegetables before cooking because a valuable layer of nutrients is stored directly beneath the skin. If necessary, scrape or pare as thin a layer as possible.

Avoid cutting produce into small pieces: The larger the surface area, the greater the nutrient loss.

Prepare vegetables as close to serving time as possible to avoid excessive exposure to light and air.

Inactivate oxidative enzymes with an acidic solution (eg, lemon juice, salad dressings) because oxidation destroys vitamins and causes fruits (eg, bananas) and vegetables to brown.

COOKING

Eat some fruits and vegetables raw.

Cook produce in as little water as possible to avoid leaching vitamins. Stir-fry, steam, microwave, or pressure-cook vegetables to retain nutrients.

Shorten cooking time as much as possible by
Cooking vegetables to the tender-crunchy, rather than to the mushy stage of doneness
Covering the pan to retain heat
Starting foods in a hot pan or hot water to speed heating time

Use aluminum, stainless steel, glass, or enamel cookware to retain vitamin C because cooking in copper pots can destroy vitamin C.

Cook vegetables in their skin whenever possible.

Don't thaw frozen vegetables before cooking.

If water is used in cooking, save and use as stock for soups, gravies, or sauces.

Cook only as much as needed at a time. Reheating vegetables causes considerable loss of vitamins.

Don't add baking soda to vegetables while cooking: Alkaline solutions destroy thiamine (vitamin B_1), riboflavin (vitamin B_2), and vitamin C.

Don't toast or brown dry rice before steaming so that the thiamine content can be retained.

Food-Borne Illness

On an average day, almost 20,000 Americans experience a food-borne illness, with approximately 25 cases ending in death daily (Schardt and Schmidt, 1995). According to the Centers for Disease Control and Prevention, 97% of the cases of food-borne illness that occurred between 1983 and 1987 could have been prevented by improved food handling practices (National Live Stock and Meat Board, 1993). Although food-borne illness can be transmitted by any food, animal products are the most frequent vehicles.

Bacteria can be blamed for almost 90% of all food-borne illness, with chemicals, viruses, and parasites causing the remaining cases. *Salmonella, Staphylococcus aureus, Clostridium botulinum*, and *Clostridium perfringens* are well known bacterial culprits that have been overshadowed by more virulent bacterial strains (eg, *Escherichia coli* 0157:H7) and by bacteria that are able to grow at low temperatures (eg, *Listeria monocytogenes*).

The most common symptoms of food-borne illness may be mistaken for the flu: diarrhea, nausea, vomiting, fever, abdominal pain, and headaches. Most cases are self-limiting and run their course within a few days. Symptoms that warrant medical attention include bloody diarrhea (possible *E. coli* 0157:H7 infection), a stiff neck with severe headache and fever (possible meningitis related to *Listeria*), excessive diarrhea or vomiting (possible life-threatening dehydration), and any symptoms that persist for more than 3 days. Infants, pregnant women, the elderly, and people with compromised immune systems (people with acquired immunodeficiency syndrome [AIDS] or cancer, organ transplant recipients, people taking corticosteroids) are particularly vulnerable to the effects of food poisoning.

The major cause of food-borne infections is unsanitary food handling. To reduce the risk of contamination (see display, Safe Food Handling), proper personal hygiene and handwashing must be practiced by all food handlers. Steps must be taken to prevent cross-contamination between raw and cooked foods and through food handlers. Because heat kills most bacteria, thorough cooking of meat and fish is vital, as is pasteurization of all milk products. Adequate refrigeration inhibits the growth of bacteria.

The majority of food-borne illness that occurs worldwide is caused by salmonellae, which are found in the intestinal tracts of humans and domestic and wild warm-blooded animals. Salmonellae can easily pass from the intestinal tract to food during preparation without proper handwashing. In the United States, there have been large increases in *Salmonella enteritidis* infections caused by eggs: Salmonellae on the shells can contaminate the egg during preparation and service. Even uncracked eggs have been implicated for the sudden increase in *S. enteritidis* infections. Salmonellae infect about half of poultry broiler carcasses, but only about 1% of beef and lamb carcasses.

Shigella bacteria are found only in human feces; no animal source is known. Infected food handlers and unsanitary conditions are responsible for most cases of infection; cold salads are most frequent source. Some people with the infection are asymptomatic, yet are carriers of the bacteria. Common symptoms include severe diarrhea that is sometimes bloody, nausea, headaches, chills, and dehydration. Children 1 to 4 years of age are most frequently affected.

Safe Food Handling

PURCHASING

- Note "sell by" and "use by" dates. Do not buy items beyond the "sell by" date. The "use by" date applies to use at home after purchase. Both dates are based on quality concerns (taste, texture, smell, appearance); they do not guarantee that a product is not contaminated, especially after the package seal is broken.
- Do not buy items with holes or tears in the packaging.
- When possible, put raw meat, fish, and poultry in a separate plastic bag before placing in the shopping cart in case the packaging leaks.
- If you don't plan to go immediately home after shopping, bring a cooler for perishable items.

HOME STORAGE

- Store perishable and frozen foods in the refrigerator and freezer as soon after shopping as possible.
- Store meat, fish, and poultry in the coldest part of the refrigerator (on a low shelf at the back). Use large cuts of meat and deli meat within 3 to 4 days; use fish and ground meats within 1 to 2 days.
- Keep meat, fish, and poultry in separate plastic bags and on plates while in the refrigerator to contain raw juices.
- Refrigerate perishable foods at 40°F or below. Freezer temperature should be at or below 0°F.
- Position items in the refrigerator so that air can freely circulate.
- Keep the interior of the refrigerator and freezer clean.
- Handle foods to be put in your home freezer as little as possible to keep bacteria at a minimum before freezing. Freezing does not kill bacteria but merely stops their growth; the bacteria then continue to multiply when the food is thawed.
- Use freezer wrap or freezer bags to preserve food quality during long-term freezing.

DEFROSTING

- Thaw frozen meat, fish, and poultry in the refrigerator in a plastic bag on a dish or pan.
- Foods defrosted in the microwave should be cooked immediately.
- Never defrost meat, fish, or poultry at room temperature.

COOKING

- Use a meat thermometer for roasts, steaks over 2″ thick, and poultry. Place thermometer in the thickest portion of the meat, being careful not to touch bone or fat. Because cooking continues after meat is removed from the oven, cook to 5° below the following recommended temperatures:

Meat

Medium rare	150°	
Medium	160°	
Well done	170°	
Ground		
meats	160°	} or until juices run clear
poultry	165°	
Poultry	180°	
Pork	160°	

- Cook stuffing to 165°F, even if cooked separately.
- Avoid using very low oven temperature roasting methods (below 300°F) and long or overnight cooking.
- Do not use paper bags for roasting.
- Cook commercially frozen stuffed poultry from the frozen state and keep it in the freezer until time to start cooking. If stuffing is made in advance at home, store it separately in the refrigerator. Stuff the bird just before putting it into the hot oven, or cook separately.
- Do not partially precook food and then finish later.
- When basting during grilling or broiling, apply sauce to cooked surfaces only. Meat and poultry can be recontaminated when brushed with bristles that have been in contact with raw or undercooked foods.
- Simmer all home-canned vegetables, meat, and poultry for 10 to 20 minutes before tasting.
- Cook eggs until whites are completely firm and yolks begin to thicken.

(continued)

Safe Food Handling (Continued)

DEFROSTING

- Microwave carefully. For a low-wattage oven, cook food longer or at a higher setting than directed. Cover and rotate food for even cooking. Let food stand outside the oven, if directed; food continues to cook as it stands.

SERVING

- Serve foods immediately after cooking or refrigerate promptly.
- When serving from a buffet, keep hot foods hot—above 140°F—and cold foods cold—below 40°F. Foods that are held for more than 2 hours at a temperature between 60°F and 125°F may not be safe to eat. When replenishing the buffet, do not mix fresh food with food that has been out for serving.
- Serve cooked food on clean plates with clean utensils.
- Do not serve baby foods directly from the jar or can to avoid contaminating any remaining food.

LEFTOVERS

- Remove the stuffing from all leftover cooked meat, poultry, or fish before storing, and store it in the refrigerator in separate container.
- Refrigerate leftover meat, fish, poultry, broth, and gravy immediately after a meal. To hasten cooling, use small, shallow containers, and cut large portions of meat into smaller pieces. Wrap leftovers before refrigerating. Use within 3 to 4 days; reheat to 160°. Freeze them if they are to be kept longer than a few days.
- Heat leftovers thoroughly; boil broths and gravies for several minutes before reusing.
- Use only containers approved for food to store leftovers.
- Never store cleaning supplies and pesticides with food or in food containers such as soda bottles and food jars.

Humans are the most important source of *S. aureus*; 40% to 50% of healthy people carry this bacteria (Ollinger-Snyder and Matthews, 1996). *Staphylococcus* is most frequently found in the nose and throat; on the skin; and in infected boils, pimples, cuts, abrasions, and burns. It is easily spread to food when sanitary food handling practices are not followed; infection occurs when a food that contains a toxin produced by *Staphylococcus* is consumed. Meat, poultry, salads containing meat or poultry, cheese, egg products, starchy salads, custards, and cream-filled desserts are most often implicated. Symptoms of vomiting and diarrhea may last 1 to 2 days; death occurs infrequently.

C. botulinum produces a toxin so potent that it is usually fatal. Home-canned, low-acid foods that have not been properly processed are a frequent cause of botulism. However, unexpected foods such as fried onions and chopped garlic have also caused outbreaks. As a precaution, cans whose clear liquids have turned milky, cans that are swollen or dented, jars with cracks or loose-fitting lids, and any can or jar that has an off-odor when opened should all be discarded.

C. perfringens, spore-forming bacteria, are pervasive in the environment—in human and animal intestines, soil, dust, insects, and sewage. Because they are anaerobic, they grow where there is little or no oxygen. Once ingested, the organism produces a chemical toxin in the GI tract if conditions are appropriate. *C. perfringens* is sometimes referred to tas "the cafeteria germ" because outbreaks frequently occur when large amounts of food cool slowly, either in the refrigerator or in chafing dishes or steam tables that fail to keep food hot enough. Symptoms are usually mild and include diarrhea that in most cases lasts less than a day; however, consequences can be serious for the elderly and people with ulcers.

E. coli, which is found in the intestinal tract of humans and warm-blooded animals and in water contaminated by human or animal feces, was once considered an infrequent cause of food-borne illness in America, but it has been responsible for traveler's diarrhea elsewhere. However, in 1982 a virulent strain, *E. coli* 0157:H7, was identified as a food-borne pathogen that is capable of causing severe and potentially fatal illness. Undercooked beef, especially ground beef, is the most frequent source, although unpasteurized milk, and plant foods that have been fertilized with raw manure, irrigated with contaminated water, or cross contaminated by human contact, have also been implicated. General symptoms include severe abdominal cramps and watery diarrhea. Hemorrhagic colitis can occur and may lead to hemolytic-uremic syndrome, which is characterized by severe anemia and renal failure. Central nervous system complications include strokes and seizures. The Centers for Disease Control and Prevention (CDC) estimates that 20,000 Americans become ill each year from *E. coli* 0157:H7, with as many as 500 cases annually ending in death (Schardt and Schmidt, 1995).

Listeria monocytogenes has been recognized as an animal pathogen for more than 50 years, but has only recently been identified as a serious food-borne pathogen that causes the illness known as listeriosis. Symptoms, which may begin from 1 day to several weeks after the onset of infection, include sudden occurrence of fever, chills, headache, backache, occasional abdominal pain, and diarrhea in adults, and respiratory distress, refusal to drink, and vomiting in infants. Septicemia, meningitis, and meningo-encephalitis are complications that may result in death. Infection can cause abortion in pregnant women. Contaminated deli-type salads, processed meats, milk, cheese, and undercooked chicken are blamed for outbreaks of listeriosis. Increased surveillance by the FDA found *Listeria* in a variety of dairy products; this resulted in numerous recalls for chocolate milk, ice cream mix, ice cream novelties, and brie and other soft-ripened cheeses. Because *Listeria* is so widespread, thrives in cold temperatures, and appears to be able to survive short-term pasteurization, it poses a serious threat to public health.

Yersinia enterocolitica, an anaerobic organism that is able to grow in normal refrigeration, is most often found in pork, but outbreaks have been linked to contaminated meat, poultry, seafood from sewage-contaminated water, milk, chocolate milk, and tofu. Symptoms of infection include diarrhea, which may be bloody, fever, and severe lower abdominal pain that mimics acute appendicitis. Young children appear to be most vulnerable. The elderly and people with compromised immune systems may develop complications of reactive arthritic or anemic conditions, heart problems, and in rare cases, meningitis.

Campylobacter jejuni has been recognized as one of the leading causes of diarrhea in the United States. In most areas of the United States, the number of cases of food-borne illness that are caused by *Campylobacter jejuni* is equal to, or exceeds, the number caused by *Salmonella* and *Shigella* combined (National Live Stock and Meat Board, 1993). *C. jejuni* is found primarily in the intestines of poultry, shellfish, livestock, and even pets; fecal excrement can contaminate foods. Undercooked poultry and meats, raw milk, and untreated water all have been vehicles for transmission. Symptoms of infection—diarrhea, muscle pain, headache, fever, nausea, and vomiting—can range from mild to severe, but they are rarely life-threatening.

A strain of *Vibrio cholerae* is responsible for mild gastroenteritis, soft-tissue infections, and septicemia. Outbreaks, which are related to eating undercooked, contaminated crabs and raw oysters or other shellfish, are generally limited in the United States to the coastal areas.

Cryptosporidium is a parasite that is found in the GI tracts of warm-blooded animals; cryptosporidiosis is the resultant illness. Although cryptosporidiosis was once rare in the United States, it is now recognized as a frequent cause of day-care and community illness, and is considered "an emerging parasite/pathogen" (National Live Stock and Meat Board, 1993). Foods of animal origin, vegetables, and contaminated water are potential carriers of the parasite. Profuse watery diarrhea, abdominal cramps, and fever, due to parasitic invasion of the intestinal cells, usually subside within 1 to 2 weeks. However, people with compromised immune systems may suffer from unremitting debilitating and wasting disease.

Vibrio vulnificus, a naturally occurring bacterium found in coastal and brackish waters of the United States, is emerging as a new food-borne pathogen (Ross et al, 1994). The most frequent source of *V. vulnificus*, which is found in high numbers in seawater that is above 20°C, is raw shellfish, especially raw oysters. Although infection occurs rarely in healthy people, immunocompromised people are at risk for infection, as are people with achlorhydria, chronic liver disease, and/or hemochromatosis. The bacteria cross the GI wall and invade the bloodstream, leading to primary septicemia. Symptoms include fever, chills, skin lesions, nausea, vomiting, diarrhea, hypotension, and shock. Mortality ranges from 46% to 75%, and near 100% in hypotensive clients (Ross et al, 1994). Prevention focuses on obtaining seafood from approved sources only, and cooking it thoroughly; *V. vulnificus* survives in both shell-stock and shucked oysters after harvest of contaminated oysters.

Naturally Occurring Toxicants in Food

"Natural" ingredients in food include the energy nutrients (carbohydrates, protein, fat, and alcohol), essential nutrients (vitamins and minerals), dietary fiber, and naturally occurring compounds like caffeine and sterols. However, certain toxins and antinutrients may also be natural ingredients in foods; therefore, "natural" foods are not synonymous with "safe" foods.

Naturally occurring toxicants are present as normal ingredients in many plant foods (Table 8-5), because plants produce these toxins to protect themselves from predators. It is estimated that we consume 10,000 times more natural toxins by weight than manmade pesticides. Still, the quantity of natural toxins consumed is generally so small that health is not endangered unless large amounts are eaten over a long period of time. A varied diet is the best assurance against untoward effects of both natural and "unnatural" toxins. Goitrogens can be classified as antinutrients because they induce goiter by their antithyroid action. Goitrogens are prevalent in members of the *Brassica* genus: cabbage, turnips, mustard greens, and radishes. Avidin, another antinutrient that destroys the vitamin biotin, is found in raw egg white.

Table 8-5
Naturally Occurring Plant Toxicants

Toxin	Effect	Food Source
Protease inhibitors	Inhibit proteolytic enzyme activity of certain enzymes	Legumes, including a trypsin inhibitor in raw soybeans Also in wheat, oats, barley, rice, and potatoes
Hemagglutinins	Agglutinate RBC; cause inflammation of GI tract, local hemorrhages	Mainly found in seeds, with lesser amounts in leaves, bark, roots, and tubers Found in soybeans, kidney beans, black beans, and wax beans Largely destroyed in the GI tract; only small amounts are absorbed
Favism	Hemolytic anemia in sensitive individuals with inherited metabolic deficiency Most common among people from Mediterranean area or Asia	Fava or broad beans
Hepatotoxins (*Senecio* alkaloids)	Delayed liver damage Potent liver toxins at low to moderate exposure	Seeds of the *Senecio* genus, which grow interspersed with grains, contaminate grains or corn during mechanical harvest
Aflatoxin	Hepatoxic and carcinogenic	Fungal mold on peanuts and corn

ECONOMIC FEASIBILITY

Consumers are faced with the challenge of selecting an adequate diet, usually within a given food budget, from approximately 12,000 different items found in the average supermarket. Suggestions for getting the most nutrition for the food dollar appear in the display, Supermarket Savvy.

Supermarket Savvy

Eat before you shop.

Shop without the children whenever possible.

Note special sales and stock up on nonperishables as much as storage space and budget will allow.

Do not go down an aisle more than once.

Read labels and compare unit prices.

Resist impulse buying.

Ask for a raincheck if the store runs out of a sale item.

Make sure items on sale are properly priced to avoid paying the regular price.

PLAN AHEAD

Make a list and stick to it.

Organize items on your list according to the store's layout to save time and energy and reduce the risk of impulse buying while looking for needed items.

(continued)

Supermarket Savvy *(Continued)*

COUPONS

Clip and use coupons only for items that you normally purchase. You don't save any money if you use a coupon to purchase something you don't use or need.

Use coupons for a competitor's brand of an item only if it saves you money and the quality is comparable. Getting a few cents off an over-priced item isn't much of a bargain.

If possible, shop at a store that doubles or triples coupons.

GENERIC BRANDS

Try various products to determine if the quality is acceptable.

Use generic brands when acceptable. Nutritionally, generic foods are similar to name brands—the difference is in the size and uniformity of the pieces. Use generic products in recipes in which appearance and uniformity are not important, such as casseroles and soups.

AVOID WASTE

Do not buy spoiled food, bulging cans, or produce that is wilted, decayed, bruised, or filled with soft spots.

Buy perishables, especially frozen foods, last and put them away first.

Avoid buying frozen food that has been partially thawed.

Check expiration dates (usually a "sell by" date).

Rotate food at home, using the oldest food first.

COMPARISON SHOP

Check unit prices to compare values.

Be aware that the economy size is not always cheaper.

Buy the economy size if it is cheaper and you can use it or store it without wasting it.

Cans of sliced or diced fruits and vegetables are generally cheaper than whole or half styles.

Frozen vegetables sold with sauces, nuts, or other ingredients cost more per serving than plain vegetables. Add your own toppings.

Compare price per serving for meats, not price per pound.

In general, the larger cuts of meat and whole chickens are cheaper than smaller pieces. If freezer space allows, buy large cuts and cut them up yourself.

Shop in a store that regularly offers lower prices instead of choosing a store that has one or two items you need on sale.

MARKED-DOWN ITEMS

Buy day-old bread that has been marked down to use for stuffing, bread crumbs, bread pudding, or casseroles.

Buy marked-down undamaged produce only if you intend to use it immediately.

BULK FOODS

Compare prices: the savings on some bulk items may be up to 50%, whereas other items (such as flour) may cost more.

Buy only as much as you need.

For added safety, look for items that are dispensed by gravity or from containers with close-fitting covers.

Avoid bins that do not have scoops attached because unattached scoops could fall on the floor or get buried in the food.

FOOD WAREHOUSES

(No-frills stores with minimal service)

Bring your own bags or boxes and be prepared to pack them yourself.

Although brand names are available, the variety is less than in a supermarket and usually is inconsistent.

FOOD CO-OPS

(Nonprofit stores run by members)

Take advantage of this opportunity if you can.

Be prepared to volunteer several hours a month in order to participate, but the savings are worth it, especially for perishables.

(continued)

Supermarket Savvy (Continued)

CHANGE YOUR EATING HABITS FOR BETTER HEALTH AND BIGGER SAVINGS

Consider using nonfat dry milk for cooking or drinking. It has all the nutrients of whole milk with none of the fat.

Eat less red meat and more poultry.

Serve an occasional meatless meal based on eggs, cheese, or dried beans and peas.

Avoid packaged items and convenience products that are often laden with salt and cost more than the homemade version.

Buy fruits and vegetables in season.

Avoid empty calorie extras such as soft drinks, candy, cakes, pies, doughnuts, sweet rolls, cookies, and traditional snack foods.

BEWARE OF SUPERMARKETING

The dairy case is usually located farthest from the front door so that people just wanting to buy milk have to walk through the entire store, giving them the opportunity to buy something else.

The prime selling area is at eye level (adult height for adult items and child height for child items). Bargains may be available at higher and lower levels.

End-of-aisle displays are not always sale items.

Checkout line goodies are obvious temptations to impulse buying: Resist the urge.

KEY CONCEPTS

- Dietary excesses play a role in five of the leading causes of death in the United States. Dietary advice from numerous health and government agencies advocate moderation and balance for disease prevention.

- The RDA are amounts of essential nutrients that are considered to be adequate to meet the nutritional needs of most healthy people. Because the RDA are set higher than actual requirements (which is the amount needed to prevent a deficiency), an individual may consume less than the RDA and not develop a deficiency.

- The purpose of the Dietary Guidelines for Americans is to help the public choose diets that are nutritionally adequate, promote health and well-being, and reduce the risk of chronic disease.

- The Food Guide Pyramid is a graphic illustration of the Dietary Guidelines for Americans. It recommends ranges of servings for each of the food groups; balance, moderation, and variety are its underlying concepts.

- The focus of nutrition labels has shifted away from avoiding nutritional deficiencies (which are now rare in the U.S.) toward avoiding nutritional excesses, namely of fat, saturated fat, cholesterol, and sodium.

- The percent Daily Value listed for fat, saturated fat, carbohydrate, and dietary fiber on food labels is based on a 2000-calorie diet; those percentages underestimate the contribution these nutrients make in diets containing fewer than 2000 calories.

- Cultural, sociodemographic, and individual variables have a much greater impact on a person's food preferences and aversions than do nutritional considerations.

- Although culture defines what is edible, how food is handled, prepared, and consumed; what foods are appropriate for particular groups within the culture; the meaning of food and eating; attitudes toward body size; and the relationship between diet and health, food habits vary considerably among individuals and families within a cultural group.

- Religion may have a greater impact on food habits than nationality or culture.

- A seemingly nutritionally adequate diet may provide suboptimal levels of certain nutrients if the food was improperly handled or overprocessed. A food begins to lose nutrients when harvesting or processing begins; the more that is done to a food, the greater the nutrient losses. Food processing has the greatest impact on water-soluble vitamins, minerals, and fiber.

- Bacteria are blamed for the majority of food-borne illnesses; viruses, parasites, and chemicals account for about 10% of cases. Unsanitary food handling is responsible for most of food-borne illness. Groups most susceptible to food-borne illness include pregnant women, infants, older adults, and people with compromised immune systems.

- Foods contain significantly more "natural" toxins than manmade chemicals, yet the risk of toxicity is small unless large amounts are eaten over a long period of time. A varied diet can minimize the risk of toxicity of both natural and manmade toxins.

 FOCUS ON **CRITICAL THINKING**

The following is a typical day's intake for Jennifer Matthews, a 20-year-old college student who is "chronically dieting" and eats a "high-protein" diet to keep her size 4 figure: (she is 5′4″ and weighs 108 pounds)

Breakfast: 2 cups coffee with Nutrasweet and heavy cream
1 banana
1 piece buttered white toast with diet jelly
Between morning classes: Diet soda
Lunch: 2 boiled hot dogs without rolls
1 raw carrot
1 bran muffin

Diet soda
After class: microwave popcorn
Diet soda
Dinner: 4 oz. skinless chicken breast salad with Italian dressing
1/2 cup broccoli
fat-free rice cakes
Bedtime: 2 oz cheddar cheese on
    4 "lite" crackers

Although her diet varies with the type of meat and vegetable eaten at dinner, she tries not to deviate from this menu, for fear of "losing control."

Evaluate Jennifer's diet according to the *Dietary Guidelines for Americans*. Specifically, what would you recommend Jennifer eat more of /eat less of to improve her diet?

Evaluate Jennifer's diet according to the Food Guide Pyramid. What groups is she deficient in? Is she consuming an excess from any group?

Plan a nutritionally adequate sample meal plan that is consistent with the *Dietary Guidelines for Americans*.

REFERENCES

Achterberg, C. (1992). A perspective: Challenges of teaching the Dietary Guidelines Graphic. Food and Nutrition News, 64(4), 23–26.

Achterberg, C., McDonnell, E., and Bagby, R. (1994). How to put the Food Guide Pyramid into practice. J Am Diet Assoc, 94(10), 1030–1035.

Allen, A. (1995). The new Nutrition Facts label in the print media: A content analysis. J Am Diet Assoc, 95(3), 348–351.

Axelson, M. (1986). The impact of culture on food-related behavior. Ann Rev Nutr, 6, 345–363.

Domel, S., Alford, B., Cattlett, H., and Gench, B. (1992). Weight control for black women. J Am Diet Assoc, 92(3), 346–347.

Food and Drug Administration (1993). Focus on Food Labeling. Read the Label, Set a Healthy Table. FDA Consumer. DHHS Publication No. (FDA)93-2262. Department of Health and Human Services, Public Health Service, Food and Drug Administration.

International Food Information Council (1994). How are Americans making food choices? IFIC Review, October 1994.

Harland, B., Smith, S., Ellis, R., O'Brien, R., Morris, E. (1992). Comparison of the nutrient intakes of blacks, Siouan Indians, and whites in Columbus County, North Carolina. J Am Diet Assoc, 92(3), 348–350.

Morreale, S., and Schwaartz, N. (1995). Helping Americans eat right: Developing practical and actionable public nutrition education messages based on the ADA Survey of American Dietary Habits. J Am Diet Assoc, 95(3), 305–308.

National Live Stock and Meat Board (1993). Safe Food Backgrounder. Chicago: National Live Stock and Meat Board.

National Research Council (1989). Recommended Dietary Allowances, 10th Edition. Washington, DC: National Academy Press.

Ollinger-Snyder, P. and Matthews, M. (1996). Food safety: Review and implications for dietitians and dietetic technicians. J Am Diet Assoc, 96(2), 163–168.

Ross, E., Guyer, L., Varnes, J., and Rodrick, G. (1994). *Vibrio vulnificus* and molluscan shellfish: The necessity of education for high-risk individuals. J Am Diet Assoc, 94(3), 312–314.

Schardt, D., and Schmidt, S. (1995). Keeping food safe. Nutrition Action Health Letter, 22(3), 4–7.

Terry, R. (1994). Needed: A new appreciation of culture and food behavior. J Am Diet Assoc, 94(5), 501–503.

United States Department of Agriculture, and United States Department of Health and Human Services (1995). Nutrition and Your Health: Dietary Guidelines for Americans. 4th ed. Home and Garden Bulletin No. 232.

United States Department of Health and Human Services, Public Health Service (1988). The Surgeon General's Report on Nutrition and Health. Summary and Recommendations. DHHS (PHS) Publication No. 88-50211.

CHAPTER 9

Assessing Nutritional Status

Chapter Outline

Key Terms

Albumin
Anthropometric Measurements
Creatinine
Creatinine Height Index
Diet History
Food Frequency Record
Food Record

Malnutrition
Midarm Circumference
Midarm Muscle Circumference
Nutrition Assessment
Percent Usual Body Weight
Percent Weight Change
Prealbumin

Retinol-binding Protein
Screening
Transferrin
Triceps Skinfold
24-hour Recall
Urea

*N*utritional status, or the state of balance between nutrient supply (intake) and demand (requirement), has a significant impact on both health and disease. For the "well" client, an optimal nutritional status helps maintain health, promotes normal growth and development, supports activity, and protects against disease. During illness, an optimal nutritional status can reduce the risk of complications and hasten recovery.

Malnutrition, a general term that literally means "bad" nutrition, may be caused by nutritional excesses (eg, obesity) or deficiencies (other variables and classifications of malnutrition are listed in Table 9-1). Severe deficiencies of specific nutrients (eg, vitamin C) can produce specific nutritional disorders (eg, scurvy); mild nutritional deficiencies can interfere with overall ability to function, quality of life, and sense of well-being. In the hospitalized population, a poor nutritional status, especially protein–calorie malnutrition (PCM), is associated with prolonged hospitalization,

Table 9-1
Variables and Classifications of Malnutrition

Variables	Classifications
Type	Overnutrition (ie, obesity) or undernutrition
Cause	Endogenous (ie, faulty metabolism) or exogenous (ie, inadequate intake)
Nutrients	Specific (ie, one nutrient) or multiple
Degree	Mild, moderate, or severe
Duration	Acute or chronic
Outcome	Reversible or irreversible

poor wound healing, lowered resistance to infection, poor clinical outcome, and death in susceptible clients (Mears, 1994). Because nutrient deficiencies progress in a sequential and predictable manner, parameters that are used to identify deficiencies vary with the stage of the disorder (see display, Sequential Development of Malnutrition/Nutrition Assessment Methods).

Nutrition assessment is the process of collecting and interpreting data for the purpose of identifying nutritional risks and poor nutritional status. Although the benefits of early recognition of malnutrition are well known, there is no universally accepted, definitive tool for use in evaluating nutritional status; assessment parameters vary among institutions, settings, and populations (Foltz et al, 1993). Often, professional judgment is as important as objective criteria.

The process of assessment is followed by planning (determining what actions are necessary to achieve nutritional goals, when and how the actions are to be taken, and who should implement the actions), implementation (putting the plan into action), and evaluation (determining the effectiveness of the plan and revising the plan as needed) (see display, Nutritional Care Process).

(text continues on page 232)

Sequential Development of Malnutrition/Nutrition Assessment Methods

Sequential Development of Malnutrition			Assessment Methods
Primary deficiency related to inadequate intake	and/or	Secondary deficiency related to altered digestion, absorption, metabolism and/or excretion	Dietary data, medical–socioeconomic data
↓			
Decreased nutrient content in cells and tissues			Laboratory data
↓			
Biochemical lesions and abnormal metabolism			Laboratory data
↓			
Anatomic lesions and signs of deficiency			Anthropometric measurement, clinical findings

Nutritional Care Process: Assessment → Planning → Implementation → Evaluation

The nutritional care process, like the nursing process, is a systematic approach used to identify the client's needs, formulate plans to meet those needs, initiate a plan or assign others to implement it, and evaluate the effectiveness of the plan. As such, it is appropriate for all clients. The following format, which is used throughout the life cycle and clinical practice units of this book, serves as a guideline for determining optimum nutritional care.

ASSESSMENT

Assessment is a two-step process that involves both the collection and interpretation of data. In addition to the general assessment criteria listed in each clinical chapter, dietary and nutritional risk factors and signs and symptoms of health disorders should be evaluated for their impact on intake and nutritional status.

Nursing Diagnosis

Nursing diagnoses may relate to nutrition either directly (ie, altered nutrition is a problem) or indirectly (ie, change in diet is one of several interventions that will help eliminate a "non-nutritional" problem). "Altered Nutrition: Less than Body Requirements" applies most obviously to people who are underweight. However, less obvious is the impact health alterations and medical treatments have on nutrient intake, digestion, absorption, metabolism, and excretion. For instance, "Altered Nutrition: Less than Body Requirements" may also be appropriate for clients with malabsorption syndrome secondary to pancreatic disease who are unable to digest and absorb adequate calories and nutrients.

Likewise, because nutrition is important all along the wellness–illness continuum, nutrition intervention may be appropriate not only for restoring health in an "ill" client, but also for maintaining or improving health status in a "well" individual. For instance, a "healthy" man with a high cholesterol level who expresses interest in a low-fat, low-cholesterol diet may have the nursing diagnosis of "Health Seeking Behaviors, related to lack of knowledge of a heart-healthy diet and a desire to learn."

Possible nutrition-related nursing diagnoses include, but are not limited to (North American Nursing Diagnosis Association, 1994):

Altered Nutrition, More than body requirements

Altered Nutrition, Less than body requirements

Altered Nutrition: Potential for more than body requirements

Risk for Infection

Constipation

Diarrhea

Fluid Volume Excess

Fluid Volume Deficit

Risk for Fluid Volume Deficit

Risk for Aspiration

Impaired Tissue Integrity

Altered Oral Mucous Membrane

Impaired Skin Integrity

Risk for Impaired Skin Integrity

Ineffective Management of Therapeutic Regimen

Noncompliance

Health Seeking Behaviors

Activity Intolerance

Fatigue

Altered Health Maintenance

Feeding Self-Care Deficit

Impaired Swallowing

Ineffective Breastfeeding

Knowledge Deficit

Dysfunctional Grieving

Throughout the clinical section of this book, only one nursing diagnosis is given as an example for each medical disorder discussed. Obviously, they represent only one way of looking at a problem; they may not be appropriate or specific for *individuals*, nor are they meant to exclude other diagnoses. In clinical practice, a nursing diagno-
(continued)

Nutritional Care Process: Assessment → Planning → Implementation → Evaluation *(Continued)*

sis is identified only after thorough analysis of the data.

PLANNING AND IMPLEMENTATION

From a nutritional perspective, client goals are objectives that may be achieved through dietary intervention; they are determined on an individual basis after priorities are established. Although planning for high-risk clients may be the responsibility of the dietitian, the nurse may do the planning for healthy clients and those with minor problems.

General short-term client goals that may be appropriate for all clients are to maintain/restore optimal nutritional status and to allow as normal an intake as possible by individualizing the diet according to the client's food habits, preferences, and tolerances. A general long-term goal is to promote good nutritional practices to reduce the risk of chronic diet-related diseases such as obesity, diabetes, hypertension, atherosclerosis, and certain kinds of cancer. Additional goals that may be appropriate for hospitalized clients are to alleviate side effects of the disease or its treatment, if possible, and to prevent complications or recurrences of the disorder, if appropriate.

Inherent in planning individual client goals are the following general considerations:

- Diet orders are not always appropriate.
- Eating behaviors and food preferences may revert to childhood patterns during illness and stress.
- It is not only important that the proper food be served, but moreso that it be consumed. The manner in which food is presented and the attitudes of the health care team members regarding the diet may have a large influence on the client's acceptance.
- Restrictive diets should be progressed as soon as possible to ensure an adequate intake and increase the client's sense of well-being.
- Communication between other members of the health care team is vital.
- Assessment and evaluation are ongoing processes.

- The optimal diet in theory may not be practical for an individual in either the clinical or home setting, depending on the client's prognosis, support systems, level of intelligence and motivation, willingness to cooperate, emotional health, financial status, religious or ethnic background, and other medical conditions.

The *Nursing Interventions* sections of this book deal with diet management, client teaching, and monitoring. *Diet management* provides general guidelines for health maintenance or restoration through general dietary changes, such as increase/decrease, limit/reduce, avoid/encourage, modify/maintain, promote, and monitor. Specific levels of nutrients or foods allowed depend on the client's condition and the physician's discretion and should be revised as needed.

Client teaching is another important facet of nursing intervention; it may be the nurse's responsibility to provide or reinforce diet instructions to the client and family. Diet instructions are generally most effective when both verbal and written instructions are provided. Clients should always be advised to eliminate any foods not tolerated and to alert the physician if a conflict exists between the diet and religious beliefs, if adverse side effects to the diet develop, or if special foods required by the diet are difficult to locate or are too costly. Compliance should be encouraged, and support and assistance offered. Ideally, teaching should occur over time.

Monitoring is done on an ongoing basis to evaluate the client's tolerance and compliance to the diet and the effectiveness of the diet interventions. Other individual-, disease-, and symptom-related criteria may be indicated.

EVALUATION

The effectiveness of the nutritional care plan is evaluated by examining the client's progress toward achieving the stated goals. Findings should be communicated to the other members of the health care team, and the nutritional plan of care should be revised as needed.

In most health care facilities, the responsibility for nutritional assessment and support is shared by the physician, the dietitian, and the nurse. By communicating and using diagnostic skills, nurses are able to obtain nutritional screening data through routine nursing histories and physical examinations. Depending on the setting and availability of personnel, the nurse may assist with and coordinate nutritional care activities, or may be responsible for identifying high-risk clients. The nurse's abilities in coordinating activities among health care team members, and maintaining close, continual interaction with the client and family place him or her in an ideal position to facilitate the nutritional care process, make referrals as needed, and initiate nutritional care.

LEVELS OF ASSESSMENT

Obviously, the more information that is obtained from a variety of sources (Table 9-2), the more accurate and reliable the assessment will be. However, comprehensive nutrition assessments are not always appropriate or necessary, depending on the purpose of the assessment and the availability of equipment, time, personnel, and funds. Assessment levels range from minimal (screening) to comprehensive (nutrition assessment); both can be "custom-made" for a particular population, medical disorder, or setting.

Screening

Screening is a simple, quick, and cost-effective process that uses a minimum amount of information to identify clients who are at moderate or high nutritional risk. In the clinical setting, clients who are found to be at moderate or high risk are followed with a nutrition assessment performed by a dietitian, with the ultimate goal of providing timely and effective nutrition care (Krasker and Balogun, 1995). Actual data obtained and definition of risk vary among settings, the population group being screened, the availability of data, and the screening objectives. Screening can be custom-designed for a particular population (eg, pregnant women) or for a specific disorder (eg, cardiac disease). Screens can be completed by a dietitian, diet technician, or other qualified health care professional (Council of Practice Quality Management

Table 9-2
Sources of Data Collection

Source	Data Collected
History	Dietary data
	Medical–socioeconomic data
Physical	Medical–socioeconomic data
	Anthropometric and physiologic measurements
	Clinical observations
Laboratory studies	Biochemical data

Committee, 1994). Often, a routine screen may occur during the initial nursing history and physical examination (Krasker and Balogun, 1995).

To be both useful and efficient in the clinical setting, screening tools must rely on data that are routinely gathered on admission to a hospital or health care facility. Much controversy exists about the accuracy and validity of screening data, especially anthropometric and biochemical data. Some studies have found that anthropometric measurements alone, such as weight loss greater than 10 pounds, are sufficient to predict mortality. Other clinical studies have shown that both anthropometric and laboratory data are necessary to evaluate the nutritional status of hospitalized clients. Most experts agree that the most accurate method of identifying future nutritional risk is a combination of both selected anthropometric and laboratory data.

Data may be recorded on a printed screening form (ie, checklist) and entered into the medical record regardless of the result, or documentation may be by exception only, so that only clients at moderate or high risk have results noted in the medical record (Krasker and Balogun, 1995). A routine hospital screen is likely to focus on height, weight, significant unintentional weight loss, and serum albumin. Other parameters that may be included in a hospital screen are listed in the display, Possible Screening Parameters. Interpretation of risk is facility-defined, based on the number of abnormal findings obtained. A sample hospital screening tool appears in Figure 9-1. Regardless of what data are gathered, the screening process is not complete until it is evaluated and a relative level of risk is assigned. Clients who are identified to be at no or mild risk may need only to be reevaluated later during their admission to monitor for any deterioration in nutritional status. A nutrition assessment is indicated for clients who are determined to be at moderate or severe risk for the purposes of quantifying the degree of malnutrition, providing effective nutrition care, and establishing a baseline for subsequent nutrition intervention.

In a wellness setting, a screening tool such as that featured in Figure 9-2 may be used to measure nutritional risk in the elderly, based on body weight, eating habits, living environment, and functional status. This screen, which may be completed by professionals in health care or social service programs, is used to identify people who may be candidates for home meal delivery, assistance with shopping or cooking, congregate meal programs, or nutrition intervention and education (NSI, 1991).

Possible Screening Parameters

Height	Food intake history
Weight	Functional status
Significant unintentional weight loss	Hemoglobin/hematocrit
Serum albumin	Total lymphocyte count
Diagnosis	Medications
Food intolerances	Ability to chew and swallow
Allergies	Diet order
Functional status	Nausea/Vomiting/Diarrhea

Nutrition Assessment Screening Sheet

1. Height   ☐ ☐ inches
2. Admission weight   ☐ ☐ ☐ pounds
3. Usual weight   ☐ ☐ ☐ pounds
4. Weight change in last 6–12 months?   ☐ yes ☐ no
5. Change in appetite or food tolerance?   ☐ yes ☐ no
     If yes, specify _____

6. Laboratory values:
     Serum albumin value   ☐ ☐ g/dl
     Hemoglobin level   ☐ ☐ g/dl
     Total lymphocyte count   ☐ ☐ ☐ ☐ cu mm
     Blood urea nitrogen   ☐ ☐ mg/dl
7. Is this patient at nutritional risk? ☐ yes ☐ no
Severity of risk: ☐ mild   ☐ moderate   ☐ severe

Patient's name _____
                             MD initials

Recorder: _____

Date: _____

Physician's name: _____

Determination of risk:

# of abnormal findings	Level of risk
0-1	no nutritional risk
2	mild
3	moderate
≥4	severe risk

Figure 9-1
A copy of the East Orange *Nutritional Screening Form.* Reprinted from March, 1983 Quality Review Bulletin.

Nutrition Assessment

Screening data that indicate a client is at moderate or severe risk for nutritional problems should be followed by a nutrition assessment. Using the screening data as a foundation, a variety of additional objective and subjective data can be analyzed to assess risk and nutritional status: medical and psychosocial data, anthropometric measurements, laboratory data, clinical findings, and dietary data. The process of nutrition assessment continues with the development of a care plan, implementation of interventions, and evaluation of progress toward goals.

Unfortunately, nutrition assessment can be costly and time-consuming, and extensively trained personnel are required to ensure accuracy of results. In the clinical setting, it is used most effectively to assess and monitor moderate- to high-risk clients who have suspected or confirmed PCM.

LEVEL 1 SCREEN

Name: _____ Date: _____

Body Weight

Measure height to the nearest inch and weight to the nearest pound. Record the values below and mark them on the Body Mass Index (BMI) scale to the right. Then use a straight edge (ruler) to connect the two points and circle the spot where this straight line crosses the center line (body mass index). Record the number below.

Healthy older adults should have a BMI between 24 and 27.

Height (in): _____
Weight (lbs): _____
Body Mass Index: _____
(number from center column)

Check any boxes that are true for the individual:

❑ Has lost or gained 10 pounds (or more) in the past 6 months

❑ Body mass index < 24

❑ Body mass index > 27

For the remaining sections, please ask the individual which of the statements (if any) is true for him of her and place a check by each that applies

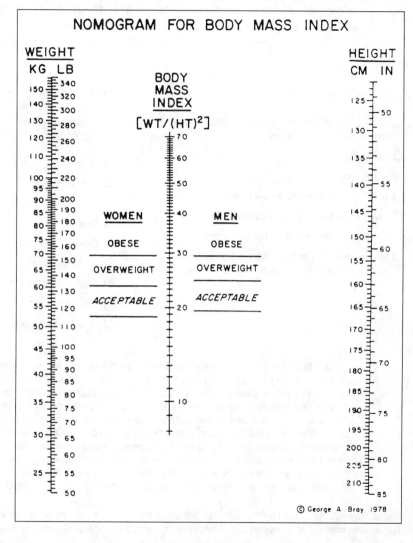

NOMOGRAM FOR BODY MASS INDEX

BODY MASS INDEX [WT/(HT)^2]

© George A Bray 1978

Eating Habits

❑ Does not have enough food to eat each day

❑ Usually eats alone

❑ Does not eat anything on one or more days each month

❑ Has poor appetite

❑ Is on a special diet

❑ Eats vegetables two or fewer times daily

❑ Drinks milk or eats milk products once or not at all daily

❑ Eats fruit or drinks fruit juice once or not at all daily

❑ Eats breads, cereals, pasta, rice, or other grains five or fewer times daily

❑ Has difficulty chewing or swallowing

❑ Has more than one alcoholic drink per day (if woman); more than two drinks per day (if man)

❑ Has pain in mouth, teeth, or gums

Figure 9-2
Level 1 Screen

A physician should be contacted if the individual has gained or lost 10 pounds unexpectedly or without intending to during the past 6 months. A physician should also be notified if the individual's body mass index is above 27 or below 24.

Living Environment

❏ Lives on an income of less than $6000 per year (per individual in the household)

❏ Lives alone

❏ Is housebound

❏ Is concerned about home security

❏ Lives in a home with inadequate heating or cooling

❏ Does not have a stove and/or refrigerator

❏ Is unable or prefers not to spend money on food (<$25–30 per person spent on food each week)

Functional Status

Usually or always needs assistance with (check all that apply):

❏ Bathing

❏ Dressing

❏ Grooming

❏ Toileting

❏ Eating

❏ Walking or moving about

❏ Traveling (outside the home)

❏ Preparing food

❏ Shopping for food or other necessities

If you have checked one or more statements on this screen, the individual you have interviewed may be at risk for poor nutritional status. Please refer this individual to the appropriate health care or social service professional in your area. For example, a dietitian should be contacted for problems with selecting, preparing, or eating a healthy diet, or a dentist if the individual experiences pain or difficulty when chewing or swallowing. Those individuals whose income, lifestyle, or functional status may endanger their nutritional and overall health should be referred to available community services: home-delivered meals, congregate meal programs, transportation services, counseling services, (alcohol abuse, depression, bereavement, etc.), home health care agencies, day care programs, etc.

Please repeat this screen at least once each year—sooner if the individual has a major change in his or her health, income, immediate family (e.g., spouse dies), or functional status.

These materials developed by the Nutrition Screening Initiative, a project of American Academy of Family Physicians, The American Dietetic Association, and the National Council on the Aging, Inc.

Figure 9-2 (Continued)

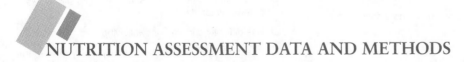

NUTRITION ASSESSMENT DATA AND METHODS

Because no single method that is currently available can assess nutritional status reliably and accurately, a combination of methods is recommended. The following descriptions of selected medical-psychosocial data, anthropometric measurements, laboratory data, clinical findings, and dietary data are intended to make the reader aware of the types of criteria that can be used to assess nutritional status; not all criteria are appropriate or useful for all situations. Possible nutrition assessment parameters appear in the display, Possible Nutrition Assessment Parameters. Exactly which parameters are evaluated is influenced by assessment objectives and other factors that were previously mentioned.

Medical-Psychosocial Data

A variety of medical-psychosocial parameters and potential risks appear in Table 9-3. All positive findings should be evaluated for their actual or potential influence on nutritional requirements secondary to alterations in intake, digestion, absorption, metabolism, or excretion.

Anthropometric Measurements

Anthropometric measurements are measurements of body dimensions, such as height, weight, skinfolds, and various body circumferences, that are used to monitor

---

Possible Nutrition Assessment Parameters

MEDICAL–PSYCHOSOCIAL FACTORS

Diagnosis

Nausea/vomiting

Treatment plan

Medications

GI integrity

Prognosis

Living situation

Socioeconomic status

ANTHROPOMETRIC MEASUREMENTS

Height

Weight

Recent weight history

Triceps skinfolds (TSF)

Mid-arm circumference (MAC)

Mid-arm muscle circumference (MAMC)

LABORATORY

Serum albumin

Total lymphocyte count (TLC)

Serum transferrin

Prealbumin

24-hour urinary creatinine excretion, creatinine height index (CHI)

Urinary urea nitrogen (UUN), state of nitrogen balance

Hemoglobin/hematocrit

Cholesterol

Lipid profile

CLINICAL OBSERVATIONS

Observe for signs and symptoms of malnutrition

DIETARY DATA

24-hour food recall

Food frequency record

Food record

Diet history, including food intolerance, past/present diet modification, vitamin/mineral use, calorie counts, who prepares food, religious impact on food choices

Table 9-3
Medical–Psychosocial Parameters and Potential Risks

Parameter	Potential Risk
Past medical history	History or evidence of
Type of disorder, treatment (including diet and drug)	Pressure ulcers, altered skin integrity cancer
Current illness or chief complaint; review of systems	AIDS or HIV infection
	GI complications (ie, dysphagia, diarrhea, anorexia, nausea, vomiting, constipation)
Surgical history: type, date, development of complications	Catabolic or hypermetabolic conditions (burns, trauma, sepsis)
	Impaired sensory function (ie, loss of taste, smell, vision)
	Chronic renal or cardiac disorders, diabetes and related complications, hypertension
	Dental problems (difficulty chewing, ill-fitting dentures, refusal to wear dentures, missing teeth, mouth or gum sores)
	Inability to communicate
	Osteoporosis or osteomalacia
	Fluid and electrolyte imbalance
	Neurologic or cognitive impairments
	Other acute and chronic disorders
	Adolescent pregnancy, closely spaced pregnancies, three or more pregnancies
	Alcohol or substance abuse
Past and present drug history	History or evidence of
Name of prescription and over the counter drugs used on a regular basis, purpose, dosage, duration of use	Chronic use (ie, laxatives)
	Multiple and concurrent use of drugs
	Drug–nutrient interactions and side effects
Psychosocial data	History or evidence of
Educational background	Illiteracy, language barriers
	Limited knowledge of nutrition, food safety
Culture	Altered/impaired intake related to culture
Religious beliefs	Altered/impaired intake related to religion
Lifestyle	Lack of caregiver/social support system
	Isolation
	Lack of/inadequate cooking arrangements
Economic status	Limited or low income
Other	Limited access to transportation to obtain food
	Limited use/knowledge of community resources
Age	Extremes in age (ie, over 80, very young (premature infant)
Activity	Impaired feeding skills, lack of ability to self-feed, feeding limitations
	Decrease in ability to perform activities of daily living
	Excessive activity

Source: Council on Practice Quality Management Committee (1994). Identifying patients at risk: ADA's definitions for nutrition screening and nutrition assessment. J Am Diet Assoc, 94(8), 838–839.

growth and development in children and to indirectly assess protein and calorie reserves in adults. Accurate equipment and standardized procedures must be used to ensure accurate and precise data collection. In addition, the data must be evaluated according to the appropriate reference standards for the client's age and sex. Potential anthropometric risk factors appear in the display, Potential Anthropometric Risk Factors. Repeated measurements taken over time can measure the degree of

Potential Anthropometric Risk Factors

Obesity

Underweight

Alterations in weight or body mass index, especially recent significant weight loss

Fat wasting; decrease in triceps skinfold

Muscle wasting; decrease in midarm muscle circumference

Amputation

Weight/(length)height (children) >95th percentile or <5th percentile; deviation of more than 2 percentile channels over time

Height(length)/age at or below 5th percentile

Source: Council on Practice Quality Management Committee (1994). Identifying patients at risk: ADA's definitions for nutrition screening and nutrition assessment. J Am Diet Assoc, 94(8), 838–839.

change in nutritional status. However, most changes are not evident until 3 to 4 weeks after they occur (CDA/SSDA, 1992).

Anthropometric measurements have the advantage of being objective, noninvasive, and relatively quick, easy, and inexpensive to obtain. In addition, when taken periodically, they can be used to monitor a client's progress. However, because changes in anthropometric measurements may be slow to occur, they are more reflective of chronic, not acute, changes in nutritional status (Table 9-4).

Inexperience on the part of the assessor, an uncooperative client, and inaccurate equipment are all frequent sources of error. However, self-reported height and weight often are inaccurate and should be used only when actual measurements cannot be obtained. Fluid retention and dehydration can skew measurements. Also, ref-

Table 9-4
Standard Values and Degree of Depletion for Anthropometric Measurements for Adults

	Standard	90% of Standard	80% of Standard	70% of Standard	60% of Standard
TRICEPS SKINFOLD (MM)					
Male	12.5	11.3	10.0	8.8	7.5
Female	16.5	14.9	13.2	11.6	9.0
MIDARM CIRCUMFERENCE (CM)					
Male	29.3	26.3	23.4	20.5	17.6
Female	28.5	25.7	22.8	20.0	17.1
MIDARM MUSCLE CIRCUMFERENCE (CM)					
Male	25.3	22.8	20.2	17.7	15.2
Female	23.2	20.9	18.6	16.2	13.9

erence standards may not be appropriate for all populations because anthropological differences may exist among races. Reference standards must also be adjusted for clients who have had amputations.

MEASURES OF GROWTH AND DEVELOPMENT/UNDER- AND OVER-NUTRITION

Height and weight are useful for assessing undernutrition and overnutrition in adults. In infants and children, length, weight, and head circumference reflect adequacy of growth and development

Length (Children) and Height (Adults)

Infants and children

Measure infants and small children while they are lying down on a measuring board with a movable footboard and an immovable headboard. The child's head is held gently against the immovable headboard while the knees are pushed against the measuring board (to fully extend the legs). The movable footboard is moved until it touches both heels. The child's feet are immediately removed and the footboard held securely so that the measurement can be read and immediately recorded.

Adults

The equipment for measuring height consists of a tape or stick that has been affixed to a vertical device or wall; a movable headpiece that slides easily is attached at a right angle to the vertical surface.

The client stands erect with feet flat on the floor and slightly apart, legs and back straight, and arms at sides. Shoulder blades, buttocks, and heels should touch the wall or surface of the measuring device. The movable headboard is lowered until it firmly touches the crown of the head. The measurement should be recorded immediately.

Weight

Infants and children

Infants and children who are too young to stand up or walk should be weighed while they are lying down on a pediatric scale with a pan.

Based on the child's age and sex, measurements should be plotted on the appropriate growth chart: length/age, weight/age, weight/length. Data can be compared to either reference standards (ie, percentile growth charts) or the child's previous measurements.

The following criteria reflect a potential problem and require further evaluation and counseling:

Weight/height at the 5th percentile or below may indicate underweight or wasting.

Height/age at the 5th percentile or below indicates a risk of growth retardation or stunting.

Weight/height at the 95th percentile or above indicates overweight or possible obesity.

Deviations in the growth pattern or the child's normal percentile channels over time (ie, falling from the 50th percentile for weight down to the 10th percentile) indicate potential abnormality.

Adults

Adults are weighed on a beam-balance scale (or a metabolic scale if client is bedridden), which is checked frequently for accuracy. Bathroom scales are inaccurate and should not be used.

Weigh the client

- On the same scale each time.
- At the same time of day, preferably before breakfast and after the client has voided.
- With the same amount of clothing on each time and without shoes.

Record the weight immediately.

Interpretation of Adult Weight

Weight for height can be compared to any of the following reference standards and evaluated accordingly:

The "rule of thumb" method to obtain estimated ideal body weight (IBW) based on gender and height:

men: 106 lb for 5 ft plus 6 lb for each additional inch

women: 100 lb for 5 ft plus 5 lb for each additional inch

Ideal body weight can be adjusted up or down by 10%, depending on body size. To evaluate a person's actual body weight according to the calculated IBW reference, the following formula is used:

$$\%IBW = (\text{actual weight} \div IBW) \times 100$$

Generally accepted standards based on %IBW are as follows:

>120% of IBW	obese
110–120% of IBW	overweight
90–110% of IBW	IBW
80–90% of IBW	mildly underweight
70–79% of IBW	moderately underweight
<70% of IBW	severely underweight

Metropolitan Life Insurance Height and Weight Tables list desirable weight for height, based on body frame size and gender (see Chapter 13). Its weights are based on mortality data that were collected over a 20-year period from healthy clients. No guidelines are offered to assess weights that deviate from standards.

The 1995 Dietary Guidelines for Americans include a weight for height table with ranges identified as "healthy," "moderate overweight," and "severe overweight." No distinctions are made for gender, age, or body frame size. This table is appropriate for general screening and teaching, but is not intended to be used for nutrition assessment.

Body mass index (BMI) is an estimate of total body mass that is highly correlated to body fat. Nomograms can be used to determine BMI (see Chapter 13), as can the following formula:

$$BMI = \text{weight (kg)/ height squared (m)}$$

Although there is no universal agreement on how to interpret BMI, the following is considered a guideline:

	Men	Women
Morbidly obese	>45.3	>44.7
Severely overweight	>31.0	>32.3
Overweight	>27.7	>27.2
Acceptable weight	20.7–27.8	19.1–27.3
Underweight	<20.7	<19.1

Interpretation of Weight Changes

Because unintentional weight loss is a risk factor for poor nutritional status, weight changes should be assessed.

Percent usual body weight compares present weight to usual weight to evaluate the degree of weight change.

$$\text{\% usual body weight (UBW)} = \text{(present weight/usual weight)} \times 100$$

For unintentional weight loss, the % UBW is evaluated as follows:

mild depletion = 85–95% UBW

moderate depletion = 75–84% UBW

severe depletion <75% UBW

Percent weight change can be calculated and evaluated to assess its significance. **Percent weight change** = (usual weight − present weight/usual weight) × 100

"Significant" weight loss is greater than:

1% to 2% loss in 1 week
5% in 1 month
7.5% in 3 months
10% in 6 months (risk factor for malnutrition)

Head Circumference (For infants up to the age of 2 years only)

Head circumference may indicate chronic undernutrition, or it may be used to screen for microcephaly or hydrocephalus.

A nonstretchable tape, preferably insertion tapes for easy reading, is placed around the middle of the forehead, making sure the ears are not under the tape and that all headwear is removed.

Interpretation

Growth in head circumference usually parallels weight gain. Two standard deviations below the mean may indicate protein–calorie malnutrition; however, head circumference is not recommended as a screening device for malnutrition because it may vary for non-nutritional reasons (eg, microcephaly and macrocephaly).

MEASURE OF BODY COMPOSITION

Although weight loss is considered an important indicator of nutritional status, it does not provide qualitative information about the type of tissue lost (ie, whether weight loss is related to a decrease in muscle or fat tissue). Also, a client can be malnourished without showing significant weight loss; conversely, the extent of weight loss does not necessarily correlate with the degree of malnutrition. Measurements that reflect body composition (fat and muscle tissue) are skinfolds, midarm circumference, and midarm muscle circumference measure.

To interpret each of the following measurements of body composition:

Compare the measurement to a previously obtained measurement to identify any change.
Compare to the reference standard (see Table 9-4).
Findings less than 90% of reference standard may indicate the need for nutritional support.

Triceps Skinfold

Triceps skinfold (TSF) measures subcutaneous fat stores and is therefore an index of total body fat, because approximately half the total body fat is directly under the skin. Studies indicate that assessments of subcutaneous body fat by skinfold measurements are accurate; they show better agreement with computed tomography results than did ultrasonographic findings (Orphanidou et al, 1994).

While the arm is hanging freely, grasp a fold of skin and subcutaneous fat between the thumb and forefinger slightly above the midpoint mark. Gently pull the skin away from the underlying muscle, apply the caliper, wait 2 to 3 seconds, and read the measurement to the nearest 1.0 mm. Repeat the procedure two more times; add the three readings, divide by 3, and record the average measurement.

Because the chance exists that fat on the arm may not accurately reflect fat in other areas of the body, taking skinfold measurements from other sites may improve validity. Other appropriate sites include the biceps, thigh, calf, and subscapular and suprailiac skinfolds.

Midarm Circumference

Midarm circumference (MAC) measures muscle mass and subcutaneous fat. Although it is not a useful measurement when used alone, it is used as part of the procedure for calculating arm muscle circumference.

A nonstretchable tape, preferably an insertion tape for easy reading (available from Ross Laboratories, Columbus, Ohio), is placed at the midpoint of the nondominant arm between the top of the acromion process of the scapula and the ole-cranon process of the ulna with the forearm flexed at 90°. With the arm in the dependent position, gently and firmly draw the tape around the mid–upper arm; do not compress the soft tissue. Record the reading to the nearest millimeter.

Midarm Muscle Circumference

Midarm muscle circumference (MAMC), which is calculated from the MAC and TSF measurements, provides an index of muscle mass (somatic protein stores). Although the measurement is not sensitive to small changes in muscle mass, it does provide a quick estimation of muscle mass and is minimally affected by edema (CDA/SSDA, 1992).

$$\text{MAMC (cm)} = \text{MAC (cm)} - [3.14 \times \text{TSF (cm)}]$$

Other less commonly used measurements of lean and fat tissue appear in the display, Other Anthropometric Measurements.

Laboratory Data

Laboratory tests, which are used to measure blood and urine levels of nutrients or to evaluate certain biochemical functions that depend on an adequate supply of essential nutrients, can objectively detect nutritional problems in their early stages before anthropometric and clinical changes occur. Most routine tests are aimed at assessing protein–calorie malnutrition (Table 9-5); specialized tests to measure vitamin, mineral, and trace element status are also available but are not routinely used (see Food for Thought, Hair Analysis: Reliable or Ridiculous?).

Unfortunately, abnormal laboratory results are not always diet or nutritionally related, and the tests do not indicate whether the cause is malnutrition, or whether the abnormality is an outcome of disease or the result of medical–surgical treat-

---

Other Anthropometric Measurements

Hydrodensitometry:	Measures body density by submerging the client underwater. Using the client's weight and the amount of water displaced when the client is submerged, body density and percent body fat are calculated from a mathematical equation.
	Although it provides an excellent measurement of body fat, it is expensive and impractical for widespread use.
Bioelectrical Impedance:	Estimates body fat using low-intensity electrical current. Electrodes placed on the wrist and ankle conduct a very low intensity electrical current through the body. Because electrolytes, which conduct an electrical current, are found primarily in lean body tissue, the leaner the client, the less resistance to the electrical current. A mathematical equation that uses the measurement of electrical resistance provides an estimate of the percent body fat.
	Although they are less expensive to use than underwater weighing, currently used equations may not be appropriate for children, the elderly, very obese people, and people who are very lean.

Table 9-5
Classification of Protein–Energy Malnutrition

ICD-9-CM* Code	Diagnosis/Description	Criteria/Characteristics
260.0	*Kwashiorkor*—nutritional edema with dyspigmentation of skin and hair	Normal anthropometrics; weight >90% of standard weight for height Depressed visceral protein concentrations; serum albumin <3.0 g/dL, transferrin <180 mg/dL Caused by acute energy and protein deficiency or as metabolic response to injury Characterized by edema, catabolism of muscle tissue, weakness, neurologic changes, loss of vigor, secondary infection, stunted growth in children, and changes in hair
261.0	*Marasmus*—nutritional atrophy, severe calorie deficiency, severe malnutrition	Depressed anthropometrics; weight <80% of standard weight for height and/or weight loss of >10% of usual weight in last 6 mo with muscle wasting Relative preservation of visceral proteins; serum albumin >3.0 g/dL Caused by chronic deficiency of energy intake Characterized by catabolism of fat and muscle tissue, generalized weakness, and weight loss
262.0	*Third-degree protein-energy malnutrition (PEM)*—nutritional edema without dyspigmentation of skin and hair	Depressed anthropometrics; weight <60% of standard weight for height Depressed visceral protein concentration; serum albumin <3.0 g/dL Occurs when a marasmic patient is exposed to stress (eg, trauma, surgery, or acute illness) Characterized by combined symptoms of marasmus and kwashiorkor, high risk of infection, and poor wound healing
263.0	*Second-degree PEM*—malnutrition of moderate degree	Depressed anthropometrics; weight 60%–75% of standard weight for height Relative preservation of visceral proteins; serum albumin 3.0–3.5 g/dL
263.1	*First-degree PEM*—malnutrition of mild degree	Depressed anthropometrics; weight 75%–90% of standard weight for height Preservation of visceral proteins; serum albumin 3.5–5.0 g/dL

*International Classification of Diseases, 9th Revision, Clinical Modification. © 1992, The American Dietetic Association. *"Manual of Clinical Dietetics."* Used by permission.

ments. Laboratory results also can be affected by genetics, sex, age, physical activity, infection, stress, and even last night's dinner; therefore, reference standards may not be appropriate for all people at all times. What's more, "normal" values for blood and urine constituents vary depending on which laboratory is performing the test and what method is used.

Because the body can store some nutrients, a low serum level may not necessarily reflect a deficiency (eg, the level of vitamin A may be low in the bloodstream but liver stores may be adequate). Also, there is not a definite value for a laboratory test that distinguishes between a deficient and a nondeficient state (eg, is less than 95% of normal considered deficient?).

Cost burden, lack of availability, and the invasive nature of blood tests may be disadvantages. Abnormal laboratory values that are potential risk factors for poor nutritional status appear in the display, Abnormal Lab Value Risks.

MEASURES OF PROTEIN STATUS

Because the primary objective of nutritional therapy is to preserve or restore body protein, assessment of this nutritional component is essential. Laboratory tests can be used to measure byproducts of protein catabolism (eg, urea, creatinine) and products of protein anabolism (eg, albumin, transferrin, prealbumin, retinol-binding protein); from these measurements, the adequacy of body protein stores can be inferred (Simko et al, 1995).

Measures of Protein Catabolism

Urinary Urea Nitrogen

Urea, a byproduct of amino acid deamination, circulates in the blood (BUN) and is excreted in the urine (UUN). Urea accounts for 60% to 90% of urine nitrogen and is reflective of current protein intake. Mean daily excretion of urea is 15.0 to 49.0 g; both blood and urine values of urea decrease during protein deficiency.

The state of nitrogen balance can be determined by comparing nitrogen intake (grams of protein divided by 6.25) to nitrogen output over a 24-hour period. Total nitrogen output equals g of UUN collected over 24 hours plus 4 g; approximately 4 g of nitrogen is lost daily through the lungs, hair, skin, and feces, and nonurea nitrogen, which is a component of the urine. A positive nitrogen balance (anabolism) exists when intake exceeds nitrogen output; conversely, negative nitrogen balance (catabolism) is indicated when output exceeds nitrogen intake. For UUN to be valid, protein intake must be accurately recorded and kidney function must be normal.

Abnormal Lab Value Risks

History or evidence of the following abnormal lab values may be a potential risk, depending on the client's age (ie, infant, child, adult, elderly)

Serum albumin, transferrin

Lipid levels, triglycerides

Hemoglobin, hematocrit, iron

BUN, creatinine, serum electrolytes

Fasting blood glucose levels

Other laboratory values, as appropriate

Source: Council on Practice Quality Management Committee (1994). Identifying patients at risk: ADA's definitions for nutrition screening and nutrition assessment. J Am Diet Assoc, 94(8), 838–839.

Urinary Creatinine

Every day, about 2% of the creatine phosphate in muscle tissue undergoes an irreversible conversion to **creatinine**. Creatinine circulates in the blood and is excreted in the urine at a constant rate that depends on the amount of muscle mass; the more muscle mass, the greater the excretion of creatinine. Urinary creatinine is considered a measure of long-term protein intake; usual ranges for adults are 20 to 26 mg/kg/24 hr for men and 14 to 22 mg/kg/24 hr for women (Simko et al, 1995). Urinary creatinine excretion varies considerably from day to day; therefore, a 3-day average calculation is more reliable than measurement of a single day's collection. Factors that influence urinary creatinine excretion include protein intake, exercise, age, renal function, and thyroid function.

Creatinine–Height Index

Creatinine–height index (CHI; %) = creatinine collected (mg/24 hr) divided by expected amount of creatinine to be excreted by reference individual of same height (mg/24 hr) × 100

   CHI combines an anthropometric measurement (height) and a biochemical value (creatinine) to assess chronic protein status in adults. After collection of a 24-hour urine sample, the amount of creatinine can be measured and compared to normal ranges based on height and sex (Table 9-6). Values less than 90% are considered abnormal and may indicate protein malnutrition and loss of lean body mass (muscle protein depletion). However, creatinine excretion tests may be invalid if renal func-

Table 9-6
Ideal Urinary Creatinine Values

Height (cm)	Ideal Creatinine for Men (mg)	Ideal Creatinine for Women (mg)
147.3		830
149.9		851
152.4		875
154.9		900
157.5	1288	925
160.0	1325	949
162.6	1359	977
165.1	1386	1006
167.6	1426	1044
170.2	1467	1076
172.7	1513	1109
175.3	1555	1141
177.8	1596	1174
180.3	1642	1206
182.9	1691	1240
185.4	1739	
188.0	1785	
190.5	1831	
193.0	1891	

tion is altered because they require a 24-hour urine collection (eg, impaired urine output secondary to renal disease causes a low urinary creatinine excretion, and thus CHI would not be a valid measure of protein status). Although creatinine excretion decreases with increasing age, there are no age-adjusted reference standards for the elderly.

Measures of Protein Anabolism

Ideally, serum proteins that are used to assess protein synthesis should have a short half-life, should respond to a protein-deficient diet, and should be decreased in the bloodstream only in response to calorie and protein deficiency. However, studies indicate that concentrations of serum proteins show significant decline only after protein deficiency is prolonged and severe. In addition, they are not specific indicators of protein deficiency because other factors, like zinc deficiency, energy deficiency, liver disease, renal disease, and systemic infection, may also contribute to their decline.

Serum Albumin

Normal value: 3.5 to 5.0 g/dL (Table 9-7)

Albumin, the most abundant form of protein in the blood, helps maintain oncotic pressure and transport other nutrients, drugs, and hormones through the blood. Albumin synthesis depends on functioning liver cells and an adequate supply of amino acids.

Malnutrition and depletion of visceral protein stores are reflected in low serum albumin concentrations. However, because albumin is degraded slowly (it has a half-life of 18 to 20 days) and because the body has a large extravascular pool that can be mobilized to maintain serum concentrations during periods of protein depletion, serum albumin concentrations are preserved until malnutrition is in a chronic stage.

Besides resulting from malnutrition, a low serum albumin may also be caused by liver disease, renal disease, congestive heart failure, and excessive protein losses (eg, those that occur in response to burns, major surgery, infection, and cancer).

Serum Transferrin

Normal levels: >200 mg/dL (see Table 9-7)

Transferrin is a transport protein that binds and carries iron from the intestine through the serum. Because it has a shorter half-life than albumin (8 to 9 days), transferrin is likely to respond more quickly to protein depletion than albumin. Although serum transferrin levels fall in severe protein–calorie malnutrition, it is not known whether they are sensitive indicators of less severe or chronic malnutrition.

A decrease in transferrin levels may be associated with malnutrition; it also may be related to liver disease, nephrotic syndrome, anemia, or neoplastic disease. Furthermore, transferrin levels are inversely related to iron status: As iron storage increases, amounts of transferrin decrease because the body requires that less iron be absorbed. Conversely, iron deficiency causes an increase in serum transferrin. Because it is influenced by other variables, transferrin alone is not a reliable indicator for evaluating protein status (Simko et al, 1995).

Table 9-7		
Serum Proteins Used To Assess Protein Synthesis		
Serum Protein (Normal Value)	**Advantages**	**Disadvantages**
Albumin (3.5–5.0 g/dL)	Readily available. May be best single indicator of nutritional status	During the acute phase following injury, infection, or active chronic disease, levels decrease regardless of nutritional status. Large body pool and long half life (20 days) cause it to have a slow response (ie, 3–4 wk) to nutritional repletion. Low levels also caused by liver and renal disease, congestive heart failure, and excessive protein losses (ie, burns, major surgery, infection, cancer).
Serum transferrin (>200 mg/dL)	More sensitive to nutritional repletion than albumin because of its shorter half-life (8–10 days), smaller body pool, and more rapid response to short-term changes in protein status	Direct measurement is expensive. Like albumin, levels decrease during acute response. Levels increase from iron deficiency, pregnancy, hyposia, and chronic blood loss. Levels decrease from pernicious anemia, chronic infection, liver disease, iron overload, and protein-losing enteropathies.
Prealbumin (20–50 mg/dL)	More sensitive than albumin because of its short half-life (2 days). Response to nutritional repletion seen in 2–3 days. Reliable measurement during acute response.	May reflect protein intake rather than protein status. Levels decrease from liver disease, surgical trauma, stress, and inflammation. Not reliable for clients with chronic renal failure on dialysis (level may appear falsely normal or elevated).
Retinol-binding protein (3–7 mg/dL)	Responds quickly to nutritional repletion due to small body pool and short half-life (10–12 hr)	Levels decrease from vitamin A deficiency, hyperthyroidism, cystic fibrosis

Prealbumin

Normal levels: 20–50 mg/dL (see Table 9-7)

Prealbumin (PAB), also known as thyroxine-binding prealbumin and transthyretin, transports thyroxine through the blood and is also a carrier for retinol-binding protein, which is the transport protein of vitamin A. Because it has a short half-life (2 days) and the body pool is small, it is an extremely sensitive indicator of nutritional status, much more so than either albumin or transferrin (Mears, 1994).

PAB levels quickly decline in protein–calorie malnutrition and return to normal with repletion, in as few as 3 days (Mears, 1994). However, tests to assess prealbumin levels are not often available in the standard hospital laboratory. Renal disease and iron can alter serum prealbumin levels.

Retinol-Binding Protein

Normal levels: 3 to 7 mg/dL

With a shorter half-life (12 hours) and smaller body pool than prealbumin, **retinol-binding protein** may be a better means of monitoring short-term acute changes in protein status. Serum concentration of retinol-binding protein quickly declines in response to both calorie and protein deficiency; however, it may also decline secondary to vitamin A deficiency, hyperthyroidism, chronic liver disorders, zinc deficiency, and cystic fibrosis.

Retinol-binding protein testing is not routinely available from most hospital laboratories.

MEASURES OF IMMUNE FUNCTION STATUS

Malnutrition has a serious effect on immunocompetence; in fact, it is recognized to be the most common cause of secondary immune deficiency. The following tests may be used to test the body's immunocompetence.

Total Lymphocyte Count

$$\text{TLC (cells/mm}^3) = \text{WBC} \times \% \text{ lymphocytes}$$

Normal levels: 1500 mm to 1800 mm

Total lymphocyte count (TLC) is obtained from samples that are collected for evaluation of complete blood count (CBC) and differential; therefore, the TLC value is usually available for hospitalized clients. Malnutrition, especially that resulting from inadequate intakes of calories and protein, decreases the total number of lymphocytes, which impairs the body's ability to fight infection. However, total lymphocyte count is of limited value because it is affected by numerous medical conditions and fluctuates widely.

Delayed Cutaneous Hypersensitivity Reaction

Cellular immunity can be evaluated by placing small quantities of recall antigens, such as *Candida*, mumps, purified protein derivative of tuberculin (PPD), and streptokinase-streptodornase (SKSD), under the skin. Clients who are immunocompetent exhibit a positive reaction within 24 to 48 hours, that is, a red area of 5 mm or more appears around the test site. Because malnutrition delays antibody synthesis and antibody response to stimulation, clients with malnutrition may experience a delayed reaction, a reaction to only one of the antigens, or no reaction (anergy). A limitation of using delayed cutaneous hypersensitivity reaction is that anergy can occur secondary to other conditions (eg, blunt trauma, cancer, acute blood loss, surgery, sepsis, age, recent anesthesia, fever, medications) and therefore is not a specific or often used measure of protein status.

Clinical Findings

Physical signs and symptoms of malnutrition may be visually apparent on inspection (Table 9-8). Abnormal findings should be closely scrutinized to determine whether or not they are caused by, or related to, a nutritional deficiency.

Obtaining clinical findings is a noninvasive and inexpensive procedure. However, it involves a subjective evaluation of "normal" versus "abnormal" findings. Most signs cannot be considered diagnostic but must, rather, be viewed as suggestive of malnutrition. Confirmation of malnutrition should be made using laboratory and dietary data.

Unfortunately, signs of malnutrition may be nonspecific. For instance, dull, dry hair may be related to kwashiorkor (severe protein depletion) or to overexposure to the sun. Also, the intensity of symptoms can vary among population groups because of genetic and environmental differences. Another disadvantage of using clinical findings is that they cannot detect subclinical malnutrition, which occurs more frequently than clinical (overt) malnutrition, because it does not produce any physical signs or symptoms.

Dietary Data

Dietary data can be collected by a variety of methods, depending on the scope of the assessment. Data can be evaluated to determine the sources and amounts of nutrients consumed, which can help to identify potential and actual nutritional problems and then to classify them as primary (caused by a poor intake) or secondary (caused by alterations in digestion, absorption, metabolism, or excretion of nutrients). As with any information that is gotten by means of an interview, the data are highly subjective and may not be reliable or precise. In addition, acute or chronic debilitating disease may make data collection difficult.

Potential risks that are based on food and nutrient intake patterns appear in the display, Food and Nutrient Intake Risk Factors.

24-HOUR FOOD RECALL

A **24-hour food recall**, which can be obtained through questionnaire or by interview, asks the client to recall the quantity and quality of all food and beverages that were consumed during the previous or any typical 24-hour period (see Figure 9-3, 24-Hour Food Recall). Food models may help to define portion sizes, and probing is often needed to obtain specific details, such as how the food was prepared, and what the client put in his coffee (Thompson and Byers, 1994). Open-ended questions, such as questions that begin with "what," "when," "how," "where," "why," or "who," usually provide more information than questions that can be answered with a simple "yes" or "no."

The data thus obtained usually are evaluated according to the Food Guide Pyramid to estimate overall adequacy (see Chapter 8); the data generally are considered incomplete or too imprecise to evaluate according to the RDA. However, this is the easiest and quickest method of evaluating dietary intake, and it is a good screening tool for assessing the average intake of a group of people.

Table 9-8
Clinical Observations for Nutritional Assessment

Body Area	Signs of Good Nutritional Status	Signs of Poor Nutritional Status
General appearance	Alert, responsive	Listless, apathetic, and cachexic
General vitality	Endurance, energetic, sleeps well, vigorous	Easily fatigued, no energy, falls asleep easily, looks tired, apathetic
Weight	Normal for height, age, body build	Overweight or underweight
Hair	Shiny, lustrous, firm, not easily plucked, healthy scalp	Dull and dry, brittle, loss of color, easily plucked, thin and sparse
Face	Uniform skin color; healthy appearance, not swollen	Dark skin over cheeks and under eyes, flaky skin, facial edema (moon face), pale skin color
Eyes	Bright, clear, moist, no sores at corners of eyelids, membranes moist and healthy pink color, no prominent blood vessels	Pale eye membranes, dry eyes (xerophthalmia); Bitot's spots, increased vascularity, cornea soft (keratomalacia), small yellowish lumps around eyes (xanthelasma), dull or scarred cornea
Lips	Good pink color, smooth, moist, not chapped or swollen	Swollen and puffy (cheilosis), angular lesion at corners of mouth or fissures or scars (stomatitis)
Tongue	Deep red, surface papillae present	Smooth appearance, beefy red or magenta colored, swollen, papillae hypertrophy or atrophy
Teeth	Straight, no crowding, no cavities, no pain, bright, no discoloration, well-shaped jaw	Cavities, mottled appearance (fluorosis), malpositioned, missing teeth
Gums	Firm, good pink color, no swelling or bleeding	Spongy, bleed easily, marginal redness, recessed, swollen and inflamed
Glands	No enlargement of the thyroid, face not swollen	Enlargement of the thyroid (goiter), enlargement of the parotid (swollen cheeks)
Skin	Smooth, good color, slightly moist, no signs of rashes, swelling, or color irregularities	Rough, dry, flaky, swollen, pale, pigmented, lack of fat under the skin, fat deposits around the joints (xanthomas), bruises, petechiae
Nails	Firm, pink	Spoon-shaped (koilonychia), brittle, pale, ridged
Skeleton	Good posture, no malformations	Poor posture, beading of the ribs, bowed legs or knock-knees, prominent scapulas, chest deformity at diaphragm
Muscles	Well developed, firm, good tone, some fat under the skin	Flaccid, poor tone, wasted, underdeveloped, difficulty walking
Extremities	No tenderness	Weak and tender, presence of edema
Abdomen	Flat	Swollen
Nervous system	Normal reflexes, psychological stability	Decrease in or loss of ankle and knee reflexes, psychomotor changes, mental confusion, depression, sensory loss, motor weakness, loss of sense of position, loss of vibration, burning and tingling of the hands and feet (paresthesia)
Cardiovascular system	Normal heart rate and rhythm, no murmurs, normal blood pressure for age	Cardiac enlargement, tachycardia, elevated blood pressure
GI system	No palpable organs or masses (liver edge may be palpable in children)	Hepatosplenomegaly

(Adapted from Christakis G [ed]: Nutritional Assessment in Health Programs. Washington, DC: American Public Health Association, 1973; and Williams SR: Nutrition and Diet Therapy. 5th ed. St. Louis: Times Mirror/Mosby, 1985.)

Food and Nutrient Intake Risk Factors

History or evidence of any of the following may be a potential risk:

Intake less or greater than standard for age and for calories, protein, and activity

Intake less or greater than standard for nutrients (ie, vitamins and minerals)

Unusual food habits, such as pica, faddism, and meal skipping

Inappropriate use of supplements (vitamins, minerals, fortified food products)

A physician's order for NPO or a clear liquid diet for more than 3 days without enteral or parenteral nutrition

Inadequate transitional feeding, enteral support, or parenteral support

Minimal or no intake from a major food group

Fluid intake less than output

Eating or feeding disorders

Food allergies

Restricted diet

Source: Council on Practice Quality Management Committee (1994). Identifying patients at risk: ADA's definitions for nutrition screening and nutrition assessment. J Am Diet Assoc, 94(8), 838–839.

Unfortunately, the 24-hour recall relies on memory and accurate interpretation of portion sizes; underreporting of food that was consumed may occur. The underlying assumption in using the 24-hour recall method is that a single day closely represents the usual pattern of intake over an extended period of time. However, numerous studies have shown that it does not, and that a 24-hour recall is not an appropriate tool for assessing the usual diet of an individual.

FOOD FREQUENCY RECORD

A **food frequency record** is a checklist that indicates how often specific foods or general food groups are eaten; that is, times/day, times/week, times/month, or frequently, seldom, never. It provides information about the types of foods eaten, but does not usually report the quantities. A selective food frequency record may focus on specific foods or nutrients that are suspected of being deficient or excessive in the diet. Figure 9-4 is an example of a self-administered, self-scoring food questionnaire that focuses on fat and fruit, vegetable, and fiber intake. Figure 9-5 is a general tool that serves as a food frequency record based on major food groups. Questionnaires may be completed relatively quickly and easily by the client, or the clinician may complete them using an interview technique; thus, they are often used in large-scale epidemiologic studies.

Because portion sizes are generally not emphasized, a food frequency record may be less intimidating than a 24-hour recall. When they are used together, a food frequency record and a 24-hour recall complement each other and present a more complete dietary intake picture than either method used alone. The major limitation of the food frequency record is that many details of dietary intake are not measured (Thompson and Byers, 1994). Also, this method relies on memory.

Name: _____   Date: _____
Day of week of recall: _____

24-Hour Food Recall Record

Directions: In the space provided below, record all food and beverages consumed in the previous 24-hour period or in any typical 24-hour period. Include estimated amounts and the time and place when they were eaten.

Food and Beverage Consumed

Type	Amount	Method of Preparation*	Time	Place

Was this a typical day?   Yes _____   No _____
If not, why not?

Do you take a vitamin or
mineral supplement (pill)?   Yes _____   No _____

If yes, how often? _____
             what kind? (i.e., multivitamin, iron, potassium. Give brand name if
known.)

*Fried, baked, broiled, boiled, creamed, toasted.

Figure 9-3
24-Hour Food Recall.

FOOD RECORD

A **food record** is a detailed diary of all food and beverages consumed and measurements of portion sizes taken during a specified period of time, usually 3 to 7 days, depending on the regularity of food habits. In theory, an average daily intake can be calculated by totaling the nutrients that were consumed during the entire period and dividing by the total number of days. In practice, food records appear to be relatively valid for obtaining the mean intakes of nutrients consumed by groups of people;

FOOD QUESTIONNAIRE

Think about your eating habits over the past year or so. About how often do you eat each of the following foods? Mark and "x" in one box for each food.

	(0) Less than once per MONTH	(1) 2–3 times per MONTH	(2) 1–2 times per WEEK	(3) 3–4 times per WEEK	(4) 5+ times per WEEK	Points Score
Hamburgers or cheeseburgers	❑	❑	❑	❑	❑	_____
Beef, such as steaks, roasts	❑	❑	❑	❑	❑	_____
Fried chicken	❑	❑	❑	❑	❑	_____
Hot dogs, franks	❑	❑	❑	❑	❑	_____
Cold cuts, lunch meats, ham, etc.	❑	❑	❑	❑	❑	_____
Salad dressings, mayo (not diet)	❑	❑	❑	❑	❑	_____
Margarine or butter	❑	❑	❑	❑	❑	_____
Eggs	❑	❑	❑	❑	❑	_____
Bacon or sausage	❑	❑	❑	❑	❑	_____
Cheese or cheese spread	❑	❑	❑	❑	❑	_____
Whole milk	❑	❑	❑	❑	❑	_____
French fries	❑	❑	❑	❑	❑	_____
Potato chips, corn chips, popcorn	❑	❑	❑	❑	❑	_____
Ice cream	❑	❑	❑	❑	❑	_____
Doughnuts, pastries, cake cookies	❑	❑	❑	❑	❑	_____

Meat/Snacks Score = _____

	(0) Less than once per WEEK	(1) About 1 time per WEEK	(2) 2–3 times per WEEK	(3) 4–6 times per WEEK	(4) Every day	Points Score
Orange juice	❑	❑	❑	❑	❑	_____
Not counting juice, about how often do you eat any fruit?	❑	❑	❑	❑	❑	_____
Green salad	❑	❑	❑	❑	❑	_____
Potatoes	❑	❑	❑	❑	❑	_____
Beans, such as baked beans, pintos, kidney beans or in chili	❑	❑	❑	❑	❑	_____
About how often do you eat any other vegetables?	❑	❑	❑	❑	❑	_____
High-fiber or bran cereal	❑	❑	❑	❑	❑	_____
Dark bread, such as whole wheat, rye	❑	❑	❑	❑	❑	_____
White bread, including french, italian, biscuits, muffins	❑	❑	❑	❑	❑	_____

Fruit/Vegetable/Fiber Score = _____

Figure 9-4A
Block Screening Questionnaire for Fat and Fruit/Vegetable/Fiber Intake (Complete).

To score:

For each food, write the number that is at the top of the column you checked, in the box at the far right. Add up the numbers in the boxes to get your total scores for Meat/Snacks and Fruit/Vegetable/Fiber.

For Meat/Snacks Score:

If Your Score Is:

more than 27	Your diet is high in fat. There are many ways you can make your eating pattern lower in fat. You should look at your higheast scores above to find areas in which to begin.
25–27	Your diet is quite high in fat. To make your eating pattern lower in fat, you may want to begin in the areas where you scored highest.
22–24	You are generally eating a typical American diet, which could be lower in fat.
18–21	You are making better low-fat food choices.
17 or less	You are making the best low-fat food choices. Keep up the great work!

If you scored 17 or less, you're doing well! This is the desirable score on this screener.

For Fruit/Vegetable/Fiber Score:

If Your Score Is:

30 or more	You're doing very well! This is the desirable score on this screener.
20 to 29	You should include more fruits, vegetables and whole grains.
less than 20	Your diet is probably low in important nutrients. You should find ways to increase the fruits and vegetables and other fiber rich foods you eat every day.

Figure 9-4B
Scoring for Block Screening Questionnaire for Fat and Fruit/Vegetable/Fiber Intake.

however, individual food records tend to become unreliable after the first few days because accuracy of recording deteriorates. Another disadvantage is that the client may modify usual intake during the recording period.

DIET HISTORY

In the general sense, a diet history is any assessment of a client's past diet. In practice, a **diet history** is a comprehensive assessment of a client's usual food intake over time, including characteristics of foods usually eaten, and the frequency and amount of food consumed (Thompson and Byers, 1994). A diet history may include a detailed interview that may comprise a 24-hour recall, a food frequency list that includes amounts of food eaten, and a food record that was obtained over several days. In the clinical setting, medical and psychosocial factors may be included and evaluated for their impact on nutritional requirements and food habits, choices, and attitudes (see display, Components of Diet History). Dietary data that are collected through a diet history can be evaluated according to the Food Guide Pyramid or the

Food Frequency Checklist

Directions: Indicate how often you eat each food item listed below, in terms of number of times consumed per week, number of times per month, seldom, or never. List the type of food, where appropriate.

Food Item	Type	How often
Meat		
Fish		
Poultry		
Eggs		
Lunch meats		
Pizza		
Peanut butter		
Dried peas and beans		
Nuts		
Milk		
Yogurt		
Cheese		
Milk desserts		
Citrus fruit or juice		
Dried fruit		
Other fruit		
Leafy green vegetables		
Dark yellow vegetables		
Potatoes		
Other vegetables		
Bread		
Cereal		
Pasta		
Rice		
Other grains		
Butter/margarine		
Oil/salad dressing		
Bacon and sausage		
Fried foods		
Cream (sweet or sour)		
Sweets		
Sugar/sugar substitute		
Snack foods		
Salt/salt substitute		
Carbonated beverages/fruit drinks		
Alcoholic beverages		
Coffee/tea		
Other foods not listed that you eat regularly		

Figure 9-5
General food frequency record.

Components of Diet History

Collect	Evaluate
DATA BASE	
Age, sex	Effect on nutritional requirements
Position in family; number in family; lifestyle	Outside support systems; social aspects of eating
Occupation; frequency and intensity of physical exercise; usual number of hours of sleep/day	Effect on calorie requirements and meal timing
Religious affiliation, cultural and ethnic background	Effect on food choices and aversions
Educational background	Ability to comprehend diet instruction; appropriate teaching materials and methods
Use of alcohol and tobacco	Effect on food intake, food budget, and nutrient requirements
DIETARY DATA	
24-hour recall of typical food and fluids consumed, including	Adequacy according to
Usual portion sizes	Food Guide Pyramid
Usual meal and snack patterns	U.S. Dietary Guidelines
Usual meal timing	Recommended Dietary Allowances (RDA)
Place where most meals are eaten	
Food frequency record	
Present intake, if different from usual intake	Reason for change, for example: loss of appetite, changes in smell, appetite, or taste, difficulty chewing and swallowing, hospitalization, modified diet
Food likes, dislikes, intolerances, allergies	Impact on food choices
Information on who does the food shopping and preparation	Responsible person's nutrition knowledge, need for diet instruction
Information on food preparation and storage facilities	Impact on intake; need for social assistance
Present and past use of therapeutic diets	Client compliance and knowledge; effectiveness of the diet; need for diet revisions or follow-up teaching
Present and past use of food fads, such as fad dieting, health foods, self-prescribed vitamin/mineral supplements	Rationale; potential risks/benefits
MEDICAL–SOCIOECONOMIC DATA	
Past medical history: type of disorder, treatment (including diet and drug)	Effect on intake, digestion, absorption, metabolism, and excretion of nutrients
Current illness or chief complaint	The need for diet modifications
Family medical history	
Past surgical history: type, date, length of hospitalization, development of complications	
Past and present drug history: name of prescription and nonprescription drugs used on a regular basis, purpose, dosage, duration of use	Potential or actual effects on nutritional status; need for diet modification
History of drug dependence; drug abuse	
Ability to chew and swallow (Does the client have missing teeth? Full or partial dentures? Do the dentures fit?)	Impact on food intake
Appetite, bowel habits	Normal pattern, recent changes, impact on intake and nutritional status, need for diet modification
Source of income	Reliability and adequacy; eligibility for social assistance
Food budget	Adequacy

FOOD *for* THOUGHT

Hair Analysis: Reliable or Ridiculous?

Although hair analysis has limited applications as a screening tool for heavy metal exposure, many commercial laboratories are promoting hair analysis to health food stores, beauty shops, chiropractors, and "nutrition consultants" as a method of evaluating a person's mineral status and managing a wide variety of illnesses.

The results of a study that sent hair samples from two healthy teenagers to 13 commercial laboratories showed that there was little agreement between laboratories regarding the mineral levels present in identical samples of hair. Even more interesting is that two identical samples sent to the same lab yielded different results. The laboratories surveyed also disagreed as to what are the "normal" or "usual" levels of many minerals. Most reports were extensive computerized interpretations of absurd and potentially frightening findings. Six of the laboratories recommended food supplements, but the types and amounts varied from report to report and from laboratory to laboratory. Needless to say, commercial hair analysis is at best unscientific, a waste of money, and possibly even illegal.

Dietary Guidelines for Americans (see Chapter 8). More precise information can be obtained, using pen and paper or computer, by calculating calorie and nutrient intake and comparing results with the RDA that are appropriate for the client's age and sex; alternatively, estimated requirements based on the client's condition may be used.

Diet histories are a time-consuming method of assessment. They require an extensive interview by a trained nutritionist or dietitian; however, in the community setting, automated diet histories may be obtained by way of a computer program that orally asks questions, participates in dialogue, and displays pictures of food (Thompson and Byers, 1994). Food data are translated into nutrient equivalents using computerized nutrient analysis programs (Slattery et al, 1994). Computerization of diet history questionnaires has proven to be an efficient method of collecting and processing dietary intake data in large studies (Slattery et al, 1994).

Diet histories appear to be a reliable method of nutrition assessment; however, it is not possible to know whether they are precise or accurate, because validation is so difficult and because food habits are not static.

KEY
CONCEPTS

- Nutritional assessment is a process of gathering and analyzing data to evaluate a person's nutritional status and nutritional risks. There is not a universally agreed upon tool to assess all groups in all settings.

- Screening uses a minimum amount of information to identify people at moderate or high risk. To be effective, it must use data that is normally available upon admission to a hospital or health care facility, such as height, weight, recent weight change, and serum albumin. Nurses may be responsible for nutritional screening in some facilities.

- People identified through the screening process to be at nutritional risk receive a nutritional assessment, from which a nutritional care plan is formulated, implemented, and evaluated. Nutritional assessments are usually the responsibility of the dietitian.

- A variety of data can be collected and analyzed for the purpose of nutritional assessment; actual data collected varies with the population and the scope of the assessment.

- Anthropometric data are measurements of body dimensions, such as height, weight, and skinfolds. These measurements are objective, noninvasive, and relatively easy to obtain; the results are evaluated according to the appropriate reference standards for the client's age and sex.

- Laboratory data can objectively identify nutritional problems before changes occur in anthropometric measurements. However, laboratory results can be altered from nonnutritional causes, such as diseases, treatments, genetics, infection, and hydration status.

- Assessment of physical signs of malnutrition apparent upon visual inspection is highly subjective; thus, positive clinical findings are considered "suggestive" of malnutrition, not a definitive diagnosis.

- Dietary data obtained through interviews is highly subjective; however, it can be used to help classify nutritional problems as primary (related to intake) or secondary (related to altered nutrient digestion, absorption, metabolism, or excretion). To increase reliability, more than one method of dietary data collection should be obtained (eg, 24-hour recall, food-frequency record, food record).

 FOCUS ON **CRITICAL THINKING**

Conduct a 24-hour recall on a friend or family member (Fig 9-3). With that same person, complete a general food frequency record (Fig 9-5).

Are the results comparable? Which method appears more valid? Why?

Complete and score the Block Screening Questionnaire for Fat and Fruit/Vegetable/Fiber Intake according to your own diet.

Do you agree with the results? Why or why not?

REFERENCES

Chicago Dietetic Association and the South Suburban Dietetic Association (1992). Manual of Clinical Dietetics. 4th ed. Chicago: American Dietetic Association.

Council of Practice Quality Management Committee (1994). Identifying patients at risk: ADA's definitions for nutrition screening and nutrition assessment. J Am Diet Assoc, 94(8), 838–839

Foltz, M., Schiller, R., and Ryan, A. (1993). Nutrition screening and assessment: Current practices and dietitians' leadership roles. J Am Diet Assoc, 93(12), 1388–1395.

Krasker, G., and Balogun, L. (1995). 1995 JCAHO standards: Development and relevance to dietetics practice. J Am Diet Assoc, 95(2), 240–243.

Mears, E. (1994). Prealbumin and nutrition assessment. Dietetic Currents, 21(1), 1–4.

North American Nursing Diagnosis Association (1994). Nursing Diagnoses: Definitions and Classification 1995–1996. Philadelphia: North American Nursing Diagnoses Association.

Nutrition Screening Initiative (1991). Nutrition Screening Manual for Professionals Caring for Older Americans. Washington, DC: Greer, Margolis, Mitchell, Grunwald & Associates, Inc.

Orphanidou, C., McCargar, L., Birminghan, L., Mathieson, J., and Goldner, E. (1994). Accuracy of subcutaneous fat measurement: Comparison of skinfold calipers, ultrasound, and computed tomography. J Am Diet Assoc, 94(8), 855–858.

Simko, M, Cowell, C., and Gilbride, J. (1995). Nutrition Assessment. A Comprehensive Guide for Planning Intervention. 2nd ed. Gaithersburg, MD: Aspen Publishers, Inc.

Slattery, M., Caan, B., Duncan, D., Berry, T., Coates, A., and Kerber, R. (1994). A computerized diet history questionnaire for epidemiologic studies. J Am Diet Assoc, 94(7), 761–766.

Thompson, F., and Byers, T. (1994). Dietary Assessment Resource Manual. Supplement to The Journal of Nutrition, 124(11S), 2245S–2317S.

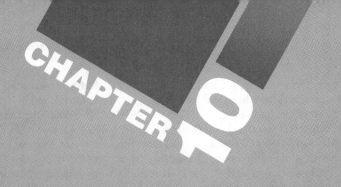

Pregnancy and Lactation

Chapter Outline

Key Terms

Colostrum
Fetal alcohol syndrome
  (FAS)

Gynecologic age
Low birth weight (LBW)
Mature milk

Pica
Preterm milk

*T*he role of nutrition in the progression and outcome of pregnancy has not always been appreciated, partly because changes that occur during pregnancy, their influence on nutritional requirements, and the effects of long-term nutritional status on reproductive health are not fully understood (Worthington-Roberts and Williams, 1993). However, proper nutrition during pregnancy promotes fetal growth and development and maternal well-being (Mikode and White, 1994). Women who begin pregnancy with adequate nutrient reserves and good eating habits are better prepared for pregnancy and lactation. Women who consume an adequate diet during pregnancy provide the fetus, placenta, and maternal tissues with the nutrients necessary for normal growth and development.

Indeed, fetal and infant morbidity and mortality are significantly more frequent among women who are malnourished. The effects of maternal malnutrition on fetal growth and development have been examined in three types of studies: 1) natural experiments (eg, study of effects of famine); 2) measurements of organ size and cell numbers in infants involved in stillbirths and neonatal deaths; and 3) epidemiologic studies. Study of the effects of unnatural famine (*ie*, that caused by war) on pregnancy outcome shows that malnutrition that occurs in the early months of pregnancy affects embryonic development and the capacity of the embryo to survive, whereas poor nutrition in the latter part of pregnancy affects fetal growth (Table 10-1). Organ studies correlate undernutrition with prenatal growth retardation in infants from low-income families. Undernutrition appears to affect the size of the placenta; a small placenta is associated with intrauterine growth failure, possibly because a small placenta may not be able to nourish the fetus adequately. Epidemiologic studies indicate that maternal body size (height and prepregnancy weight) and the amount of weight gained during pregnancy are consistently associated with infant birth weight. It appears that underweight women may reduce their risk of adverse pregnancy outcome by attaining a higher prepregnancy weight and/or by gaining extra weight during pregnancy.

Gestational weight gain, especially during the second and third trimesters, is an important indicator of fetal growth. Studies show that low weight gain at 20 weeks' gestation increases the chances of delivering a **low-birth-weight** (**LBW**) infant (a baby weighing less than 2500 g or 5.5 lbs). Low-birth-weight babies tend to be malnourished, especially if born full-term, and they have a high incidence of postnatal complications and mortality. In fact, birth weight may be the most important predictor not only of mortality, but also of subsequent development.

Table 10-1
Stages of Fetal Growth

Stage	Duration	Characteristics
Implantation Stage	Two-week period following conception	Fertilized egg undergoes cell division, differentiates into three distinct germinal layers, and implants itself into the uterine wall. During this critical period preceding growth, insults, including malnutrition, can cause birth defects or prevent implantation.
Organogenesis	Six-week period following implantation	Differentiation and development of various organs and tissues occur. Adequate nutrient reserves established before conception can be used by the embryo for nourishment if maternal intake is impaired because of nausea and vomiting. Maternal intake is more important if preconceptual reserves are marginal.
Growth Stage	The remaining 7 months of pregnancy	The most intense period of anabolism in the life cycle, characterized by the extensive growth and development of tissues. During this period, the placenta nourishes the fetus by transferring nutrients and oxygen from maternal circulation. The placenta also removes fetal wastes. Inadequate nutrient intake impairs growth.

However, adequate weight gain during pregnancy cannot by itself ensure the delivery of a normal-birth-weight infant. A growing body of evidence shows that prepregnancy weight for height influences fetal growth beyond the effect of gestational weight gain; that is, women who are thinner before pregnancy tend to have smaller babies compared to their heavier counterparts with the *same* gestational weight gain. Current recommendations for weight gain during pregnancy stress the importance of individualizing weight gain goals based on an accurate assessment of prepregnancy weight.

NUTRITION AND PREGNANCY

Nutrient requirements increase during pregnancy to support optimal fetal growth and development, and to maintain maternal homeostasis despite physiologic changes that involve all body systems. Alterations in metabolism, body composition, and gastrointestinal function, and an expanded blood volume account for some of the maternal changes that have nutritional implications (Table 10-2).

Table 10-2
Maternal Physiologic Changes of Pregnancy With Nutritional Significance

Physiologic Change	Rationale
ALTERED METABOLISM	
Basal metabolic rate increases	Increased oxygen consumption related to the increase in maternal cardiac output and the oxygen needs of the placenta and fetus. The rate usually increases by the fourth month of gestation and rises to 15% to 20% above normal by term.
Fat becomes the major source of fuel	To conserve glucose for the fetus: Glucose is the fetus' primary fuel for meeting its energy requirements.
Decrease in insulin efficiency develops during the latter part of pregnancy	May be a compensatory mechanism to provide the growing fetus with an adequate supply of glucose.
Total body water increases throughout pregnancy: It is estimated that 62% of weight gain at term is from the increase in water	Minor edema may be considered normal if not accompanied by hypertension and proteinuria.
GASTROINTESTINAL CHANGES	
Nausea and vomiting are common in the first trimester; so are increases in appetite and thirst	Hypoglycemia, decreased gastric motility, relaxation of the cardiac sphincter, or anxiety may contribute to nausea and vomiting.
Decreased tone and motility of the smooth muscles of the GI tract may lead to esophageal reflux with heartburn and constipation	Increased progesterone production slows GI motility. Displaced stomach and intestines are related to enlarging uterus.
Nutrient absorption increases	Increased progesterone production slows GI motility.
BLOOD VOLUME CHANGES	
Physiologic anemia of pregnancy	The increase in blood volume exceeds the increase in red blood cell production, resulting in hemodilution.

Recommended Dietary Allowances for Pregnancy

With the exception of vitamins A and K, the requirements for all nutrients with defined RDA increase during pregnancy over those for nonpregnant women aged 25 to 50 (Table 10-3). However, the degree and timing of changing needs vary considerably among nutrients. For instance, the RDA for iron triples during pregnancy, yet only 10% more vitamin B_{12} is needed. Likewise, the RDA for calories is specified for each trimester; no other RDA makes such a distinction for nutritional needs across trimesters. The 10th edition of the *Recommended Dietary Allowances* lists absolute amounts of nutrients required during pregnancy, instead of additional amounts needed. For instance, the previous allowance for calcium during pregnancy was +400 g; in the 10th edition, the RDA is a total of 1200 g. The change reflects the precision with which the additional needs of pregnancy are known (National Research Council, 1989). However, calories are listed in incremental amounts.

Because calorie needs increase relatively little compared to the increased requirements for other nutrients, like calcium, iron, and folic acid, nutrient density is important. Table 10-4 outlines the sources and functions of calories and selected nutrients that are important during pregnancy (see display, Food for Thought).

Table 10-3
Recommended Dietary Allowances for Pregnancy and Lactation

| | Nonpregnant Women | | | Lactation | |
	Ages 19–24	Ages 25–50	Pregnancy	1st 6 months	2nd 6 months
Calories	2200	2200	1st tri: +0 / 2nd tri: +300 / 3rd tri: +300	+500	+500
Protein, g	46	50	60	65	62
Vit A, µg	800	800	800	1300	1200
Vit D, µg	10	5	10	10	10
Vit E, mg	8	8	10	12	11
Vit K, µg	60	65	65	65	65
Vit C, mg	60	60	70	95	90
Thiamine, mg	1.1	1.1	1.5	1.6	1.6
Riboflavin, mg	1.3	1.3	1.6	1.8	1.7
Niacin, mg	15	15	17	20	20
Vit B_6, mg	1.6	1.6	2.2	2.1	2.1
Folate, µg	180	180	400	280	260
Vit B_{12}, µg	2.0	2.0	2.2	2.6	2.6
Calcium, mg	1200	800	1200	1200	1200
Phosphorus, mg	1200	800	1200	1200	1200
Magnesium, mg	280	280	320	355	340
Iron, mg	15	15	30	15	15
Zinc, mg	12	12	15	19	16
Iodine, µg	150	150	175	200	200
Selenium, µg	55	55	65	75	75

Table 10-4
Sources and Functions of Calories and Selected Nutrients During Pregnancy

Nutrient and Sources	% Increase in RDA Above Nonpregnant Adult Female Aged 25–50	Rationale for Increase	Possible Outcome of Deficiency
Calories (It is recommended that CHO supply approximately 50% of total calories, mostly in the form of complex CHO)	1st trimester: no increase 2nd & 3rd trimesters: 14% increase	To spare protein for tissue synthesis; to meet increased BMR and increased energy expenditure related to increased body weight; to store calorie reserves for lactation	Inadequate weight gain increases the risk of low birthweight, fetal growth retardation, and fetal and neonatal death
Protein High biologic sources: eggs, milk, yogurt, cheese, meat, poultry, seafood Low biologic sources: nuts, seeds, grains, legumes	20%	Fetal growth and development; formation of the placenta and amniotic fluid; growth of breast and uterine tissue; expanded blood volume	Associated with toxemia, anemia, poor uterine muscle tone, abortion, decreased resistance to infection, and shorter, lighter infants with low Apgar scores
Folic acid Liver Beef Legumes Wheat germ Enriched cereals Dark green leafy vegetables	122%	Important for DNA and RNA synthesis, and therefore cell proliferation related to growth and development; plays a role in the maturation of RBC	Maternal megaloblastic anemia, nausea, third trimester bleeding; may be related to congenital malformations or impaired fetal growth
Vit D Sunlight Vitamin D–fortified milk Margarine Breakfast cereals Liver Egg yolks	100%	Needed for fetal bone mineralization and normal calcium metabolism	Associated with neonatal hypocalcemia, tetany, and tooth enamel hypoplasia; may lead to maternal osteomalacia
Iron Liver Red meat Dried fruit Egg yolk Enriched and whole-grain breads and cereals Leafy vegetables Nuts Legumes (The absorption of iron from plant sources is greatly enhanced when a rich source of vitamin C is eaten at the same meal.)	100%	Increased maternal blood volume and hemoglobin; fetal iron storage	Maternal iron deficiency anemia: infants born to anemic mothers have decreased iron reserves and are more prone to anemia in the first year of life. Effect of maternal iron deficiency on infant birth weight is controversial; maternal iron deficiency may increase the incidence of prematurity.

(continued)

Nutrient and Sources	% Increase in RDA Above Nonpregnant Adult Female Aged 25–50	Rationale for Increase	Possible Outcome of Deficiency

Calcium
  Milk
  Yogurt
  Cheese
  Ice cream
  Green leafy vegetables
  Legumes
	50%	Formation of fetal skeleton and teeth; maintenance of maternal serum and bone calcium	Decreased maternal bone density → osteomalacia; decreased infant bone density → congenital rickets; may be a major factor in the development of toxemia

Table 10-4 (Continued)
Sources and Functions of Calories and Selected Nutrients During Pregnancy

Although the RDA for pregnancy may help health care professionals assess, plan, and evaluate dietary data, especially for a high-risk client, the following limitations must be considered:

- The RDA represents allowances, not requirements. Actual requirements during pregnancy vary among individuals and are influenced by previous nutritional status and health history, including chronic illnesses, multiple pregnancies, and closely spaced pregnancies.
- The requirement for one nutrient may be altered by the intake of another (ie, protein requirements increase if calorie needs are not met).
- Nutrient needs are not constant throughout the course of pregnancy.
- The evaluation of a client's diet using the RDA is complex and time-consuming. Many daily food guides for pregnancy have been developed for simple, quick, routine assessments and client teaching.

The Food Guide Pyramid Approach for Pregnancy and General Dietary Suggestions

Numerous federal, state, and private agencies have published sound daily food guides for choosing a healthy diet that promotes adequate weight gain during pregnancy. Most food guides are based on the food group approach to eating, with additional information provided regarding weight gain, meal frequency, water intake, and the use of vitamins, salt, alcohol, caffeine, and artificial sweeteners (March of Dimes Birth Defects Foundation, IFIC, 1991).

There are relatively few differences between the Food Guide Pyramid recommendations for nonpregnant adults and the Daily Food Guide recommendations for pregnancy (Table 10-5). One notable distinction is that the recommended number of servings from the milk group doubles during pregnancy; milk is an excellent source of protein, vitamin D, calcium, and other minerals. In fact, two additional glasses of 2% milk supply 240 calories (an extra 300 calories/day is recommended during the

FOOD *for* **THOUGHT**

Folic Acid: An Effective Weapon Against Birth Defects

Neural tube defects (NTD) occur when the neural tube, which develops into the spinal cord 18 to 26 days after conception, fails to close (Liebman, 1995). Errors at the top of the tube cause the infant to be born without a brain, causing infant death soon after birth. Spina bifida, the second most common birth defect in the United States, results when the error occurs further down the spinal cord: It is characterized by the incomplete closing of the bone casing surrounding the spinal cord. Two thirds of infants born with NTD survive into childhood; many of its victims lack bowel and bladder control, or suffer paralysis from the waist down. In some cases, mental retardation results from the excess accumulation of fluid in the brain.

Numerous studies have shown that women with diets low in folic acid are at increased risk of NTD, and conversely, women supplemented with folic acid during the first 6 weeks of pregnancy have a decreased incidence of babies born with NTD. Although researchers aren't exactly sure how folic acid prevents NTD, it is most likely related to its role in DNA formation, and thus cell division. The evidence is so convincing that the Centers for Disease Control and Prevention estimates that 50% to 70% of NTD could be prevented if all women of childbearing age consumed adequate amounts of folic acid.

Because NTD occur before many women even realize they are pregnant, adequate folic acid before conception and during the first critical weeks of pregnancy are imperative. This is why the U.S. Public Health Service recommends that all women of childbearing age consume 400 µg of folic acid daily, even though the current RDA for nonpregnant women is only 180 µg (International Food Information Council, 1994). The March of Dimes advises all women who are capable of becoming pregnant to eat a balanced diet and to take a daily multivitamin that contains folic acid.

Because folic acid is so important and yet many women fail to consume adequate amounts, especially minority and low-income women, policymakers are debating whether cereal grains should be fortified with folic acid, and if so, at what level (International Food Information Council, 1995). The benefits of fortification must be weighed against the potential risk: Folic acid can mask vitamin B_{12} deficiency, which, if left untreated, can result in permanent neurologic damage.

In the meantime, women who are planning to become pregnant should modify their diets to include more folate, which can be found in leafy, dark green vegetables, legumes, citrus fruits and juices, peanuts, whole grains, and fortified cereals. Also, a multivitamin that provides 100% of the recommended daily value of folic acid is a good idea.

second and third trimesters of pregnancy) and 16 g of protein (the RDA for protein increases by only 10 g during pregnancy). Obviously, little more is needed to fulfill the requirement for extra calories; however, milk does not supply adequate amounts of *all* essential nutrients. Consequently, wise food selections from the remaining food groups are needed to ensure nutritional adequacy.

WEIGHT GAIN

Women who begin pregnancy while underweight and poorly nourished are at higher risk for delivering LBW infants and for experiencing preterm labor of small, under-

Table 10-5
Daily Food Guide for Pregnancy and Lactation

Food Group	Serving Size of Representative Foods	No. of Servings Recommended for Adults (Food Guide Pyramid)	No. of Servings Recommended for Pregnancy	No. of Servings Recommended for Lactation
Bread, Cereal, Rice, and Pasta	1 slice bread ½ hamburger bun or English muffin 3–4 small or 2 large crackers ½ cup cooked cereal, pasta, or rice 1 oz ready-to-eat cereal	6–11	6–11	6–11
Vegetable	½ cup cooked or chopped raw vegetables 1 cup leafy raw vegetables ¾ cup vegetable juice	3–5	3–5 (Include at least 2 servings of dark green leafy, yellow, or orange vegetables	3–5 (Include at least 2 servings of dark green leafy, yellow, or orange vegetables
Fruit (Include at least one citrus fruit or juice)	¾ cup juice 1 medium apple, banana, or other fruit ½ cup fresh, cooked, or canned fruit	2–4	2–4	2–4
Milk, Yogurt, and Cheese	1 cup milk 1 cup buttermilk 8 oz yogurt 1½ oz natural cheese 2 oz processed cheese	2–3	4	4
Meat, Poultry, Fish, Dry Beans, Eggs, and Nuts	Total of 5–7 oz cooked lean meat/poultry/fish/other protein sources daily 1 oz = 1 egg ½ cup cooked beans 2 tablespoons peanut butter	2–3 (5–7 oz)	2–3 (6–7 oz)	2–3 (5–7 oz)
Fats, Oils, and Sweets	1 tsp butter or margarine 1 tbsp mayonnaise or salad dressing 2 tbsp sour cream 1 oz cream cheese 1 tsp jelly or jam 12 oz soft drink 1 oz chocolate bar ½ cup sherbet, gelatin, or sorbet Alcohol	Use sparingly	Limit fats and sweets; avoid alcohol	

Source: March of Dimes Birth Defects Foundation, International Food Information Council: *Healthy Eating During Pregnancy, 1991* and USDA, prepared by Human Nutrition Information Service: USDA's Food Guide Pyramid *Home and Garden Bulletin* number 249. Hyattsville, MD, 1992.

developed infants. Inadequate weight gain during pregnancy also increases the risk of giving birth to a low-birth-weight infant. Conversely, very high weight gain during pregnancy increases the incidence of high birth weight, which is associated with some increase in the risk of fetopelvic disproportion and other complications. The effect seems to be greatest in women who are shorter than 62 inches. Some studies also indicate that excessive weight gain during pregnancy contributes to maternal obesity.

Since 1970, there has been a shift away from recommending limited weight gain during pregnancy. Currently, the Weight Gain Subcommittee of the Institute of Medicine sets forth desirable ranges of total weight gain based on prepregnancy weight status, which can be evaluated by calculation of body mass index (BMI) (Table 10-6). Body mass index is defined as weight/height squared × 100, and it can be calculated using either English or metric units. For women of normal prepregnancy weight who are carrying a single fetus, a total gain of 25 to 35 lbs is recommended; optimal weight gain for underweight women may be 28 to 40 lbs, and obese women should gain at least 15 lbs (Subcommittee on Nutritional Status and Weight Gain During Pregnancy, 1990). Within each weight category, adolescent and black mothers should be encouraged to strive for weight gains toward the upper range. The Weight Gain Subcommittee of the Institute of Medicine recommends women carrying twins gain 35 to 45 lbs; however, some studies suggest gains of 40 to 45 pounds by 35 to 38 weeks gestation for ideal twin outcome (Luke and Leurgans, 1996). Length of gestation, BMI, and weight have been shown to be positive factors in twin birthweight (Luke and Leurgans, 1996).

The pattern of weight gain can also be an indicator of increased risk during pregnancy. Adult women who fail to gain 10 pounds by 20 weeks' gestation appear to be at greater risk for delivering a LBW infant (Springer et al, 1992). During the first trimester, a 2- to 5-lb weight gain is considered normal. Thereafter, recommended weight gain for normal-weight women is approximately 1 lb/week. Underweight women should gain slightly more than 1 lb/week, overweight women should gain about 0.66 lb/week, and women pregnant with twins should be encouraged to gain at

---

Table 10-6
Recommended Weight Gain During Pregnancy Based on Body Mass Index (BMI)

Prepregnancy BMI	Classification	Recommended Total Weight Gain Range
<19.8	Underweight	28–40 pounds
19.8–26.0	Normal weight	25–35 pounds
>26.0–29.0	Overweight	15–25 pounds
>29.0	Obese	At least 15 pounds

Source: Subcommittee of Nutritional Status and Weight Gain During Pregnancy, Food and Nutrition Board, National Academy of Sciences; *Nutrition During Pregnancy.* Washington, DC: National Academy Press, 1990.

least 1 lb/week. The rate of weight gain for severely obese women should be determined on an individualized basis; however, weight reduction should never be undertaken during pregnancy. Although slightly higher or lower rates of weight gain can be considered normal, obvious or persistent deviations warrant further investigation. For example, after the 20th week of gestation, a sudden sharp weight gain, accompanied by generalized edema and an elevated blood pressure, may signal preeclampsia.

MEAL FREQUENCY

Fasting, especially after midgestation, can result within 24 hours in hypoglycemia, hyperketonemia, acetonuria, and other signs of metabolic acidosis. Although the fetus can metabolize ketones to some degree, the effect of chronic maternal ketosis is not completely understood (Worthington-Roberts and Williams, 1993). Some studies concluded that children whose mothers had acetonuria during pregnancy had impaired intellectual and mental development, but more recent studies have failed to confirm these results. It appears that ketonuria and acetonuria occur normally in pregnancy (eg, after overnight fasting), and under normal circumstances, they probably do not threaten the fetus. However, the more serious condition of ketoacidosis, which results from severe calorie restriction, may pose a risk for the developing fetus. Therefore, women are advised to avoid periods of hunger by eating three meals and two to three nutritious snacks each day. Small, frequent meals may also help to alleviate nausea in the first trimester and heartburn during the second half of the pregnancy.

WATER INTAKE

Women are encouraged to drink six to eight glasses of fluid daily in the form of either water, fruit juice, or milk. Empty-calorie drinks like carbonated beverages and fruit-ades provide little more than calories.

VITAMIN SUPPLEMENTS

The Subcommittee on Dietary Intake and Nutrient Supplements During Pregnancy considers food to be the ideal source of required nutrients. The Committee states that the use of supplements "should be based on evidence of a benefit as well as a lack of harmful effects." They recommend that multivitamin and mineral supplements not be used routinely, nor should they replace food. However, supplements may be appropriate for certain nutrients and certain population groups. For instance, a low-dose multivitamin–mineral supplement is recommended for pregnant women in high-risk categories (eg, heavy smokers, drug abusers, and those carrying twins) and for those unlikely to consume an adequate diet despite dietary advice or counseling. Other indications for supplements are outlined in Table 10-7.

Based on dietary intake studies, the Subcommittee determined that iron is the only nutrient for which requirements *cannot* be met by diet alone. A daily supplement of 30 mg of ferrous iron is recommended for all women during the second and third trimesters, preferably taken between meals or at bedtime on an empty stomach to maximize absorption.

Table 10-7
Recommendations for Nutrient Supplements During Pregnancy

Supplement	Indications
Iron	30–60 mg of ferrous iron is recommended for all pregnant women during the second and third trimesters. Absorption is enhanced on an empty stomach; however, it may be better tolerated with food. Vitamin C does not improve absorption of ferrous iron supplements.
Folic acid	300 μg/day may be used when dietary intake appears inadequate.
Multivitamin and mineral supplements	Indicated beginning at the second trimester for women with inadequate intakes and for high-risk women: heavy cigarette smokers, alcohol and drug abusers, or women carrying more than one fetus. Supplements are better absorbed on an empty stomach.
Vitamin D	10 μg (400 IU) are recommended for complete vegans and others who do not consume adequate amounts of vitamin D–fortified milk. Adequate dietary/supplement intake is especially important for women with minimal exposure to sunlight.
Calcium	600 mg/day is recommended for women under 25 years of age who consume less than 600 mg of calcium/day. Calcium supplements should be taken with meals to enhance absorption and reduce interaction with iron supplements.
Vitamin B_{12}	2.0 μg/day is recommended for complete vegans.
Zinc and copper	Because iron can interfere with their absorption and utilization, 15 mg of zinc and 2 mg of copper are recommended for women who take more than 30 mg of iron/day for the treatment of anemia.

Source: Subcommittee on Nutritional Status and Weight Gain During Pregnancy, Food and Nutrition Board, National Academy of Sciences: *Nutrition During Pregnancy.* Washington, DC: National Academy Press, 1990.

SALT

Sodium needs increase during pregnancy to maintain normal sodium levels in the expanded blood volume and tissues. Restricting sodium intake may adversely affect both mother and fetus; therefore, a moderate intake of iodized salt is recommended.

ALCOHOL

Because alcohol is a potent teratogen and a "safe" level of consumption is not known, women are advised to avoid alcohol during pregnancy (March of Dimes Birth Defects Foundation, International Food Information Council, 1991). Alcohol may cause damage by dehydrating fetal cells, leaving them dead or functionless, or by causing secondary nutrient deficiencies related to poor intake, decreased absorption, altered metabolism, or increased excretion.

Chronic alcohol consumption can result in **fetal alcohol syndrome (FAS)**, a condition that is characterized by varying degrees of physical and mental growth failure and birth defects. Unlike other small-for-gestational-age infants, infants with FAS do not experience normal "catch-up" growth. Some degree of intellectual impairment is also frequently reported in children with FAS.

Not all alcoholic mothers deliver FAS infants, yet even alcoholics who abstain during pregnancy have a higher incidence of LBW infants than women who do not have a history of alcoholism. Although chronic alcohol abuse clearly increases the risks of growth failure and birth defects, and the effects of alcohol appear to be dose-related, there are no established guidelines to indicate when consumption is safe and how much alcohol can be consumed safely. Studies on the effects of low doses of alcohol on fetal growth have been limited and inconsistent. Although an occasional drink may not cause damage, abstinence is recommended.

CAFFEINE

Studies show no association between moderate caffeine consumption and adverse pregnancy outcomes such as miscarriage, low birth weight, and short gestation (IFIC, 1994). Moderate use of coffee and caffeine (the equivalent of 2–3 cups of coffee daily) does not appear to pose any risk.

ARTIFICIAL SWEETENERS

The use of artificial sweeteners during pregnancy has been extensively studied. Because saccharin can cross the placenta, excessive use should be avoided during pregnancy, even though there is no evidence that saccharin is harmful to the fetus (ADA, 1993b). With the exception of women with phenylketonuria, aspartame is safe during pregnancy, even at extremely high intakes. Of its three metabolites, aspartate crosses the placenta only when enormous amounts are consumed; phenylalanine crosses the placenta, but in amounts far below the neurotoxic level; and the amount of methanol present in the compound is very small, although little is known about placental transfer and its fetal effects (ADA, 1993b). Studies have also concluded that acesulfame K is safe for use during pregnancy. Prudent use of aspartame or acesulfame K during pregnancy allows women to satisfy their taste for "sweets" without consuming extra calories.

NURSING PROCESS

Initial assessment of anthropometric, biochemical, dietary, and clinical data, including medical–socioeconomic information, should be performed to identify clients who are at risk for poor nutritional status during pregnancy (see display, Risk Factors for Poor Nutritional Status During Pregnancy) and also to establish baseline data. Ongoing nutritional assessment and dietary evaluation, performed regularly throughout the course of pregnancy, provide continuing surveillance and help to identify clients in need of dietary counseling or community assistance (see display, General Pregnancy and Lactation Assessment Criteria).

Assessment

In addition to general pregnancy and lactation assessment criteria, assess for the following factors:

Risk Factors for Poor Nutritional Status During Pregnancy

ANTHROPOMETRIC DATA

Prepartum weight <85% or >120% of ideal weight

Inadequate weight gain: <10 lb weight gain during the first 20 weeks of pregnancy; <2 lb weight gain/month after the first trimester

Excessive weight gain: >2 lb/week

BIOCHEMICAL DATA

Low or deficient hemoglobin and hematocrit

DIETARY DATA

Use of a therapeutic diet for a chronic disease

Substance abuse: tobacco, alcohol, drugs

Food faddism, unbalanced diet, pica (ingestion of nonfood items)

MEDICAL–SOCIOECONOMIC DATA

Age ≤15 years or ≥35 years

Poor obstetric history (LBW, stillbirth, abortion, and fetal anomalies), high parity, multipara

Repetitive pregnancies at short intervals

Economically deprived

Chronic preexisting medical problems, such as hypertension, diabetes, heart disease, pulmonary disease, renal disease, maternal phenylketonuria

Current weight, projected and actual quantity and rate of weight gain. Figures 10-1, 10-2, and 10-3 are provisional weight gain graphs based on prepregnancy body mass.

Usual 24-hour intake according to the Daily Food Guide for Pregnancy, including foods from the "Fats, Oils, and Sweets" group and fluids consumed. A food frequency record or food record is obtained to provide more specific information. Pay particular attention to total quantity of food consumed, as well as the

ASSESSMENT CRITERIA

General Pregnancy and Lactation Assessment Criteria

Prepregnancy weight, preferably from a previously recorded measure

Height

Present weight

BMI

Blood pressure

Hemoglobin, hematocrit to detect preexisting anemia. (Many laboratory values change during pregnancy because of normal adjustments in maternal physiology, and therefore laboratory tests during pregnancy cannot be validly compared to nonpregnancy standards. Biochemical norms have not been established for lactating

women; hence laboratory tests are not indicated for routine assessments.)

Severe dependent edema

Other clinical signs that may occur during pregnancy (ie, bleeding gums) may be related to normal physiologic changes, not to nutritional deficiencies. However, a general examination of the skin, mucous membranes, gums, teeth, tongue, eyes, and hair that reveals abnormal findings may indicate potential nutritional problems that warrant further investigation.

History of chronic illness, use of medications

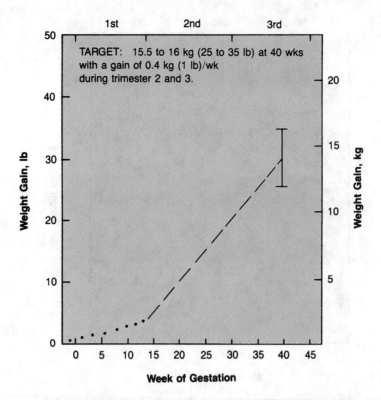

Assumes a 1.6-kg (3.5-lb) gain in first trimester and the remaining gain at a rate of 0.44 kg (0.97 lb) per week.

Figure 10-1
Provisional weight gain graph for normal weight women with BMI of 19.8 to 26.0 (metric)

number of servings consumed from each of the food groups. Because low intakes of iron, and folic acid are common in the average American diet, assess food sources of these nutrients (see Table 10-4). Other nutrients that are often consumed in suboptimal amounts by the general population include vitamin B_6 (chicken, fish, peanuts, oats, pork, organ meats, egg yolk, whole grains), and zinc (meat, oysters, seafood, milk, egg yolks, legumes, whole grains). Determine what interventions are required to improve intake.

Gastrointestinal (GI) side effects of pregnancy (nausea, vomiting, constipation, heartburn, increased appetite); assess onset, frequency, causative factors, severity, interventions attempted, and the results of these interventions.

Dietary changes made in response to pregnancy or diet-related complications of pregnancy (ie, foods avoided, foods preferred) (see display, Nutrition-Related Problems and Complications During Pregnancy). Determine foods best and least tolerated.

The frequency of eating; assess for periods of fasting.

Cultural, familial, religious, and ethnic influences on eating habits. Determine what specific beliefs the client has regarding diet during pregnancy, including the practice of **pica,** and how they affect intake and the need for diet counsel-

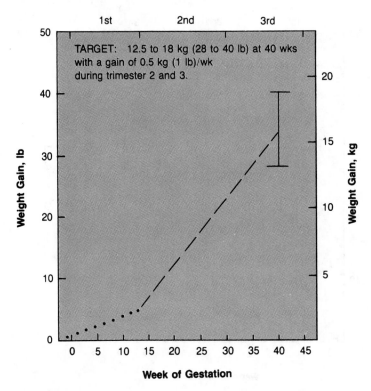

Assumes a 2.3-kg (5-lb) gain in first trimester and the remaining gain at a rate of 0.49 kg (1.07 lb) per week.

Figure 10-2

Provisional weight gain graph for underweight women with BMI less than 19.8 (metric)

ing (Carruth and Skinner, 1991) (see display, Common Myths About Nutrition During Pregnancy).

The use of vitamin and/or mineral supplements—type, amount, and frequency. Evaluate their safety and effectiveness; determine if they are being used appropriately or whether they are being used as a substitute for a healthy diet.

History of food intolerances (especially lactose intolerance) or allergies; evaluate their impact on overall intake.

The client's nutritional knowledge and ability and/or willingness to implement dietary changes.

The client's knowledge and plans regarding breast-feeding; consider whether the client is carrying more than one fetus.

The client's use of alcohol, tobacco, caffeine, drugs, and artificial sweeteners.

Financial status. Women who are determined to be at nutritional risk because of inadequate nutrition and inadequate income may be eligible for Women, Infants and Children (WIC), a supplemental food program for pregnant and postpartum women (provided up to 1 year if breast-feeding, up to 6 months if bottle-feeding), infants, and children up to age 5 years. WIC provides nutritional counseling and vouchers for specified foods of high nutritional quality.

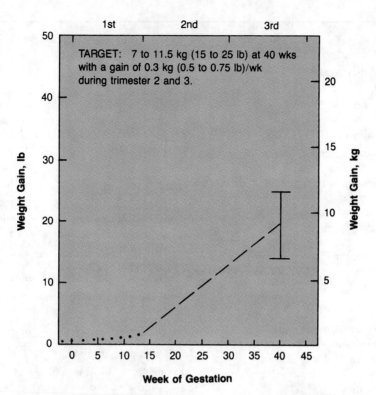

Assumes a 0.9-kg (2-lb) gain in first trimester and the remaining gain at a rate of 0.3 kg (0.67 lb) per week.

Figure 10-3
Provisional weight gain graph for overweight women with BMI of more than 26.0 to 29.0 (metric).

Nursing Diagnosis

Health Seeking Behaviors, as evidenced by a lack of knowledge of appropriate diet for pregnancy and a desire to learn.

Planning and Implementation

Nutritional counseling is an essential component of prenatal care. For optimal impact on maternal and infant health, nutritional counseling ideally should begin before conception. However, before counseling can begin, it is necessary to identify the client's emotional needs by talking with her to learn about her attitudes, beliefs, and fears.

The most effective approach to nutritional counseling begins with a dietary assessment to determine usual intake and food preferences and aversions, and to identify potential nutritional problems. Individualized nutritional counseling, initiated during the first prenatal visit and continued throughout the course of pregnancy, should stress the maintenance of good dietary habits and should recommend

(text continues on page 283)

Nutrition-Related Problems and Complications During Pregnancy

COMMON GASTROINTESTINAL DISCOMFORTS

Nausea and Vomiting

Nausea and vomiting, common during the first trimester, may be related to hypoglycemia, decreased gastric motility, relaxation of the cardiac sphincter, or anxiety.

Nursing Interventions
Encourage the client

- To eat small frequent meals every 2 to 3 hours
- To increase CHO intake; in addition to leaving the stomach quickly, CHO also raise blood glucose levels
- To eat CHO before rising, like dry crackers, melba toast, dry cereal, hard candy
- To avoid drinking liquids with meals
- To avoid coffee, tea, and spicy foods
- To avoid high-fat foods because they delay gastric emptying time
- To eliminate individual intolerances

Constipation

Constipation during pregnancy may be caused by relaxation of GI muscle tone and motility related to elevated progesterone levels, or may result from pressure of the fetus on the intestines. Other contributing factors may include a decrease in physical activity and an inadequate intake of fluid and fiber. Constipation is also a common side effect of iron supplements.

Nursing Interventions
Encourage the client

- To increase fiber intake, especially whole-grain breads and cereals high in bran (see Chap. 16)
- To drink at least eight glasses of liquid daily
- To try hot water with lemon or prune juice on waking to help stimulate peristalsis

Recommend regular exercise. Reduce the dosage or frequency, if possible, if iron supplement is contributing to constipation.

Heartburn

A decrease in gastric motility, relaxation of the cardiac sphincter, and pressure of the uterus on the stomach are contributing factors to heartburn.

Nursing Interventions
Encourage the client

- To eat small frequent meals and eliminate liquids immediately before and after meals to avoid gastric distention
- To avoid coffee, high-fat foods, and spices
- To eliminate individual intolerances

Advise the client not to lie down or bend over after eating.

NUTRITIONAL COMPLICATIONS

Iron Deficiency Anemia

Although iron absorption increases during pregnancy and losses through menstruation cease, maternal stores and diet are not likely to be sufficient to meet the increased demands for iron related to expanded blood volume and fetal requirements.

Nursing Interventions
Advise the client that

- Liver and red meats are the best sources of iron.
- Iron absorption from plant sources can be maximized by eating them with a rich source of vitamin C or with red meat.
- Iron absorption from plant sources is impaired when food is consumed with coffee and tea.

Encourage the client to take iron supplements as prescribed. See *Drug Alert* for possible adverse side effects and nursing actions related to iron supplements.

Inadequate Weight Gain

Inadequate weight gain may occur secondary to a poor appetite related to nausea, vomiting, heartburn, or smoking, or from an inadequate intake

Nutrition-Related Problems and Complications During Pregnancy *(Continued)*

related to lack of knowledge, fear of gaining weight, or an inadequate food budget. Women who mistakenly believe that the fetus is a perfect parasite and will be adequately nourished regardless of maternal intake may also experience inadequate weight gain.

Although a short-term goal is to promote weight gain, the timing and the source of the weight gain are equally important. On a long-term basis, an improvement in overall eating habits will benefit both the health of the family and any subsequent pregnancies.

Nursing Interventions

Encourage the client to continue good eating practices and recommend specific ways to improve other habits.

Set mutually agreeable weight gain goals.

Depending on the cause, make appropriate diet modifications to improve appetite. Advise the client to quit smoking, not only to improve appetite, but because smoking is detrimental to both maternal and infant health.

Counsel the client on the recommended rate and quantity of weight gain associated with optimal maternal and infant health and the ability to successfully breast-feed. Explain how the weight gain is distributed between the fetus, placenta, and maternal tissues. Encourage the client to ask questions and verbalize feelings. Advise the client that extra weight gained during pregnancy is quickly lost during lactation or through dieting *after* pregnancy.

Advise the client that

- If her diet is inadequate in calories, it also probably is inadequate in other nutrients.
- All nutrient requirements increase during pregnancy to support the growth of the fetus, placenta, and maternal tissues.
- Although the fetus can utilize maternal nutrient stores if her diet is inadequate, many nutrients are not stored by the body and a daily dietary intake is necessary.

- An inadequate intake can adversely affect maternal health (ie, poor iron intake → anemia, poor calcium intake → increased chance of bone loss later in life) and infant health (low birth weight, anemia, other postnatal complications)

Refer the client to social services; determine if the client is eligible for WIC.

Excessive Weight Gain

After the 20th week of gestation, rapid weight gain may be a sign of fluid retention and preeclampsia.

Women who overeat may do so because they lack knowledge concerning recommended weight gain, or may believe that a pregnant woman must "eat for two." Stress may add to overeating; a decrease in physical activity can contribute to weight gain.

Although it is prudent to prevent excessive weight gain, weight reduction diets should *never* be undertaken because of the risk of ketonemia and its potential damage to the fetus. Also, counting calories may take priority over the nutritional value of foods and result in a nutrient-poor diet. Again, a long-term objective of diet counseling is to improve eating habits for family health and any subsequent pregnancies.

Nursing Interventions

Notify the physician if signs of preeclampsia are observed: hypertension, fluid retention, albuminuria, complaints of headaches, blurred vision or visual disturbances.

Counsel the client on the recommended rate and quantity of weight gain associated with optimal maternal and infant health and the ability to successfully breast-feed. Explain how the weight gain is distributed between the fetus, placenta, and maternal tissues. Set mutually agreeable weight gain goals. Recommend specific ways to limit the rate of weight gain without compromising nutrient intake.

(continued)

Nutrition-Related Problems and Complications During Pregnancy *(Continued)*

Substitute skim or low-fat milk for whole milk.

Bake, broil, or steam foods instead of frying.

Eliminate empty calories: carbonated beverages, candy, rich desserts, traditional snack foods.

Limit portion sizes to those recommended by the Daily Food Guide for pregnancy.

Use fats and oils sparingly.

Inadequate Intake of Vitamin B₁₂, Calcium, Vitamin D, Riboflavin, and Possibly Calories Related to Pure Vegetarianism/Veganism (Elimination of All Animal Products)

Vegan diets are lacking in vitamin B_{12} because it is found only in animal products (and fortified soybean milk). Also, diets lacking in milk and dairy products are likely to be deficient in calcium, vitamin D, and riboflavin, particularly during pregnancy. In addition, vegetarian diets tend to be lower in calories than normal mixed diets.

Nursing Interventions
Explain the importance of obtaining adequate amounts of vitamin B_{12}, calcium, vitamin D, riboflavin, and calories during pregnancy, and the difficulty in obtaining these nutrients through a vegan diet.

Encourage the client

- To include milk, dairy products, and eggs in her diet during pregnancy and lactation
- To eat a variety of foods
- To take vitamin B_{12}, calcium, and vitamin D supplements if milk and dairy product intake is deficient
- To replace sea salt with iodized salt, if appropriate.

Inadequate Intake of Calcium, Vitamin D, Riboflavin, and Possibly Protein Related to Lactose or Milk Intolerance

Clients with lactose or milk intolerance avoid milk because they experience gas, distention, cramping, and diarrhea to some degree after ingesting lactose (milk sugar). Diets lacking in milk and dairy products are likely to be deficient in calcium, vitamin D, and riboflavin.

Nursing Interventions
Obtain a history to determine the extent of milk or lactose intolerance.

Many people with milk intolerance (milder form of lactose intolerance) can tolerate milk if it is consumed slowly and with food. Encourage the maximum intake of milk tolerated.

Advise the client of the importance of an adequate calcium intake during pregnancy (and lactation) and suggest other dairy products that may be tolerated: Lactaid milk (commercially treated to reduce the lactose content), yogurt, buttermilk. (Other sources of calcium are listed in Appendix 12; see Chap. 16 for more information on lactose intolerance.)

Provide a calcium supplement, if appropriate.

Pica

Pica is a psychobehavioral disorder characterized by the ingestion of nonfoodstuffs—dirt, clay, starch, and ice are the most common items ingested. Eating these items may displace the intake of nutritious foods or interfere with nutrient absorption. Other potential complications vary with the items ingested and include lead poisoning, fecal impaction, parasitic infections, prematurity, and toxemia.

Iron deficiency may be a risk factor for pica; however, studies suggest it is more likely a consequence. Pica can be a strongly rooted social tradition and is more prevalent among blacks and rural residents. Other suggested risk factors include low socioeconomic status, inadequate nutritional status, and a childhood or family history of pica. Pica is surrounded by misconceptions about pregnancy and childbirth.

Some women who practice pica claim that it "helps" babies, cures swollen legs, relieves nausea and vomiting, ensures beautiful children, helps infants "slide out" more easily, and prevents birth marks. Pica may also be used to relieve tension or hunger, and some women claim they are merely satisfying cravings for clay or starch.

Nutrition-Related Problems and Complications During Pregnancy (Continued)

Some studies indicate anemia, iron deficiency, and toxemia are the most common outcomes in mothers with pica; dysfunctional labor related to fecal impaction, maternal death, premature birth, perinatal mortality, low birth weight, and anemia in the infant have also been reported.

Nursing Interventions

Determine what is being ingested and why. Refer the client to social services or WIC if appropriate.

Remain nonjudgmental but stress the importance of an adequate diet during pregnancy and the potential dangers of pica.

Offer economical ways to obtain an adequate diet.

Provide an iron supplement if appropriate.

Encourage a high-fiber, high-fluid diet if the client experiences constipation.

Observe for diarrhea and vomiting, which may indicate a parasitic infection or lead poisoning.

MEDICAL COMPLICATIONS

Maternal Phenylketonuria

Phenylketonuria (PKU) is an inborn error of phenylalanine (an essential amino acid) metabolism that results in retardation and physical handicaps in newborns, if not treated with a low-phenylalanine diet shortly after birth. Women who have PKU and who consume a normal diet during pregnancy have a high risk of delivering an infant with microcephaly, mental retardation, and LBW, even though the infant does not have PKU. The incidence of spontaneous abortion also increases.

Animal studies indicate that the fetus is more vulnerable to phenylalanine than the PKU mother and that a safe maternal intake may be harmful to the fetus. Also, low-phenylalanine diets initiated after conception may be of little value; in order to prevent mental and physical handicaps, rigid diets may be necessary before conception.

Nursing Interventions

Obtain a complete history to determine if the client has PKU. Many adults may not be aware of their history of PKU if the diet was discontinued early in childhood. Maternal PKU may present a bigger problem for adolescents with unexpected pregnancies who may hide the pregnancy until late in gestation.

Advise the client

- That complete understanding and strict adherence to the diet are vital.
- That protein foods are high in phenylalanine and must be eliminated: meat, fish, poultry, eggs, dairy products, and nuts.
- That the special PKU formula is expensive and often offensive to adult palates, but must be consumed in adequate amounts both to support fetal growth and to prevent maternal tissue breakdown, which would have results similar to those from cheating on the diet.
- That an adequate calorie intake is necessary for normal protein metabolism.
- On the importance of close monitoring and periodic evaluations.

Diabetes Mellitus

Diabetes mellitus, which is characterized by abnormal glucose tolerance, requires dietary management, whether it was present before conception (established diabetes) or develops during gestation (gestational diabetes) as a result of the metabolic changes of pregnancy. Diabetes increases the risk of infection, especially urinary tract infection, preeclampsia, and eclampsia. The incidence of spontaneous abortion, hydramnios, extrauterine and neonatal deaths, and congenital abnormalities is higher among established diabetic patients. Gestational diabetes doesn't usually produce maternal complications or birth defects, but it can make delivery difficult because babies born to gestational diabetics are usually large, which may increase the risk of postpartum hemorrhage.

(continued)

Nutrition-Related Problems and Complications During Pregnancy (Continued)

Diabetic management during pregnancy includes diet therapy and, possibly, multiple daily doses of insulin.

Nursing Interventions

Monitor the progress and course of pregnancy of established diabetics. Screen all women for gestational diabetes between 24 and 28 weeks of pregnancy. Check for ketonuria regularly.

Advise the client

- That pregnant diabetics require the same nutrients and weight gain as nondiabetic pregnant women.
- That she is not on a "diet"; weight loss and fasting should never be undertaken during pregnancy.
- That calorie requirements are based on prepregnancy weight (Fagen et al., 1995):

    30 cal/kg for women of normal weight prior to conception

    24 cal/kg for women weighing >120% desirable weight before conception

    36–40 cal/kg for women weighing <90% desirable weight before conception.

- That adequate food intake prevents ketone formation and promotes proper weight gain. The individualized meal plan should be high in complex CHO and fiber, and limited in fat and sugar.
- That three meals plus three snacks daily may promote better glycemic control.
- That close monitoring (ie, daily urine ketone testing for gestational diabetics, blood monitoring for established diabetics) and periodic evaluations are necessary throughout the course of pregnancy to meet nutritional needs and to control blood glucose levels.
- That glucose tolerance returns to normal in gestational diabetics after delivery, although they are at increased risk to develop diabetes later in life (Jonaitis, 1995).

Pregnancy-Induced Hypertension

Pregnancy-induced hypertension (PIH or toxemia) is a hypertensive syndrome occurring in approximately 6% to 7% of all pregnancies. Severe cases are associated with an increased risk of maternal, fetal, and neonatal deaths.

Preeclampsia is characterized by hypertension accompanied by proteinuria, edema, or both. A sudden weight gain (>2 lb/week after the 20th week of gestation) may indicate preeclampsia.

Eclampsia develops with the occurrence of one or more convulsions resulting from preeclampsia.

Although the exact cause is unknown, the development of PIH is strongly correlated to poverty and malnutrition, especially inadequate intakes of calories, protein, sodium, and possibly calcium. Good nutrition can prevent toxemia, and prevention is far more effective than treatment. Women at risk include those who are poorly nourished, primigravida, economically deprived, very young or very old, obese and gain too much weight, or underweight and fail to gain enough weight.

Nursing Interventions

Screen women at risk for toxemia and monitor for signs and symptoms: Hypertension, facial edema, proteinuria (especially albumin), headaches, blurred vision or visual disturbances.

Obtain a 24-hour recall and evaluate the diet according to the Daily Food Guide for Pregnancy, paying particular attention to calorie, protein, calcium, and sodium intakes.

Advise clients at risk for preeclampsia to consume a liberal intake of calories, protein, and calcium, and to salt their food to taste. Sodium-restricted diets and diuretics are not advised.

Recommend ways to improve the diet that are acceptable to the client.

Identify and refer women who are eligible for social service programs or WIC.

Common Myths About Nutrition During Pregnancy

You can eat anything you want because you're eating for two.

You can eat double portions because you're eating for two.

You should eat whatever you're craving; your body must need it.

If you take prenatal vitamins, you don't have to worry about what you eat.

You must take vitamins to have a healthy baby.

The baby gets what he or she needs first, the rest goes to the mother.

If you breast-feed, you can lose all the weight you gain in pregnancy.

Obese women don't need to gain weight during pregnancy.

It doesn't matter what you eat because the baby will take what it needs from your body.

As long as you take vitamins, it's all right to skip meals.

When you are pregnant, you will crave pickles and ice cream.

Gaining lots of weight makes a healthy baby.

You lose a tooth with every baby if you don't drink milk.

Beets build red blood.

Food cravings during pregnancy will determine your child's likes and dislikes later in life.

Give in to your cravings, or you will mark the baby.

Do not eat fish and milk at the same meal.

Do not eat egg yolks because they will rot the uterus.

If you crave sweets, the baby will be a girl; if you crave pickles, the baby will be a boy.

Source: Carruth BR, Skinner JD: Practitioners beware: Regional differences in beliefs about nutrition during pregnancy. J Am Diet Assoc 91:435, 1991.

realistic ways to improve intake. A variety of teaching materials are available; select those appropriate for the client's level of understanding.

Because the risk of low gestational weight gain is higher among unmarried women, adolescents, black and Hispanic women, cigarette smokers, and women with low levels of education, these women should receive additional nutritional counseling to ensure an adequate weight gain during pregnancy (Subcommittee on Nutritional Status and Weight Gain During Pregnancy, 1990).

Breast-feeding promotion should begin early and continue throughout gestation.

CLIENT GOALS

The client will:

Explain the importance of diet for her health and for fetal growth and development.

Plan ___ days' menus that are nutritionally adequate, using the Daily Food Guide for Pregnancy.

Consume an adequate, varied, and balanced diet based on the Daily Food Guide for Pregnancy.

Avoid periods of fasting by consuming three meals per day plus two to three nutritious snacks.

Gain weight within the recommended range and rate, as determined by her assessment data.

Have an absence of nutrition-related problems or complications of pregnancy (see display, Nutrition-Related Problems and Complications During Pregnancy).

NURSING INTERVENTIONS

Diet Management

Set a mutually agreeable weight gain goal (range), based on the client's prepregnancy weight for height.

Promote the intake of a varied, nutrient-dense diet based on the Daily Food Guide for Pregnancy (see Table 10-5). Although the actual nutrient content of the diet will vary with the foods chosen, using the Guide will help ensure an average adequate intake.

Modify the diet as needed, to avoid or alleviate nutrition-related problems or complications of pregnancy.

Client Teaching

Instruct the client and family:

About the importance of adequate nutrition and weight gain for maternal and infant health. Describe the optimal rate of weight gain. Explain that weight gain during pregnancy is not synonymous with "getting fat," and that weight reduction should never be undertaken during pregnancy, even by overweight women. Overweight women who require less weight gain than normal should be instructed on how to choose a nutrient-dense diet for a controlled amount of high-quality weight gain.

About how to achieve nutritional adequacy by using the Daily Food Guide for Pregnancy. Stress the principles of variety, balance, and moderation; items from the "Fats, Oils, and Sweets" group should be used sparingly. Counsel the client on meal frequency, fluid requirements, and the use of salt, alcohol, caffeine, and artificial sweeteners.

To take supplements only as prescribed by the physician. Discourage the use of supplements that are not prescribed by the physician and stress the importance of taking only the prescribed dosage, because megadoses of some vitamins and minerals may cause fetal malformations. Advise against the use of dolomite and bone meal as calcium supplements; they may contain high levels of lead and other heavy metals, which pose a hazard to both mother and fetus.

To avoid alcohol, tobacco, and drugs during pregnancy because of the actual or potential adverse health effects on both mother and baby (Yu and Jackson, 1995).

That although coffee, caffeine, and artificial sweeteners are not necessarily contraindicated during pregnancy, they should be used in moderation.

That cravings during pregnancy do not appear to have a physiologic basis; rather, they are likely to be influenced by culture, geography, social traditions, the availability of foods, and previous experience. Satisfying cravings for foods is relatively harmless, as long as the overall impact on nutrient intake is not negative (eg, an occasional dill pickle is okay; eating an entire jar of them is not). Cravings for nonfood items should be investigated (see display, Nutrition-Related Problems and Complications During Pregnancy, for discussion of pica). Dispel myths about diet during pregnancy (see display, Common Myths About Nutrition During Pregnancy).

About how to modify her diet to alleviate or avoid nutrition-related problems and complications of pregnancy (see display, Nutrition-Related Problems and Complications During Pregnancy), as appropriate.

To avoid all medications unless approved by the physician.

That once labor begins, no food or liquids should be consumed in order to prevent aspiration if anesthesia is used.

Monitoring Progress

Monitor for the following signs or symptoms:

Monthly weight gain. Weight gains of less than 1 pound per month by obese women or less than 2 pounds for all other women warrant further investigation.

Food intolerances, especially lactose intolerance, and the overall impact on diet adequacy.

Ongoing compliance and tolerance of diet; evaluate adequacy and the need for further diet counseling or WIC participation.

Evaluation

Evaluation is ongoing. Assuming that the plan of care has not changed, the client will achieve the goals as stated above.

DRUG
ALERT   *Iron Supplements*

USE

Prevention and treatment of iron deficiency anemia

POSSIBLE ADVERSE SIDE EFFECTS

May cause diarrhea, constipation, dark-colored stools, and GI upset. Although better absorbed when taken between meals, iron supplements are less irritating to the GI tract when taken with food.

ACTIONS

Observe for diarrhea and constipation. If constipation is not alleviated with a high-fiber diet, consider reducing the dosage or frequency.

If supplements are irritating to the GI tract when taken between meals, advise the client to take them with food.

Advise the client that a change in stool color is to be expected.

ADOLESCENT PREGNANCY

Each year, 10% of American females between the ages of 15 and 19 become pregnant, with half choosing to keep their infants (ADA, 1994). Compared to infants born to adults, infants of adolescent mothers are more likely to be preterm, have low birth weight, require intensive care, or die at birth. They are also more likely to have physical problems or to die just after the newborn period (ADA, 1994).

Adolescent pregnancies are at increased risk for complications because of psychosocial and economic factors. In addition, adolescents with a **gynecologic age** (age at conception minus age of menarche) of less than 4 years are at high nutritional risk; gynecologic age less than 2 years has the highest risk for pregnancy complications. Preterm births, pregnancy-induced hypertension, anemia, and sexually transmitted disease are the most common problems seen in pregnant adolescents under the age of 16 (ADA, 1994). Compared to adult women, pregnant adolescents:

- Are more likely to be physically, emotionally, financially, and socially immature. Low socioeconomic status may be the major reason for the high incidence of LBW infants and other complications of adolescent pregnancy (ADA, 1994).
- May not have adequate nutrient stores because they need large amounts of nutrients for their own growth and development. Although female adolescent growth is usually complete by age 15, physical maturity is not reached until 4 years after menarche, which usually occurs by age 17 (Dunn et al, 1994).
- Have dietary practices that do not provide adequate nourishment to support their own growth, pregnancy, and fetal development. Voluntary calorie restriction to control weight, erratic eating patterns, reliance on fast foods and convenience foods, and meal skipping are common adolescent practices.
- Must gain weight early and steadily in order to maximize the chance of giving birth to an optimal-weight infant (ADA, 1994). The National Academy of Science recommends that pregnant adolescents gain 25 to 40 pounds, depending on their prepregnancy BMI.
- Give low priority to nutrition. In one study, pregnant teens frequently reported drinking three to four cans of soda per day and substituting chips, candy, and soda for a meal (Schneck et al, 1990). More than 40% of teens studied indicated that they did not make any dietary changes while pregnant, and other studies indicate much higher percentages of teens reporting similar behavior (Schneck, 1990).
- Are more reluctant to take supplements, making adequate dietary intake essential.
- Seek prenatal care later and have fewer total visits.

Nutritional Requirements

The RDA for pregnancy are not categorized according to maternal age. For instance, the RDA for calcium for nonpregnant women aged 11 to 24 is 1200 mg, the same amount that is recommended for pregnant women. Obviously, teenagers require more than their normal RDA during pregnancy; however, actual nutrient needs depend more on gynecologic age than chronologic age and should be determined on an individual basis.

Nutrient requirements during pregnancy also are influenced by preconception nutritional status. Nutrients most often lacking in female adolescent diets are calcium; iron; zinc; vitamins A, D, and B_6; riboflavin; folic acid; and calories (ADA, 1994). Like pregnant adults, adolescents need supplements of iron in addition to a nutritious diet. It is recommended that adolescents at risk of poor intakes take supplements containing calcium, vitamins B_6 and D, and folate (ADA, 1994).

Diet Counseling

Proper nutrition is one of the most important controllable factors that determine the overall outcome of pregnancy; it has the potential to decrease the incidence of LBW infants and to improve the health of infants born to adolescents (ADA, 1994). In addition, nutritional counseling can influence the outcome of subsequent pregnancies and improve the nutrition of families headed by adolescents (ADA, 1994).

The diet management and client teaching procedures outlined earlier are appropriate for adolescent pregnancies as well. However, to maximize the effectiveness of nutritional counseling for adolescents, it is particularly important to establish a rapport in a relaxed, nonthreatening, nonjudgmental environment. In addition to assessing the client's nutritional needs, her social, emotional, and economic needs, as well as psychosocial status and ethnicity, must also be evaluated. Many teens have limited reading skills; therefore, teaching materials must be appropriate for their level of understanding. The Daily Food Guide for Pregnancy is useful both in assessing dietary strengths and weaknesses and in providing a framework for implementing dietary changes in a way the teenager can understand.

Set mutually agreeable realistic goals for weight gain and food intake. Diet recommendations must be concrete, reasonable, and achievable within the client's financial status and lifestyle. Because teens living with one or more parents may have little control over what food is available to them, parents and significant others should also be encouraged to attend counseling sessions.

Ideally, the client should be counseled early in the pregnancy and monitored frequently throughout gestation to evaluate the effectiveness of the nutritional care plan and to redefine needs as the pregnancy progresses. Prenatal counseling should also include information about infant and child feeding practices.

LACTATION

Breast-feeding is widely believed to be the method of feeding that provides optimal health and well-being for most infants (Sciacca et al, 1995). Because it imparts benefits to both mother and infant, exclusive breast-feeding is recommended for all normal, full-term infants for the first 5 to 6 months of life (ADA, 1993a) (see display, Advantages and Disadvantages of Breast-feeding). The benefits of breast-feeding are especially important to infants born of low-income mothers because they are at

Advantages and Disadvantages of Breast-feeding

ADVANTAGES

For the infant:

- "Breast is best"—breast milk contains all essential nutrients in optimal amounts and in forms the infant can easily tolerate and digest, and it changes to match the needs of a growing infant. Breast milk is recommended as the sole source of nutrition for the first 5 to 6 months of life.
- Breast milk is a "natural" food that contains no artificial colorings, flavorings, preservatives, or additives.
- Breast-feeding is associated with significant decreases in the incidence and duration of both GI and non-GI infections, such as otitis media, pneumonia, bacteremia, and meningitis (ADA, 1993).
- Breast milk is sterile, is at the proper temperature, and is readily available.
- Breast-feeding promotes better tooth and jaw development than bottle-feeding because the infant has to suck harder.
- Breast-feeding avoids nursing-bottle caries.
- Breast-feeding is protective against food allergies.
- Overfeeding is not likely with breast-feeding.
- Breast-feeding is associated with decreased frequency of certain chronic diseases later in life, such as NIDDM, lymphoma, and Crohn's disease.

For the mother:

- Breast-feeding promotes optimal maternal–infant bonding.
- Breast-feeding can mobilize fat stores to help women lose weight, particularly in the lower body (Kramer, et al., 1993).
- Early breast-feeding stimulates uterine contractions to help control blood loss and regain prepregnant size.
- Breast milk is readily available and requires no mixing or dilution.
- Breast-feeding may be less expensive than purchasing bottles, nipples, sterilizing equipment, and formula.
- Breast-feeding may decrease the risk of thromboembolism, especially after operative deliveries.
- Childbirth and breast-feeding may be protective against breast cancer.
- Although not reliable, breast-feeding affords some contraceptive protection.

DISADVANTAGES

Others cannot share in feeding the infant until successful lactation is established.

Breast-feeding may be uncomfortable, particularly in women with inverted nipples.

Drugs and environmental contaminants can be transmitted through breast milk.

Vegan mothers may produce milk that is deficient in vitamin B_{12} and vitamin D.

Breast-feeding is contraindicated when

- The infant has an inborn error of metabolism (ie, galactosemia, phenylketonuria).
- The mother has a chronic illness or must use medications that can harm the infant.
- The mother has a serious psychiatric disorder.
- The mother has cancer and is being treated with chemotherapeutic drugs or radiotherapeutics.
- The mother's milk is contaminated with environmental pollutants.
- The mother becomes pregnant, because the combined demands of pregnancy and lactation on maternal tissues are great.
- The mother is infected with HIV.
- The mother uses addictive drugs (eg, cocaine, PCP) or consumes more than a minimal amount of alcohol.

higher risk for health problems that could be minimized by breast-feeding. Unfortunately, a large percentage of American women, especially low-income, minority, and younger women, do not breast-feed their babies, or do so for only a short period of time (Sciacca et al, 1995).

Although almost all women have the potential to breast-feed successfully, lactation may fail because of inadequate knowledge, lack of adequate support, or conflict with lifestyle and career. Studies show that the feeding method preferred by the baby's father was one of the most important variables influencing WIC women to breast-feed (Sciacca et al, 1995). To provide the greatest chance for success, counseling about the benefits of breast-feeding and how best to initiate and continue lactation should begin early in pregnancy and should actively involve the baby's father.

Composition of Breast Milk

Breast milk is ideally formulated to promote normal infant growth and development (see display, Composition of Breast Milk). Human milk, which differs from milk of other mammals, is unique in its types and concentrations of macronutrients (carbohydrates, protein, fat), micronutrients (vitamins and minerals), enzymes, hormones, growth factors, host resistance factors, inducers/modulators of the immune system, and anti-inflammatory agents.

The composition of breast milk may vary not only among individuals but also with the time of day, maternal age, and parity. Other significant variables include the stage of lactation, maternal diet, and the duration of the feeding.

STAGE OF LACTATION

Breast milk varies considerably with the stage of lactation. **Preterm milk**, which is secreted in small amounts before delivery, is higher in nitrogen (protein) than milk produced after a term delivery.

Colostrum, which is secreted during the first few postpartum days, is a thick, yellowish fluid that is higher in protein and lower in sugar, fat, and calories than mature milk. Colostrum is also rich in antibodies and anti-infective factors that protect the infant against various GI and non-GI infections (ADA, 1993a).

Colostrum begins to change to transitional milk about 3 to 6 days post partum as the protein content decreases and the CHO and fat content increase. Major changes in the milk take place by the 10th day, and **mature milk** is stable by the end of the first month.

MATERNAL DIET

Almost all women are capable of producing enough high-quality breast milk to promote infant growth and development. In well-nourished women, neither the volume nor caloric density of breast milk is affected by excessive or inadequate intake of calories. Likewise, the concentrations of CHO, protein, major minerals (calcium, phosphorus, magnesium), and most trace elements in breast milk are stable, regardless of whether the maternal diet is inadequate or excessive in those nutrients. How-

Composition of Breast Milk

PROTEIN

Protein content of mature milk is 0.7–0.9 g/100 ml (4%–5% of total calories).

Content is adequate to support growth and development without contributing to an excessive renal solute load.

Provides more whey proteins (60%) than casein (40%); whey is easy to digest and therefore better tolerated.

The amino acid patterns are ideal for infants. Breast milk contains small amounts of amino acids that may be harmful in large amounts (eg, phenylalanine) and high levels of amino acids that infants cannot synthesize well (eg, taurine).

FAT

Fat content of mature milk is approximately 4.5 g/100 ml (approximately 58% of total calories).

Content is high in linoleic acid, the essential fatty acid.

Is easily digested because of fat-digesting enzymes contained in the milk.

Contains high levels of cholesterol, which may help infants develop enzyme systems to handle cholesterol later in life.

CHO

Lactose is the most abundant CHO, which stimulates the growth of friendly GI bacteria and promotes calcium absorption; trace amounts of glucose, galactose, and nitrogen-containing oligosaccharides are also present.

Lactose content of mature milk is 6.2–7.2 g/100 ml (35%–41% of total calories).

Contains amylase (a starch-digesting enzyme), which may promote glucose polymer and starch digestion in early infancy when pancreatic amylase is low or absent.

ANTIBODIES

Although more abundant in colostrum, antibodies and anti-infective factors are present in mature breast milk.

MINERALS

Content is adequate for growth and development but not excessive to the point of burdening immature kidneys with a high renal solute load.

Calcium, phosphorus, chlorine, potassium, and sodium are the major minerals in mature milk; trace amounts of iron, copper, and manganese are present. Amounts of zinc, magnesium, aluminum, iodine, chromium, selenium, and flourine are minute.

The calcium-to-phosphorus ratio is 2:1, ideal for calcium absorption.

Iron absorption is about 50%, compared to an absorption rate of about 4% for iron-fortified formulas.

Zinc absorption is better from breast milk than from either cow's milk or formula.

Low in sodium.

VITAMINS

All vitamins needed for growth and health are supplied in breast milk, but the amounts vary considerably between individuals.

The amount of biologically active Vit D is low; controversy exists over routine Vit D supplementation for exclusively breast-fed infants.

RENAL SOLUTE LOAD

Renal solute load of 10 mOsml/100 cal is half that of commercial formulas and one quarter that of cow's milk.

Low renal solute load is suited to the immature kidneys' inability to concentrate urine.

OTHER COMPOUNDS

Resistance factors, including bifidus factor, which promote the growth of friendly GI bacteria (*Lactobacillus bifidus*), which protect the infant against harmful GI bacteria.

Several enzymes (lipases, amylase).

Numerous hormones and hormonelike substances, such as melatonin, thyroid gland hormones, adrenal gland hormones, estrogen, insulin, and prostaglandins.

ever, some studies indicate that poor maternal nutrition decreases the concentrations of certain host resistance factors.

The concentrations of some nutrients in breast milk are maintained at the expense of maternal reserves when intake is inadequate. However, the concentrations of fat, fatty acids, and vitamins do vary with maternal intake.

Fat and Fatty Acids

The fat composition of breast milk varies with maternal diet; that is, a diet high in polyunsaturated fats results in a high polyunsaturated fat content in the milk. The fatty acid composition of milk produced by women on low-calorie diets (ie, women mobilizing their fat stores for energy) is similar to the fatty acid composition of stored fat. Women who consume low-calorie diets and have inadequate fat reserves may produce milk that is significantly reduced in fat content.

Vitamins

The vitamin content of breast milk depends on maternal intake and reserves, although the magnitude of this association varies among vitamins. The levels of water-soluble vitamins in human milk are more likely to reflect maternal diet or use of supplements than levels of most other ingested nutrients (Worthington-Roberts and Williams, 1993). Unusually high intakes of most vitamins, through either food or supplements, do not increase their concentration in breast milk, with the exception of vitamin D.

DURATION OF THE FEEDING

Fore-milk, the milk secreted as each feeding begins, is significantly lower in fat than hind-milk, the milk secreted at the end of each feeding. The increase in fat content may be a physiologic mechanism designed to provide satiety and to signal the infant to stop nursing.

Recommended Dietary Allowances for Lactation

The RDA for lactation are based on the nutritional content of breast milk and the nutritional "cost" of producing milk. Compared to the RDA for nonpregnant, non-lactating women, the requirements for all nutrients with established RDA (except iron) are significantly increased in lactation (see Table 10-3). In fact, the RDA for lactation are equal to, or higher than, those for pregnancy for all nutrients except vitamin B_6, folic acid, and iron.

New to the 10th edition of the *Recommended Dietary Allowances* are two separate categories for lactation: the first 6 months and the second 6 months of breast-feeding. The differences in recommendations between the two groupings reflect the variation in the average amount of milk produced (750 ml and 600 ml, respectively).

Calorie requirements while breast-feeding are proportional to the amount of milk produced. The average calorie content of breast milk that is produced by well nourished mothers is 70 cal/100 ml, and approximately 85 calories are needed by the mother for every 100 ml produced. The average woman uses approximately 640 calories/day for the first 6 months and 510 calories/day during the second 6 months to produce a normal amount of milk; women who only partially breast-feed use fewer calories.

The RDA recommends that women who gained the appropriate amount of weight during pregnancy increase their calorie intake by 500 per day for both the first and second 6 months of lactation. This allows women to mobilize fat that accumulated during pregnancy and may help them to achieve prepregnancy fat stores and weight. Women who failed to gain enough weight during pregnancy, or who have inadequate fat reserves, should consume a total of 650 additional calories per day during the first 6 months of breast-feeding. Theoretically, women who breast-feed can consume more calories and still lose weight more easily than women who do not breast-feed. In fact, women who eat self-selected diets tend to lose approximately 1 to 2 lbs/month during the first 4 to 6 months of breast-feeding. However, studies indicate that about 20% of lactating women maintain or gain weight.

Assuming that lactating women follow an eating pattern that is similar to that of nonlactating women, but with additional calories to meet their energy requirements, the nutrients most likely to be consumed in inadequate amounts are calcium, magnesium, zinc, folic acid, and vitamin B_6 (Subcommittee on Nutrition During Lactation, 1991). Women who voluntarily restrict their calorie intake to promote weight loss may obtain less than optimal amounts of other nutrients as well.

The Food Group Approach for Lactation and General Dietary Suggestions

Although actual nutrient content of the diet varies with the foods chosen, using the Daily Food Guide for Lactation helps ensure an adequate intake (see Table 10-5). Compared with the guidelines for pregnancy, there are few changes during lactation. Again, the most notable difference is that four or more servings of milk are suggested in order to meet calcium requirements. The extra servings of milk also provide the extra protein to meet the increased requirements. Liberal amounts of fruits and vegetables, whole-grain breads and cereals, and protein-rich foods are encouraged to meet the additional requirements that are imposed by lactation.

Another nutritional consideration during lactation is fluid intake. It is suggested that women drink 2 to 3 quarts of fluid daily, preferably in the form of water, milk, and fruit juices instead of carbonated beverages, sweetened fruit drinks, and caffeine-containing beverages. Thirst is a good indicator of need; fluids consumed in excess of thirst quenching do not increase milk volume.

NURSING PROCESS

The reliability and validity of using anthropometric and biochemical methods for assessing the nutritional status of lactating women have not been proven. Therefore, the only criteria recommended for routine screening for nutritional problems are maternal weight and dietary intake.

Assessment

In addition to the general pregnancy and lactation assessment criteria (see display, General Pregnancy and Lactation Assessment Criteria), assess for the following factors:

Weight. Studies on American women indicate that weight is the only anthropometric measurement that is useful for monitoring ongoing nutritional status during lactation. It is suggested that after lactation is established in overweight women, moderate dieting should strive to achieve a weight loss that does not exceed 2 kg/month (Dewey and McCrory, 1994).

Usual 24-hour intake; a food frequency record or food record is also collected for additional information. Intakes below 1500 calories/day are not recommended any time during lactation, and women consuming fewer than 1800 calories/day may not be getting adequate amounts of certain nutrients. Even at intakes greater than 1800 calories/day, multivitamin and mineral supplements may be necessary, depending on actual foods consumed. Key nutrients that may be marginal include calcium, magnesium, zinc, folate, and vitamin B_6 (see Table 10-4) (Dewey and McCrory, 1994).

Usual intake of milk and other calcium-rich dairy products, compared to the Daily Food Guide for Lactation. Also of particular importance are the use of vitamin D–fortified foods and the intake of vitamin-rich fruits and vegetables.

Strict vegetarianism, or the elimination of whole food groups from the diet (eg, milk because of lactose intolerance).

Cultural, familial, religious, and ethnic influences on eating habits.

Use of a modified diet to treat a disease.

Adequacy of sunlight exposure.

The client's use of alcohol, tobacco, caffeine, drugs, and artificial sweeteners.

Nursing Diagnosis

Health Seeking Behaviors, as evidenced by a lack of knowledge of diet during lactation and a desire to learn.

Planning and Implementation

Lactating women should be encouraged to consume at least 1800 calories per day to obtain adequate amounts of essential nutrients. Because the vitamin content of the mother's diet influences the concentration of vitamins in breast milk, women should be encouraged to choose a varied diet and to eat fresh fruits and vegetables with a minimal amount of preparation.

Multivitamin and mineral supplements are not recommended for routine use. However, specific supplements may be indicated when maternal intake is inadequate. For instance, a balanced multivitamin and mineral supplement may be necessary for women who consume fewer than 1800 calories. Women who are lactose-intolerant or who do not consume enough milk and other calcium-rich foods may require a calcium supplement. Supplemental vitamin D may be indicated for women who avoid vitamin D–fortified foods (eg, milk and cereals) and have limited exposure to the sun. Strict vegans need supplemental vitamin B_{12} if they do not regularly consume vitamin B_{12}–fortified plant products.

Ideally, preparation for breast-feeding should begin prenatally with counseling, guidance, and support that are provided for both the woman and her partner throughout the gestational period. Postpartum teaching has been shown to have a significant impact on both the ability to breast-feed successfully and the duration of lactation. Individual or small group counseling sessions should first assess the couple's attitudes, fears, expectations, misperceptions, and knowledge, before providing information on how milk is produced and secreted, factors that impair lactation (see display, Factors That Impair Lactation), breast care, feeding positions, how to express milk manually, how to stimulate the infant, and how to prevent and manage various breast-feeding problems (Sciacca et al, 1995).

Some studies show that the most vulnerable period for lactation is the immediate postpartum period. To establish lactation and promote the best chance of success, the infant should be offered the breast as soon as possible after birth and at frequent intervals thereafter. Hospital procedures should allow for immediate maternal–infant contact after delivery and true demand feedings (Karra et al, 1993). Effective ways that hospitals can promote and support breast-feeding appear in the display, "Ten Steps to Successful Breast-feeding."

Allergy to breast milk occurs infrequently, and some researchers believe it may not even exist. However, the infant may develop an allergic reaction to breast milk if the mother ingests a protein that enters the breast milk intact; if this occurs, the protein can be identified and eliminated from the mother's diet.

Few foods are contraindicated during lactation. It is generally not necessary to eliminate any particular foods while breast-feeding unless the infant shows an intolerance, except for freshwater fish from water contaminated with dioxin, PCB, or other chemicals. Women should contact their State Health Department for recom-

Factors That Impair Lactation

FAILURE TO ESTABLISH LACTATION RELATED TO

Delayed or infrequent feedings

Weak infant sucking because of anesthesia during labor and delivery

Nipple discomfort or engorgement

Lack of support, especially from baby's father

DECREASED DEMAND RELATED TO

Supplemental bottles of formula or water

Introduction of solid food

The infant's lack of interest

IMPAIRED LET-DOWN RELATED TO

Embarrassment or stress

Fatigue

Negative attitude, lack of desire, lack of family support

Excessive intake of caffeine or alcohol

Smoking

Drugs

The "Ten Steps to Successful Breast-feeding"

Every facility providing maternity services and care for newborn infants should:

1. Have a written breast-feeding policy that is routinely communicated to all health care staff.
2. Train all health care staff in the skills necessary to implement this policy.
3. Inform all pregnant women about the benefits and management of breast-feeding.
4. Help mothers initiate breast-feeding within a half-hour of birth.
5. Show mothers how to breast-feed and how to maintain lactation even if they are separated from their infants.
6. Give newborn infants no food or drink other than breast milk unless medically indicated.
7. Practice rooming-in. Allow mothers and infants to stay together 24 hours a day.
8. Encourage breast-feeding on demand.
9. Give no artificial teats or pacifiers (eg, dummies, soothers) to breast-feeding infants.
10. Foster the establishment of breast-feeding support groups and refer mothers to them on discharge from hospital or clinic.

Source: Karra, M., Auerback, K., Olson, L., and Binghay, E. (1993). Hospital feeding practices in metropolitan Chicago: An evaluation of five of the "Ten Steps to Successful Breastfeeding." J Am Diet Assoc, 93(12), 1437–1439.

mendations regarding fish consumption during lactation. It may also be prudent to avoid saccharin while breast-feeding.

Garlic and onion oils may flavor the taste of breast milk. However, they need not be eliminated from the mother's diet unless the taste of the milk is objectionable to the infant.

Breast-feeding is contraindicated when the mother is being treated with certain drugs or uses addictive drugs (see display, Drugs Contraindicated During Lactation). Medications that have the potential to enter breast milk and harm the infant should be avoided, if possible, and replaced with safer, more acceptable ones. Although tobacco, caffeine, alcohol, and artificial sweeteners are not absolutely contraindicated, they should be used as little as possible. Women who have been exposed to high levels of environmental toxins should have their milk analyzed for contaminants.

Studies show that colostrum and breast milk can efficiently transmit human immunodeficiency virus (HIV) from infected mothers to their infants. The Centers for Disease Control recommends that infected women be advised against breast-feeding to avoid postnatal HIV transmission. However, in developing countries where infants are at high risk of dying from infectious disease and malnutrition, breast-feeding is always recommended, regardless of HIV status (Black, 1996).

CLIENT GOALS

The client will:

Explain the importance of diet for her health and for infant growth and development.

Drugs Contraindicated During Lactation

Drugs	Radiotherapeutics	Street Drugs
Bromocriptine	Gallium-67	Amphetamine
Cyclophosphamide	Indium-111	Cocaine
Cyclosporine	Iodine-125	Heroin
Doxorubicin	Iodine-131	Marijuana
Ergotamine	Radioactive sodium	Nicotine
Lithium	Technetium-99m	Phencyclidine (PCP)
Methotrexate		
Phenindione		

Source: Worthington-Roberts, B. and Williams, S. (1993). Nutrition in Pregnancy and Lactation (5th ed.). St Louis: Mosby.

Plan ___ days' menus that are nutritionally adequate, using the Daily Food Guide for Lactation.

Consume an adequate, varied, and balanced diet based on the Daily Food Guide for Lactation.

Attain/maintain normal weight.

NURSING INTERVENTIONS

Diet Management

Promote the intake of a varied, nutrient-dense diet based on the Daily Food Guide for Lactation (see Table 10-5). Although the actual nutrient content of the diet will vary with the foods chosen, using the Guide will help ensure an average adequate intake.

Individualize the diet as much as possible to correspond with the client's likes, dislikes, and eating pattern. Special attention should be given to calcium intake among women who are lactose-intolerant.

Encourage fluid intake to satisfy thirst.

Limit caffeine and alcohol intake, and use of artificial sweeteners

Client Teaching

Principles of Breast-feeding

Instruct the client:

About the benefits of breast-feeding for both mother and infant.

That providing even a short period of breast-feeding is better than not nursing at all.

About the normal physiology of lactation, the role of hormones, and the factors that may inhibit lactation (see display, Factors That Impair Lactation).

That all women have the ability to breast-feed if given proper instruction and encouragement.

That the infant should be allowed to nurse for 5 minutes on each side on the first day in order to achieve let-down and milk ejection. By the end of the first week, the infant should be nursing up to 15 minutes per side.

That the supply of milk is equal to the demand; the more the infant sucks, the more milk is produced. Six- and 12-week-old infants who suck more are probably experiencing a growth spurt and hence need more milk.

That once the milk supply is established and let-down is functioning, the infant will be able to virtually empty the breast within 5 to 10 minutes. However, the infant needs to nurse beyond that point to satisfy his need to suck and to receive emotional and physical comfort.

That both feeding the infant more frequently and manually expressing milk will help increase the milk supply.

That a warm bath, gentle massages, and a relaxed atmosphere may help achieve let-down.

That because breast milk is easier to digest than formula, breast-fed babies usually need to nurse at shorter intervals than bottle-fed babies.

That early substitution of formula or introduction of solid foods may decrease the chance of maintaining lactation.

That breast pumps are available for manual expression of milk. Milk that is expressed into a sanitary bottle should be refrigerated or frozen immediately. Milk should be used within 24 hours if refrigerated, within 3 months if stored in the freezer compartment of the refrigerator, and within 2 years if maintained at 0°F.

Role of Nutrition in Lactation

Instruct the client:

About the importance of eating a diet that is adequate in calories, fluid, calcium, and vitamins, and how to use the Daily Food Guide for Lactation in meal planning.

That even if a mother has adequate fat stores, calorie intake should increase during lactation because fat is mobilized slowly.

That lactating women may experience a 1- to 2-lb weight loss per month, although some women may lose up to 4 lbs/month. Normal weight loss does not adversely affect milk production; however, lean women may be at risk for impaired lactation if calorie intake is restricted (Dewey and McCrory, 1994). Excessive maternal weight gain during pregnancy increases the likelihood of postpartum weight retention despite breast-feeding.

That appetite and thirst are generally good indicators of need; consuming excesses of either food or liquid will not produce "better" or more milk.

To avoid freshwater fish and saccharin. Other foods may be eliminated if the infant appears to develop an intolerance.

That although moderate amounts of alcohol may help let-down, large amounts can enter breast milk and should be avoided.

To avoid large amounts of caffeine because it also enters breast milk, although at very low levels. However, infants are unable to metabolize caffeine as well as adults, and over time, caffeine can accumulate in the infant's bloodstream.

General Information Related to Lactation

Instruct the client:

Not to take drugs or medications unless approved by the physician.

About breast care, positioning of the infant, ways to stimulate the infant, and how to end a feeding, and provide suggestions of methods for weaning.

That the La Lèche League is an international organization that was founded for the purpose of helping nursing mothers. The League prints a bimonthly newsletter, holds conventions and monthly group meetings, and is available as a source of information and advice 24 hours a day.

That numerous instructional materials and books on breast-feeding are available from community organizations and bookstores.

Monitoring Progress

Monitor for the following signs or symptoms:

Weight changes

Food intolerances, especially lactose intolerance, and the overall impact on diet adequacy

Ongoing compliance to diet; evaluate adequacy and the need for further diet counseling

Evaluation

Evaluation is ongoing. Assuming that the plan of care has not changed, the client will achieve the goals as stated above.

KEY CONCEPTS

- Although proper nutrition before and during pregnancy cannot guarantee a successful pregnancy outcome, it does profoundly affect fetal development and birth.
- A woman's prepregnancy weight status and weight gain during pregnancy are correlated to infant birth weight. Underweight women should gain weight before conception or gain more weight during pregnancy to reduce their risk of adverse pregnancy outcomes.
- Except for vitamins A and K, the RDA for all nutrients increase during pregnancy. Because calorie requirements increase relatively little compared to the increased requirements for other nutrients, a nutrient-dense diet is vital to meeting nutrient needs without exceeding calorie requirements.
- Because diet alone cannot supply enough iron during pregnancy, supplemental iron is recommended for all pregnant women. Women in high-risk categories (smokers, drug abusers, women carrying twins) and those who do not consume an adequate diet should take a multivitamin and mineral supplement.

- Nutritional counseling should be initiated early in prenatal care and continue throughout the pregnancy. It should stress the importance of weight gain, ways to improve overall intake, the adverse effects of smoking, and the benefits of breast-feeding.

- Proper nutrition may help reduce the incidence of preterm births, pregnancy-induced hypertension, and anemia, three problems common to adolescent pregnancies.

- Breast-feeding is recommended as the sole source of nutrition for the first 5 to 6 months of life. In addition to being uniquely suited to infant growth and development, it imparts other significant benefits to both infant and mother.

- Almost all women are capable of breast-feeding. Maternal diet does influence the concentrations of fat, fatty acids, and vitamins; the concentration of some nutrients in breast milk is maintained at the expense of maternal stores when the mother's diet is inadequate. Neither the volume nor caloric density of breast milk is influenced by an excessive or inadequate intake of calories.

- Except for iron, folic acid, and vitamin B6, the RDA for lactation are equal to or greater than those for pregnancy for all nutrients, including calories. In theory, lactating women can still lose weight during lactation while consuming a higher calorie intake.

FOCUS ON **CRITICAL THINKING**

Ann Wilson is 22 years old and 6 weeks pregnant with her first child. She is 5'10" tall and her prepregnancy weight was 130 pounds. Ann now weighs 134 pounds. She is complaining of a voracious appetite despite periodic nausea and vomiting throughout the day. Her typical intake is as follows:

Breakfast: 2 fried eggs, 2 pieces of toast with butter, 2 pieces of bacon, 3 cups of coffee with cream and sugar

Snack: jelly doughnut with 1 cup of coffee with cream and sugar

Lunch: 1/2 tuna fish submarine sandwich with potato chips and cola

Snack: 2 to 3 cookies with cola

Dinner: hamburger on a bun with ketchup, french fries, cola, cake or cookies for dessert

Snack: chips or pretzels

Evaluate Ann's diet based on the Daily Food Guide for pregnancy. In what food groups is she deficient? What nutrients may she be lacking in her diet?

From what food groups is she consuming too much? What nutrients may she be consuming in excess of need?

What recommendations would you make to help her improve her intake? Design a meal plan, using her typical pattern of 3 meals with 3 snacks.

What interventions would you suggest to help relieve nausea and vomiting?

How much weight should she gain throughout the course of her pregnancy? Evaluate her weight gain thus far.

REFERENCES

American Dietetic Association (1993). Position of The American Dietetic Association: Promotion and support of breast-feeding. J Am Diet Assoc, 93(4), 467–469.

American Dietetic Association (1993b). Position of The American Dietetic Association: Use of nutritive and nonnutritive sweeteners. J Am Diet Assoc, 93(7), 816–821.

American Dietetic Association (1994). Position of The American Dietetic Association: Nutrition care for pregnant adolescents. J Am Diet Assoc, 94(4), 449–450.

Black, R. (1996). Transmission of HIV-1 in the breast-feeding process. J Am Diet Assoc, 96(3), 267–274.

Carruth, B. and Skinner, J. (1991). Practitioners beware: Regional differences in beliefs about nutrition during pregnancy. J Am Diet Assoc, 91(4), 435–440.

Dewey, K. and McCrory, M. (1994). Effects of dieting and physical activity on pregnancy and lactation. Am J Clin Nutr, 59(suppl), 446S–453S.

Dunn, C., Kolasa, K., Dunn, P., and Ogle, M. (1994). Dietary intake of pregnant adolescents in a roral southern community. J Am Diet Assoc, 94(9), 1040–1041.

Fagen, C., King, J., and Erick, M. (1995). Nutrition management in women with gestational diabetes mellitus: A review by ADA's Diabetes Care and Education dietetic practice group. J Am Diet Assoc, 95(4), 460–467.

International Food Information Council (1995). Folic acid: Powerful tool against birth defects. Food Insight, July/Aug, 6.

International Food Information Council (1994). Healthy beginnings: Nutrition's role in preventing birth defects. Food Insight, Jan/Feb, 2–3.

Jonaitis, M. (1995). Diabetes 2000. Complications during pregnancy. RN, 58(10), 40–44.

Karra, M., Auuerbach, K, Olson, L, and Binghay, E. (1993). Hospital feeding practices in metropolitan Chicago: An evaluation of five of the "Ten Steps to Successful Breastfeeding." J Am Diet Assoc, 93(12), 1437–1439.

Kramer, F., Stunkard A., Marshall, K., McKinney, S., and Liebschutz, J. (1993). Breast-feeding reduces maternal lower-body fat. J Am Diet Assoc, 93(4), 429–433.

Liebman, B. (1995). Folic acid: For the young and heart. Nutrition Action Health Letter, 22(7), 1, 4–6.

Luke, B. and Leurgans, S. (1996). Maternal weight gains in ideal twin outcomes. J Am Diet Assoc, 96(2), 178–181.

March of Dimes Birth Defects Foundation, International Food Information Council (1991). Healthy Eating During Pregnancy. White Plains, NY.

Mikode, M. and White, A. (1994). Dietary assessment of middle-income pregnant women during the first, second, and third trimesters. J Am Diet Assoc, 94(2), 196–199.

National Research Council (1989). Recommended Dietary Allowances (10th ed.). Washington, DC: National Academy Press.

Schneck, M., Sideras, K., Fox, R., et al (1990). Low-income pregnant adolescents and their infants: Dietary findings and health outcomes. J Am Diet Assoc 90(4), 555–558.

Sciacca, J., Phipps, B., Dube, D., and Ratliff, M. (1995). Influences on breast-feeding by lower-income women: An incentive-based, partner-supported educational program. J Am Diet Assoc, 95(3), 323–328.

Springer, N., Bischoping, K., Sampselle, C., Mayes, F., and Petersen, B. (1992). Using early weight gain and other nutrition-related risk factors to predict pregnancy outcomes. J Am Diet Assoc 92(2), 217–219.

Subcommittee on Nutrition During Lactation, Food and Nutrition Board, National Academy of Sciences (1991). Nutrition During Lactation. Washington, DC: National Academy Press.

Subcommittee on Nutritional Status and Weight Gain During Pregnancy, Food and Nutrition Board, National Academy of Sciences (1990). Nutrition During Pregnancy. Washington, DC: National Academy Press.

Worthington-Roberts, B. and Williams, S. (1993). Nutrition in Pregnancy and Lactation (5th ed.). St Louis: Mosby.

Yu, S. and Jackson, R. (1995). Need for nutrition advice in prenatal care. J Am Diet Assoc, 95(9), 1027–1029.

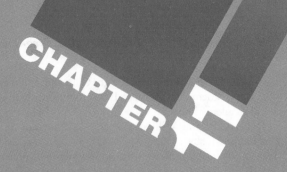

CHAPTER 11

Growth and Development: Infancy Through Adolescence

Chapter Outline

Key Terms

Development
Growth

Hypoallergenic
Nursing bottle caries

302

RELATIONSHIP BETWEEN GROWTH, DEVELOPMENT, AND NUTRITION

*G*rowth is defined as an increase in the number and size of cells. **Development** is the increase in function and complexity that occurs through growth, maturation, and learning. Mental, emotional, social, and physical growth and development occur throughout the life cycle. The timing and rate of growth and development are influenced by genetic, hormonal, behavioral, and environmental factors, including diet.

An optimal diet provides adequate amounts of all the nutrients essential for growth and development. Early in life, nutrition is important for enabling a child to reach his genetic potential for physical and mental growth and development. Average increases in height (length) and weight can be predicted according to the child's age (Table 11-1). Actual assessment of an individual's physical growth and growth pattern should be done periodically by measuring and plotting height (length), weight, and weight for height (length) on the National Center for Health Statistics (NCHS) growth grids (Appendix 9). Normally, an individual's percentile status for height (length) and weight remains fairly constant throughout childhood. A devia-

Table 11-1
Average Increases in Weight and Height (Length) Based on Age

Age	Average Weight Gain	Average Height Gain (inches)
Birth–6 months	140–200 g/week (5–7 oz) Birthweight doubles between 4–6 months.	2.5 cm (1 in)/month
6–12 months	85–140 g/week (3–5 oz) Birthweight triples by the end of the first year.	1.25 cm (½ in)/month Birth length increases by about 50% by the end of the first year.
1–3 years	2–3 kg (4.4–6.6 lb)/year Birthweight quadruples by age 2½.	12 cm (4.8 in) during second year; 6–8 cm (2.4–3.2 in) during third year. Height at 2 years is about 50% of eventual adult height.
3–6	2–3 kg (4.4–6.6 lb/year)	6–8 cm (2.4–3.2 in)/year
6–pubertal growth spurt	2–3 kg (4.4–6.6 lb)/year	5 cm (2 in)/year after age 7
Pubertal growth spurt	7–25 kg (15–55 lb)	5–25 cm (2–10 in)
Females between 10–14 years old	Mean = 17.5 kg (38.1 lb)	Mean = 20.5 cm (8.2 in) Approximately 90% of mature height is attained by onset of menarche or skeletal age of 13 years.
Males between 11–16 years old	7–30 kg (15–65 lb) Mean = 23.7 kg (52.1 lb)	10–30 cm (4–12 in) Mean = 20.5 cm (8.2 in) Approximately 95% of mature height is attained by skeletal age of 15 years.

Adapted with permission from Whaley LF, Wong DL: *Nursing Care of Infants and Children*, 4th ed., St. Louis: Mosby–Year Book, 1991

tion of more than 2 percentile channels warrants a more in-depth assessment of growth and nutritional status. An increase in weight percentile may suggest the development of obesity; a decrease may indicate undernutrition, an undiagnosed chronic disease, or the onset of emotional problems.

Another reason to provide proper nutrition for healthy children is that diet has a role in the prevention of chronic diseases that are related to nutritional excesses (ADA, 1995). Variety, balance, and moderation in food choices during childhood promote health and vigor, help prevent nutrition-related problems that occur frequently among the healthy pediatric population (see display, Nutrition-Related Problems Among the Healthy Pediatric Population), and may help prevent nutrition-related chronic diseases that occur with aging.

(text continues on page 307)

Nutrition-Related Problems Among the Healthy Pediatric Population

IRON DEFICIENCY ANEMIA

Iron stores of formula-fed infants become depleted between 3 and 6 months after birth if not supplemented.

Six-month to 2½year-old may develop "milk" anemia related to excessive milk intake (ie, >32 oz/day), displacing other iron-rich foods.

In childhood, iron deficiency anemia is commonly related to finicky eating habits; there are relatively few rich sources of iron that are acceptable to children.

Adolescent boys can develop iron deficiency quickly after the onset of puberty because of the increased need for iron related to expanding blood volume and muscle mass.

Adolescent girls tend to develop iron deficiency slowly after puberty related to poor eating habits, chronic fad dieting, and menstrual losses.

Nursing Implications and Considerations

To prevent iron deficiency among infants, encourage mothers

- To give iron-fortified formula to breast-fed infants who are weaned before 1 year of age; iron-fortified formula should be used until the infant is 1 year old.

- To use iron-fortified infant cereals until the infant is 12 to 18 months old because its iron is absorbed more readily than the iron in other cereals.
- To limit milk consumption to amounts recommended in the infant feeding schedule or daily food guide (for toddlers) because milk can displace iron-rich food from the diet.

To prevent iron deficiency in children and adolescents, encourage

- A liberal intake of high-iron foods: liver, organ meats, dried fruit, iron-fortified cereals, whole grains.
- A rich source of vitamin C at every meal to enhance iron absorption from plant sources.

Nursing Considerations

Studies suggest that hemoglobin alone may not be sensitive enough to identify iron deficiency; iron supplements given to babies whose hemoglobin was normal but whose total iron-binding capacity was elevated resulted in improved attention span and performance on mental development tests. Because iron deficiency is so prevalent and may affect learning ability, iron status should be carefully monitored.

Cow's milk should not be given to infants younger than 1 year of age because it is a poor

(continued)

Nutrition-Related Problems Among the Healthy Pediatric Population (Continued)

source of iron, and may promote occult blood loss.

Infants born to iron-deficient mothers may have inadequate iron stores.

Once anemia develops, diet alone cannot cure anemia, and supplements are needed (see Chap. 7).

OBESITY

Obesity is loosely defined as weight above the 95th percentile for age, or BMI >85th percentile. It develops when calorie intake exceeds energy expenditure.

The causes of obesity may be multifactorial and difficult to determine; genetic, physiologic, environmental, psychological, behavioral, or a combination of factors may be implicated. Children from low socioeconomic backgrounds tend to become overweight before adolescence, whereas children from higher socioeconomic backgrounds tend to become overweight during or after the onset of adolescence.

According to NHANES III data, the prevalence of overweight among 12 to 19 year olds is 22% for females and 20% for males, an increase of 6% over previous data collected.

Nursing Implications and Considerations

Before a child is labeled as obese or overweight, assess

- The age of onset. Obesity in infants younger than 1 year old is not predictive of obesity later in life; however, childhood fatness does predict adolescent fatness. In most studies, 25% to 50% of obese children and adolescents become obese adults (Dietz and Robinson, 1993). Because obesity may be easier to prevent than treat, overweight children (who are likely to become obese adolescents and adults) should be identified and treated.
- The degree and duration of the obesity. Fat stores that increase before puberty in preparation for the adolescent growth spurt may cause

transient excess body weight and resolve themselves as the child grows taller while maintaining body weight.
- Family history for genetic or endocrine problems that may be the cause of obesity.
- Health status for medical complications. In children, obesity is the major cause of hypertension, and increases the risk of cardiovascular disease, diabetes mellitus, joint diseases, and other chronic illnesses.
- Family dynamics and attitudes toward body weight. Unresolved crisis and conflicts within the family may contribute to eating problems and complicate weight control. Tolerance toward body weight varies considerably among families; weight status acceptable to one family may not be tolerated by another. Children with two normal-weight parents have a 10% chance of becoming obese; one obese parent increases the chance of obesity to 40%; and if both parents are obese, children have an 80% chance of becoming obese.

The social and psychological impact of obesity is greater on children than on adults. Overweight or obese children

- Tend to have poorer academic performance than normal-weight children of the same intellectual ability.
- May be teased and psychologically abused by peers and adults, which leads to social isolation, depression, and low self-esteem.
- May actually consume fewer calories than their thin counterparts, but because they are social outcasts, a perpetuating cycle of weight gain → inactivity → weight gain makes weight control difficult.
- May be discriminated against in school, and later in college and at work. Studies have found that most preschoolers believe a fat child is ugly, stupid, mean, sloppy, lazy, dishonest, forgetful, naughty, sad, lonely, and poor at sports. Both children and adults

(continued)

Nutrition-Related Problems Among the Healthy Pediatric Population (Continued)

ranked a chubby child lower on a scale of preference than a child with crutches and a brace, a child in a wheelchair, a child missing the left hand, or a child with a facial disfigurement.

To prevent obesity

- Parents should recognize the infants cry for reasons other than hunger and should not be fed every time they cry. Overfeeding is one of the biggest hazards of formula feeding.
- Infant formula should be properly diluted; concentrated formulas are a source of concentrated calories.
- Infants should not be forced to finish their bottle.
- Solid foods should not be introduced before the infant is developmentally ready (4 to 6 months old).
- Children should be allowed to eat at their own pace in a relaxed atmosphere.
- Children should be allowed to stop eating whey they are full and should not be made to eat until their "plate is clean."
- Healthy "thin" eating habits should be learned by parental example, because young children tend to imitate their parents.
- Lower fat intake, increase complex CHO.
- Children should not be given food rewards for good behavior, denied food as punishment, bribed with food, or given food for comfort.
- Encourage activity.

To treat obesity

- Assess the child's normal daily intake, eating behaviors and attitudes, and activity patterns.
- Individualize the plan of care for the child and the family.
- Reduce total fat intake, increase intake of complex CHO.
- Reduce television time; increase level of activity.
- If possible, it is best to allow children to "outgrow" obesity by maintaining their weight as they grow taller, rather than actually losing weight.

- Children should not be put under pressure to lose weight; resentment and rebellion may cause extreme behavior, resulting in anorexia nervosa, bulimia, or compulsive eating. Subtle changes such as limiting portion sizes, eating baked instead of fried foods, substituting fresh fruits and nutritious desserts for pies, cakes, and cookies, and eliminating traditional empty-calorie snack foods is more effective than measuring food and counting calories.
- Encourage exercise that an obese child will feel comfortable doing, for example, exercise that does not require a lot of skill or a change of clothes, such as walking and bowling.
- Contractual agreements between parents and children may be highly effective; positive reinforcement must be immediate, frequent, and consistent (Dietz and Robinson, 1993).
- Group support is most effective at achieving and maintaining weight loss in overweight adolescents.

DENTAL CARIES

Sugar (sucrose, lactose, fructose) plus bacteria found in plaque produce acids that destroy tooth enamel, leading to tooth decay (dental caries). A high intake of CHO, especially between meals, increases the risk of caries. Although on an ounce-for-ounce basis sticky foods are more likely to cause caries than liquids, the frequency and quantity of soft drinks consumed may make them equally as damaging. "Nursing bottle caries" occur when infants or children are put to bed with a bottle of milk, juice, or any other sweetened liquid.

Nursing Implications and Considerations

Protein, calcium, vitamins A, C, D, and fluoride are important for dental health. Fluoride has been shown to prevent tooth decay by incorporating itself into the structure of the teeth as they form during infancy and childhood. Sources of fluoride include fluoridated water; concentrated liquid or powdered formula mixed with fluoridated water; and fluoride supplements. Breast milk and ready-

(continued)

Nutrition-Related Problems Among the Healthy Pediatric Population (Continued)

to-use formulas may be inadequate sources of fluoride. The American Academy of Pediatrics recommends fluoride supplements be given to formula-fed infants living in areas with unfluoridated water and breast-fed infants.

Advise parents

- That only bedtime bottle feedings of plain water should be given to infants after the teeth erupt.
- Not to give their infants more than the prescribed dose of fluoride, because it may cause spots to form on the teeth.

- That because young children tend to swallow toothpaste, avoid giving fluoridated toothpaste to children under age 3.
- That if sweets are consumed, they are less damaging when eaten with other foods and liquids than when eaten alone.
- That so-called "healthy" snacks may be high in sugar: granola, dried fruit, anything made with molasses or honey.
- That a good diet must also be accompanied by good dental hygiene to be most effective against dental caries.

Nutrient requirements and eating behaviors vary according to health status, activity patterns, and growth rate; the greater the rate of growth, the more intense the nutritional needs. A child's growth pattern is individualized; however, using age as the standard, predictions can be made about the sequence, characteristics, and rate of growth and development; this provides a basis from which to assess nutritional needs. The RDA are based on age from birth through age 10; thereafter, they are grouped according to age and sex (Table 11-2). At best, the RDA are rough esti-

Table 11-2
RDAs of Selected Nutrients for Infants, Children and Adolescents

Age (Years)	Protein (g)	Vitamin A (µg RE)	Vitamin D (µg)*	Vitamin C (mg)	Calcium (mg)	Iron (mg)	Zinc (mg)
Birth–0.5	13	375	7.5	30	400	6	5
0.5–1.0	14	375	10	35	600	10	5
1–3	16	400	10	40	800	10	10
4–6	24	500	10	45	800	10	10
7–10	28	700	10	45	800	10	10
Males							
11–14	45	1000	10	50	1200	12	15
15–18	59	1000	10	60	1200	12	15
Females							
11–14	46	800	10	50	1200	15	12
15–18	44	800	10	60	1200	15	12

* As cholecalciferol. 10 µg cholecalciferol = 400 IU vitamin D. (Food and Nutritional Board, National Academy of Sciences–National Research Council: *Recommended Daily Dietary Allowances*. Revised 1989)

Table 11-3
The Food Guide Pyramid Daily Food Guide for Children and Adolescents

Group	Number of Servings (based on age) 1–5	6–11	Teen	Adult
Bread, Cereal, Rice, and Pasta	6–11 (¼ to ½ adult size)	6–11*	6–11*	6–11
Vegetable	3–5†	3–5*	3–5*	3–5
Fruit	2–4†	2–4*	2–4*	2–4
Milk, Yogurt, and Cheese	2 cups	2 cups	4 cups	2–3 servings
Meat, Poultry, Fish, Dry Beans, Eggs, and Nuts‡	2–3 oz	2–3 oz	4–5 oz	5–7 oz

* Serving sizes for 6–11-year-olds and teens are about the same as those of an adult.
† Serving sizes for ages 1–5 years are about 1 level tablespoon per year of age; e.g., 1 serving is 3 tablespoons for a 3-year-old, 5 tablespoons for a 5-year-old.
‡ Nuts are not recommended for children under 4 because they are a choking hazard.
Source: Dray J: *Mealtime Family Time.* Manhattan, Kansas: Cooperative Extension, 1992.

mates of actual needs; recommended nutrient allowances are less precise for children than adults because of individual variations in growth rate and activity patterns. A more appropriate nutrition teaching tool is the Food Guide Pyramid, which recommends the number of servings from each food group that children at various ages should eat daily (Table 11-3).

INFANT NUTRITION (BIRTH TO 1 YEAR)

Growth Characteristics and Nutritional Implications

Physical and Physiologic Growth	Nutritional Implications
Excluding fetal growth, growth in the first year of life is more rapid than at any other time in the life cycle (see Table 11-1).	Although the total amount recommended for most nutrients during infancy is less than adult requirements, the amount needed per unit of body weight is greater than at any other age.

EXAMPLE

	174 lb Adult Male (79 kg)	13 lb Infant (6 kg)
Calories		
Per kg:	37 cal/kg	108 cal/kg
Total:	2900 cal	650 cal
Protein		
Per kg:	0.8 g	2.2 g
Total:	63 g/day	13 g/day

(continued)

Physical and Physiologic Growth	Nutritional Implications
Birthweight doubles in 4 to 6 months and triples by age 1. Length increases 50% during the first year. The percentages of both lean body mass and body fat increase.	Nutritional deficits can impair growth and development.
Muscular control of the head, neck, jaw, and tongue develops, as well as hand-eye coordination, and the ability to sit, grasp, chew, drink, and self-feed.	Because of inborn reflexes, the most appropriate feeding for an infant is milk (breast milk or commercial formulas). Between 4 to 6 months, reflexes disappear, head control develops and the infant is able to sit, making spoon-feeding possible. (See Table 11-8 for developmental landmarks and the introduction of solids.)
At birth, the kidneys are immature and unable to concentrate urine; by 4 to 6 weeks of age, urine concentrating ability approximates adult levels.	Excess protein and mineral intake (eg, cow's milk) can tax kidney function and lead to dehydration. Infants need more water per unit of body weight (150 ml/kg) than adults related to their immature renal function and the high percentage of body weight from water.
Stomach capacity is limited to about 90 ml at birth. Emptying time is short (about 2½ to 3 hours), and peristalsis is rapid. The GI tract is sterile at birth.	Initially, small frequent feedings are necessary; the amount of food/feeding increases with age and increased stomach capacity. Lack of gut bacteria that synthesizes Vit K necessitates an IM injection of Vit K shortly after birth to prevent hemorrhagic disease.
Decreased quality and quantity of pancreatic amylase (starch-digesting enzyme), pancreatic lipase (fat-digesting enzyme) and bile (fat digestion) limits digestion and absorption of nutrients.	Infants are unable to digest starch (cereal) until about 3 months of age; bile composition reaches maturity around 6 months of age.
Susceptibility to food allergies decreases between 4 and 6 months as the immune system matures. Teeth erupt.	Introducing solid foods (beikost) before 4 to 6 months increases the risk of food allergies. The texture of food progresses from strained to mashed to chopped fine to regular as the ability to chew improves.

Infant Feeding

BREAST-FEEDING

Because of the advantages of breast-feeding for both mother and infant, the American Academy of Pediatrics recommends that infants should be breast-fed for the full first year of life (see Chapter 10). Even low-birth-weight (LBW) infants weighing less than 1250 g have been shown to tolerate breast milk better than formula. However, formula feeding is an acceptable alternative if lactation is contraindicated or the mother is unwilling or unable to breast-feed.

FORMULA FEEDING

Infant formulas are designed to resemble breast milk and provide comparable nutritional benefits (Table 11-4). Standards for levels of nutrients in formulas

Table 11-4

Comparison Between Breast Milk and Cow's Milk, and How Cow's Milk Is Modified in the Production of Milk-Based Formula

Nutrient	Mature Breast Milk	Whole Cow's Milk	How Cow's Milk Is Modified To Resemble Breast Milk
Protein (g/L)	7–9	35	Total protein control is reduced.
Whey:casein	60:40	18:82	Milk is homogenized and treated with heat to reduce curd tension and increase digestibility. Some formulas combine demineralized whey with nonfat milk to approximate the whey/casein ratio of breast milk. Taurine (an amino acid that infants cannot efficiently synthesize) is being added to many milk-based and soy formulas to approximate the levels found in breast milk.
Fat (g/L)	45	38	Butterfat is removed (difficult to digest) and replaced with vegetable oils to increase polyunsaturated fat, which is more easily digested by infants.
P:S ratio	0.32	0.06	
% Lineolic acid calories	4	1	
Lactose (g/L)	62–72	49	Lactose is added.
Minerals (mg/L)			Total mineral content is reduced. Calcium:phosphorus ratio is adjusted to be no less than 1.1 and no greater than 2.0.
Sodium	150	506	
Calcium	280 ± 26	1200	
Phosphorus	140 ± 22	940	
Ca:P ratio	2.4	1.3	
Iron	0.4	0.5	Formulas may be fortified with additional iron.
Cal/L	690	660	Standard formulas contain the same amount of calories as cow's milk.

have been established by the Infant Formula Act and are based mostly on recommendations of the Committee on Nutrition of the American Academy of Pediatrics. With the exception of fluoride, supplements are not necessary for infants who are given iron-fortified formula. Milk-based and whey-adjusted formulas are available for full-term infants. Infants who are intolerant of the protein or lactose in cow's milk may be given formulas made with soy isolates or casein hydrolysates (Table 11-5).

Incomplete formulas are also available for infants with inborn errors of metabolism, such as phenylketonuria (PKU) and maple syrup urine disease. These specialized formulas are intentionally lacking or deficient in one or more nutrients and therefore do not supply adequate nutrition for normal infants; they must be supplemented with small amounts of regular formula.

A variety of formulas have been developed for infants with special needs, such as LBW infants. Numerous physiologic and developmental problems may make feeding the premature infant difficult (see display, Feeding the Premature Infant). Studies indicate that the nutrient needs of premature infants differ from those of full-term infants with regard to rate of growth, body composition, and physiologic maturity;

Table 11-5
Comparison Between Various Types of Formulas

Type of Formula	Source of Protein	Source of Fat	Source of Carbohydrate
REGULAR Milk-based (Manufacturer): Intended for routine use. Provide 67–68 cal/100 ml (normal dilution)			
Similac (Ross)	Casein	Soy oil, coconut oil, corn oil	Lactose
Enfamil (Mead)	Reduced mineral whey, casein	Soy oil, coconut oil	Lactose
SMA (Wyeth)	Demineralized whey, casein	Oleo; soybean, safflower, and coconut oils	Lactose
Gerber (Gerber)	Nonfat milk	Soy oil, coconut oil	Lactose
Good Start (Carnation)	Hydrolyzed reduced mineral whey	Palm, safflower, and coconut oils	Lactose, corn syrup
SOY-BASED (Uses: Lactase deficiency, galactosemia; infants born to vegetarian families and for infants recovering from diarrhea. Provide 67–68 cal/100 ml [normal dilution].)			
Prosobee (Mead)	Soy protein	Soy oil	Corn syrup solids
Isomil (Ross)	Soy protein	Coconut oil, soy oil	Sucrose, corn syrup solids
CASEIN HYDROLYSATE (Uses: For infants who do not tolerate either cow's milk or soy.)			
Nutramigen (Mead)	Casein hydrolysate	Corn oil	Modified tapioca, sucrose
Pregestimil (Mead)	Casein hydrolysate	Corn oil, medium chain triglycerides	Corn syrup solids, modified tapioca starch
INCOMPLETE FORMULAS (must be supplemented with regular formula)			
Lofenalac (Mead) (Use: Phenylketonuria [PKU])	Hydrolyzed casein with most of the phenylalanine removed	Corn oil	Corn syrup solids and modified tapioca starch
MSUD Diet Powder (Mead) (Use: Maple syrup urine disease [disorder of branched chain amino acid metabolism])	Amino acids without any branched-chain amino acids	Corn oil	Corn syrup solids and modified tapioca starch

thus, the nutritional requirements of LBW infants are not precisely defined. Compared to routine formulas for full-term infants, LBW formulas generally contain more calories (24 cal/oz instead of 20 cal/oz), more whey protein, more vitamins and minerals (except iron, which can interfere with vitamin E absorption and result in hemolytic anemia), and less lactose; they also comprise medium-chain triglyceride (MCT) oil as part of the fat source.

Formula feeding offers the advantage of allowing others to share in infant feeding, which gives the mother more freedom. In addition, the supply of formula is unlimited.

Although they have been designed to resemble breast milk, formulas lack the unique nutrient, enzyme, and hormone content; ease of digestibility; and anti-infective properties of breast milk. There is also a greater chance of overfeeding when formulas are used, and they must be properly prepared; too dilute → failure to

(text continues on page 314

Feeding the Premature Infant

POTENTIAL PROBLEM/RATIONALE

Failure to achieve adequate "catch-up" growth related to high nutrient requirements combined with limited tolerance to feedings. Premature infants are usually expected to "catch up" to normal weight by 24 months of age and to height by 36 months.

Normally, weight gain between 26 to 36 weeks of gestation is greater than at any other time in the life cycle; the earlier the infant is born before term, the greater the impact on nutritional status and requirements. Calorie requirements are higher than normal because of the following:

Most of the fat stores are laid down during the last 6 weeks of pregnancy. In a premature infant, fat may comprise less than 1% of total body weight, compared to 16% of total body weight in a term infant. A lack of fat stores leaves the infant dependent on exogenous sources of calories.

Glycogen stores are usually deposited during the last 4 weeks of a term pregnancy. Without adequate glycogen reserves, the infant does not have a readily available source of stored energy and is at risk of hypoglycemia.

Even labored breathing related to an immature respiratory function can increase calorie requirements.

Nursing Interventions and Considerations

Individualize the diet according to the infant's physiologic and developmental status. Most preterm infants are unable to tolerate enteral feedings in the early neonatal period and are therefore given intravenous fluid, glucose, and electrolytes to maintain fluid balance and promote metabolic homeostasis. Partial or total parenteral nutrition may be necessary until GI tolerance is established, especially in preterm infants with limited metabolic reserves. Usually enteral feedings can begin after the initial acute treatment of respiratory distress, perinatal sepsis, or other stressful events.

Although breast milk has numerous benefits (low renal solute load, anti-infective properties, easily digested fat, a high nitrogen content, unique amino acid composition, and a high whey/casein ratio), some researchers believe that even if consumed in high-volume amounts, preterm breast milk lacks sufficient amounts of calcium, phosphorus, and, possibly, some essential vitamins. Further compounding the problem is the inability of many preterm infants to consume enough milk to meet their nutritional needs.

To boost its nutritional value, calcium, phosphorus, and vitamins can be added to breast milk through nasogastric or bottle feedings; however, GI intolerance often results because of the increase in osmolarity. Another option, alternating breast milk feedings with premature formula, falls short of providing adequate amounts of calcium and phosphorus; although preterm milk formula provides adequate amounts of calcium and phosphorus when used as the sole source of nutrition, it cannot compensate for their low content in breast milk when it is used as a supplemental feeding. Relatively new to the market are human milk fortifiers (Enfamil Human Milk fortifier powder and liquid Similac Natural Care Low Iron Human Milk Fortifier), designed to supplement breast milk given to preterm infants whose tolerance for enteral feedings has been established. Along with calcium and phosphorus, the human milk fortifiers also provide protein, carbohydrates, fat, vitamins, and minerals. Because they may lack sufficient quantities of some nutrients (ie, vitamin D) and have the potential to contribute excessive amounts of other nutrients when consumed in large quantities (ie, potassium), their use should be closely monitored. Human milk fortifiers are not necessary for every preterm infant and are not used once the infant weighs 2 kg.

Although exact nutritional requirements are unknown, a premature infant receiving enteral nutrition may need

3.5–4.0 grams of protein/kg of body weight/day. Even if premature infants need more protein than this, they should not receive more than 4 to 5 g of protein/kg because their immature kid-

Feeding the Premature Infant (Continued)

neys are unable to handle large amounts of nitrogenous waste generated from protein metabolism.

A whey-to-casein ratio of 60:40, which is typical of breast milk and LBW formulas. This ratio is easily digested and provides adequate amounts of the nonessential amino acids cystine and methionine, which premature infants may have difficulty synthesizing. In addition, the nonessential amino acids taurine and tyrosine may be essential for premature infants.

120 to 130 cal/kg of body weight to promote growth. After the first week of life, the calorie requirements of premature infants are greater than those of term infants. Standard LBW formulas supplying 24 cal/oz are indicated until the infant weighs 2 kg.

Thirty percent to 55% of total calories in the form of fat. Linoleic acid should provide at least 3% of total calories to meet essential fatty acid requirements.

Adequate amounts of essential fatty acids in a form of fat that the infant can easily absorb. Because of premature infants' impaired fat digestion, premature formulas contain a combination of MCT oil and vegetable oil; excessive intake of PUFA should be avoided because they increase the risk of vitamin E deficiency and hemolytic anemia.

Vitamin and mineral supplements. Compared to term infants, preterm infants have notably higher vitamin and mineral requirements, especially for calcium, phosphorus, iron, vitamin E, vitamin C, and folic acid. Iron supplements may be initiated as early as 2 weeks after birth, but not later than 2 months of age.

Monitor nutritional status for several years after birth, basing the assessment on the infant's corrected age (chronologic age minus the number of weeks the infant was born prematurely). Neonates' postnatal growth should parallel in utero growth at term, that is, a weight gain of approximately 14 to 36 g/day.

POTENTIAL PROBLEM/RATIONALE

Maldigestion or malabsorption related to an insufficient amount or potency of digestive enzymes. Inadequate lactase, amylase, and lipase may cause maldigestion of lactose, starch, and lipids and the fat-soluble vitamins, respectively.

Nursing Interventions and Considerations

Observe for signs of maldigestion/malabsorption, such as diarrhea and steatorrhea.

POTENTIAL PROBLEM/RATIONALE

Aspiration, which may be related to delayed or incomplete gastric emptying, leading to gastric residuals and abdominal distention. Immature sucking or swallowing reflexes (if less than 32 to 34 weeks of gestation) also increase the risk of aspiration.

Nursing Interventions and Considerations

If possible, premature infants are given small, frequent feedings by mouth. Gavage feedings by continuous infusion or bolus may be needed for very small premature infants. Check for gastric residuals before administering a feeding to avoid distention and possible aspiration.

Parenteral nutrition is required if enteral feedings are contraindicated or if growth falls below established minimum standards.

POTENTIAL PROBLEM/RATIONALE

Vitamin E deficiency leading to hemolytic anemia. Vitamin E deficiency may occur secondary to fat malabsorption (vitamin E is a fat-soluble vitamin) and/or to excessive iron supplementation, which interferes with vitamin E absorption.

Nursing Interventions and Considerations

Vitamin E deficiency can be prevented by giving water-soluble supplements of vitamin E orally and by avoiding excess iron supplementation.

Monitor the infant for signs of vitamin E deficiency (hemolytic anemia is the first sign), especially at 6 to 10 weeks of age.

(continued)

<hr>

Feeding the Premature Infant *(Continued)*

POTENTIAL PROBLEM/RATIONALE

Dehydration related to immature renal function and a low renal solute tolerance. In particular, the high osmolalities of concentrated LBW formulas (24 cal/oz) increase the risk of dehydration.

Nursing Interventions and Considerations

Fluid requirements vary with the infant's condition and treatment. Initially, 100 ml/kg/day may be given and adjusted as needed.

Monitor the infant's intake and output and serum BUN levels. Observe for signs and symptoms of hypernatremia and dehydration.

POTENTIAL PROBLEM/RATIONALE

Hypoglycemia, which may be related to (1) immature hepatic function → inadequate enzymes for glycogenolysis and gluconeogenesis → tendency toward hypoglycemia; (2) inadequate glycogen reserves; (3) respiratory distress syndrome; or (4) hypothermia, which occurs due to inadequate brown fat reserves.

Nursing Interventions and Considerations

Monitor the infant's serum glucose levels.

To prevent hypoglycemia, frequent and adequate feedings containing a readily utilized source or carbohydrate are needed.

<hr>

thrive, too concentrated → excess weight gain, obesity. Depending on the form of formula used, it may be expensive or require refrigeration (Table 11-6).

Formula Preparation

Most parents prepare formula a single bottle at a time, using the clean technique, which if done properly, may be as safe as sterilization. Care must be taken to prepare formulas to the proper level of dilution: Formulas that are made too dilute can result in inadequate growth and water intoxication; formulas that are made too concentrated may cause hypernatremia, tetany, and excessive weight gain (see display, Formula Preparation).

Table 11-6
Formula Varieties

	Advantages	Disadvantages
Powder	Unprepared powder does not require refrigeration; can be stored in a cool, dry place Least expensive form of formula	Requires proper dilution with water
Liquid concentrate	Less expensive than ready-to-use formula	Must be refrigerated after opening Requires proper dilution with water
Ready-to-use	Convenient: no preparation, no dilution with water Easy: poured directly into clean bottles	Most expensive form of formula Must be refrigerated after opening

Formula Preparation

"CLEAN" TECHNIQUE; (Prepare one bottle at a time, immediately before each feeding):

Wash hands thoroughly.

Wash and rinse all equipment to be used thoroughly: Formula can, bottles, nipples

Open can with a clean opener; cover and refrigerate remaining liquid formula

For ready-to-use formula: Pour directly into clean bottle.

For liquid concentrate formula: Pour directly into clean bottle and add equal amounts of water.

For powdered concentrate formula: Pour proper amount of water into clean bottle or container and add correct amount of powdered concentrate. Allow the formula to settle for a few minutes before shaking to mix.

After the formula has been warmed and the infant fed, discard any formula remaining in bottle.

NURSING PROCESS

Assessment

In addition to the general growth and development assessment criteria, assess for the following factors:

Length of gestation. Determine whether there were complications during pregnancy, labor, or delivery.

Growth rate, weight status, and weight fluctuations.

Sleeping habits; determine whether the infant is given a bottle at bedtime, and if so, what it contains.

Type of feeding (formula, breast milk, use of solids).

The use of vitamin/mineral supplements—type, amount, and frequency. Determine if the local water is fluoridated.

For breast-fed infants, assess the mother's prepregnancy nutritional status, weight gain pattern, and food allergies, as well as adequacy of present intake. Assess maternal use of alcohol, tobacco, caffeine, and drugs.

For formula-fed infants, assess the type of formula used, the frequency of feeding, and the method of formula preparation. Determine if the formula is iron-fortified.

For infants who are receiving solid foods, determine what is given, at what age each item was introduced in the diet, the frequency of eating these foods, and whether they are age-appropriate. Determine if any untoward side effects, such as diarrhea, fussiness, or skin rash, occurred after eating.

Familial attitudes about food, eating, and body weight.

Whether the infant has received immunizations.

Nursing Diagnosis

Health Seeking Behaviors, as evidenced by the lack of knowledge of infant nutritional requirements and feeding practices, and the desire to learn.

Planning and Implementation

The primary objective of diet intervention for infants is to promote normal growth and development. Breast-feeding should be encouraged as the only source of nutrition for the first 5 to 6 months of life. If breast-feeding is contraindicated or has failed because of maternal anxiety or misconceptions, the mother should be assured that infant formula will supply adequate nutrition (see Chapter 10).

The amount of formula provided per feeding and the frequency of feeding depend on the infant's age and individual needs. Feeding guidelines are listed in Table 11-7. Evaporated milk is not recommended as a substitute for breast milk because it does not meet the minimum standards set by the Infant Formula Act. Even when it is correctly diluted and mixed with carbohydrates, additional vitamins and some minerals are required. Also, the only source of fat in evaporated milk is butterfat, which is poorly tolerated by infants, and the concentration of some minerals is too great.

Infants generally are not developmentally ready for solid foods until 4 to 6 months of age (Table 11-8); feeding solids before the infant is ready may contribute to overfeeding, may increase the chance of food allergies, and may frustrate both the mother and the infant. There is no evidence to support the belief that solids help the infant sleep through the night. The early introduction of cow's milk and solid foods should be discouraged. Conversely, the introduction of solids should not be delayed beyond 7 to 9 months of age in order to provide a nutritionally adequate intake and promote normal development.

Breast milk or formula intake should decrease after 6 months of age to avoid displacing the intake of other iron- and nutrient-rich foods. Iron-fortified infant rice cereal is recommended as the first solid because it is not likely to cause an allergic reaction (**hypoallergenic**). The cereal may be mixed with breast milk, formula, or water. New foods, in plain and simple forms, should be introduced one at a time for a period of 5 to 7 days each to observe for possible allergic reactions, which may be exhibited as rash, fussiness, vomiting, diarrhea, or constipation. The amount of solids taken at a feeding may vary from 1 to 2 teaspoons initially, to one-quarter to one-half cup as the infant gets older.

Table 11-7
Guidelines for Formula Feeding*

Age	Feedings/ 24 Hours	Amount/Feeding	Amount/Day
1 week–1 month	6–8	4–5 oz	21–24 oz
1–3 months	5–6	5–7 oz	24–32 oz
3–6 months	4–5	6–7 oz	24–32 oz
6–12 months (feedings from the cup and bottle if the infant is not completely weaned)	3–4	6–8 oz	16–24 oz

* Actual number of feedings and amount/feeding depend on the infant's rate of growth and size. Never force infants to finish a bottle.

Table 11-8		
Introduction of Solid Foods Based on Development		

Age (Months)	Feeding Skills	Appropriate Foods to Introduce
0–3	Sucking reflex Rooting reflex Swallowing reflex Tonic head reflex	Breast milk; formula
4–6	Sucking, rooting, and biting (clamps down on spoon) reflexes disappear between 3 and 5 months. Head and neck control develop. Can transfer food to the back of the mouth for swallowing Can sit with support	Introduce iron-fortified infant cereals between 4 and 6 months for formula-fed infants; after 6 months for exclusively breast-fed infants.

5–8	Brings hand to mouth
	Grasps and reaches for objects in sight; can feed self finger foods
	At 7 months, grasps spoon, nipple, cup rim
	Drinks from cup when held to lips
	Interested in biting and chewing: begins chewing movements
	Sits alone
		5–7 months
		  Strained vegetables, fruits, and fruit juices (noncitrus)
		  Sips of water, juice, formula, from cup
		6–8 months
		  Ready for finger foods between 24 to 28 weeks of age: arrowroot biscuits, crackers, dry toast
		  Begin protein foods: strained meats, egg yolk, cheese, yogurt
		  Rice, noodles, potatoes
		  Citrus juices
		  Plain desserts: pudding, custards, ice cream, plain cookies

9–12	Increased ability to chew Improved pincer grasp	Gradually increase texture by replacing strained foods with finely chopped, mashed, or soft vegetables, fruit, and meat. Prefer finger foods: can give smaller-sized finger foods Can drink from cup alone
12	Chewing more refined, especially after molars erupt Increasingly independent Drinks from cup without sucking; blows bubbles in cup	Limit milk to 16–24 oz/day, all by cup. Because the risk of allergy is diminished, egg white may be added. Using molars, can eat regular solid foods and teething crackers Continue iron-fortified infant cereal until 18 months old, if possible.

Because cow's milk is a poor source of iron, may cause occult blood loss (possibly from an allergic response to the protein), and provides an unsuitably high potential renal solute load related to its protein, phosphorus, and electrolyte composition, it is an undesirable choice when feeding infants. Many experts recommend delaying the introduction of cow's milk until after the age of 1 year; intakes of milk between ages 1 and 4 years average 1 to 2½ cups per day (Pipes and Trahms, 1993). Skim and 2% milks do not provide adequate fat and sufficient calories for the amount of protein they contain; they should not be used before the age of 2 years.

Adequacy of growth is the best indicator of whether an infant is receiving sufficient nutrition. However, it should be noted that breast-fed infants usually have a slower growth rate than formula-fed infants. Also, infants who have suffered impaired growth related to undernutrition or illness experience "catch-up" growth, which usually is completed by 2 years of age. When this occurs, weight gain increases rapidly until the child reaches his normal weight percentile; thereafter, weight and height increase together at a slower rate. However, depending on the timing, severity, nature, and duration of the malnutrition, growth may or may not be permanently affected.

Iron is the nutrient that is most frequently deficient during infancy. The American Academy of Pediatrics recommends that iron-fortified formula be used for formula-fed infants. The long-standing belief that the addition of iron to formula increases the incidence of gastrointestinal problems (colic, constipation, cramping, diarrhea, gas, regurgitation) or that it interferes with the absorption of other minerals has not been proven in case studies.

Although approximately one third to one half of infants over 6 months of age receive nutrient supplements, their use is controversial. From birth to 6 months of age, breast-fed infants may be given fluoride and vitamin D; iron may be given after 4 months of age. Formula-fed infants may be given iron, if the formula is not iron-fortified, and fluoride, if the local water supply is not fluoridated. The American Academy of Pediatrics has stated that vitamin and mineral supplements are "usually not required" by normal, healthy infants during the second 6 months of life; however, it is important that vitamin D–fortified milk be used, that the diet provide adequate vitamin C, and that iron be supplied from iron-fortified formula or infant cereals. High-risk infants may be given a multivitamin or multimineral supplement.

Vegan diets (no animal products) are not recommended for infants and young children because certain vitamins and minerals are likely to be deficient if not properly supplemented, namely riboflavin, vitamin D, calcium, iron, zinc, and vitamin B_{12}. In addition, the intake of protein, fat, and calories may be inadequate, and the high-fiber content may increase satiety (further reducing calorie intake) or interfere with the absorption of some vitamins and minerals.

CLIENT GOALS

The caretaker will:

> Describe the principles and rationale of infant feeding, and practice age-appropriate feeding.
> Delay the introduction of solids until the infant is 4 to 6 months old.

The infant will:

> Experience normal growth and development.
> Avoid nursing bottle caries, if formula-fed.
> Consume an age-appropriate intake.

NURSING INTERVENTIONS

Diet Management

Provide the RDA for protein, calories (see Table 11-2), and nutrients for infancy. These can be obtained through either breast milk or formula; breast-feeding is recommended as the exclusive source of nutrition for the first 5 to 6 months of life.

Delay the introduction of solids until the infant is developmentally ready, usually between 4 and 6 months of age. Introduce one new food at a time and observe for an allergic response.

Advance the diet according to the infant's feeding skills (see Table 11-8).

Client Teaching

Instruct the family

On Formula Feeding

Infants should not be given supplements unless prescribed by the physician.

Formula may be given at room temperature, slightly warmed, or directly from the refrigerator; however, it should always be given at approximately the same temperature.

Each feeding should last 20 to 30 minutes.

Hold the infant closely and securely. Position the infant so that his head is higher than the rest of his body.

Avoid jiggling the bottle and making extra movements that could distract the infant from feeding.

Never prop the bottle or put the infant to bed with a bottle. Giving the infant a bottle of anything but plain water at bedtime can cause tooth decay (**nursing bottle caries**) once the teeth erupt.

Check the flow of formula by holding the bottle upside down. A steady drip from the nipple should be observed. If the flow is too rapid because of too large a nipple opening, the infant may overfeed and develop indigestion. If the flow rate is too slow because of too small a nipple opening, the infant may tire and fall asleep without taking enough formula. Discard any nipples with holes that are too large; enlarge holes that are too small with a sterilized needle.

There is no danger of "spoiling" an infant by feeding him when he cries for a feeding.

Burp the infant halfway through the feeding, at the end of the feeding, and more often if necessary, to help get rid of air that is swallowed during the feeding. An infant can be burped by gently rubbing or patting his back as he is held on the shoulder, laying over the lap, or sitting in an upright position.

One of the greatest hazards of formula feeding is overfeeding. Never force the infant to finish a bottle or take more than he wants. Signs that an infant is finished include biting the nipple, puckering the face, and turning away from the bottle.

Discourage the misconception that a "fat baby = a healthy baby = good parents."

During hot weather the baby may want supplemental bottles of water.

Spitting up a small amount of formula during and after a feeding is normal. Feeding the infant more slowly and burping more frequently may help alleviate spitting up.

On Proper Handling and Storage of Formulas

Before beginning, wash hands thoroughly with soap and hot water.

Prepare formula one bottle at a time by the clean technique.

Use standard measuring devices to ensure accuracy.

Fill bottles with just the amount of formula the infant will need at one feeding; discard formula that is left over after a feeding.

Use formula immediately after preparation, or store it in the refrigerator. Formula in a bottle or can that is left at room temperature for more than an hour should be discarded (bacteria thrive on warm formula).

Maintain the refrigerator temperature between 32°F and 40°F.

Discard opened, refrigerated cans of formula if they are not used within 2 days.

On Adding Solids to the Infant's Diet

Always feed the infant in an upright position; do not feed the infant solids from a bottle.

Infant rice cereal is recommended as the first solid feeding; follow with other iron-fortified infant cereals.

Before giving cereal the first few times, give the infant a small amount of formula or breast milk to take the edge off hunger and increase the likelihood of acceptance. After the infant is accustomed to solids, introduce new foods at the beginning of the feeding (when the infant is most hungry) and with a familiar favorite.

Infants differ in the amount of food they want or need at each feeding; let the baby determine how much food he needs.

Respect the infant's likes and dislikes; rejected foods may be reintroduced at a later time.

If there is a positive family history for food allergies, delay introducing milk, eggs, wheat, and citrus fruits, which tend to cause allergic reactions in susceptible infants.

Infants can be given the same plain, pure fruit juices as the rest of the family instead of expensive infant juices. Avoid sweetened fruit drinks.

For young infants, limit the serving size of high-nitrate vegetables (beets, carrots, collard greens, spinach, turnips) to 1 to 2 tablespoons per feeding. Nitrates can be converted to nitrites, which can bind with iron in the blood, decreasing its oxygen-carrying ability.

Except for mixed dinners (little meat content) and desserts (highly sweetened), commercially prepared baby food is nutritious and safe for infant use (sodium was removed in 1976). Read the label to determine if sugar or fillers have been added.

Homemade baby food can be prepared by blending, mashing, or grinding food to the proper consistency for the infant's stage of development. However:

- Do not salt the food or use spicy or high-fat foods.
- Do not use canned vegetables because of the high sodium content, possibility of lead contamination, and generally lower water-soluble vitamin content than fresh and frozen vegetables.
- Do not give honey to infants under 1 year of age because of the risk of infant botulism.

Between 6 to 8 months of age, the infant may be ready for three meals with three planned snacks.

When the infant is ready for finger foods, try ripe banana, Cheerios, toast strips, graham or soda crackers, cubes of cheese, noodles, and chunks of peeled apple, pears, or peaches.

To decrease the risk of choking:

- Avoid foods that are most often the cause of choking: hot dogs, candy, nuts, and grapes. Other offenders include raw carrots, tough meat, watermelon with seeds, celery, biscuits, cookies, popcorn, and even peanut butter.
- Always supervise meals and snacks.
- Do not allow the infant to eat or drink from a cup while lying down, playing, or strapped in a car seat.
- Cook foods well and serve in small pieces.
- Do not give a child food he cannot chew, or food you are not sure he can chew.
- Topical teething anesthetics that numb the gums can interfere with the ability to swallow foods that require chewing.

Avoid foods that may be difficult to digest: bacon, sausage, fatty or fried foods, gravy, spicy foods, and whole-kernel corn.

How to avoid common nutrition-related problems of iron deficiency, obesity, and dental caries (see display, Nutrition-Related Problems Among the Healthy Pediatric Population).

Monitoring Progress

Monitor:

Growth and development; weight status
Diet progressions (ie, what foods are eaten and in what form)
The development of food allergies
The need for follow-up family diet counseling

Evaluation

Evaluation is ongoing. Provided the plan of care has not changed, the client will achieve the goals as stated above.

NUTRITION FOR PRESCHOOL-AGE CHILDREN (1 TO 6 YEARS OF AGE)

Growth Characteristics and Nutritional Implications

Physical and Physiologic Growth	Nutritional Implications
Growth rate decreases dramatically (see Table 11-1).	Appetite decreases dramatically; becomes erratic. Interest in food declines → "physiologic anorexia"
Maturation of biting, chewing, and swallowing abilities continues.	Can eat a variety of textures, table food
Develops greater mobility, coordination, and autonomy	Self-feeding skills improve, can completely self-feed by the end of the second year
	Can seek food independently
	May use food to express autonomy and manipulate parents; finicky food habits and food jags may begin around 15 months
Muscle mass and bone density increase.	Need adequate amounts of protein, calcium, and phosphorus to support normal bone growth
Language skills increase.	Between the ages of 1 and 3, associate food with taste and name; between the ages of 4 and 6 begin verbalizing food dislikes and preferences
Between the ages of 3 and 5, develop attitudes about food and eating	Inappropriate use of food (eg, to reward, punish, convey love, bribe) may lead to inappropriate food attitudes.

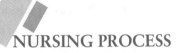

NURSING PROCESS

Assessment

In addition to the general growth and development assessment criteria, assess for the following factors:

Growth rate, weight status, and weight fluctuations

Pattern of meals and snacks

Adequacy of intake based on the Daily Food Guide (see Table 11-3), paying particular attention to variety, and the intake of meat, fruits, vegetables, and sweets

Feeding skills and "feeding problems"

Pica. If the child or family practices pica, determine what items are consumed, how frequently, and the rationale

Dental health

The frequency and intensity of physical activity

Nursing Diagnosis

Health Seeking Behaviors, as evidenced by a lack of knowledge of age-appropriate eating behaviors and nutritional requirements, and the desire to learn.

Planning and Implementation

Parents are the primary gatekeepers and role models of their young children's food intake and habits; they influence the variety, frequency, and macronutrient composition of their diet through food purchasing decisions, food preparation, and food accessibility. Although parents should be encouraged to set a good example, they must also realize that children's individual food preferences have an important impact on their actual intake (Fisher and Birch, 1995).

Young children eat an average of five to seven times a day (Pipes and Trahms, 1993). Snacks have been noted to contribute one fourth to one third of total calories, over one third of total sugar, and one fifth of total protein consumed by children.

Milk intake decreases to about 16 oz/day by 2 years of age, which is adequate. Excessive milk intake can contribute to iron deficiency anemia by displacing iron-rich foods in the diet (see display, Nutrition-Related Problems Among the Healthy Pediatric Population). Liquids should be withheld until halfway through the meal or until the end of the meal to avoid replacing the intake of nutrient-rich foods.

Appetite fluctuates widely because of erratic growth patterns. Children eat to satisfy hunger and should not be forced to overeat. Although there are individual differences, usually a larger child eats more than a smaller one, an active child eats more than a quiet one, and a happy, content child eats more than an anxious one.

The most frequent concerns of parents include a limited variety of foods eaten; dawdling while eating; a limited intake of fruits, vegetables, and meat; and consumption of too many sweets (Pipes and Trahms, 1993). However, feeding problems tend to be a product of culture, economic status, and parental nutrition knowledge, and they often occur because parents overestimate the amount of food children need and force them to overeat. Assure parents that if the child's growth chart shows a consistent and reasonable rate of growth, nutritional intake is probably adequate.

Nutrients that are most likely to be received in inadequate amounts are iron and zinc; calcium, vitamin A, and vitamin C are also frequently consumed in less than recommended amounts (Pipes and Trahms, 1993). However, supplements are generally not needed unless the child has a chronic illness or is a particularly poor eater. Studies show that children of heavier parents are more likely to have strong preferences for high-fat foods and are more likely to have a high total fat intake (Fisher and Birch, 1995).

All children over 2 years of age are advised to follow the same heart-healthy diet as adults: 30% calories from fat, less than 10% calories from saturated fat, and less than 300 mg of cholesterol/day (see Food for Thought: Heart Smarts Kids Can Live With).

FOOD *for* **THOUGHT**

Heart Smarts Kids Can Live With

Compelling evidence suggests that atherosclerosis and hypertension begin before the second decade of life (Anding et al, 1996). Like American adults, American children eat too much fat, saturated fat, cholesterol, and sodium, and not enough fruits and vegetables, characteristics that place them at increased risk for cardiovascular disease (Kotz and Story, 1994).

Because adult risk factors are believed to apply to children and adolescents, several expert panels and health organizations have reached a consensus and issued dietary recommendations directed at the general population, including all healthy children over the age of 2 years (Kotz and Story, 1996). The Expert Panel on Blood Cholesterol Levels in Children and Adolescents recommends that nutritional adequacy be achieved by eating a wide variety of foods; that calories be adequate to support growth and development and to reach or maintain desirable body weight; and that intake follow the pattern of no more than 30% calories from fat, less than 10% calories from saturated fat, and less than 300 mg/day of cholesterol daily.

Practical tips include:

- Start your day with breakfast.
- Snack smart.
- Balance your food choices—don't eat too much of any one thing.
- Eat more grains, fruits, and vegetables.
- Foods aren't good or bad

Studies show that kindergartners understand the relationship between diet, body fat, and health; nutrition education can begin with children as early as preschool and kindergarten. Basic principles can be presented, nutrition terms may be introduced, and positive experiences with healthful foods can be provided (Murphy et al, 1995).

Children younger than 6 years are at significant risk for lead poisoning related to their higher rate of intestinal absorption of lead, rapidly developing nervous system, and frequent exposure to lead from mouthing objects (Pipes and Trahms, 1993). Lead poisoning can cause permanent growth stunting, cognitive deficits, and other neurologic problems. It appears that inadequate intakes of calories, calcium, phosphorus, iron, and zinc may increase susceptibility to the effects of lead poisoning; the CDC recommends that children eat at regular intervals (more lead is absorbed on an empty stomach) and that they consume adequate amounts of iron and calcium.

CLIENT GOALS

The child will:

Experience normal growth and development; maintain optimal nutritional status.
Avoid common nutrition-related problems: iron deficiency anemia, obesity, and dental caries (see display, Nutrition-Related Problems Among the Healthy Pediatric Population).

Avoid milk anemia.
Begin to establish lifelong healthy eating patterns.
Engage in regular physical activity.

NURSING INTERVENTIONS

Diet Management

Provide a varied, nutrient-dense diet, based on the Daily Food Guide for Childhood (see Table 11-3).
Provide three meals daily plus two to three planned snacks.
Modify the diet, as needed, to avoid frequent nutrition-related problems (see display, Nutrition-Related Problems Among the Healthy Pediatric Population).
Limit milk intake to 16 oz/day.
After 2 years of age, limit fat intake to no more than 30% of calories, saturated fat to less than 10% of calories, and cholesterol to less than 300 mg/day (see Food for Thought: Heart Smarts Kids Can Live With).
Allow children to choose their own food likes and dislikes, and to regulate their own intake according to appetite.

Client Teaching

Instruct the family

On Eating Behaviors Characteristic of This Age

Food "jags" are a normal expression of autonomy as the child develops a sense of independence. As long as the diet is adequate but not excessive in water, calories, and all essential nutrients, food jags should not be a cause of concern.
Foods most commonly rejected are as follows:
- Meats (with the exception of chicken, hamburger, and hot dogs). The iron status of children who refuse animal sources of iron may require monitoring.
- Cooked vegetables. Serve vegetables raw if possible, or serve more fruit.
- Casseroles or mixed dishes. Serve plain, simple foods.

Avoid encouraging the inborn preference for sweets. Sweets can displace other nutrient-rich foods and contribute to nutrient deficiencies, dental caries, and obesity.
Children may refuse to eat for the following reasons:
- Too excited or distracted. Allow the child time to calm down before eating and try to minimize mealtime commotion.
- Too tired. A brief rest or quiet time before mealtime may help.
- Not hungry. Remove the child's plate without comment. If the child wants a snack later, make it nutritious. Try spacing meals further apart and limit snacking so the child will be hungry at mealtime.

- Seeking attention. Provide attention other than at mealtimes. Do not tolerate manipulative behavior.
- Expressing independence. Accept it as a normal phase of development and do not make it an issue.

Appetite is often least at dinner.

Ritualistic eating may become apparent.

On How to Foster Good Eating Habits

Offer the proper food.

    Using the Daily Food Guide, offer a variety of nutritious foods. It is not important if a child refuses to eat a particular food (eg, spinach), as long as he has a reasonable intake from each of the major food groups.

    Encourage the child to taste new foods, but respect individual likes and dislikes.

    Introduce a small amount of a new food with a familiar favorite.

    Prepare mildly flavored foods, which children usually prefer.

    Make dessert (such as pudding, fruit, nutrient-rich cookies) a nutritious part of the meal instead of using it as a bribe, reward, or routine bedtime snack.

    Serve nutritious planned snacks (see display, Heart-Healthy Snacks).

    Offer child-sized servings. Generally, a serving size equals 1 tablespoon of food/year of age (eg, the serving size for a 3-year-old is 3 tablespoons). It is better to serve seconds than to overwhelm the child with too much food. Parents should decide *what* the child should eat; the child should decide *how much*. Instead of "clean your plate," the rule should be "try a little bit of everything."

    Offer foods the child can easily chew and digest.

Use child-sized utensils and small, unbreakable cups and plates.

Serve colorful foods (red tomatoes, orange slices, green peas) of various textures (smooth mashed potatoes, crunchy raw vegetables, tender meats) that are attractively presented (shaped sandwiches made with cookie cutters, carrot curls).

Children prefer finger foods. Allow children to explore foods by touching. Children who are learning to use utensils often place the food on the utensil by hand.

Provide an enjoyable atmosphere.

    Never force a child to eat; if a healthy child is hungry, he will eat.

    Do not use food to reward, punish, bribe, or convey love.

    Mealtime should be relaxed, pleasant, and unhurried. Allow 20 to 30 minutes per meal.

    Eat with the child.

    Provide comfortable, child-sized tables and chairs.

    Minimize confusion and excess noise at mealtime. Keep mealtime conversation pleasant; do not use mealtime as a time for discipline.

Heart-Healthy Snacks

SNACKS

Are an excellent way to provide additional protein, calories, and essential nutrients to children who cannot eat a lot at mealtime.

Should be offered at least 1.5 hours before mealtime to avoid interfering with appetite.

Should be based on the child's appetite, preferences, and ability to chew and digest.

SUGGESTIONS

Unsweetened cereal, with or without milk

Meat or cheese on whole-grain bread or crackers

Graham crackers, fig bars

Whole-grain cookies or muffins made with oatmeal, dried fruit, or iron-fortified cereal

Quick breads like banana, date, pumpkin

Raw vegetables, vegetable juices

Fresh, dried, or canned fruit without sugar

Pure fruit juice as a drink or frozen on a stick

Low-fat yogurt, with or without fresh fruit added

Air-popped popcorn (not before age 3), pretzels

Peanut butter on bread, crackers, celery, apple slices

Milk shakes made with fruit and ice milk or frozen yogurt

Low-fat ice cream, frozen yogurt, ice milk, sherbet, sorbet, fruit ice

Animal crackers, ginger snaps

Angel food cake

Skim or 1% milk

Low-fat cheese, low-fat cottage cheese

Expect occasional table accidents as a part of growing up.

Encourage children to participate in food preparation and clean-up.

Praise good eating behaviors and do not scold children for not eating.

On how to avoid common nutrition-related problems of healthy children (see display, Nutrition-Related Problems Among the Healthy Pediatric Population)

Monitoring Progress

Monitor:

Growth and development, and weight status
Overall intake according to the Daily Food Guide
Iron status
Dental health
The development of food allergies
The need for follow-up family diet counseling

Evaluation

Evaluation is ongoing. Provided the plan of care has not changed, the client will achieve the goals as stated above.

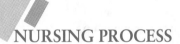

NUTRITION FOR SCHOOL-AGE CHILDREN (6 TO 12 YEARS OF AGE)

Growth Characteristics and Nutritional Implications

Physical and Physiologic Growth	Nutritional Implications
Latent period of growth, characterized by a consistent, slow rate of growth	Nutrient needs per unit of body weight continue to decline; dietary intake is regular and appetite gradually increases in preparation for the adolescent growth spurt.
Wide variations in growth rates among individuals	
Digestive system matures; can handle larger meals and eat less frequently	Meal pattern: 3 meals with 2 snacks
Permanent teeth erupt.	Nutrients important for dental health include fluoride, vitamin A, vitamin D, calcium, and phosphorus.
Increased socialization, growing sense of independence	Parents' role as gatekeepers declines; advertising has an impact on food choices; variety of food increases.
Reserves are laid down for upcoming adolescent growth spurt. By the end of this period, girls are usually well into puberty.	Toward the end of the school-age period, nutrient needs increase in preparation for the adolescent growth spurt.

NURSING PROCESS

Assessment

In addition to the general growth and development assessment criteria, assess for the following factors:

Growth rate, weight status, and weight fluctuations

Pattern of meals and snacks

Adequacy of intake based on the Daily Food Guide for the child's age, paying particular attention to the sources of calories, and fruit and vegetable intake. It is estimated that 91% of children 6 to 11 years of age do not consume the recommended minimum of five servings of fruits and vegetables per day (Nicklas et al, 1995).

The use of vitamin or mineral supplements—type, amount, and frequency

Frequency and intensity of physical activity

Nursing Diagnosis

Health Seeking Behaviors, as evidenced by a lack of knowledge of normal nutritional requirements of children, and a desire to learn.

Planning and Implementation

According to NHANES III data, 6- to 11-year-olds consume 53% of total calories from carbohydrates, 14% from protein, and 34% from fat; 75% of children consume more fat, saturated fat, and cholesterol than is recommended (Nicklas, 1995). School lunch and breakfast together provide approximately 50% of the day's total intake of calories, protein, cholesterol, carbohydrates, and sodium, and 40% of total fat. Zinc is likely to be consumed in inadequate amounts (CDC, 1994).

Nutrients that are most likely to be consumed in less than recommended amounts are calcium, iron, vitamin B_6, vitamin A, and vitamin C (Pipes and Trahms, 1993).

School-age children maintain a relatively constant intake in relation to their age group—that is, children who are considered big eaters in second grade are also big eaters in sixth grade.

A child's genetic potential for growth is reached only if nutrient needs are met. A calorie deficit of as little as 10 cal/kg can result in malnutrition.

Generally, eating is still a ritual for 6- and 7-year-olds; 8-year-olds tend to have large appetites, and 9-year-olds have firmly established likes and dislikes. Although some children increase the variety of foods that they eat, many continue to reject vegetables (typically their least favorite food), mixed dishes, and some meats (Pipes and Trahms, 1993).

School-age children typically eat less frequently than younger children, usually 4 to 5 times per day, with snacks contributing about one third of their total calorie intake.

Health assessments of school-age children have identified several nutrition-related concerns. These include the following: (1) low intake of fruits and vegetables; (2) obesity; (3) consumption of snacks with low nutrient density; (4) the tendency to skip breakfast; (5) limited understanding of fiber in foods; (6) lack of variety in food choices; (7) the need to moderate sugar intake; (8) inability to identify foods that are low in fat, saturated fat, or cholesterol; (9) lack of knowledge about food composition; and (10) consumption of too much fat and saturated fat (Murphy, et al 1995).

Breakfast skipping is a concern of parents of school-age children. Studies suggest that skipping breakfast alters brain function, particularly that concerned with the speed and accuracy of information retrieval in working memory. The impact appears to be greatest in 9- to 11-year-olds, who are at nutritional risk based on history and anthropometric measurements (Pollitt, 1995). Normally, breakfast adds significantly to a child's total intake of calories, protein, carbohydrate, and micronutrients, and increases the likelihood of meeting nutritional requirements (Pollitt, 1995).

Another concern of parents and nutrition professionals is the effect of advertising on children's food choices. One study showed that 43.6% of all commercials that were featured during children's Saturday morning television were for foods high in fat and/or sugar, many with low nutritional value. The most frequently advertised product was high-sugar cereals. The most frequent explicit messages used to sell food products involved taste, fun, and the promise of a free toy (Kotz and Story, 1994).

Food additives are a concern of parents with hyperactive children. Although the term is difficult to define objectively, common characteristics of hyperactivity (or attention deficit disorder [ADD] with or without concurrent hyperactivity) include specific learning deficits, impulsivity, hyperkinesis, short attention span, motor and coordination deficits, and aggression. In the 1970s, the late Dr. Ben Feingold proposed that food additives and salicylates may be responsible for about 25% of cases of hyperactivity with learning disability among school-age children (Feingold, 1974). Numerous studies indicate that the Feingold diet (a diet that is devoid of artificial colors, flavors, BHT, BHA, and salicylate-containing fruits, vegetables, and spices) rarely helps control hyperactivity. However, the Feingold diet is probably not nutritionally harmful (as long as fruits and vegetables containing vitamin C are allowed) and may have a placebo effect on behavior.

Food allergies, which are usually caused by protein substances in food (ie, the protein component of milk, wheat, eggs, corn), are influenced by a variety of environmental, emotional, genetic, and physical factors. Introducing solids into the diet before the immune system matures increases the likelihood of food allergies. Fortunately, most children tend to outgrow food allergies as they get older. Because allergies may be difficult to diagnose, foods should be introduced in the diet one at a time for 5 to 7 days each so that if a reaction occurs, the offending item can be identified easily (see display, Allergic Reactions). Older children who are suspected of having food allergies may benefit from eliminating common allergens from the diet (Table 11-9). If the food allergy persists, it may be necessary to use skin testing or elimination diets to diagnose the offending item. Children who are placed on elimination diets initially receive foods that are relatively hypoallergenic (rice, tapioca), after which other foods are introduced singly and the child is observed for a reaction.

CLIENT GOALS

The child will:

Experience normal growth and development, and maintain optimal nutritional status.

Avoid common nutrition-related problems: iron deficiency anemia, obesity, and dental caries.

Continue to establish lifelong healthy eating patterns.

Engage in regular physical activity.

Allergic Reactions

- May be immediate (within 1 hour) or delayed (within 24 to 48 hours)
- May be cyclical (not always occurring after the offending item is eaten) or fixed (always occurring after the offending item is eaten)
- May produce skin, GI, respiratory, or CNS symptoms

Table 11-9
Common Food Allergens

Bacon	Peanut butter
Chocolate	Pineapple
Citrus fruit	Pork
Cocoa	Seafood
Eggs	Strawberries
Milk and milk products	Tomatoes
Nuts	Wheat

NURSING INTERVENTIONS

Diet Management

Provide a varied, nutrient-dense diet, based on the Daily Food Guide for Childhood (see Table 11-3).

Modify the diet, as needed, to avoid common nutrition-related problems (see display, Nutrition-Related Problems Among the Healthy Pediatric Population).

Limit fat intake to no more than 30% of calories, saturated fat to less than 10% of total calories, and cholesterol to less than 300 mg/day (see Food for Thought: Heart Smarts Kids Can Live With).

Allow children to choose their own food likes and dislikes, and to regulate their own intake according to appetite.

Client Teaching

Instruct the child and family

On the importance of nutrition in normal growth and development, and overall health and well-being.

On the principles and rationale of the Daily Food Guide, and how to choose an adequate diet.

How to modify the diet, as needed, to avoid common nutrition-related problems (see display, Nutrition-Related Problems Among the Healthy Pediatric Population).

On the relationship between nutrition, physical activity, and health status. Encourage regular physical activity.

Monitoring Progress

Monitor:

Growth and development, and weight status

Overall intake according to the Daily Food Guide for childhood

Iron status

Dental health

The need for follow-up family diet counseling

Evaluation

Evaluation is ongoing. Provided the plan of care has not changed, the client will achieve the goals as stated above.

ADOLESCENT NUTRITION (12 TO 18 YEARS OF AGE)

Growth Characteristics and Nutritional Implications

Physical and Physiologic Growth	Nutritional Implications
Rapid period of physical, emotional, social, and sexual maturation	To support adequate growth and development, nutritional needs increase, especially for calories, protein, calcium, iron, and zinc.
Growth begins at different times in different individuals; therefore, physiologic age is a more valid indicator of need than chronologic age.	Because the RDA are based on chronologic, not physiologic age, they may be invalid for some or many adolescents, depending on when the growth spurt begins (the increase in nutritional requirements is dependent on the timing and duration of the growth spurt).
Generally, the growth spurt begins in females around age 10 to 11, peaks at age 12, and is completed by age 15.	Nutritional needs increase earlier for girls than boys.
Menstruation begins.	To replace monthly losses, the requirement for iron increases and remains high until menopause.
Girls experience fat deposition, especially in the abdomen and pelvic girdle; the pelvis widens in preparation for childbearing.	Fat requires fewer calories to be maintained than does lean body tissue; therefore, girls have lower calorie requirements than boys and may have difficulty meeting nutrient needs without exceeding calorie needs.
Girls experience less growth of lean body tissue and bones than boys.	Girls tend to become weight and figure conscious and often voluntarily restrict the amount and types of food eaten.
Generally, the growth spurt begins in males around age 12 to 13, peaks at age 14, and is completed by age 19.	Nutritional needs increase later for boys than girls.
Boys experience an increase in muscle mass, lean body tissue, and bones.	Lean body tissue requires more calories to be maintained than fat tissue; therefore, boys have higher calorie needs than girls.
	During the growth spurt, adolescent males need the same amount of iron as menstruating females because of the increase in muscle mass and blood volume; iron need decreases to below female requirement after the growth spurt is complete.
Period of intense psychosocial growth, family conflict, social and peer pressures.	Nutritional needs may be difficult to meet because Fewer meals are eaten at home Of strong peer influence Of busy schedules Adolescents may express their independence through the diet.

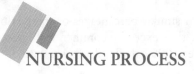

NURSING PROCESS

Assessment

In addition to the general growth and development assessment criteria (see display, General Growth and Development Assessment Criteria), assess for the following factors:

Growth rate, weight status, and weight fluctuations

Pattern of meals and snacks

Adequacy of intake based on the Daily Food Guide for Adolescents, paying particular attention to iron and protein intake

The use of vitamin or mineral supplements—type, amount, and frequency

The use of alcohol, tobacco, and drugs

Familial attitude toward weight, thinness, and the client's weight

The use of any fad diets; assess the age at which dieting began and elicit associated events, methods and patterns of dieting that have been used, and the client's feelings and beliefs about food and dieting.

The frequency and intensity of physical activity

Nursing Diagnosis

Health Seeking Behaviors, as evidenced by a lack of knowledge of normal nutritional requirements for adolescents, and the desire to learn.

Planning and Implementation

Because of varying growth rates, a wide range of weights is considered normal during adolescence.

General Growth and Development Assessment Criteria

Age

Height (length in infants)

Weight

Weight for height and head circumference (for infants)

Hemoglobin

Hematocrit

Clinical observations: skin color, pallor, turgor; gross deformities; subcutaneous fat; dental caries

Chronic illness, family history of chronic illness

Use of medication for chronic illness

Allergies, nature of allergic reactions

Socioeconomic status

Developmental status

Frequency and intensity of physical activity

Use of alcohol, tobacco, street drugs

Studies show that adolescents and children eat similar percentages of total calories from carbohydrates, protein, and fat; that is, they exceed recommended intakes for fat. The intake of all vitamins and minerals per 1000 calories decreases with age, with the exception of sodium (Nicklas, 1995).

Childhood nutritional problems tend to intensify during adolescence. Mild nutrient deficiencies occur frequently; for example, laboratory values may indicate a deficiency but overt clinical symptoms are not apparent. Nutrients that are most likely to be consumed in inadequate amounts are vitamin A, vitamin B_6, iron, calcium, zinc, and magnesium in females; and zinc in males (CDC, 1994).

Peer and social pressures and enjoyment often have a greater impact on adolescent food choices than the nutritional quality of the food and dietary health implications.

In high school, students tend to have several options available to them in addition to the United States Department of Agriculture (USDA) school lunch meals, although these do not include many healthful or low-fat alternatives. One study found that more than half of school vending machines had potato, corn, or taco chips, but only a quarter had pretzels (low-fat alternative) (Story et al, 1996). Also, carbonated beverages were more prevalent and less expensive than fruit juice. Emphasis should be placed on making healthful, low-fat alternatives available and affordable for students in schools.

Effective adolescent nutrition education programs are those that allow adolescents to express their attitudes, beliefs, concerns, and feelings regarding food, food choices, eating, and diet; they are also tailored to meet the needs and interests of the individual or group. Effective programs encourage self-direction and responsibility for food choices based on an adequate knowledge base, and allow the educator to be a facilitator of learning, not a "teacher." Nutrition education programs should also encourage physical activity for overall well-being.

Nutritional concerns of parents and nutrition professionals regarding this age group include the following:

- *Meal skipping:* The number of meals missed and eaten away from home increases from early to late adolescence. Girls are more likely to skip meals than boys, often because they think skipping breakfast and/or lunch will help them control their weight. In one recent poll of 9- to 15-year-olds, 51% of respondents said they skip breakfast and 28% skip lunch (IFIC, 1995).
- *Snacking:* Snacks may contribute 30% or more of adolescents' total calorie intake each day. Unfortunately, snacks are often high in fat, sugar, or sodium, and may increase the risk of obesity and dental caries. Adolescents should be encouraged to take responsibility for choosing healthy snacks.
- *Reliance on fast foods:* Although fast foods can be incorporated into a healthy diet, there is cause for concern when they become a mainstay in the diet. Fast foods tend to be high in fat, calories, and sodium and low in folic acid, fiber, and vitamin A. They are also low in calcium and riboflavin (except when milk or a milkshake is ordered). See display, Foods in the Fast Lane for fast food selection suggestions.

Foods in the Fast Lane

Here are some tips on fast foods to choose:

- Order a small hamburger instead of a larger one. Try the extra lean hamburger.
- Order roast beef for a leaner choice than most burgers.
- Order a baked potato instead of french fries. Be careful of high-fat toppings like sour cream or cheese.
- Order grilled, broiled, or baked fish and chicken.
- Order skim or 1% milk instead of a shake. Try the low-fat frozen yogurt.
- Order a salad. Use vinegar and oil or low-calorie dressing more often than creamy salad dressing.

- Create a salad at a salad bar. Choose any raw vegetables, fruits, or beans. Limit high-saturated fat toppings of cheese, fried noodles, bacon bits, and some salads made with mayonnaise. Also limit salad dressings high in saturated fat and cholesterol.
- For sandwich toppings, try lettuce, tomato, and onion, pickles, mustard, and ketchup instead of high saturated fat toppings like cheese, bacon, special sauces, or butter.
- Order pizza with vegetable toppings like peppers, mushrooms, or onions instead of extra cheese, pepperoni, or sausage.

Credit to: NIH/NHLBI National Cholesterol Education Program, USDHHS Publication #92-3101-1992.

- *Dieting:* Many adolescents are preoccupied with dieting because of concerns about their appearance. Also, many girls do not understand that increases in fat tissue during puberty are necessary for normal growth and development; boys may have the mistaken belief that dieting will improve athletic performance. Adolescents should be counseled on realistic views of desirable weight, and on the importance of regular physical activity. For a discussion of extreme eating disorders, see the section on anorexia and bulimia (Chapter 13).
- *Adolescent pregnancy:* Adolescent pregnancy is associated with increased medical, nutritional, social, and economic risks depending on biologic maturity, ethnic background, economic status, prenatal care, and lifestyle (see Chapter 10).
- *Acne:* There is no scientific evidence to correlate any dietary factors with the appearance or severity of acne. Although vitamin A is important for normal skin integrity, vitamin A supplements are not effective in treating acne and are toxic in large amounts. A compound related to vitamin A (13-*cis*-retinoic acid or Accutane) has been approved for treatment of severe cystic acne but is available only through prescription and must be used with caution.
- *The use of alcohol, tobacco, marijuana, oral contraceptives:* Alcohol, especially in growing adolescents, can produce nutritional deficiencies related to decreased food intake, decreased absorption, increased excretion, decreased storage, and altered metabolism of nutrients. Likewise, tobacco and marijuana can alter food intake. The effect of substance abuse on nutritional status depends on the nature of the substance; the amount, duration, and frequency of use; previous health and nutritional status; stage of physical growth; and the nutritional adequacy of the diet consumed (Pipes and Trahms, 1993). Oral

contraceptives alter serum levels of some nutrients and may increase the requirement for folic acid and vitamin B_6, although clinical observations of deficiencies are rare and vitamin supplements are usually unnecessary.

- *Nutrition for the growing athlete:* Diet guidelines for growing athletes suggest a balanced, varied diet with adequate fluid and calories to meet increased needs. During training, the diet should be composed of about 15% protein, 55% carbohydrate, and 30% fat. Young athletes may develop a transient low hemoglobin value that is related to a greater increase in plasma volume than in red blood cell mass, or from true iron deficiency anemia. Amenorrhea is common among adolescent female athletes and may be related to the stress of physical training and competition, or to a reduction in body fat. Regular menstrual activity returns after intense training is reduced and body fat level increases. Misconceptions regarding the role of nutrition and diet in athletic competition should be dispelled (see display, Misconceptions About Sports Nutrition).

CLIENT GOALS

The client will:

Consume adequate calories, protein, and nutrients to support the adolescent growth spurt.

Prevent or correct nutritional deficiencies.

Avoid common nutrition-related problems: iron deficiency anemia, obesity, and dental caries.

Engage in regular physical activity.

Continue to establish lifelong healthy eating patterns.

NURSING INTERVENTIONS

Diet Management

Provide a varied, nutrient-dense diet based on the Daily Food Guide for Adolescents (see Table 11-3).

Modify the diet, as needed, to avoid common nutrition-related problems.

Limit fat intake to no more than 30% of total calories, saturated fat to less than 10% of total calories, and cholesterol to less than 300 mg/day.

Client Teaching

Instruct the client

On the principles and rationale of the Daily Food Guide, and how to choose an adequate diet.

On the relationship between diet, health, weight control, and physical fitness. Explain that an increase in fat tissue before the adolescent growth spurt is a normal physiologic occurrence. Encourage regular physical activity.

On how to modify the diet, as needed, to avoid common nutrition-related problems.

Fallacy: Extra protein builds muscles.

Fact: Muscle mass increases only through repeated exercise, providing that a sufficient supply of calories is available. According to the American Dietetic Association, the RDA for protein may be inadequate for adult endurance athletes, who may actually need 1.0 g of protein/kg, instead of the RDA of 0.8 mg/kg. However, because most American diets provide more protein than is needed, young athletes are probably consuming enough. Protein taken in excess of need is not magically converted to muscle, rather it is converted to and stored as fat, just like an excess intake of CHO or fat.

Fallacy: Carbohydrate foods are fattening and should be avoided by athletes.

Fact: The primary muscle fuel during exercise is carbohydrates, in the form of blood glucose or stored glycogen. When low-CHO diets are consumed during training, the body's storage of fuel may not be adequate to sustain an athlete through prolonged competition, resulting in weakness, the inability to perform, or "hitting the wall." Carbohydrates also provide the same amount of calories as an equivalent amount of protein and less than half the calories in an equal measure of fat.

Fallacy: CHO loading can be used routinely to increase athletic performance.

Fact: CHO loading is based on the idea that glycogen stores can be maximized, and, therefore, endurance improved, in a step-by-step process involving training and diet. Traditionally, CHO loading involved depleting glycogen stores followed by loading, in which the athlete exercised to a minimum and ate a high-CHO intake to supersaturate the muscles with glycogen.

Unfortunately, carbohydrate loading is beneficial only to athletes participating in long-duration endurance or multiple-event competitions. Also, it is now recommended that athletes follow a high-CHO diet throughout training and begin a tapered rest approximately 7 days before the competition, with complete rest the day before the event. CHO loading is not recommended for growing athletes.

Fallacy: The less body fat, the better the athlete.

Fact: Different sports require different amounts of body fat for optimum performance; for example, the ideal percentage of body weight as fat for male distance runners is 4% to 8%, and for male tennis players, 14% to 16%. While it is true that too much body fat means excess body weight and interferes with the body's ability to dissipate heat, too little fat should also be avoided. Adjusting body weight is a gradual process; rapid weight loss results in a greater loss of lean body tissue than fat tissue, can impair performance, may endanger health, and could adversely effect growth. Likewise, rapid weight gain usually means fat gain, not an increase in lean body tissues.

Fallacy: Salt tablets are needed to replace sodium lost through perspiration.

Fact: Salt tablets are not recommended; sodium chloride taken without adequate amounts of water can further aggravate intracellular dehydration caused by sweating. Dehydration can impair physical performance, and thirst is not always a reliable indicator of need. Plain water is probably the most important substance for replacing fluid loss. Prepubescent athletes are particularly susceptible to heat stroke or heat-induced collapse because of their inability to produce sweat effectively and, thus, cool the body through evaporation.

Fallacy: Supplements of vitamin B_6 and other vitamins will improve performance.

Fact: An increase in calorie intake does warrant a higher intake of vitamins used to metabolize calories, namely thiamine, riboflavin, and niacin. However, sufficient amounts of these vitamins can easily be obtained by the increase in calorie (food) intake. These and other water-soluble vitamins taken in excess of need do not enhance energy metabolism but are excreted in the urine. Megadoses of the fat-soluble vitamins and some water-soluble vitamins can cause toxic or adverse effects and should not be used.

Fallacy: The precompetition meal should be high in protein.

Fact: High-protein meals can lead to mild dehydration because the kidneys must excrete the nitrogenous wastes resulting from protein metabolism. In addition, high-protein meals may also be high in fat, which delays gastric emptying. A meal high in complex CHO should be eaten 3.5 to 4 hours before competition to ensure gastric emptying and to avoid discomfort and cramping. Although the meal may contain between 300 to 1000 calories, generally, the lighter the better.

On the importance of not skipping meals, especially breakfast.
To choose nutritious snacks.
That limiting fat intake may help prevent heart disease later in life.

Monitor Progress

Monitor:

Growth and development, and weight status
Overall intake according to the Daily Food Guide for Adolescents
Iron status
Dental health
The need for follow-up family diet counseling

Evaluation

Evaluation is ongoing. Provided the plan of care has not changed, the client will achieve the goals as stated above.

Nursing Interventions and Considerations for Disorders of Infancy and Childhood

FAILURE TO THRIVE

Failure to thrive is generally defined as an inadequate gain in weight and/or height compared to growth and development standards. It may be caused by clinical diseases, such as CNS disorders, endocrine disorders, congenital defects, or intestinal obstructions, or it may occur secondary to an inability to suck, chew, or swallow related to neuromuscular problems. An inadequate calorie intake related to inappropriate formula selection, improper formula dilution, or alterations in digestion or absorption (ie, lactose intolerance) can lead to failure to thrive. Family problems, such as inadequate nurturing and infant stimulation, may also be implicated.

Nursing Interventions and Considerations

To develop a plan of care, the cause(s) of failure to thrive must first be identified.

Diet interventions depend on the infant's age and stage of development. Generally, a high-calorie, high-protein diet is indicated.

Physical, emotional, and intellectual growth may be permanently affected if failure to thrive becomes a chronic problem.

COLIC

Colic is characterized by intermittent periods of profuse crying lasting 3 hours or more per day. It is generally accompanied by symptoms of irritability, GI distention, and abdominal cramping (Lust et al, 1996). It most often affects the first-born child, is more common in formula-fed infants than breast-fed infants, and usually resolves itself by the time the infant is 3 months old. The exact cause of colic is unknown, but it may be related to overfeeding, underfeeding, feeding too quickly, swallowed air, or maternal or infant anxiety. Although conclusive evidence is lacking, some studies suggest cruciferous vegetables (broccoli, cauliflower, Brussel's sprouts), cow's milk, onion, and chocolate in the diets of women who exclusively breast-feed may be related to colic symptoms in infants (Lust et al, 1996).

Nursing Interventions and Considerations

Assess feeding practices: frequency of burping, type of feeding used, volume, concentration, frequency of feedings, and size of nipple opening

(continued)

Nursing Interventions and Considerations for Disorders of Infancy and Childhood *(Continued)*

(formula-fed infants). Assess maternal diet for intake of cruciferous vegetables, cow's milk, onion, and chocolate; advise the mother to eliminate these and observe for improvement. Women who eliminate cow's milk may need supplemental calcium. If no feeding problems are identified, assure the parents that colic is transient and not indicative of health problems or parental ineptness.

CLEFT PALATE

Numerous combinations of developmental defects involving the lip and palate may occur, resulting in an opening in the roof of the mouth or incompletely formed lips. Feeding difficulties begin at birth. The cause may be hereditary or unknown.

Nursing Interventions and Considerations

Depending on the type of defects, infants with a cleft palate may be unable to suck. Squeezable cleft lip/palate nurser and cross-cut nipple with rigid bottle are effective methods of feeding.

Infants with cleft palate may achieve normal growth when parents are educated about feeding techniques, formula volume goals, and use of energy-dense solids (Brine et al, 1994). Advise parents to

- Feed the infant in an upright position and direct the formula to the side of the mouth to prevent formula from entering the nasal passage.
- Feed the infant slowly and burp the infant frequently. Feeding may be a long and tiring process for both the infant and parents.
- Follow the normal diet progression and introduction of solids based on the child's development and nutritional needs. Assure the parents that children with a cleft palate can handle solids better than liquids.

PYLORIC STENOSIS

Pyloric stenosis is characterized by an obstructive narrowing of the pyloric opening, resulting in projectile vomiting within 30 minutes after feed-

ing, weight loss, dehydration, and poor nutritional status. It is caused by excessive thickening of the pyloric muscle or hypertrophy and hyperplasia of mucosa and submucosa.

Nursing Interventions and Considerations

The major goal of nutritional therapy is to achieve fluid and electrolyte balance so that the infant can undergo surgery.

After surgery, the infant is given glucose water and is advanced to full-strength formula as tolerated, after which the infant can be breast-fed, if desired.

VOMITING

Vomiting, characterized by the ejection of stomach contents through the mouth, may occur secondary to viral infections, formula contamination, food poisoning, or intestinal obstructions.

Nursing Interventions and Considerations

Food intake is unimportant. The major nutritional concern for prolonged vomiting is fluid and electrolyte replacement.

Advise parents

- To withhold solid food and offer the child small amounts of clear liquids.
- To progress the diet as tolerated after the vomiting subsides.

MILD DIARRHEA (1 TO 4 DAY'S DURATION)

Mild diarrhea may be related to numerous causes, such as viral infections, formula contamination, food poisoning, overfeeding, excessive fat intake, excessive fiber intake, and food allergies. Sorbitol (sugar alcohol used as a sweetener) may cause osmotic diarrhea if consumed in large amounts. In infants, a frequent cause of mild diarrhea is the introduction of solid food (cereal) before enzyme levels are adequate, leading to CHO fermentation within the GI tract.

Nursing Interventions and Considerations

Diarrhea may cause intestinal inflammation, resulting in the loss of the enzyme lactase.

(continued)

Nursing Interventions and Considerations for Disorders of Infancy and Childhood (Continued)

Decreased lactase → lactose intolerance → increased bowel aggravation and permeability of the GI wall → possibility of protein leakage through the bowel into the bloodstream, setting up an allergic reaction. An allergy to protein and impaired ability to digest lactose (milk) may persist for a few days after diarrhea subsides.

Obtain a diet history to rule out diet-related causes.

Prolonged or severe diarrhea can be serious in infants and young children; hospitalization may be required to correct fluid and electrolyte imbalances parenterally.

Advise parents

- To withhold all food for 12 to 24 hours, then offer small amounts of clear liquids (avoid iced liquids). However, clear liquids lack the proper balance of electrolytes; therefore, a commercial electrolyte solution (Pedialyte, Resol, Lytren) may be indicated for electrolyte replacement. It is recommended that a total of 1 cup of commercial oral rehydration mixture be given between each loose bowel movement, perhaps 1 teaspoon at a time if necessary, until diarrhea subsides, to prevent dehydration.
- That it may be necessary to withhold milk and lactose-containing formulas for at least a week if diarrhea is severe. Soy or casein formulas are used until the infant is able to tolerate lactose.
- That when milk-based formula is reintroduced, it should be diluted and gradually progressed to full strength (ie, 1 part formula to 3 parts water for one day, followed by 1:2 → 1:1 → full strength).
- That older children should be given foods high in pectin to help firm the stools: firm Bananas; plain Rice; Applesauce; white Toast (BRAT diet).

CONSTIPATION

Formula that is too concentrated or inadequate in CHO may contribute to constipation in formula-fed infants; constipation is rare in breast-fed infants. In older children, constipation may be caused by an excessive milk intake, inadequate fluid and fiber intake, or irregular bowel habits, or it may be labeled psychogenic constipation related to toilet-training trauma.

Nursing Interventions and Considerations

Daily bowel movements are not necessary as long as the stools are easily passed.

Obtain a diet history to determine the cause of constipation.

Advise parents how to modify the diet to prevent constipation, such as

- Properly diluting the formula. Some physicians recommend adding corn syrup to formula to increase the CHO content. Honey should never be added because of the risk of infant botulism.
- Limiting milk intake to the recommended amount for the child's age.
- Adding fiber to the diet, whole-grain breads and cereals, fresh fruits and vegetables, and dried peas and beans. The American Health Foundation suggests that fiber intake during childhood be approximately equivalent to the child's age plus 5 g/day to promote normal laxation (Williams, 1995) (see Chap. 16 for more on high-fiber diet).

PHENYLKETONURIA

Phenylketonuria (PKU) is an inborn error of metabolism (autosomal recessive hereditary trait) characterized by a defect in phenylalanine (an essential amino acid) metabolism that prevents the conversion of phenylalanine to tyrosine (a nonessential amino acid), which is normally converted to thyroxine, melanin, and catecholamines. Tyrosine becomes an essential amino acid. Phenylketonuria causes the accumulation of toxic phenylalanine in the tissues, bloodstream, and CNS, resulting in mental retardation and urinary excretion of phenylketones.

(continued)

Nursing Interventions and Considerations for Disorders of Infancy and Childhood (Continued)

Nursing Interventions and Considerations

Because early diagnosis and initiation of the diet can prevent mental retardation, all infants should be tested for PKU immediately after birth. Diet cannot reverse brain damage after it occurs.

The diet for PKU is low in phenylalanine, not phenylalanine free. Because phenylalanine is an essential amino acid, it must be supplied in the diet for tissue growth and repair to occur. If the phenylalanine content of the diet is inadequate, the body will catabolize its own body protein to supply the missing amino acid; the effect is the same as cheating on the diet, namely an increase in blood and urine phenylalanine levels. Therefore, the phenylalanine content of the diet, as well as the child's blood and urine phenylalanine levels and physical and mental growth and development, must be closely monitored and evaluated. The diet is continuously modified to provide enough phenylalanine to support growth and development without causing a build-up of phenylketones.

The diet must be adequate in protein-sparing calories to prevent the use of protein for energy, which would also result in body protein catabolism.

The age at which the diet can be discontinued is controversial. From a practical standpoint, some physicians recommend discontinuing the diet when the child enters school (4 to 6 years of age) because brain growth is at least 90% completed. However, a study of school-age children who followed the diet from the first few weeks of life until age 6 showed that although discontinuing the diet did not affect baseline IQ, the children performed less well in school, which could be as damaging to the child's overall development as a decrease in IQ. Some researchers are recommending that the diet be followed to adolescence or even later.

Women with PKU have a high incidence of aborted pregnancies and infants born with mental handicaps, unless they follow a low-phenylalanine diet during pregnancy or possibly before conception (see Chap. 10).

Lofenelac (Mead), the formula specially prepared for infants with PKU, has 95% of the phenylalanine removed. It may need to be supplemented with small, controlled amounts of formula or milk to supply the proper amount of phenylalanine. Unfortunately, it is expensive, and older children and adults find the taste objectionable, although it is usually well accepted by infants.

Once solid foods are added to the infant's diet (at 4 to 6 months of age), parents may be given meal patterns and exchange lists of foods grouped according to their phenylalanine content to aid in diet planning.

Comprehensive and frequent diet counseling is necessary to assess the child's intake, monitor progress, and allay the parents' fears.

Advise parents

- That following the diet is essential to prevent mental retardation and other problems of PKU.
- That although other infant formulas or milk may *supplement* Lofenalac, they cannot *replace* Lofenalac in the infant's diet.
- That the diet is low in phenylalanine, not phenylalanine-free, and must provide adequate calories.
- That phenylalanine is an amino acid and, therefore, is found in greatest concentrations in high-protein foods such as meat, fish, poultry, milk, dairy products, and eggs. These products are eliminated or restricted.
- That vegetables, fruits, some cereals, breads, and other starches are low in phenylalanine and are used in measured amounts.
- That label reading is essential; for example, aspartame (NutraSweet) is not appropriate for phenylketonurics because it contains phenylalanine.

(continued)

Nursing Interventions and Considerations for Disorders of Infancy and Childhood (Continued)

CYSTIC FIBROSIS

Cystic fibrosis (CF), inherited as a recessive trait, is a metabolic disease characterized by excessive exocrine secretions (especially mucous) that form plugs. The sites most commonly affected by mucous plugs are the bronchi, leading to chronic pulmonary infections and fibrosis of the lung tissue; the intestines, creating problems with nutrient absorption; and the pancreatic and bile ducts, which impairs pancreatic enzyme secretion and results in protein and fat malabsorption (streatorrhea), secondary nutrient deficiencies, malnutrition with possible growth retardation, and glucose intolerance related to impaired insulin secretion. In addition, sweat gland secretions contain excessive amounts of sodium and chloride. Nutrition interventions should begin as soon as CF is diagnosed.

Nursing Interventions and Considerations

Monitor fluid and electrolyte balance, and growth and development.

Fat malabsorption, leading to steatorrhea, malabsorption syndrome, and malnutrition, is the greatest nutritional problem of CF. Fat tolerance varies considerably among individuals.

Clients with CF need to take pancreatic enzyme supplements with all meals and snacks to enhance fat digestion and absorption.

Because protein requirements are greatest during the first year of life, infants are particularly susceptible to protein deficiency and malnutrition. Energy requirements may be 120% to 150% of RDA.

Anorexia, nausea, and early satiety may occur during periods of decreased pulmonary function and infection and impair intake (Hayes et al, 1994).

Clients with CF excrete high concentrations of sodium in their sweat. Additional table salt to formula or food may be needed to prevent hyponatremia, especially in summer months.

Protein–calorie malnutrition impairs immune function and increases the risk of pulmonary infection. Increasing calorie intake and weight seems to improve clinical and respiratory status (Hayes et al, 1994).

Advise parents

- That good nutritional status can influence long-term survival and quality of life (Cannella et al., 1993).
- That a high-protein, high-calorie diet is necessary to replace losses. The Daily Food Guide can be used to plan a varied, balanced diet.
- That although fats are a concentrated source of calories and are needed for the essential fatty acid, fat may not be well tolerated and may need to be restricted; medium-chain triglycerides (MCT) are readily absorbed and may be given for additional calories (see Chap. 3).
- That simple sugars are better tolerated than starches.
- To give the child water-soluble supplements of the fat-soluble vitamins and a multivitamin, as prescribed.
- To give the child pancreatic enzyme supplements with all meals and snacks.
- That children with CF need more fluid and sodium; encourage a liberal intake of both.
- When cystic fibrosis is complicated by diabetes, the diet is adjusted. Nutrition guidelines recommend adequate calories (100%–200% RDA) with 30% to 40% total calories from fat. Simple sugars are not restricted. Carbohydrate counting may be used to achieve glycemic control without limiting calories or sacrificing preferences (Hayes et al, 1994).

KEY CONCEPTS

- An optimal diet is necessary to support normal growth and development.
- The concepts of moderation, balance, and variety are appropriate for children. A heart-healthy diet that limits total fat to 30% of calories and saturated fat to less than 10% of calories is recommended for children over the age of 2 years.
- Because of varying rates of growth and activity, nutritional requirements are less precise for children than they are for adults.
- Breast-feeding is the preferred method of infant feeding up to the age of 1 year. Formula feeding is an acceptable alternative.
- Adequacy of growth is the best indicator of whether an infant's intake is nutritionally adequate.
- Solid foods should not be introduced before 4 to 6 months of age. New foods should be introduced one at a time for a period of 5 to 7 days so that if an allergic reaction occurs, it can be easily identified.
- Parents of preschoolers are frequently concerned that their children lack variety in their diets; that they don't eat enough fruits, vegetables, and meat; and that they eat too many sweets. Feeding problems often occur because parents overestimate how much food their young children should eat.
- School-age children often do not eat enough fruits and vegetables; eat nonnutritious snacks, lack variety in their diets; eat too much fat and cholesterol; have a tendency to skip breakfast; lack adequate nutrition knowledge; and may consume excess sugar. Obesity is a health concern.
- Childhood nutrition problems often intensisfy during adolescence. Common concerns include meal skipping, snacking, heavy use of fast foods, dieting, adolescent pregnancy, acne, substance abuse, and optimal diet for athletics.

FOCUS ON **CRITICAL THINKING**

Karen Thomas is 10 years old, is 4'10" tall, and weighs 101 pounds. Karen has consistently been above the 95th percentile for height and weight since birth. She is concerned that she weighs too much, which prompted her mother to bring her to the pediatrician, for fear her daughter may develop an eating disorder.

What dietary information would you gather to assess Karen's nutritional status and growth?

What is an appropriate weight for Karen?

Develop a nutritionally adequate meal plan for Karen, based on the Daily Food Guide.

What would you tell Karen's mother about:
a) her growth record
b) her concerns about snacking
c) activity
d) substituting low-fat foods for high-fat foods
e) weight loss diets for 10-year-olds
f) Karen's upcoming adolescent growth spurt

REFERENCES

American Dietetic Association (1995). Timely statement of The American Dietetic Association: Dietary guidance for healthy children. J Am Diet Assoc, 95(3), 370.

Anding, J., Kubena, K., McIntosh, A., and O'Brien, B. (1996). Blood lipids, cardiovascular fitness, obesity, and blood pressure: The presence of potential coronary heart disease risk factors in adolescents. J Am Diet Assoc, 96(3), 238–242.

Brine, E., Rickard, K., Brady, M., et al. (1994). Effectiveness of two feeding methods in improving energy intake and growth of infants with cleft palate: A randomized study. J Am Diet Assoc, 94(7), 732–738.

Cannella, P., Bowser, E., Guyer, L., and Borum, P. (1993). Feeding practices and nutrition recommendations for infants with cystic fibrosis. J Am Diet Assoc, 93(3), 297–300.

Centers for Disease Control and Prevention (1994). Advance Data. Dietary intake of vitamins, minerals, and fiber of persons ages 2 months and over in the United States: Third National Health and Nutrition Examination Survey, Phase 1, 1988–1991. DHHS Publication No. (PHS) 95-1250.

Dietz, W. and Robinson, T. (1993). Assessment and treatment of childhood obesity. Pediatr Rev, 14(9), 337–343.

Feingold, B.F. (1974). Why your child is hyperactive. New York: Random House.

Fisher, J., and Birch, L. (1995). Fat preferences and fat consumption of 3- to 5-year-old children are related to parental adiposity. J Am Diet Assoc, 95(7), 759–764.

Hayes, D., Sheehan, J., Ulchaker, M., and Rebar, J. (1994). Management dilemmas in the individual with cystic fibrosis and diabetes. J Am Diet Assoc, 94(1), 78–80.

International Food Information Council (1995). The healthy attitude of today's kids. Food Insight, May/June, 1, 4–5.

International Food Information Council (1993). Advertising, Nutrition, and Kids. A Practical Guide for Parents. New York: Council of Better Business Bureaus, Inc., Children's Advertising Review Unit.

Kotz, K., and Story, M. (1994). Food advertisements during children's Saturday morning television programming: Are they consistent with dietary recommendations? J Am Diet Assoc, 94(11), 1296–1300.

Lust, K., Brown, J., and Thomas, W. (1996). Maternal intake of cruciferous vegetables and other foods and colic symptoms in exclusively breast-fed infants. J Am Diet Assoc, 96(1), 46–48.

Murphy, A., Youatt, J., Hoerr, S., Sawyer, C., and Andrews, S. (1995). Kindergarten students' food preferences are not consistent with their knowledge of the Dietary Guidelines. J Am Diet Assoc, 95(2), 219–223.

National Institutes of Health/National Heart, Lung, and Blood Institute (1992). Cholesterol in Children. Healthy Eating is a Family Affair. NIH Publication No. 92-3099.

Nicklas, T. (1995). Dietary studies of children: The Bogalusa Heart Study experience. J Am Diet Assoc, 95(10), 1127–1133.

Nicklas, T., Farris, R., Myers, L., and Berenson, G. (1995). Dietary fiber intake of children and young adults: The Bogalusa Heart Study. J Am Diet Assoc, 95(2), 209–214.

Pipes, R., and Trahms, C. (1993). Nutrition in Infancy and Childhood. 5th ed. St Louis: Mosby.

Pollitt, E. (1995). Does breakfast make a difference in school? J Am Diet Assoc, 95(10), 1134–1139.

Story, M., Hayes, M., and Kalina, B. (1996). Availability of foods in high schools: Is there cause for concern? J Am Diet Assoc, 96(2), 123–126.

United States Department of Health and Human Services, Public Health Service, National Institutes of Health (1991). National Cholesterol Education Program. Report of the Expert Panel on Blood Cholesterol Levels in Children and Adolescents. NIH Publication No. 91-2732.

Williams, C. (1995). Importance of dietary fiber in childhood. J Am Diet Assoc, 95(10), 1140–1146, 1149.

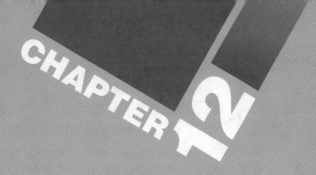

CHAPTER 12

Adult Health Issues and Nutrition Considerations for Older Adults

Chapter Outline

Key Terms

Aging
Frail elderly

Nutrition Screening
   Initiative (NSI)

*W**ith* the exceptions of Chapter 10 (Pregnancy and Lactation) and Chapter 11 (Growth and Development), this book implicitly addresses nutrition as it pertains to adults. All Chapters in Section I, Principles of Nutrition, and Chapter 8 provide background on what constitutes a "healthy" diet and why; in-depth discussion on the role of nutrition in the treatment of various disorders is reserved for Section III. It is the intent of this chapter to increase awareness about health issues that concern "well" adult women and men. The second part of this chapter deals with nutrition as it specifically relates to elderly adults.

WOMEN'S HEALTH ISSUES

It has long been recognized that women have more health problems than men, even though women live longer. Biologic, social, and political factors place women at unique risk for nutrition-related diseases, such as cardiovascular disease, certain cancers, osteoporosis, diabetes, and weight-related problems (ADA, 1995). Generally, women are more likely to develop acute symptoms and chronic health problems and disabilities than men. Some diseases, like uterine and ovarian cancers, are unique to women. Other diseases, like osteoporosis, affect women much more often than they do men (ADA, 1995).

Minority women are at even greater risk for health problems secondary to higher rates of poverty, lack of education, and limited or no access to health care. Minority women have shorter life expectancies, higher rates of maternal and infant mortality, and a higher incidence of chronic disease, such as hypertension and diabetes (ADA, 1995).

Women's health issues have recently emerged as both a political and public health concern, with the realization that women are often not included in clinical health studies and that predominantly female diseases are less likely to be studied than predominantly male diseases (ADA, 1995). In 1990, the National Institutes of Health established an Office of Research on Women's Health to bring women's health issues to the forefront of the health research agenda.

Leading causes of morbidity and mortality among North American women appear in the display, Women's Health Concerns. Although each disorder is distinctly different and a woman's risk for each is determined on an individual basis, dietary recommendations to reduce their risk are remarkably similar from disease to disease (ADA, 1995): Eat less fat and more fruits and vegetables, and avoid obesity. Balance, moderation, and variety are recurrent concepts. Messages that are detailed in the Food Guide Pyramid and Dietary Guidelines for Americans, many of which are reiterated in the Healthy People 2000 report (see display, Healthy People 2000: Risk Reduction Objectives for Nutrition), should serve as the foundation of a diet that promotes health and helps avoid disease.

MEN'S HEALTH ISSUES

Men have shorter life spans than women, partly because men are greater risk-takers. Rates of accidental death and disability are greater among men, and such outcomes are associated with both voluntary activities (eg, driving) and involuntary activities (eg, serving in combat). Nutrition intervention can do little to change these risks.

In terms of health issues, at most stages of life, men are 88% more likely to die of heart disease, 45% more likely to die of cancer, 18% more likely to die of stroke, 69% more likely to die of pneumonia or influenza, and almost 8 times more likely to die of acquired immunodeficiency syndrome (AIDS) than women (Schardt, 1995).

Women's Health Concerns

CARDIOVASCULAR DISEASE

- Cardiovascular disease is the number one cause of illness and death among American women, even though it usually appears 10 to 15 years later in women than in men.
- One in ten women 45 to 64 years old has some form of heart disease; over age 65 the incidence increases to one in four (NIH, NHLBI, 1992).
- Black women are 24% more likely to die of coronary heart disease than white women, and their death rate for stroke is 83% higher (NIH, NHLBI, 1992).
- Women with heart disease do not fare as well as men: women are much more likely than men to die within a year of having a heart attack, and their mortality from coronary bypass surgery is twice that of men (ADA, 1995).
- In women, a low level of high-density lipoprotein (HDL) cholesterol appears more predictive of CVD risk than a high-LDL cholesterol.
- Menopause and declining estrogen levels cause total cholesterol, low-density lipoprotein (LDL) cholesterol, and triglyceride levels to rise and HDL levels to stay the same or decline. The increased ratio of total cholesterol to HDL cholesterol increases the risk of cardiac vascular disease.
- More than half of American women will develop high blood pressure at some time in their lives; at greatest risk are women who are black, are overweight, have "high-normal" blood pressure, and have a positive family history (NIH, NHLBI, 1992).

CANCER

- Breast cancer will affect 1 out of 9 North American women; data implicating high-fat diets and obesity are inconsistent. Alcohol appears to increase the risk of breast cancer, and high intakes of fruits and vegetables may be protective.
- Colorectal cancer is the third most common cancer among women. A high-fat diet, and possibly red meat, have been implicated in its promotion.
- A diet high in fat and low in antioxidants (vitamins C, E, and beta-carotene) may contribute to ovarian cancer. Overweight women have a higher incidence of endometrial cancer.

OSTEOPOROSIS

- In North America, osteoporosis affects 25 million women over the age of 45.
- Osteoporosis cannot be cured, but may be prevented or delayed by maximizing bone density during preadolescence through young adulthood with weight-bearing exercise and adequate calcium intake, both of which are important for bone health throughout a woman's life.

WEIGHT

- More women are overweight than men, with estimates of one quarter to one third of North Americans. Excess weight, especially when located in the abdominal area, increases the risk of coronary heart disease, hypertension, hyperlipidemias, diabetes, gallstones, and reproductive cancers.
- The dismal success rate of treating obesity necessitates the need for prevention and early intervention for the whole family (ADA, 1995).
- Cultural pressures on women to be thin and unrealistic body images increase the risk of disordered eating patterns, such as compulsive eating, binge eating, purging, severe dieting, and fasting (ADA, 1995). Women comprise 95% of cases of anorexia nervosa and bulimia nervosa.

DIABETES MELLITUS

- Diabetes increases the risk of heart disease 5 to 7 times in women compared to 2 to 3 times in men (Liebman, 1995).
- Some studies suggest diabetes increases blood pressure more in women than in men (Liebman, 1995).
- Diabetes may lower HDL cholesterol more in women than men; the protective effects of premenopausal estrogen are almost eliminated by diabetes (ADA, 1995).
- Diabetes in women is complicated by hypertension more than it is in men.
- Diabetes increases a woman's risk of endometrial cancer and increases the risk of maternal and fetal complications during pregnancy.

Healthy People 2000: Risk Reduction Objectives for Nutrition

Healthy People 2000 represents the thinking of over 300 private and public organizations, led by the U.S. Public Health Service. As the sequel to Healthy People, published by the Surgeon General in the 1980s, its purpose is to increase the span of healthy life for Americans, reduce disparities among Americans, and provide all Americans with access to preventative services. Nutrition is one of the public health priorities identified; measurable goals for the year 2000 are to:

2.5 Reduce dietary fat intake to an average of 30% of calories or less and average saturated fat intake to less than 10% of calories among people 2 years of age and older.

2.6 Increase complex carbohydrate and fiber-containing foods in the diets of adults to 5 or more daily servings for vegetables (including legumes) and fruits, and to 6 or more daily servings for grain products.

2.7 Increase to at least 50% the proportion of overweight people 12 years of age and older who have adopted sound dietary practices combined with regular physical activity to attain an appropriate body weight.

2.8 Increase calcium intake so at least 50% of youth 12 through 24 years of age and 50% of pregnant and lactating women consume three or more servings daily of foods rich in calcium, and at least 50% of people 25 years of age and older consume two or more servings daily.

2.9 Decrease salt and sodium intake so at least 65% of home meal preparers prepare foods without adding salt, at least 80% of people avoid using salt at the table, and at least 40% of adults regularly purchase foods modified or lower in sodium.

2.10 Reduce iron deficiency to less than 3% among children 1 through 4 years of age and among women of childbearing age.

2.11 Increase to at least 75% the proportion of mothers who breast-feed their babies in the early postpartum period and to at least 50% the proportion who continue breast-feeding until their babies are 5 to 6 months old.

2.12 Increase to at least 75% the proportion of parents and caregivers who use feeding practices that prevent baby bottle tooth decay.

2.13 Increase to at least 85% the proportion of people 18 years of age and older who use food labels to make nutritious food selections.

Interestingly, men live as long as women among some groups of Mormons, which points to lifestyle, not biology, as the basis for gender differences in longevity.

As for women, heart disease and cancer among men are the number one and two killers, respectively. Adding to their risk is that men are more likely to be long-term smokers and heavy drinkers. Also, men's diets tend to be lower in fruits and vegetables and higher in meat (fat). Men's health issues and their nutritional implications appear in the display, Men's Health Concerns.

HEALTH ISSUES OF OLDER ADULTS

The elderly, especially those over 85 years of age, represent the fastest-growing segment of the American population. By the year 2005, approximately 25% of Americans will be 65 or older, and the number of people 85 and older will double (ADA,

Men's Health Concerns

CARDIOVASCULAR DISEASE

- Men in their 40s are 4 times more likely to die from coronary heart disease than women of the same age; by age 70, this ratio decreases to a factor of 2 (NCEP, 1993).
- Up until 1990, most of the studies done on heart disease almost exclusively involved men. Risks are similar among men and women, except that high-LDL cholesterol is more predictive of risk in men than in women; low-HDL cholesterol levels are less significant.
- Strokes are more common in men than women; similar risk factors exist for stroke as for coronary heart disease. Both may be linked to intakes high in fat and low in fruits and vegetables.

CANCER

- After lung cancer, colon and prostate cancers are the most frequent cause of cancer deaths in men; both are linked to high intakes of red meat. It is not known if the risk is related to the fat content of the red meat intake, or to what is missing from a high-meat diet (like fruits and vegetables).
- The incidence of lower esophageal and lower stomach cancer is rising, with men the leading victims of both (Schardt, 1995). Lower esophageal cancer appears to be related to obesity and inadequate intake of fruits and vegetables.

WEIGHT

- Although a greater percentage of women are overweight than men, the prevalence of overweight between 1960 and 1980 increased more for men than women: 6% for white men compared to 3% for white women, and 28% in black men compared to 7% in black females (Williamson, 1993).

1993). Currently, life expectancy is 72 years for men and 77 years for women, compared to 45 years in 1900. The increase can be attributed to improved health care, greater use of immunizations, better hygiene, and the development of nutrition practices that promote well-being.

Aging is a gradual, inevitable, complex process of progressive physiologic, cellular, cultural, and psychosocial changes that begin at conception and end at death. As cells age, they undergo degenerative changes in structure and function, which eventually impair organ, tissue, and body functioning. Exactly how and why aging occurs is unknown, although most theories are based on either genetic or environmental causes (Table 12-1).

Despite the misconceptions and stereotypes that people have of elderly adults, they are a heterogeneous group that vary in age, marital status, social background, financial status, living arrangements, and health status. Only 5% of the elderly are institutionalized. Eighty percent of adults over 65 suffer from arthritis, hypertension, heart disease, or diabetes, with 35% suffering from three or more of these disorders (Administration on Aging, DHHS, 1994). Yet the majority of elderly people consider their health to be good to excellent, possibly because they define wellness and illness differently as they age, and they accept changes in health as a normal aspect of aging (ADA, 1993). Certainly, differences exist between the "well" elderly and the **"frail" elderly** (those with defined needs for support for activities of daily living). Genetic and environmental "life advantages," such as genetic potential for longevity,

Table 12-1 **Theories of Aging**	
Proposed Cause of Aging	**Theory**
Genetic	Genes fail to function normally, possibly because of radiation or faulty selection of amino acids for protein synthesis, which leads to defective replication, transcription, or translation of DNA.
Immunologic	As immune function decreases with age, the incidence of autoimmune reactions increases; that is, the body makes antibodies against its own tissue. It is speculated that the process of aging can be delayed by manipulating the immune system through diet modification, temperature regulation, or avoidance of illness.
Free radical	Because of a force on the polyunsaturated fats in the cell, unstable free radicals are released and peroxidized, resulting in destruction of cell structure. Vitamin E, vitamin C, and selenium (antioxidants) may all inhibit the production of free radicals and thus delay aging.
Cross linkage	Aging molecules link together to form complexes that cannot function normally. This theory has been observed in collagen in aging organisms.
Biologic clock	Each cell is believed to be programmed, through DNA, to self-destruct; that is, certain cells are known to multiply and divide a fixed number of times and then self-destruct.
Aging pacemakers	Pacemakers in the brain initiate a neurohormonal response, possibly through serotonin, dopamine, norepinephrine, or tryptophan, that results in aging.

intelligence, motivation, curiosity, good socialization, religious affiliation, marriage and family, physical activity, avoidance of substance abuse, availability of health care, adequate sleep, sufficient rest and relaxation, and good eating habits, have a positive effect on both the length and quality of life.

Throughout the life cycle, nutrition has a significant impact on health and the quality of life. Studies suggest that good eating habits that are established early in life promote health maintenance in old age. Clearly, the development and progression of certain degenerative disorders that are associated with aging, such as diabetes mellitus, atherosclerosis, hypertension, and obesity, are influenced by lifelong eating habits. Although dietary modifications that are initiated late in life may not prevent or delay the development of disease, they may influence disease progression and improve the quality of life.

NUTRITIONAL IMPLICATIONS OF AGING

Predictable changes in physiology and function, income, health, and psychosocial well-being are associated with aging, although the rate and timing at which they occur vary among individuals. Changes with a potential impact on diet and nutritional status include the following.

Changes in Physiology and Function	Nutritional Implications

BODY COMPOSITION AND ENERGY EXPENDITURE

Energy expenditure decreases related to the following:
   Decrease in REE of about 20% from age 20 to 90
   Decrease in physical activity related to retirement or physical impairments (cardiovascular or pulmonary disorders, arthritis, bone fracture, poor vision)

Calorie requirements decrease in response to the decrease in REE, decrease in physical activity, and change in body composition. Studies show that people tend to eat less as they get older.

Changes in body composition:
   Loss of lean body mass. Muscle mass is replaced by fat and connective tissue.
   Increase in adipose tissue, which requires fewer calories to be maintained than muscle tissue

Loss of muscle mass → loss of muscle strength → loss of range of motion and mobility → impaired ability to purchase, prepare, and eat food

ORAL AND GI CHANGES

Difficulty chewing related to loss of teeth and periodontal disease. One-third of Americans have lost all their teeth by age 65. Jaw bone deterioration may be related to osteoporosis.
Decreased saliva occurs in 20% of elderly as a side effect of some diseases and medications.

If intake is limited to soft, easy-to-chew foods, some essential nutrients may be deficient. Meat is the food most commonly eliminated by people who have difficulty chewing.
People with dry mouth may have difficulty wearing dentures, and may have altered taste and difficulty eating.

Constipation is 5 to 6 times more frequent in the elderly than in younger adults, and may be related to the following:
   Decreased peristalsis related to loss of abdominal muscle tone
   Inadequate fluid and fiber intake
   Secondary to drug therapy: antihypertensives, diuretics, sedatives, laxative dependence
   Decrease in physical activity

40% to 50% of the elderly reportedly use laxatives. A high-fiber diet with an adequate fluid intake can help relieve constipation.

Digestive disorders may develop related to the following:
   Decreased secretion of hydrochloric acid (stomach) and digestive enzymes (pancreatic and intestinal)
   Decreased GI motility
   Decreased organ function
Nutrient absorption may decrease because of decreased mucosal mass and decreased blood flow to and from the mucosal villi.

Diet modification may be necessary if food intolerances or impaired nutrient absorption develops.

METABOLIC CHANGES

Altered glucose tolerance. The underlying reason is unclear; may be due to a decrease in insulin secretion or a decrease in tissue sensitivity to insulin.

Nutritional implications are not clear.

CNS CHANGES

Tremors, slowed reaction time, short-term memory deficits, personality changes, and depression may be related to a decrease in the number of brain cells or the decrease in blood flow to the brain and nervous system. Between 1% and 6% of people over 65 have severe dementia, another 2% to 15% have mild dementia.

Food purchasing, preparation, and eating may all be impaired.

(continued)

Changes in Physiology and Function	Nutritional Implications

RENAL CHANGES

Decreased ability to excrete nitrogen and other metabolic wastes related to: Decreased capillary blood flow Decreased glomerular filtration rate (GFR) Inability to regenerate nephrons	If renal failure develops, protein, sodium, and other nutrients may need to be restricted in the diet.
Urinary incontinence may develop related to impaired bladder sphincter function.	The elderly may voluntarily restrict fluid intake to cope with incontinence.

SENSORY LOSSES

Gradual progressive sensory losses may be related to impaired nerve cell function. Hearing loss begins around age 30.	Socialized eating may be difficult or intimidating: Lack of socialization can significantly impair appetite and intake in the elderly.
Loss of visual acuity, visual accommodation, ability to see in low light, ability to distinguish color intensities, and decrease in depth perception begins at age 50.	Food purchasing and preparation may be impaired.
Sensory losses can cause a decrease in salivation, gastric secretion, pancreatic enzyme secretion, and pancreatic hormone secretion, which could alter nutrient utilization.	
As many as 50% of the elderly experience major olfactory impairment. Loss of taste begins between 50 and 55 years of age and may be related to: A decrease in the number of taste buds and papilla. Sweet and salty tastes are lost first, followed by bitter and sour. Oral infections, poor hygiene, decreased flow of saliva Decreased sensation of thirst, which may be due to changes in the thirst center in the hypothalamus.	Studies show that the elderly have elevated odor thresholds, lower perceived odor intensities, lower ability to identify odors and olfactory food flavors, and inability to detect spice in a food (Duffy et al, 1995). Changes in olfaction cause food to be less flavorful and less enjoyable. Many elderly subsequently change their eating habits; elderly women may compensate by eating more, especially more fat and sugar. The elderly are prone to dehydration.

Change in Income Related to Retirement

More than 50% of the elderly population are estimated to be economically deprived; as many as 40% have annual incomes under $6,000.	The first items sacrificed when food budget is limited are milk and meats, which are rich sources of calcium, protein, zinc, iron, and B vitamins. The lower the income, the less likely an adequate and varied diet will be consumed.

Changes in Health

Degenerative diseases like diabetes, atherosclerosis, hypertension, and cancer are more common among the elderly, as are disabling disorders like bone fractures, arthritis, and strokes.	May affect nutrient requirements, intake, digestion, absorption, metabolism, and excretion. Disabling disorders may impair food purchasing, preparation, or eating.

(continued)

Changes in Physiology and Function	Nutritional Implications
Reliance on drugs. The elderly, who comprise 11% of the population, account for approximately 25% of all drugs used. Compared to younger adults, the elderly are more likely to use drugs, to use a combination of drugs, and to take drugs over a longer period of time.	Drugs may affect nutritional status by altering appetite, the ability to taste and smell, or the digestion, absorption, metabolism, and excretion of nutrients (Appendix 5). Likewise, food intake can increase or decrease the effectiveness of some drugs by altering the rate of absorption. If a large percentage of a fixed income is spent on medication, less money is available for food.

Alcohol abuse. Some segments of the elderly population may rely on alcohol to relieve boredom, loneliness, depression, or pain.	Alcohol abuse may cause nutrient deficiencies, particularly of folic acid and thiamine, by altering
	    Food intake through a decrease in appetite, food budget, or alertness
	    Nutrient digestion, absorption, metabolism, and excretion

Psychosocial Changes	

Social isolation related to
  Death of spouse; death of friends
  Living alone
  Impaired mobility
	The elderly frequently complain that they do not like to cook for one person or eat alone, either at home or in a restaurant. Studies indicate that elderly living alone do not make poorer food choices than those living with a spouse, but they do eat fewer calories.

Poor self-esteem related to
  Change in body image
  Lack of productivity
  Feelings of aimlessness
	Poor self-esteem may lead to lack of interest in eating.

Institutionalized	Generally, elderly who are institutionalized are more likely to have an inadequate diet than those living independently. Thirty percent to 50% of elderly in nursing home residences are estimated to be underweight; up to 50% may exhibit clinical signs of protein–calorie malnutrition (ADA, 1993).

NUTRITION FOR THE ELDERLY

Although the nutritional needs of the elderly have been studied with more frequency within the last 20 years, there are limited data available on the nutritional requirements of relatively healthy people over 70 years of age. Most large-scale national surveys on food consumption have had few participants over the age of 74, and most studies on the nutritional status of older adults have focused on people confined to nursing homes or hospitals. Overall, 5% to 15% of elderly adults may have nutrient deficiencies, such as protein–calorie malnutrition, or clinically detrimental levels of certain vitamins or minerals (ADA, 1993).

Recommended Dietary Allowances

The current RDA divide the mature adult population into two age groups: those who are 25 to 50 years old and those 51 years of age and older. However, one would expect the nutritional requirements of 51-year-olds to be different from those of 60-, 70-, 80-, and 90-year-olds. Unfortunately, there are insufficient data available to break down recommendations and requirements further into more precise age groupings.

Compared with the recommendations for adults from 25 to 50 years of age, the only RDA that differ for older adults are those for calories, certain B vitamins, and iron (for women only) (Table 12-2). The RDA of all other essential nutrients remain constant from age 25 throughout adulthood.

However, for any elderly individual, the RDA may be inappropriate because they are not based on studies of nutrition in the elderly but are, instead, extrapolated from studies of younger adults; the elderly differ from younger adults in the way they absorb some nutrients, their gastric acidity, and in their overall nutrient utilization. Also, the RDA are intended to meet the needs of healthy people and do not take into account the effects that chronic diseases or use of medications may have on nutritional needs.

CALORIES

Beginning in early adulthood, lean body mass (muscle and bone) declines and the proportion of fat increases, resulting in a decrease in resting energy expenditure (REE). Physical activity also declines with aging, although this is neither desirable nor inevitable. Together, the decline in REE and the reduced physical activity result in decreased energy requirements. However, because these changes occur at varying times among individuals, chronologic age is not a good predictor of energy requirements.

The RDA for calories for men and women of "reference size" over 50 years of age are 2300 and 1900, respectively, or 30 cal/kg of body weight (see Table 12-2). The NAS-NRC Subcommittee notes that the calorie requirements of people over 75 years of age are likely to be lower because of the decrease in lean body mass, REE,

Table 12-2
Adult RDA for Calories, Certain B Vitamins, and Iron

	Men		Women	
	Age 25–50	*Age 51+*	*Age 25–50*	*Age 51+*
Total calories	2900	2300	2200	1900
Thiamine (mg)	1.5	1.2	1.1	1.0
Riboflavin (mg)	1.7	1.4	1.3	1.2
Niacin (mg N.E.)	19	15	15	13
Iron (mg)	10	10	15	10

and physical activity (National Research Council, 1989). However, no specific recommendations were made. As calorie intake declines, it becomes increasingly difficult to consume adequate amounts of all essential nutrients.

THIAMINE, RIBOFLAVIN, AND NIACIN

Because these B vitamins are involved in energy metabolism, lesser amounts are needed when calorie intake is reduced. Only minor reductions are suggested in the RDA for people over 51 years of age (see Table 12-2).

IRON (FOR WOMEN)

Physiologic data (such as cessation of growth and menstruation) and measurements of body iron stores in the elderly indicate that iron requirements are lowest in old age. The RDA for iron in women decreases from 15 mg (23- to 50-year-olds) to 10 mg (51+-year-olds) (see Table 12-2).

However, some segments of the older adult population may be at risk for developing iron deficiency and iron deficiency anemia because of a decrease in iron availability or absorption. Compared with younger adults, the elderly often eat less red meat, which is the best source of heme iron in the diet. Chewing difficulties and economic factors are often to blame. Iron absorption may be impaired by the decrease in gastric HCl secretion that occurs with aging, or deficits in absorption may occur secondary to partial or complete gastrectomy, malabsorption syndrome, or chronic use of antacids. Reliance on "tea and toast" may also be a factor—tea is a potent inhibitor of iron absorption. Finally, chronic blood loss due to hemorrhoids, ulcers, renal disease, neoplasms, or medications such as aspirin, anticoagulants, and drugs for arthritis may result in iron deficiency anemia.

The RDA for the elderly are especially controversial with regard to protein and calcium.

PROTEIN

The process of protein metabolism changes with aging, and there is little agreement on protein requirements in the elderly. Whereas some studies have shown that the elderly require more protein based on nitrogen balance studies, other studies indicate decreased protein requirements resulting from the reduction in muscle mass and the decrease in renal function that characterize the aging process. The most recent studies suggest that the elderly may need more protein than the current recommendation of 0.8 g/kg, and that a safe intake for people over 65 years of age may be 1.0 to 1.25 g/kg/day (Campbell et al, 1994). Although the NAS-NRC Subcommittee acknowledges that aging may alter protein requirements, the RDA for people 51 years of age and older are not different than those for younger adults.

CALCIUM

The elderly are at risk for calcium deficiency because both calcium intake and efficiency of calcium absorption decrease with age. Studies suggest a strong relationship between calcium deficiency and the development of osteoporosis, a metabolic bone disease of the elderly that is characterized by a negative calcium balance and loss of bone mass.

Some researchers believe that the current RDA for calcium (800 mg) may be too low to maintain normal calcium balance, especially for postmenopausal women and men 65 and older. In fact, the National Institutes of Health Consensus Development Panel on Optimal Calcium Intake recommends that postmenopausal women (from 50 to 64 years of age) who are on estrogen replacement therapy consume 1000 mg of calcium daily. All women 50 and older who are not on estrogen, and all men 65 and older are urged to consume 1500 mg calcium/day, an amount that is almost double the current RDA (IFIC, 1994). However, because prevention is far more effective than treatment, good eating habits and weight-bearing exercise should be encouraged early in life so that maximum bone density may be attained (see Chapter 20 for more information on osteoporosis).

Recommendations for the Aged

Recognizing that the elderly are the fastest-growing segment of the population and account for 30% of all health care expenditures in the United States, the U.S. Department of Health and Human Services has identified maintenance of the health and functional independence of older persons as a priority in its report, Healthy People 2000 (ADA, 1993). Specific objectives for improving the health of older people include reducing the incidence of morbidity and mortality associated with both acute and chronic disease, increasing the number of years of healthy and independent life, decreasing disability, improving access to and use of supportive social and health care services, decreasing alcohol and tobacco use, and increasing physical activity (see Food for Thought: Do and Diet). In terms of nutrition, the report recommends improving dietary intake by reducing the intake of fat, saturated fat, and sodium and increasing the consumption of fiber and complex carbohydrates. The report also advocates reducing the prevalence of obesity.

Similar suggestions appear in the Dietary Guidelines for Americans, which provide advice for all healthy Americans 2 years of age and older about food choices that promote health and prevent disease. Certainly, to "eat a variety of foods," "choose a diet with plenty of grain products, vegetables, fruits," and "if you drink alcoholic beverages, do so in moderation" is good advice for people of all ages. However, the applicability of other guidelines to the elderly population is less obvious, especially the frail elderly. Because the focus of diet modification for the frail elderly is on improving the quality of life and maintaining the person's ability to function, the guidelines must be assessed for their relevance to each individual. No single dietary prescription can be applied to all older adults; this makes individualization of dietary interventions essential (ADA, 1993).

For some individuals, there may be little value in adopting the guidelines late in life, and abiding by some of the guidelines may even adversely affect the health of older adults. For instance, lowering fat and saturated fat may not be appropriate for older adults who are at risk for malnutrition because of the potential negative impact on overall calorie and nutrient intake. Some epidemiologic evidence indicates that

FOOD *for* THOUGHT

Do and Diet

While diet may help prevent or delay chronic diseases associated with aging-heart disease, diabetes, hypertension, and osteoporosis, it's not the whole story. Beginning at twenty-something, our bodies lose muscle and gain fat every day . . . neither a high-protein nor low-fat diet alters the rate of muscle loss. With the loss of muscle comes a decrease in metabolic rate, loss of strength, loss of bone mass, and decreased aerobic capacity; loss of strength causes people to become less active, which in turn, contributes to loss of muscle. Thus the spiral of "normal aging" continues regardless of our best laid dietary interventions.

But there is hope on the horizon—a way to not only keep from losing muscle, but also to restore what's already gone, in effect, reversing the aging process. The modern-day fountain of youth may very well be exercise; the motto for the nineties: "use it or lose it." Aerobic exercise (repeated muscle contraction with little or no resistance) is credited with increasing HDL cholesterol, decreasing the risk of heart disease, lowering blood pressure, protecting against non–insulin-dependent diabe-

tes, slowing the rate of bone loss, and possibly lowering the incidence of colon cancer, but it doesn't prevent loss of muscle mass. The only way to achieve that is through strength-training exercise, which means contracting muscles a few times against a heavy load. Not only does strength training maintain or restore muscle mass, and thus boost metabolic rate (causing the body to burn more calories at rest), it also increases bone density and helps improve range of motion in seniors with arthritis. If you're sedentary, any regular exercise of moderate intensity will allow you to live longer (Liebman, 1995). While the fittest people live the longest, exercise causes the biggest gain in life expectancy when sedentary people become moderately active (Liebman, 1995). And it's never too late to begin; even people in their 60s and 70s can increase their life expectancy by exercising.

According to William Evans, Director of the Noll Physiological Research Center at Pennsylvania State University, "there is nothing else you can do that has as great an effect on extending life. It's extraordinarily powerful" (Liebman, 1995).

Source: Liebman, B. (1995). Exercise. Use it or lose it! Nutrition Action Health Letter, 22(10):1, 4–6.

serum cholesterol levels as a risk factor for chronic heart disease become less important after age 64. Also, overly-restrictive diets may actually contribute to malnutrition (Administration on Aging, DHHS, 1994).

Another controversial recommendation for the elderly calls for reduced sodium intake. Younger adults are advised to reduce their intake of sodium because excessive sodium may increase the risk for hypertension. Sodium restriction may not be appropriate for older adults, however, because studies indicate that the risk of stroke from hypertension is less in the elderly than in other age groups. Also, a diet that is low enough in sodium to lower blood pressure effectively (2 to 3 g sodium) would limit food choices and may make the diet less palatable; this would complicate meal planning for someone who is underweight or has a poor appetite. In addition, because taste sensitivity for salt decreases with age, compliance is difficult.

Encouraging weight loss in the elderly should also be approached with caution. Healthy body weight and ideal percentage of body fat have not yet been determined for older adults. The assumption that excess weight reduces longevity may be true for younger adults but is not necessarily true for the elderly. Some studies suggest that among people aged 70 and older, the highest risk of mortality is among those whose BMI is in the lowest quintile (Losonczy et al., 1995). The inverse relationship between weight and mortality appears to reflect illness-related weight loss from a heavier weight in middle age (Losonczy et al., 1995). Except for clients with medical conditions that are aggravated by obesity (eg, debilitating arthritis), weight reduction may not be prudent in elderly people who are moderately overweight. Older adults who are underweight should be encouraged to gain weight.

The Food Guide Pyramid and Daily Food Guide

Because few RDA change with aging except those for calories, it is important for the elderly to choose a nutrient-dense diet that includes a variety of foods from the major food groups. Although the Food Guide Pyramid is still appropriate, older adults may need to limit the number of servings from each major food group to the least amount recommended, so as not to exceed calorie requirements (Table 12-3). Elderly people who require more calories should eat more foods from the major food groups and not fill up on "Fats, Oils, and Sweets."

NURSING PROCESS

A large portion of elderly Americans are at greater risk for nutritional problems than the general population, and many have poor nutritional status that requires nutrition intervention. Studies suggest that specific nutritional deficiencies exist in as many as 50% of independently living elderly people in the United States, and that as many as 20% of the elderly skip meals almost daily. Two major indicators that are highly predictive of mortality and morbidity in older adults are low body weight and rapid unintentional weight loss (see display, Risk Factors and Major and Minor Indicators of Poor Nutritional Status Among the Elderly).

For the noninstitutionalized elderly, nutrition screening may be used to quickly and cost-effectively identify clients who are at risk, before they become malnourished. The **Nutrition Screening Initiative (NSI)**, a joint effort of the American Acad-

Table 12-3
Daily Food Guide for the Elderly

Food Group	Number of Servings Recommended in the Food Guide Pyramid	Number of Servings Appropriate for the Elderly (about 1600 calories)
Bread, Cereal, Rice, and Pasta Group	6–11	6
Vegetable Group	3–5	3
Fruit Group	2–4	2
Milk, Yogurt, and Cheese Group	2–3	2–3
Meat, Poultry, Fish, Dry Beans, Eggs, and Nuts Group	2–3 (5–7 ounces)	2 (5 ounces)
Fats, Oils, and Sweets	Use sparingly	Use sparingly

Risk Factors and Major and Minor Indicators of Poor Nutritional Status Among the Elderly

The following are the risk factors, as well as the major and minor indicators, of poor nutritional status:

Risk Factors	Major Indicators	Minor Indicators
Inappropriate food intake	Weight loss	Alcoholism
Poverty	Under-/overweight	Cognitive impairment
Social isolation	Low serum albumin	Chronic renal insufficiency
Dependency/disability	Change in functional status	Multiple concurrent medications
Acute/chronic diseases or conditions	Inappropriate food intake	Malabsorption syndromes
Chronic medication use	Midarm muscle circumference <10th percentile	Anorexia, nausea, dysphagia
Advanced age (80+)	Triceps skinfold <10th percentile or >95th percentile	Change in bowel habit
	Obesity	Fatigue, apathy, memory loss
	Nutrition-related disorders	Poor oral/dental status, dehydration
	Osteoporosis	Poorly healing wounds
	Osteomalacia	Loss of subcutaneous fat and/or muscle mass
	Folate deficiency	Fluid retention
	B_{12} deficiency	Reduced iron, ascorbic acid, zinc

emy of Family Physicians, The American Dietetic Association, and the National Council on Aging, has developed the DETERMINE Checklist as a public awareness tool to be used as the first step in identifying older adults who may be at nutritional risk so that the appropriate referral can be made (Fig. 12-1). The second step (the Level I screen to be used by professionals in health care and social services) and the third step (the Level II screen used in medical settings) are used for elderly people who have been referred for evaluation and for those with potential serious nutritional or medical problems.

Unfortunately, assessment data for use in evaluating the elderly may be unreliable or invalid because of age-related changes. For instance, accurate anthropometric measurements and dietary information may be difficult to obtain because of illness or cognitive changes. Also, normal laboratory test standards that are used for younger adults may not be appropriate for the elderly. Standards of nutritional assessment that have been specifically developed for the elderly must be defined. Problems that are specifically associated with assessing the nutritional status of the elderly are listed in the display, Problems With Nutritional Assessment of the Elderly.

Assessment

In addition to the general geriatric assessment criteria (see display, General Geriatric Assessment Criteria), assess the following factors:

Significant undesirable weight loss, which is defined as weight loss equal to or greater than 5% in one month, or equal to or greater than 10% in 6 months.

(text continues on page 362)

The Warning Signs of poor nutritional health are often overlooked. Use this checklist to find out if you or someone you know is at nutritional risk.

Read the statements below. Circle the number in the yes column for those that apply to you or someone you know. For each yes answer, score the number in the box. Total your nutritional score.

DETERMINE YOUR NUTRITIONAL HEALTH

	YES
I have an illness or condition that made me change the kind and/or amount of food I eat.	2
I eat fewer than 2 meals per day.	3
I eat few fruits or vegetables, or milk products.	2
I have 3 or more drinks of beer, liquor, or wine almost every day.	2
I have tooth or mouth problems that make it hard for me to eat.	2
I don't always have enough money to buy the food I need.	4
I eat alone most of the time.	1
I take 3 or more different prescribed or over-the-counter drugs a day.	1
Without wanting to, I have lost or gained 10 pounds in the last 6 months.	2
I am not always physically able to shop, cook and/or feed myself.	2
	TOTAL

Total Your Nutritional Score. If it's —

0–2   **Good!** Recheck your nutritional score in 6 months.

3–5   **You are at moderate nutritional risk.** See what can be done to improve your eating habits and lifestyle. Your office on aging, senior nutrition program, senior citizen center or health department can help. Recheck your nutritional score in 3 months

6 or more   **You are at high nutritional risk.** Bring this checklist the next time you see your doctor, dietitian or other qualified health or social service professional. Talk with them about any problems you may have. Ask for help to improve your nutritional health.

These materials developed and distributed by the Nutritional Screening Initiative, a project of:

 AMERICAN ACADEMY OF FAMILY PHYSICIANS

 THE AMERICAN DIETETIC ASSOCIATION

 NATIONAL COUNCIL ON THE AGING, INC.

Remember that warning signs suggest risk. but do not represent diagnosis of any condition. Turn the page to learn more about the Warning Signs of poor nutritional health.

Figure 12-1
Public awareness tool.

**The Nutrition Checklist is based on the Warning Signs described below.
Use the word <u>DETERMINE</u> to remind you of the Warning Signs.**

Disease

Any disease, illness or chronic condition which causes you to change the way you eat, or makes it hard for you to eat, puts your nutritional health at risk. Four out or five adults have chronic diseases that are affected by diet. Confusion or memory loss that keeps getting worse is estimated to affect one out of five or more of older adults. This can make it hard to remember what, when or if you've eaten. Feeling sad or depressed, which happens to about one in eight older adults, can cause big changes in appetite, digestion, energy level, weight and well-being.

Eating Poorly

Eating too little and eating too much both lead to poor health. Eating the same foods day after day or not eating fruit, vegetables, and milk products daily will also cause poor nutritional health. One in five adults skip meals daily. Only 13% of adults eat the minimum amount of fruit and vegetables needed. One in four older adults drink too much alcohol. Many health problems become worse if you drink more than one or two alcoholic beverages per day.

Tooth Loss/Mouth Pain

A healthy mouth, teeth and gums are needed to eat. Missing, loose or rotten teeth or dentures which don't fit well or cause mouth sores make it hard to eat.

Economic Hardship

As many as 40% of older Americans have incomes of less than $6,000 per year. Having less—or choosing to spent less—than $25–30 per week for food makes it very hard to get the foods you need to stay healthy.

Reduced Social Contact

One-third of all older people live alone. Being with people daily has a positive effect on morale, well-being and eating.

Multiple Medicines

Many older Americans must take medicines for health problems. Almost half of older Americans take multiple medicines daily. Growing old may change the way we respond to drugs. The more medicines you take, the greater the chance for side effects such as increased or decreased appetite, change in taste, constipation, weakness, drowsiness, diarrhea, nausea, and others. Vitamins or minerals when taken in large doses act like drugs and can harm. Alert your doctor to everything you take.

Involuntary Weight Loss/Gain

Losing or gaining a lot of weight when you are not trying to do so is an important warning sign that must not be ignored. Being overweight or underweight also increases your chance of poor health.

Needs Assistance in Self Care

Although most older people are able to eat, one of every five have trouble walking, shopping, buying and cooking food, especially as they get older.

Elder Years Above Age 80

Most older people lead full and productive lives. But as age increases, risk of frailty and health problems increase. Checking your nutritional health regularly make good sense.

The Nutrition Screening Initiative, 2626 Pennsylvania Avenue, NW, Suite 301, Washington, DC 20037

The Nutrition Screening Initiative is funded in part by a grant from Ross Laboratories, a division of Abbott Laboratories.

Figure 12-1 (Continued)

Problems With Nutritional Assessment of the Elderly

ANTHROPOMETRIC MEASUREMENT

Accurate weights may be difficult to obtain if the client

- Is bedridden.
- Has edema.

Accurate heights may be difficult to obtain if the client

- Is bedridden.
- Has curvature of the spine (kyphosis).

Accurate skinfold thickness may be difficult to obtain because of changes in compressibility of subcutaneous fat with aging.

BIOCHEMICAL DATA

Not all normal laboratory values for the elderly have been defined; therefore, interpretation of results is difficult.

CLINICAL OBSERVATIONS

Nonspecific signs of malnutrition (eg, anorexia, fatigue) may be attributed to other causes, for example, aging, chronic diseases, secondary to drug therapy.

Age-related changes in physiology and function may mimic signs of a nutritional deficiency (eg, loss of visual acuity in dim light occurs with aging and may not indicate a deficiency of vitamin A).

Most malnutrition in the United States is subclinical; that is, a deficiency may exist but physical signs are not apparent.

DIETARY ASSESSMENT

A 24-hour recall or food frequency record may be unreliable if the client has short-term memory deficits, confusion, or is hard of hearing.

Significant weight loss is one of the most important and sensitive indicators of malnutrition (Administration on Aging, DHHS, 1994).

Dentition and ability to swallow.

Acute or chronic illness and its impact on nutrient intake, digestion, metabolism, and excretion.

Usual 24-hour intake, including the frequency and pattern of eating, as well as the method of food preparation. A food record or food frequency questionnaire may provide additional intake data. If malnutrition is suspected, intake and output may be carefully monitored to calculate actual nutritional intake.

Adequacy of the client's usual intake based on the Food Guide Pyramid/Daily Food Guide for the Elderly (see Table 12-3); pay particular attention to nutrient density and the intake of foods from the "Fats, Oils, and Sweets" group, which supply little more than calories.

Appetite. Determine if there have been any recent significant changes in eating patterns and, if so, why.

The use of a modified diet and, if so, its appropriateness and duration of use; evaluate also the client's ability to understand and comply with the diet.

Cultural, familial, religious, and ethnic influences on eating habits.

The use of vitamin or mineral supplements. Evaluate their safety and appropriateness.

The use of prescribed medications and over-the-counter drugs. Determine if any food–drug interactions are affecting nutritional status or drug effectiveness.

ASSESSMENT CRITERIA

General Geriatric Assessment Criteria

Weight, weight status (see example, Evaluating Weight Status). For the nonambulatory client, a bed or wheelchair scale is needed to accurately assess weight.

Hemoglobin, hematocrit

Serum albumin, lipids, glucose

Urinalysis for glucose, ketones, protein, occult blood

Skin turgor and appearance

Bowel and bladder function

Past and present medical history

Use of medications, laxative abuse

Physical disabilities

Living arrangements, social life, source of income, and how income is allocated

Activity pattern and frequency

Mental health status

The client's use of alcohol, tobacco, caffeine, and drugs.

Functional disabilities, such as impaired ability to shop, cook, and eat. Frequent disabling conditions include arthritis, dementia, heart disease, hip fractures, lung disease, Parkinson's disease, and stroke.

Adequacy of food budget.

Adequacy of social support, evidence of depression or dementia.

Nursing Diagnosis

Altered Nutrition: Less than Body Requirements, related to inadequate intake as evidenced by weight loss.

Planning and Implementation

Rather than using a textbook approach, which may be appropriate for younger adults, nutritional care of older adults should be client-centered and based on the individual's physiologic, pathologic, and psychosocial condition. With any diet intervention for the elderly, overall goals are to maintain or restore maximal independent functioning, and to maintain the client's sense of dignity and quality of life by imposing as few dietary restrictions as necessary. Except in treating diet-related diseases such as severe hypertension, renal disease, ascites, brittle diabetes, and obe-

EXAMPLE

Evaluating weight status:

$$\text{Percentage of usual body weight} = \frac{\text{current weight}}{\text{usual weight}} \times 100$$

$$\text{Percent weight change} = \frac{(\text{usual weight} - \text{actual weight})}{\text{usual weight}} \times 100$$

sity in clients with debilitating arthritis, modified diets may be of little value. In fact, special diets are a major cause of malnutrition in the elderly. Therefore, dietary changes should be undertaken only when a significant improvement in the individual's health can be expected. Any necessary dietary changes should be incorporated into the client's existing food pattern, because planning a completely new approach to eating would result in decreased compliance.

Like all age groups, older adults need a balanced diet from all major food groups; however, some elderly may consume less than optimal intake from one or more food groups. Those at greatest risk are less educated, live alone, and have incomes less than 150% of poverty (Melnik et al, 1994). One study found that, with the exception of fruit intake (which was influenced by the fact that the study was conducted in summer), only one third or fewer of elderly people who were screened followed the Food Guide Pyramid recommendations for each food group; only 8% of participants met the Food Guide Pyramid recommendations for four to five groups (Melnik et al, 1994). Nutrients that are deficient in certain segments of the elderly population (when compared to the RDA) include calories, calcium, zinc, vitamin B_6, vitamin B_{12}, and vitamin D (ADA, 1993). Excessive intakes of vitamins A, D, E, and C have been noted in older adults who regularly consume vitamin supplements.

Inadequate intakes from the meat group often occur in older adults secondary to a limited food budget or difficulty chewing. Many adults avoid milk, which is another source of high-quality protein, because of its association with childhood. The intake of fruits and vegetables may be limited because they are expensive or difficult to chew. Clearly, food choices of the elderly often are based on considerations other than food preferences, such as income; the client's physical ability to shop, prepare, chew, and swallow food; and the occurrence of food intolerances that are related to chronic disease or present as side effects of medications.

Generally, food preferences in the elderly are the accumulation of a lifetime of food habits that have been influenced by cultural, social, and personal factors. To have the greatest impact on food habits and nutritional status in the elderly, nutrition education should be initiated at a young age and continued throughout life.

Older adults should be encouraged to be as physically active as possible to improve calcium balance, to help promote gastrointestinal function, and to improve their sense of well-being. Exercise also increases energy expenditure, making a greater calorie (and therefore nutrient) intake possible.

The client's need for homemaker services, shopping assistance, transportation, food stamps, congregate meals, or Meals-on-Wheels should be evaluated and the appropriate referral made. Congregate meals and Meals-on-Wheels are federally funded nutrition programs that are specifically provided for the elderly; they have been designed to provide low-cost, nutritious hot meals; education about food and nutrition; opportunities for socialization and recreation; and information on other health and social assistance programs. The congregate meal program provides a hot, balanced, midday meal and the opportunity to socialize in senior citizen centers and other public or private facilities. Those who choose to pay may do so; otherwise the meal is free. Meals-on-Wheels is a home-delivered meal program for the elderly who are unable to get to congregate meal centers, because they live in an isolated area or have a chronic illness or disability. Usually a hot meal is served at midday, and a bagged lunch is included to be used as the evening meal. Modified diets, like diabetic diets and low-sodium diets, are provided as needed.

CLIENT GOALS

The client will:

Attain/maintain "healthy" weight.
Consume, on average, the recommended number of servings from each of the major food groups.
Modify food texture, as needed, to facilitate chewing and swallowing.

NURSING INTERVENTIONS

Diet Management

- Provide a varied, nutrient-dense diet based on the Daily Food Guide for the Elderly (see Table 12-3). Although the actual nutrient content of the diet may vary with the foods chosen, using the guide helps ensure an average adequate intake. A variety of foods should be selected from each food group; limiting food choices or skipping a food group increases the risk of both nutrient deficiencies and excesses. If additional calories or protein is needed, encourage additional servings from the milk group; although two servings are recommended, five cups of milk or the equivalent may be needed to maintain calcium balance, especially in postmenopausal and osteoporotic women (see Appendix 12 for foods high in calcium).
- Limit foods that are calorically dense but provide few other essential nutrients, such as foods high in sugar, fats, and oils. As calorie requirements decline with age, nutrient density (the nutritional value of a food compared to the amount of calories it provides) becomes increasingly important in order to meet nutritional needs without exceeding calorie requirements.
- Discourage excessive or frequent use of alcohol. Small amounts of alcohol, however, such as an occasional glass of wine or beer, may help stimulate the appetite and enhance sleep. In an institutional setting, the use of alcohol may result in improved socialization and increased food intake. However, alcohol contributes little nutritional value to the diet except calories, and it may cause multiple nutritional problems if used excessively. Even moderate use can displace the intake of nutrient-dense foods, especially in the diets of older adults who have limited budgets, reduced food intakes, and decreased calorie requirements.
- Increase fiber intake to prevent or alleviate constipation and laxative dependence. Substituting whole-grain breads and cereals for refined products is a subtle way to increase the fiber content of the diet that is realistic for elderly people who have difficulty chewing or who are on a fixed income. If income and dental health allow, increasing the intake of fresh fruits and vegetables also adds fiber to the diet.
- Avoid excessive salt intake. Opinions vary as to the optimal sodium content in a healthy diet for the elderly. Recommendations on sodium intake should be

made on an individual basis according to the client's cardiac and renal status, appetite, and use of medications.

- Drink six to eight glasses of water daily to maintain hydration and normal urine and fecal output. Thirst is not a reliable indicator of need in the elderly.
- Take supplements only as prescribed by the physician. According to the National Institute on Aging (NIA), a balanced diet based on the Daily Food Guide is nutritionally adequate for most healthy elderly men and women. However, vitamin and mineral supplements are popular among the elderly. Estimates from survey populations indicate that 40% to 60% of older adults use some form of vitamin or mineral supplement, 56% of whom do so on the recommendation of family, friends, or the media. The elderly are particularly vulnerable to false nutritional claims that promise to restore youth, cure disease, and improve sense of well-being. The purchase of unnecessary and ill-advised supplements can displace the purchase of food if funds are limited or may prevent an individual from seeking sound medical advice if the supplements are used to "cure" illness.
- Modify the texture of the diet as needed, if chewing or swallowing is compromised. Meats and vegetables may be served soft-cooked, chopped, ground, or puréed. Eggs and dairy products are good substitutes for meats and are easy to consume and relatively economical. Take care to avoid overprocessing foods because this may lead to loss of nutrients and appeal. Liquids that are thickened to the consistency of honey are easier to swallow than thin liquids. Other diet modifications to help relieve eating problems that are related to aging are listed in Table 12-4.

Client Teaching

Instruct the client and family

That a balanced diet based on the major food groups can help maximize the quality of life. Stress the importance of consuming adequate protein, calcium, fiber, and fluid.

On how to modify the diet, as needed, to alleviate eating problems that occur frequently in the elderly (see Table 12-4).

That unless prescribed by a physician, taking vitamin and mineral supplements may be unnecessary and potentially dangerous. If the client is insistent about using a supplement, or if the diet appears inadequate, a multivitamin that supplies 100% of the Daily Value is recommended.

That because eating alone is a risk factor for poor nutritional status among older adults, efforts should be made to eat with friends and relatives whenever possible; encourage participation in congregate-dining programs.

That eating alone does not have to be boring if you set a pretty table and use good dishes. Meals that vary in color, texture, temperature, and flavor also add interest. Experiment with herbs and spices, or try a new recipe. Eat by a window, on the porch, or out in the yard. For company, listen to the radio or music, watch television, read, or eat with friends.

That making meals is less of a chore if you choose easy-to-prepare foods or make extra portions for homemade TV dinners that can be frozen and used later.

Table 12-4
Dietary Interventions for Eating Problems of the Elderly

Problem	Rationale	Dietary Interventions
Difficulty chewing	Missing or decayed teeth Periodontal disease Missing or ill-fitting dentures	Provide liquid, semisolid, mashed or chopped foods as tolerated. Progress liquid diet as soon as possible.
Difficulty swallowing	Paralysis related to stroke Parkinson's disease	Thickened and gelled liquids are usually better tolerated than thin liquids. Baby food can be used as a nutritious thickener. Avoid overuse of puréed foods because of the negative connotations associated with it.
Lack of appetite	Depression Acute or chronic disease Loss of sense of smell and taste Side effect of medication Loneliness Early satiety	Offer small frequent meals. Solicit food preferences. Allow plenty of time to eat. Because appetite is usually greatest in the morning, emphasize a nutritious breakfast. Encourage group eating.
Impaired ability to feed self	Poor vision Arthritis of the hands; stroke	Describe the meal and how it is arranged on the plate. Assist the client by opening packages of bread and crackers, buttering bread and vegetables, cutting meat, and opening milk cartons. Assess the client's ability to grasp utensils and guide food to the mouth. Refer the client to an occupational therapist to evaluate the need for assistive devices or retraining.
Loss of taste and smell	Normal aging Endocrine disorders secondary to drug therapy Certain nutrient deficiencies (zinc, vitamin B_{12}, niacin)	Add commercial flavors to foods to intensify smell. Add texture, when possible (ie, crunchiness, chewiness). Appearance of food becomes more important. Sour/bitter fruits and vegetables are the foods most likely to be avoided; encourage the intake of other types/forms of fruits and vegetables acceptable to the individual.

To stretch the food budget by buying only as much as needed, unless freezer and storage space is adequate. Although single-serving cans of vegetables cost more per unit of measure, they are less expensive than allowing unused portions of regular-sized cans to spoil in the refrigerator. Large bags of frozen vegetables are economical because they allow you to cook only as much as you need. Ask the butcher to wrap individual portions of meat; freeze in freezer bags until needed.

Monitor Progress

Monitor:

Compliance to the diet and the need for follow-up diet counseling
Effectiveness of the diet, and the need for additional dietary changes

Weight changes

Laboratory values, as available

Medical–social status. Periodically evaluate the need for Meals-on-Wheels or other assistance programs.

Evaluation

Evaluation is ongoing. Provided the plan of care has not changed, the client will achieve the goals as stated above.

NUTRITIONAL CONSIDERATIONS FOR THE INSTITUTIONALIZED ELDERLY

The typical long-term care resident has numerous psychosocial, functional, and medical problems that often are complicated by poor nutritional status. Anorexia and weight loss are often present upon admission to a long-term care facility; the incidence of malnutrition upon admission is greater among residents being admitted from hospitals than those admitted from their homes (Administration on Aging, DHHS, 1994). The incidence of protein–calorie malnutrition has been reported to range from 30% to 50% among nursing home residents, and 40% or more of residents are unable to feed themselves independently. One study showed that the average staff time spent feeding each resident was 6 to 10 minutes, when 30 to 45 minutes may be needed to adequately feed impaired residents (Administration on Aging, DHHS, 1994).

Institutionalization of older adults often means a loss of independence and is viewed both as a punishment and as going to a place to die. Nursing home residents generally tend to eat less food and have a greater risk of nutritional deficiencies than independently living elderly people, possibly because of limited food choices and unfamiliarity with the foods offered. Loss of favorite or familiar foods, altered meal schedules, and a change in serving style can also contribute to poor intakes. Depression, anxiety, and feelings of hopelessness contribute to anorexia. Residents with Alzheimer's disease are at increased nutritional risk (see display, Nutrition Intervention for Alzheimer's Disease).

Nutrition intervention that is aimed at preventing overt malnutrition is economically, medically, and functionally desirable. Indeed, prevention of unintentional weight loss and pressure ulcers, which are two common problems among long-term care residents, is a key component of meeting the regulation about quality of life in the Omnibus Budget Reconciliation Act (OBRA) of 1987 (Pub Law No. 101-239) (Gilmore et al, 1995). Both prevention and treatment require a high-calorie, high-protein diet; small frequent feedings or fortified supplements may help maximize intake. For clients with altered skin integrity, supplemental vitamin C and zinc may be indicated to promote healing. Frequent monitoring of the resident's intake, acceptance and tolerance of supplements, and hydration status is vital; a low serum albumin is associated with both unintentional weight loss and pressure ulcers and should also be monitored (Gilmore et al, 1995).

Nutrition Intervention for Alzheimer's Disease

Alzheimer's disease is the most common cause of dementia in the United States today and the fourth leading cause of death. Although the cause of Alzheimer's disease is unknown, there appears to be a genetic predisposition. Aluminum toxicity has been proposed as an etiologic factor. However, most researchers believe that the aluminum accumulation seen in Alzheimer's disease is not the cause of the disease but, rather, a consequence of it.

The course of Alzheimer's disease is progressive and nonreversible. Initially, the disease manifests itself with loss of memory, forgetfulness, and a decrease in social and vocational abilities. The victim may become lost in familiar surroundings, and personality changes may develop. As the disease progresses, the victim can no longer cope without assistance, and he becomes disoriented to time and place. Delusions, depression, agitation, and language difficulties are noted. Finally, severe intellectual impairment and complete disorientation are seen. Verbal skills are lost, motor skills deteriorate, and self-care activities may be impossible. Urinary and fecal incontinence are common, and clients may become bedridden. Death usually results from infection.

At present, there is no clear evidence that Alzheimer's disease alters nutritional requirements. However, it can have a devastating impact on the nutritional status. Early in the disease, impairments in memory and judgment may make shopping, storing, and cooking food difficult. The client may forget to eat or may forget that he already ate and, consequently, eat again. Changes in the sense of smell and food preferences may also develop. A preference for sweets and salty foods is noted, and unusual food choices may occur. Agitation increases energy expenditure, and calorie requirements may increase by as much as 1600/day. Weight loss is common. Choking may occur if the client forgets to chew food sufficiently before swallowing, or if he hoards food in the mouth. Eating of nonfood items may occur, and eventually self-feeding ability is lost.

Nutrition interventions that may be appropriate for clients with Alzheimer's disease include the following recommendations:

- Closely supervise mealtime; check food temperatures to prevent accidental mouth burns.
- Serve meals in the same place at the same time each day, and keep distractions to a minimum.
- Minimize confusion by providing a nonselect menu based on the resident's likes and dislikes, if known.
- Provide one food at a time; a whole tray may be overwhelming.
- Provide in-between meal snacks that are easy to consume such as sandwiches, beverages, and finger foods.
- Modify food consistency as needed, cutting food into small pieces and reminding the client to chew to avoid choking. Physical assistance (eg, light pressure applied to the underside of the chin to push up on the tongue) may be needed to promote swallowing.
- Monitor weight closely.
- Clients in the latter stage of Alzheimer's disease are not only unable to feed themselves, but also no longer know what to do when food is placed in their mouth. When this occurs, a decision regarding the use of other means of nutritional support (ie, NG or PEG tube feedings) must be made.

In contrast, rigid or unnecessary dietary restrictions can compound the client's feelings of hopelessness and depression. Therapeutic diets should be used only when a significant improvement in health can be expected, as in cases of severe hypertension, ascites, congestive heart failure, constipation, brittle diabetes, and obesity if excess weight aggravates arthritis (see appropriate chapters in the section on Nutrition in Clinical Practice for possible diet modifications). The validity of other diet modifications to prevent or delay disease in the elderly is questionable, especially if diet restrictions are viewed as a "punishment" and discourage the patient from eating.

In place of standard therapeutic diets, many clinicians recommend a more progressive approach to feeding the elderly. Clients who receive a liberal geriatric diet (see display, Liberal Geriatric Diet) similar to what they were eating at home tend to eat better, have fewer bowel problems, enjoy their meals more, are more alert, and are generally happier than clients receiving therapeutic diets.

Liberal Geriatric Diet

The Liberal Geriatric Diet is designed to meet the nutritional requirements of institutionalized elderly by offering a diet as close to the individual's usual diet as possible. It provides 1500 to 2000 cal/day using a variety of regular foods. Simple sugars are kept to a minimum and low-fat milk is used routinely. A moderate sodium intake of 3 to 4 g/day is achieved by eliminating salty foods and by using herbs and spices as alternatives to salt in many foods. An adequate fluid intake is encouraged. The fiber content of the diet is increased by emphasizing whole-grain breads and cereals, adding coarse raw bran, if needed, and offering fresh fruits and vegetables. Individual preferences should be honored whenever possible.

The Liberal Geriatric Diet can be modified as needed. For instance, texture can be altered for residents who have difficulty chewing or swallowing. Reducing portion sizes, eliminating sugar, and restricting sweets may be appropriate for clients with diabetes or obesity. For residents who require a sodium restriction, salt-containing condiments can be eliminated and salt-free breads and cereals used as needed. Residents with early satiety should receive small, frequent meals. More comprehensive modifications may be needed for residents with diet-related diseases or nutrient deficiencies.

SAMPLE LIBERAL GERIATRIC DIET

Breakfast
Orange juice
Oatmeal
1 soft-cooked egg
1 slice buttered whole-wheat toast
Low-fat milk
Coffee/tea
Salt*/pepper/sugar*

Lunch
Grilled cheese sandwich made with two slices whole-wheat bread
Cream of broccoli soup
Sliced strawberries
1/2 cup low-fat milk
Coffee/tea
Salt*/pepper/sugar*

Dinner
Baked chicken
Steamed rice
Baked acorn squash
Fresh fruit salad
Ice milk
Coffee/tea
Salt*/pepper/sugar*

Snack
1/2 cup low-fat milk
Bran muffin

* Packages of salt and sugar may be omitted if a restriction of either is appropriate.

DRUG
ALERT

Drug Considerations in the Elderly

The elderly, who make up 12% of the population, consume 25% of all prescription drugs in the United States (Administration on Aging, DHHS, 1994). It is estimated that the average noninstitutionalized older adults take three or more medications daily; those in hospitals and long-term care facilities take an average of eight to ten (Administration on Aging, DHHS, 1994). The most commonly prescribed medications for the elderly include analgesics, laxatives, cardiovascular medications, vitamins and minerals, diuretics, psycholeptics, antiflatulents, and antihistamines (Livingston and Reeves, 1993). Large numbers of older adults are also regular users of over-the-counter medications for pain, indigestion, colds, flu, sinus, constipation, gas, and diarrhea.

Because the elderly take more drugs than any other age group, they are particularly prone to nutritional problems related to drug use. Drugs may affect nutrition by inhibiting appetite, altering the sense of taste or smell, altering secretion of saliva, irritating the stomach, or causing nausea. Some drugs contribute directly to dietary deficiencies by altering nutrient absorption, utilization, or excretion. In a study of long-term care residents, of those taking one or more drugs causing anorexia, vomiting, and aversion to food, 41% lost more than 10% of their weight over 3 to 12 months (Administration on Aging, DHHS, 1994). Drugs that are frequently given to long-term care residents may cause deficiencies of vitamins B_6, B_{12}, C, D, and K, phosphate, potassium, calcium, magnesium, and zinc.

Of the 3% to 8% of all hospital admissions caused by adverse drug reactions, almost one third occur in the elderly. Drug reactions occur more frequently after the age of 60, and when five or more drugs are used daily (Administration on Aging, DHHS, 1994). Factors that contribute to an increased incidence of drug reactions in older adults include chronicity and multiplicity of diseases, inability to follow complex medication routines, interactions between prescribed and over-the-counter medications, errors in dosage due to unresolved issues of optimal doses for the elderly, prescriptions written by multiple physicians, and age-related body changes (especially in the liver) that alter drug absorption, circulation, or excretion (Administration on Aging, DHHS, 1994).

To avoid potential problems, older adults should be informed about the side effects of medications they are using—that is, how their medications interact with food, alcohol, and other medicines—and also about the proper dosage and timing of medications. They should be advised to consult their physician or pharmacist if problems arise, and should keep all their physicians informed of which prescription and over-the-counter medications they are using.

To reduce instances of nutrient–drug and drug–drug interaction in long-term care facilities, care should be taken to 1) communicate potential interactions in the resident's medical record; 2) weigh residents frequently; 3) discourage self-medication; 4) administer drugs at the appropriate time; and 5) become familiar with potential adverse side effects (Livingston and Reeves, 1993).

Aspirin may cause GI bleeding, which can result in iron deficiency, decreased serum folate levels, and an increased vitamin C requirement.

Use of *diuretics* alone may cause magnesium deficiency.

Simultaneous use of *potassium-wasting diuretics* and *laxatives* increases the risk for severe potassium deficiency.

Digoxin may cause nausea, and possibly anorexia and weight loss.

Long-term use of *anticonvulsants* may cause vitamin D deficiency, and can lead to decreased calcium absorption and osteomalacia.

Aluminum-containing antacids may cause phosphate depletion and secondary calcium malabsorption.

Commercial supplements are often given between meals to increase the calorie and protein content of a patient's diet. Although they may be temporarily useful, they are generally not well accepted or tolerated; nor are they usually effective on a long-term basis. Taste fatigue and lack of hunger for the meal that follows often occur. Compliance may be better if relatively tasteless supplements are added to foods that the client normally eats, thereby increasing the nutrient density of the diet without increasing the volume of food consumed.

To promote optimal intake in an institutional setting, the nurse should make mealtime as enjoyable an experience as possible; she should encourage independence in eating, or if necessary, provide assistance with eating. Food preferences should be honored whenever possible, and food from home should also be encouraged. Provide liberal intake of fluid and protein in clients who have, or are at risk of, decubitus ulcers. Vitamin C and zinc are also necessary for healing.

Ongoing monitoring may include intake observations or intake and output records when a problem is suspected. Because weight loss is one of the most important and sensitive indicators of malnutrition, obtaining accurate monthly weights is vital. More frequent weights may be necessary if a nutritional problem is indicated. Communicate feeding or eating problems, food intolerances, and significant weight changes to the dietitian for further assessment and intervention.

KEY CONCEPTS

- Although women live longer than men, they have more health problems, especially nutritional-related disease such as cardiovascular disease, certain cancers, osteoporosis, diabetes, and weight-control problems.
- Men have shorter life expectancies than women. This may be related to lifestyle, not simply a matter of biology.
- Aging begins at birth and ends in death. Exactly how and why aging occurs is not known.
- Good eating habits developed early in life promote health in old age. Diet modifications initiated late in life may not influence the progression of disease but may improve quality of life.
- As a group, older adults are at risk for nutritional problems because of changes in physiology (including changes in body composition, gastrointestinal tract, metabolism, central nervous system, renal system, and in the senses), changes in income, changes in health, and psychosocial changes.
- The RDA for older adults were extrapolated from studies on younger people and may not be accurate. It is difficult to generalize needs in such a heterogeneous population; individualization of diet is essential.
- Goals of diet intervention for older adults are to maintain or restore maximal independent functioning and to maintain quality of life. Except when a significant improvement in health can be expected, therapeutic diets may not be appropriate for older adults; often they are a major cause of malnutrition.
- Institutionalized elderly are at high risk for malnutrition. Preventive efforts should focus on maintaining an adequate intake: Honor special requests, encourage food from home, provide assistance with eating as needed.

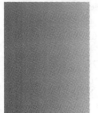

- Weight loss, low serum albumin, and altered skin integrity increase the need for calories and protein. Increasing nutrient density without increasing the volume of food served (eg, adding protein powder to fluid milk or nonfat dried milk, butter, and sugar to cooked cereal) may be the most effective method of delivering additional nutrients. However, in-between meal supplements may also be needed to maximize intake.

- As a group, the elderly are more prone to drug–nutrient interactions and drug-induced nutritional deficiencies.

 FOCUS ON **CRITICAL THINKING**

Bertha Wicks is an 86-year-old newly-admitted resident of a nursing home. She is 5' tall, weighs 103 pounds, and has recently been hospitalized for a broken hip that was surgically repaired. She has a history of glucose intolerance, although since losing 13 pounds while in the hospital, her glucose has been within normal limits. However, her doctor has ordered a 1400-calorie diet for her. Bertha is legally blind, and very unhappy about being institutionalized. She complains that the other residents are "old ladies" and refuses to eat in the dining room. She hates the food and her family is concerned that she will continue to lose weight.

Identify risk factors and major and minor indicators of poor nutritional status that are exhibited by Bertha Wicks.

Is Bertha's current diet order adequate and appropriate? Support your answers.

What diet would you recommend for Bertha?

What interventions could you try to improve Bertha's intake?

REFERENCES

Administration on Aging, DHHS (1994). Food and Nutrition for Life: Malnutrition and Older Americans. Report by the Assistant Secretary for Aging prepared by National Edlercare Institute on Nutrition.

American Dietetic Association (1993). Position of The American Dietetic Association: Nutrition, aging, and the continuum of health care. J Am Diet Assoc, 93(1), 80–82.

American Dietetic Association (1995). Position of The American Dietetic Association and The Canadian Dietetic Association: Women's health and nutrition. J Am Diet Assoc, 95(3), 362–366.

Campbell, W., Crim, M., Dallal, G., Young, V., and Evans, W. (1994). Increased protein requirements in elderly people: New data and retrospective reassessments. Am J Clin Nutr, 60, 501–509.

Duffy, V., Backstrand, J., and Ferris, A. (1995). Olfactory dysfunction and related nutritional risk in free-living, elderly women. J Am Diet Assoc, 95(8), 879–884.

Gilmore, S., Robinson, G., Posthauer, M., and Raymond, J. (1995). Clinical indicators associated with unintentional weight loss and pressure ulcers in elderly residents of nursing facilities. J Am Diet Assoc, 95(9), 984–992.

Gray-Donald, K. (1995). The frail elderly: Meeting the nutritional challenges. J Am Diet Assoc, 95(5), 538–540.

International Food Information Council (1994). Calcium: Make no bones about it. Sept/Oct, 1, 4.

Liebman, B. (1995). For women only. Nutrition Action Health Letter, 22(7), 1, 4–7.

Livingston, J., and Reeves, R. (1993). Undocumented potential drug interactions found in medical records of elderly patients in a long-term-care facility. J Am Diet Assoc, 93(10), 1168–1172.

Losonczy, K., Harris, T., Cornoni-Huntley, J., Simonsick, E., Wallace, R., Cook, N., Ostfeld, A., and Blazer, D. (1995). Does weight loss from middle age to old age explain the inverse weight mortality in old age? Am J Epidemiol, 141, 312–321.

Melnik, T., Helferd, S., Firmery, L., and Wales, K. (1994). Screening elderly in the community: The relationship between dietary adequacy and nutritional risk. J Am Diet Assoc, 94(12), 1425–1427.

National Cholesterol Education Program (1993). Second Report of the Expert Panel on Detection, Evaluation, and Treatment of High Blood Cholesterol in Adults. U.S. Department of Health and Human Services, NIH Publication No. 93-3095.

National Institutes of Health, National Heart, Lung, Blood Institute (1992). The Healthy Heart Handbook for Women. NIH Publication No. 92-2720.

National Research Council (1989). Recommended Dietary Allowances, 10th ed. Washington, DC: National Academy Press.

Nutrition Screening Initiative (1991). Nutrition Screening Manual for Professionals Caring for Older Americans. Washington, DC: Greer, Margolis, Mitchell, Grunwald & Associates, Inc.

Schardt, D. (1995). For men only. Nutrition Action Health Letter, 22(5), 1, 4–5.

Spangler, A., and Eigenbrod, J. (1995). Field trial affirms value of DETERMINE-ing nutrition-related problems of free-living elderly. J Am Diet Assoc, 95(4), 489–490.

Stolley, J. (1994). When your patient has Alzheimer's Disease. AJN 94(8), 34–40.

United States Department of Agriculture, and United States Department of Health and Human Services (1995). Nutrition and Your Health: Dietary Guidelines for Americans. 4th ed. Home and Garden Bulletin No. 232.

Williamson, D. (1993). Descriptive epidemiology of body weight and weight changes in US adults. Ann of Intern Med, 119(7, part 2), 646–649.

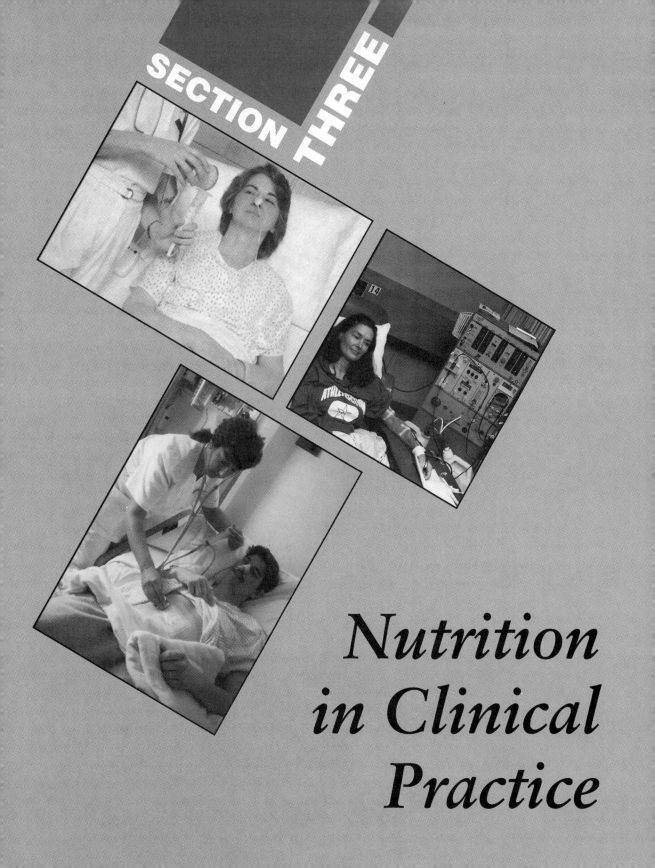

Nutrition
in Clinical
Practice

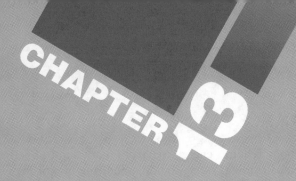

Energy Balance and Weight Control

Chapter Outline

Key Terms

Anorexia nervosa
Basal metabolic rate (BMR)
Body mass index (BMI)
Bulimia nervosa
Kilocalorie

Kilojoule
Obesity
Overweight
Resting energy expenditure
    (REE)

Specific dynamic action
    (SDA)
Weight cycling

ENERGY BALANCE

*T*he body requires energy to carry on any kind of activity—whether voluntary, such as reading, eating, talking, and running, or involuntary, such as inflating the lungs, secreting enzymes, and beating the heart. The body derives energy in the form of calories from carbohydrates, protein, fat, and also from alcohol. By comparing energy intake with output, a person's state of energy balance can be determined (Table 13-1).

Energy Intake

UNITS OF MEASURE

Kilocalorie

A **kilocalorie** represents the amount of heat that is needed to raise the temperature of 1 g of water from 15°C to 16°C. It is the only unit of measure that is used in nutrition, and it is commonly abbreviated as kcal, calorie, cal, or c. In this text, kilocalories are abbreviated to "calories" and "cal." However, a kilocalorie actually is 1000 times larger than a true *calorie*, which is a unit of measure that is used only in chemistry and physics.

Kilojoule

Although calorie is the unit of measure that is used in food composition tables and on food labels, the Committee on Nomenclature of the American Institute of Nutrition recommended in 1970 that the unit *kilojoule* replace kilocalorie as soon as feasible. A kilojoule is a metric measurement defined as the amount of mechanical energy that is required when a force of 1 newton (N) moves 1 kilogram (kg) by a distance of 1 meter (m). One kilojoule equals 1000 joules and may be abbreviated as j, kJ, or KJ. Because 1 calorie equals 4.18 kilojoules, calories can be converted to kilojoules by multiplying the number of calories by 4.18.

Table 13-1
State of Energy Balance

Balance	Description	Weight Status
Neutral	Calorie intake = calorie expenditure	Stable
Positive	Calorie intake > calorie expenditure	Increasing
Negative	Calorie intake < calorie expenditure	Decreasing

FOOD ENERGY

To measure the calorie content of a food, a device known as a bomb calorimeter is used. In carefully controlled laboratory settings, a sample of food is burned in the calorimeter and its energy value is determined by measuring the rise in temperature of the surrounding water (Fig. 13-1). Although a similar process takes place in the body when food is oxidized for energy, food actually produces less energy in the body than in the calorimeter because small amounts of the energy nutrients are not absorbed but rather are excreted in the feces. Also, digestion, absorption, and metabolism are energy-requiring processes, and thus, some energy is used to produce energy. For instance, 20% of the total calories available from carbohydrates are used

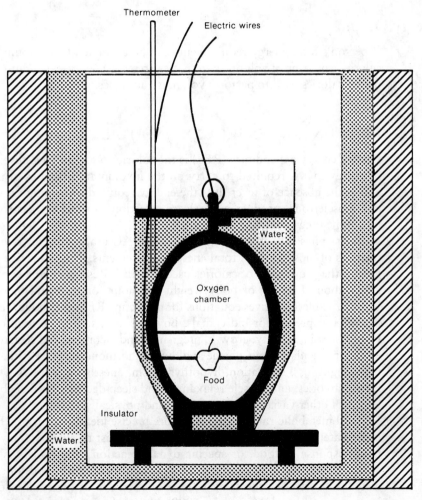

Figure 13-1
Sketch of a bomb calorimeter.

to digest, absorb, and convert carbohydrate to energy; the "cost" of processing fat is much lower at about 6% of the total energy available from fat (Butterfield and Gates, 1994) (see Food for Thought: A Calorie is a Calorie is a Calorie . . . Or Is It?). In addition, any nutrients that are incompletely oxidized yield less than the optimal amount of available energy.

The amount of energy that is available to the body from the metabolism of food has been determined to be 4 cal/g of carbohydrates, 4 cal/g of protein, 9 cal/g of fat, and 7 cal/g of alcohol. The total number of calories in a food or diet can be calculated if the total amount of carbohydrate, protein, fat, and alcohol is known (see display, Sample Calculation). The calorie amounts and nutritional compositions of selected foods are listed in Appendix 1.

Energy Output

A person's total energy requirements can be estimated by combining the estimated calories spent on involuntary activities (resting energy expenditure) and the estimated calories used to perform voluntary activities.

INVOLUNTARY ENERGY EXPENDITURE

Resting energy expenditure (REE) is the caloric cost of staying alive, or the amount of energy that is required to carry on the involuntary activities of the body at rest and in the absence of fever. It is the energy required to maintain body temperature and muscle tone, produce and release secretions, propel the gastrointestinal tract, inflate the lungs, and beat the heart.

Unless physical activity is unusually high, REE accounts for two thirds to three quarters of most people's total energy requirements. The less active a person is, the greater the proportion of calories used for REE. Resting energy expenditure is generally about 1 cal/kg of body weight per hour for men and 0.9 cal/kg/hour for women. Table 13-2 gives equations for predicting REE from body weight. These values are not precise for individuals, however, and should be used only as a guide. Hyperthermia, anxiety, growth, pregnancy and lactation, and elevated levels of hormones, particularly epinephrine and thyroid hormone, increase REE. Prolonged fasting, weight loss, starvation, hypothyroidism, anesthesia, paralysis, drugs (barbiturates, narcotics, and muscle relaxants), and sleep decrease REE. Table 13-3 lists the effects of other variables on both REE and physical activity.

Basal metabolic rate (BMR) is a more precise measurement of REE that is taken immediately after waking and after a 12-hour fast to eliminate any residual metabolic response to food, or **specific dynamic action (SDA)**. SDA is the amount of energy that is required to digest, absorb, and metabolize food. In a normal mixed diet, the "cost" of processing food is about 10% of the total calorie intake. For instance, people who consume 1800 calories/day use about 180 to process their food. Therefore, REE and BMR differ by less than 10%, and the terms are generally used interchangeably.

FOOD *for* THOUGHT

A Calorie Is a Calorie Is a Calorie . . . or Is It?

Compared to the turn of the century, Americans are eating fewer calories but average weight continues to climb. True, our lifestyle is generally more sedentary because an increase in mechanization has caused us to burn fewer calories at work and at play. But we are also eating a greater percentage of our calories from fat, and research has shown that the more fat calories are consumed, the greater the tendency to gain weight, regardless of total calorie intake.

It appears that the body uses only 6% of the calories in fat to convert dietary fat into fat deposits, compared to using 23% of calories in carbohydrates to convert carbohydrate into adipose. In addition, carbohydrates appear to require more energy to be digested than previously thought, so actual available calories from carbohydrates are less. Simply stated, if two people with the same calorie requirements adhere to a 1200-calorie reduction diet, the one eating the fewest fat calories will lose weight faster. So it is not just how *much* we eat, but *what* we eat that determines body weight. And strike up another plus for complex carbohydrates.

PHYSICAL ACTIVITY

Unfortunately, mental activity requires little energy, although it may increase REE if it increases tension—and people may be *busy* without being physically active. Since the turn of the century, work-related energy expenditure has declined for most Americans because of the increase in mechanization and the proliferation of labor-saving devices.

The actual amount of energy that is expended on voluntary physical activity depends on the intensity and duration of the activity—the more intense and prolonged the activity, the greater the energy expended. Another factor is the weight of the person performing the activity. Heavier people, who have more weight to move, use more energy than lighter people to perform the same activity.

Numerous methods are available for estimating energy expenditure based on activity level (ie, sedentary, light, moderate, or heavy). Table 13-4 gives calories

Sample Calculation of the Number of Calories in a Food Based on Its CHO, Protein, and Fat Content

A piece of pumpkin pie containing 32 g CHO, 5 g protein, and 15 g fat contains

$$32 \text{ g CHO} \times 4 \text{ cal/g CHO} = 128 \text{ cal of CHO}$$
$$5 \text{ g pro} \times 4 \text{ cal/g pro} = 20 \text{ cal of protein}$$
$$\underline{15 \text{ g fat} \times 9 \text{ cal/g fat} = 135 \text{ cal of fat}}$$
$$283 \text{ total calories}$$

Table 13-2
Equations for Predicting Resting Energy Expenditure From Body Weight*

Sex and Age Range (years)	Equation to Derive REE in kcal/day	Sex and Age Range (years)	Equation to Derive REE in kcal/day
MEN		**WOMEN**	
0–3	(60.9 × wt†) − 54	0–3	(61.0 × wt) − 51
3–10	(22.7 × wt) + 495	3–10	(22.5 × wt) + 499
10–18	(17.5 × wt) + 651	10–18	(12.2 × wt) + 746
18–30	(15.3 × wt) + 679	18–30	(14.7 × wt) + 496
30–60	(11.6 × wt) + 879	30–60	(8.7 × wt) + 829
>60	(13.5 × wt) + 487	>60	(10.5 × wt) + 596

* From WHO (1985). These equations were derived from BMR data.
† Weight of person in kilograms.
(National Research Council: Recommended Dietary Allowances. 10th ed. Washington, DC: National Academy of Sciences, 1989)

expended per minute by the "average" man and woman for various activity levels. A quick method of estimating daily energy expenditure for voluntary (muscular) activities is to calculate the percent increase above REE based on the intensity of activity. For people who are mostly sedentary (mostly sitting), REE multiplied by 0.4 to 0.5 equals the number of calories spent on activity. The following values are used for more active people:

Table 13-3
The Impact of Variables on REE and Physical Activity

Variable	Effect on REE	Effect on Activity
Age	The amount and composition of active tissue is influenced by age. Lean body mass decreases after early adulthood by 2% to 3% per decade; REE declines proportionately.	Children are typically active. Activity generally decreases with age.
Sex	After maturity, men have a greater amount of lean body mass than women, which accounts for approximately 10% difference in REE between the sexes.	Due to an increase in the number of women in the workplace, work-related activity requirements are now similar for men and women.
Body Size	REE is higher for people with large body size compared to smaller people of the same sex and age.	The more a person weighs, the more calories are expended per unit of time performing activities.
Climate		
Cold	Exposure to cold that induces shivering results in an increase in REE.	Calorie expenditure may increase modestly as a result of carrying extra weight of cold weather clothing and footwear.
Heat	Environmental temperatures greater than 99°F increase REE by requiring more energy be spent to regulate body temperature.	Extreme heat may result in a voluntary reduction in physical activity.

Table 13-4
The Amount of Calories Expended/Minute Based on Activity and Weight

Activity	Cal/Min	
	70-kg Men	58-kg Women
Sleeping, reclining	1.0–1.2	0.9–1.1
Very light activity: seated and standing activities, painting, auto and truck driving, laboratory work, typing, playing musical instruments, sewing, ironing, walking slowly	Up to 2.5	Up to 2.0
Light activity: level walking at 2.5 mph to 3 mph, tailoring, pressing, garage work, electrical trades, carpentry, restaurant trades, cannery workers, washing clothes, shopping with light load, golfing, sailing, table tennis, volleyball	2.5–4.9	2.0–3.9
Moderate activity: walking 3.5 mph to 4 mph, plastering, gardening, loading and stacking bales, scrubbing floors, shopping with heavy load, cycling, skiing, tennis, dancing	5.0–7.4	4.0–5.9
Heavy activity: walking with load uphill, tree felling, working with pick and shovel, basketball, swimming, climbing, football, jogging, chopping wood	7.5–12.0	6.0–10.0

(Previte JJ: Human Physiology. New York: McGraw-Hill, 1983)

Lightly active: multiply REE by 0.55 − 0.65
Moderately active: multiply REE by 0.65 − 0.7
Heavy activity: multiply REE by .75 − 1.0

Total energy requirements can then be estimated by adding REE and calories for voluntary activity (see display, Estimating Total Calorie Needs). Although they are highly variable and individualized, average calorie requirements have been set by the National Research Council of the National Academy of Sciences (Table 13-5). Generally, calorie requirements are higher among men than among women, because men have a higher proportion of body weight that is muscle, which requires more energy to be maintained than fat tissue. Calorie requirements increase during periods of

Estimating Total Calorie Needs

To determine the total energy requirements for a lightly active 143-pound (65 kg) person:

Male	Female
1. CALCULATE REE:	
65 kg × 1 cal/kg × 24 h = 1560 cal/d	65 kg × 0.9 cal/kg × 24 h = 1404 cal/d
2. DETERMINE CALORIES FOR ACTIVITY:	
1560 × .55 = 858 cal	1404 × .55 = 772 cal
3. TOTAL REE AND ACTIVITY NEEDS:	
1560 + 858 = **2418 cal/d**	1404 + 772 = **2176 cal/d**

Table 13-5
Median Heights and Weights and Recommended Energy Intake

Category	Age (years) or Condition	Weight (kg)	Weight (lb)	Height (cm)	Height (in)	REE* (kcal/day)	Average Energy Allowance (kcal)† Multiples of REE	per kg	per day‡
INFANTS	0.0–0.5	6	13	60	24	320		108	650
	0.5–1.0	9	20	71	28	500		98	850
CHILDREN	1–3	13	29	90	35	740		102	1300
	4–6	20	44	112	44	950		90	1800
	7–10	28	62	132	52	1130		70	2000
MEN	11–14	45	99	157	62	1440	1.70	55	2500
	15–18	66	145	176	69	1760	1.67	45	3000
	19–24	72	160	177	70	1780	1.67	40	2900
	25–50	79	174	176	70	1800	1.60	37	2900
	51+	77	170	173	68	1530	1.50	30	2300
WOMEN	11–14	46	101	157	62	1310	1.67	47	2200
	15–18	55	120	163	64	1370	1.60	40	2200
	19–24	58	128	164	65	1350	1.60	38	2200
	25–50	63	138	163	64	1380	1.55	36	2200
	51+	65	143	160	63	1280	1.50	30	1900
PREGNANT	1st trimester								+0
	2nd trimester								+300
	3rd trimester								+300
LACTATING	1st 6 months								+500
	2nd 6 months								+500

* Calculation of REE (Resting Energy Expenditure) based on FAO equations, then rounded.
† In the range of light to moderate activity, the coefficient of variation is ±20%.
‡ Figure is rounded.
(National Research Council: Recommended Dietary Allowances. 10th ed. Washington, DC: National Academy of Sciences, 1989)

growth (infancy, childhood, adolescence, pregnancy, and lactation) and during periods of stress, illness, and recovery.

WEIGHT STANDARDS

Ideal Body Weight

"Ideal body weight" has yet to be conclusively defined; it is an imprecise term that is used to describe optimal weight for optimal health. Standards for ideal body weight are often controversial: Overweight people may regard them as overly harsh, whereas people who are underweight may argue that they are inflated. Because most Americans are overweight and gain weight as they age, the Fourth Edition of the *Dietary Guidelines for Americans* has initiated a change in terminology regarding weight recommendations (USDA, USDHHS, 1995). Instead of the previous "maintain healthy weight," Americans are now urged to "maintain or improve your weight." The "healthy" weight ranges that appear in Table 13-6 apply to men and

Table 13-6
Healthy Weight Ranges for Men and Women

Height*	Weight in Pounds†
4'10"	91–119
4'11"	94–124
5'0"	97–128
5'1"	101–132
5'2"	104–137
5'3"	107–141
5'4"	111–146
5'5"	114–150
5'6"	118–155
5'7"	121–160
5'8"	125–164
5'9"	129–169
5'10"	132–174
5'11"	136–179
6'0"	140–184
6'1"	144–189
6'2"	148–195
6'3"	152–200
6'4"	156–205
6'5"	160–211
6'6"	164–216

* Without shoes.
† Without clothes.
Source: Derived from National Research Council, 1989, for adults.

women of all ages. Weights at the higher end of each range represent people with more muscle and bone; the higher weights within any given range are not values intended to encourage people to gain weight.

The following guidelines for determining ideal body weight are generally accepted as appropriate for populations; they may or may not be appropriate for individuals, depending on muscle mass, body frame, other physiologic factors, and age.

Infants: Based on weight/age or weight/length (see growth charts in Appendix 9)
Children: Based on weight/age (see Chapter 11)
The standard "rule-of-thumb" formula (also known as the Hamwi formula) to determine ideal body weight (IBW) for adults over 5 feet tall:
  Adult Women:
  Allow 100 lb for 5 ft of height
  Add 5 lb for each additional inch over 5 ft
  Subtract 10% for small frame; add 10% for large frame
  Adult Men:
  Allow 106 lb for 5 ft of height
  Add 6 lb for each additional inch over 5 ft
  Subtract 10% for small frame; add 10% for large frame

E X A M P L E

IBW for a 5'6" adult is

	Female	Male
5' of height:	100 lb	106 lb
Per additional inch:	6" × 5 lb/" = 30 lb	6" × 6 lb/" = 36 lb
IBW equals:	130 lb ± 13 lb	142 lb ± 14 lb
	depending on frame size	depending on frame size

Metropolitan Life Insurance Tables

Initially, life insurance weight tables presented average weights of policyholders. As they were periodically updated, the tables developed into "ideal" weight tables based on mortality statistics. Although the weights indicated in the most recent edition (1983) of the *Metropolitan Life Insurance Tables* are associated with the lowest mortality rate (Table 13-7), they are not labeled "ideal" and are heavier values than were included in previous tables. A guide for estimating body size has also been included (Table 13-8).

EVALUATING BODY WEIGHT: BODY MASS INDEX

Body mass index (BMI), which is defined as weight in kilograms divided by height in meters squared, is the most frequently used measure of body fatness (Robinson et al, 1993). Because BMI has a low correlation with height, it allows comparison of weights between people of differing heights. Except for the complicated and impractical direct measurement of body fat, BMI is considered the best method of measuring obesity (Atkinson, 1993). For people of average height, one BMI unit equals approximately 3.1 kg (6.8 pounds) in men and 2.6 kg (5.8 pounds) in women (Williamson, 1993). Nomograms have been developed for men and women to make BMI a quick and easy assessment method (Fig. 13-2). Notice that women are expected to have smaller BMI than men because they have smaller bones and less muscle.

Using BMI to evaluate body weight is inexpensive, nonthreatening, and noninvasive to clients, and requires minimal equipment and skill. The major disadvantage of using BMI is that weight can be elevated for reasons other than excess fat, such as large muscle mass or edema.

So far, experts have not achieved a consensus on exact cutoff values for defining overweight, underweight, and obesity. The National Center for Health Statistics has defined overweight as a BMI of 27.8 or more in men and of 27.3 or more in women (Williams, 1993). These cutoffs correspond to approximately 20% above the desireable weights listed in the 1983 Metropolitan Life Insurance Tables. A BMI that is less than 20 for men and 19 for women is considered underweight. See display, Classification of Weight Status based on BMI.

Table 13-7
1983 Metropolitan Life Insurance Co. Height and Weight Tables

Height	Small Frame	Medium Frame	Large Frame
		lb	
MEN*			
5'2"	128–134	131–141	138–150
5'3"	130–136	133–143	140–153
5'4"	132–138	135–145	142–156
5'5"	134–140	137–148	144–160
5'6"	136–142	139–151	146–164
5'7"	138–145	142–154	149–168
5'8"	140–148	145–157	152–172
5'9"	142–151	148–160	155–176
5'10"	144–154	151–163	158–180
5'11"	146–157	154–166	161–184
6'0"	149–160	157–170	164–188
6'1"	152–164	160–174	168–192
6'2"	155–168	164–178	172–197
6'3"	158–172	167–182	176–202
6'4"	162–176	171–187	181–207
WOMEN†			
4'10"	102–111	109–121	118–131
4'11"	103–113	111–123	120–134
5'0"	104–115	113–126	122–137
5'1"	106–118	115–129	125–140
5'2"	108–121	118–132	128–143
5'3"	111–124	121–135	131–147
5'4"	114–127	124–138	134–151
5'5"	117–130	127–141	137–155
5'6"	120–133	130–144	140–159
5'7"	123–136	133–147	143–163
5'8"	126–139	136–150	146–167
5'9"	129–142	139–153	149–170
5'10"	132–145	142–156	152–173
5'11"	135–148	145–159	155–176
6'0"	138–151	148–162	158–179

* Weights at ages 25 to 59 based on lowest mortality. Weight in pounds according to frame (in indoor clothing weighing 5 lb, shoes with 1" heels).
† Weights at ages 25 to 59 based on lowest mortality. Weight in pounds according to frame (in indoor clothing weighing 3 lb, shoes with 1" heels).
(Courtesy of Metropolitan Life Insurance Company)

Table 13-8
How to Determine Your Body Frame by Elbow Breadth*

To make a simple approximation of your frame size:

Extend your arm and bend the forearm upwards at a 90° angle. Keep the fingers straight and turn the inside of your wrist toward the body. Place the thumb and index finger of your other hand on the two prominent bones on either side of your elbow. Measure the space between your fingers against a ruler or a tape measure. Compare this measurement with the measurements shown below.

These tables list the elbow measurements for men and women of medium frame at various heights. Measurements lower than those listed indicate that you have a small frame, while higher measurements indicate a larger frame.

Height (in 1" heels)	Elbow Breadth (in.)	Height (cm) (in 2.5-cm heels)	Elbow Breadth (cm)
MEN			
5'2"–5'3"	2½–2⅞	158–161	6.4–7.2
5'2"–5'7"	2⅝–2⅞	162–171	6.7–7.4
5'8"–5'11"	2¾–3	172–181	6.9–7.6
6'0"–6'3"	2¾–3⅛	182–191	7.1–7.8
6'4"	2⅞–3¼	192–193	7.4–8.1
WOMEN			
4'10"–4'11"	2¼–2½	148–151	5.6–6.4
5'0"–5'3"	2¼–2½	152–161	5.8–6.5
5'4"–5'7"	2⅜–2⅝	162–171	5.9–6.6
5'8"–5'11"	2⅜–2⅝	172–181	6.1–6.8
6'0"	2½–2¾	182–183	6.2–6.9

* Source of basic data: Data tape, HANES I. (Courtesy of Metropolitan Life Insurance Company)

EVALUATING BODY COMPOSITION AND DISTRIBUTION

Although weight standards provide a general guideline for ideal or desirable weight for height, they do not take into consideration body composition. A football player, for instance, may greatly exceed the average ideal weight range for his height because of a large muscle mass, not because he is too fat.

Weight standards also do not consider the distribution of body fat, which may be an important indicator of health risk. Within the last decade, the significance of body fat distribution has been studied. It appears that the location of excess fat deposition may be a more important and reliable indicator of health risk than the degree of total body fatness. People with a high distribution of abdominal fat (ie, "apples") have a greater health risk than people with lower body fatness (ie, "pears") (Fig. 13-3). Increased abdominal fat increases risks for coronary heart disease, hypertension, insulin resistance, hyperinsulinemia, diabetes mellitus, hyper-

Body mass index = (Weight [kilograms]/height [meters]^2).
Weights and heights shown are for adults without shoes and clothing.

FEMALES

Height, m (in.)

Weight kg (lb)	1.47 (58)	1.50 (59)	1.52 (60)	1.55 (61)	1.57 (62)	1.60 (63)	1.63 (64)	1.65 (65)	1.68 (66)	1.70 (67)	1.73 (68)	1.75 (69)	1.78 (70)	1.80 (71)	1.83 (72)	1.85 (73)	1.88 (74)	1.90 (75)	1.93 (76)
39 (85)	17.8	17.2	16.6	16.1	15.5	15.1	14.6	14.1	13.7	13.3	12.9	12.6	12.2	11.9	11.5	11.2	10.9	10.6	10.3
41 (90)	18.8	18.2	17.6	17.0	16.5	15.9	15.4	15.0	14.5	14.1	13.7	13.3	12.9	12.6	12.2	11.9	11.6	11.2	11.0
43 (95)	19.9	19.2	18.6	18.0	17.4	16.8	16.3	15.8	15.3	14.9	14.4	14.0	13.6	13.2	12.9	12.5	12.2	11.9	11.6
45 (100)	20.9	20.2	19.5	18.9	18.3	17.7	17.2	16.6	16.1	15.7	15.2	14.8	14.3	13.9	13.6	13.2	12.8	12.5	12.2
48 (105)	21.9	21.2	20.5	19.8	19.2	18.6	18.0	17.5	16.9	16.4	16.0	15.5	15.1	14.6	14.2	13.9	13.5	13.1	12.8
50 (110)	23.0	22.2	21.5	20.8	20.1	19.5	18.9	18.3	17.8	17.2	16.7	16.2	15.8	15.3	14.9	14.5	14.1	13.7	13.4
52 (115)	24.0	23.2	22.5	21.7	21.0	20.4	19.7	19.1	18.6	18.0	17.5	17.0	16.5	16.0	15.6	15.2	14.8	14.4	14.0
54 (120)	25.1	24.2	23.4	22.7	21.9	21.3	20.6	20.0	19.4	18.8	18.2	17.7	17.2	16.7	16.3	15.8	15.4	15.0	14.6
57 (125)	26.1	25.2	24.4	23.6	22.9	22.1	21.5	20.8	20.2	19.6	19.0	18.5	17.9	17.4	17.0	16.5	16.0	15.6	15.2
59 (130)	27.2	26.3	25.4	24.6	23.8	23.0	22.3	21.6	21.0	20.4	19.8	19.2	18.7	18.1	17.6	17.2	16.7	16.2	15.8
61 (135)	28.2	27.3	26.4	25.5	24.7	23.9	23.2	22.5	21.8	21.1	20.5	19.9	19.4	18.8	18.3	17.8	17.3	16.9	16.4
64 (140)	29.3	28.3	27.3	26.5	25.6	24.8	24.0	23.3	22.6	21.9	21.3	20.7	20.1	19.5	19.0	18.5	18.0	17.5	17.0
66 (145)	30.3	29.3	28.3	27.4	26.5	25.7	24.9	24.1	23.4	22.7	22.0	21.4	20.8	20.2	19.7	19.1	18.6	18.1	17.7
68 (150)	31.4	30.3	29.3	28.3	27.4	26.6	25.7	25.0	24.2	23.5	22.8	22.2	21.5	20.9	20.3	19.8	19.3	18.7	18.3
70 (155)	32.4	31.3	30.3	29.3	28.4	27.5	26.6	25.8	25.0	24.3	23.6	22.9	22.2	21.6	21.0	20.4	19.9	19.4	18.9
73 (160)	33.4	32.3	31.2	30.2	29.3	28.3	27.5	26.6	25.8	25.1	24.3	23.6	23.0	22.3	21.7	21.1	20.5	20.0	19.5
75 (165)	34.5	33.3	32.2	31.2	30.2	29.2	28.3	27.5	26.6	25.8	25.1	24.4	23.7	23.0	22.4	21.8	21.2	20.6	20.1
77 (170)	35.5	34.3	33.2	32.1	31.1	30.1	29.2	28.3	27.4	26.6	25.8	25.1	24.4	23.7	23.1	22.4	21.8	21.2	20.7
79 (175)	36.6	35.3	34.2	33.1	32.0	31.0	30.0	29.1	28.2	27.4	26.6	25.8	25.1	24.4	23.7	23.1	22.5	21.9	21.3
82 (180)	37.6	36.4	35.2	34.0	32.9	31.9	30.9	30.0	29.1	28.2	27.4	26.6	25.8	25.1	24.4	23.7	23.1	22.5	21.9
84 (185)	38.7	37.4	36.1	35.0	33.8	32.8	31.8	30.8	29.9	29.0	28.1	27.3	26.5	25.8	25.1	24.4	23.8	23.1	22.5
86 (190)	39.7	38.4	37.1	35.9	34.8	33.7	32.6	31.6	30.7	29.8	28.9	28.1	27.3	26.5	25.8	25.1	24.4	23.7	23.1
88 (195)	40.8	39.4	38.1	36.8	35.7	34.5	33.5	32.4	31.5	30.5	29.6	28.8	28.0	27.2	26.4	25.7	25.0	24.4	23.7
91 (200)	41.8	40.4	39.1	37.8	36.6	35.4	34.3	33.3	32.3	31.3	30.4	29.5	28.7	27.9	27.1	26.4	25.7	25.0	24.3
93 (205)	42.8	41.4	40.0	38.7	37.5	36.3	35.2	34.1	33.1	32.1	31.2	30.3	29.4	28.6	27.8	27.0	26.3	25.6	25.0
95 (210)	43.9	42.4	41.1	39.7	38.4	37.2	36.0	34.9	33.9	32.9	31.9	31.0	30.1	29.3	28.5	27.7	27.0	26.2	25.6
98 (215)	44.9	43.4	42.0	40.6	39.3	38.1	36.9	35.8	34.7	33.7	32.7	31.8	30.8	30.0	29.2	28.4	27.6	26.9	26.2
100 (220)	46.0	44.4	43.0	41.6	40.2	39.0	37.8	36.6	35.5	34.5	33.5	32.5	31.6	30.7	29.8	29.0	28.2	27.5	26.8
102 (225)	47.0	45.4	43.9	42.5	41.2	39.9	38.6	37.4	36.3	35.2	34.2	33.2	32.3	31.4	30.5	29.7	28.9	28.1	27.4
104 (230)	48.1	46.5	44.9	43.5	42.1	40.7	39.5	38.3	37.1	36.0	35.0	34.0	33.0	32.1	31.2	30.3	29.5	28.7	28.0
107 (235)	49.1	47.5	45.9	44.4	43.0	41.6	40.3	39.1	37.9	36.8	35.7	34.7	33.7	32.8	31.9	31.0	30.2	29.4	28.6
109 (240)	50.2	48.5	46.9	45.3	43.9	42.5	41.2	39.9	38.7	37.6	36.5	35.4	34.4	33.5	32.6	31.7	30.8	30.0	29.2
111 (245)	51.2	49.5	47.8	46.3	44.8	43.4	42.1	40.8	39.5	38.4	37.3	36.2	35.2	34.2	33.2	32.3	31.5	30.6	29.8
113 (250)	52.3	50.5	48.8	47.2	45.7	44.3	42.9	41.6	40.4	39.2	38.0	36.9	35.9	34.9	33.9	33.0	32.1	31.2	30.4
116 (255)	53.3	51.5	49.8	48.2	46.6	45.2	43.8	42.4	41.2	39.9	38.8	37.7	36.6	35.6	34.6	33.6	32.7	31.9	31.0
118 (260)	54.3	52.5	50.8	49.1	47.6	46.1	44.6	43.3	42.0	40.7	39.5	38.4	37.3	36.3	35.3	34.3	33.4	32.5	31.6
120 (265)	55.4	53.5	51.8	50.1	48.5	46.9	45.5	44.1	42.8	41.5	40.3	39.1	38.0	37.0	35.9	35.0	34.0	33.1	32.3
122 (270)	56.4	54.5	52.7	51.0	49.4	47.8	46.3	44.9	43.6	42.3	41.1	39.9	38.7	37.7	36.6	35.6	34.7	33.7	32.9
125 (275)	57.5	55.5	53.7	52.0	50.3	48.7	47.2	45.8	44.4	43.1	41.8	40.6	39.5	38.4	37.3	36.3	35.3	34.4	33.5
136 (300)	62.7	60.6	58.6	56.7	54.9	53.1	51.5	49.9	48.4	47.0	45.6	44.3	43.0	41.8	40.7	39.6	38.5	37.5	36.5
159 (350)	73.2	70.7	68.4	66.1	64.0	62.0	60.1	58.2	56.5	54.8	53.2	51.7	50.2	48.8	47.5	46.2	44.9	43.7	42.6
181 (400)	83.6	80.8	78.1	75.6	73.2	70.9	68.7	66.6	64.6	62.6	60.8	59.1	57.4	55.8	54.3	52.8	51.4	50.0	48.7

☐ Underweight ☐ Overweight
☐ Acceptable weight ☐ Severe overweight
☐ Marginal overweight ☐ Morbid obesity

Figure 13-2
Nomograms for BMI.

(continued on next page)

MALES

Height, m (in.)

Weight kg (lb)	1.47 (58)	1.50 (59)	1.52 (60)	1.55 (61)	1.57 (62)	1.60 (63)	1.63 (64)	1.65 (65)	1.68 (66)	1.70 (67)	1.73 (68)	1.75 (69)	1.78 (70)	1.80 (71)	1.83 (72)	1.85 (73)	1.88 (74)	1.90 (75)	1.93 (76)
39 (85)	17.8	17.2	16.6	16.1	15.5	15.1	14.6	14.1	13.7	13.3	12.9	12.6	12.2	11.9	11.5	11.2	10.9	10.6	10.3
41 (90)	18.8	18.2	17.6	17.0	16.5	15.9	15.4	15.0	14.5	14.1	13.7	13.3	12.9	12.6	12.2	11.9	11.6	11.2	11.0
43 (95)	19.9	19.2	18.6	18.0	17.4	16.8	16.3	15.8	15.3	14.9	14.4	14.0	13.6	13.2	12.9	12.5	12.2	11.9	11.6
45 (100)	20.9	20.2	19.5	18.9	18.3	17.7	17.2	16.6	16.1	15.7	15.2	14.8	14.3	13.9	13.6	13.2	12.8	12.5	12.2
48 (105)	21.9	21.2	20.5	19.8	19.2	18.6	18.0	17.5	16.9	16.4	16.0	15.5	15.1	14.6	14.2	13.9	13.5	13.1	12.8
50 (110)	23.0	22.2	21.5	20.8	20.1	19.5	18.9	18.3	17.8	17.2	16.7	16.2	15.8	15.3	14.9	14.5	14.1	13.7	13.4
52 (115)	24.0	23.2	22.5	21.7	21.0	20.4	19.7	19.1	18.6	18.0	17.5	17.0	16.5	16.0	15.6	15.2	14.8	14.4	14.0
54 (120)	25.1	24.2	23.4	22.7	21.9	21.3	20.6	20.0	19.4	18.8	18.2	17.7	17.2	16.7	16.3	15.8	15.4	15.0	14.6
57 (125)	26.1	25.2	24.4	23.6	22.9	22.1	21.5	20.8	20.2	19.6	19.0	18.5	17.9	17.4	17.0	16.5	16.0	15.6	15.2
59 (130)	27.2	26.3	25.4	24.6	23.8	23.0	22.3	21.6	21.0	20.4	19.8	19.2	18.7	18.1	17.6	17.2	16.7	16.2	15.8
61 (135)	28.2	27.3	26.4	25.5	24.7	23.9	23.2	22.5	21.8	21.1	20.5	19.9	19.4	18.8	18.3	17.8	17.3	16.9	16.4
64 (140)	29.3	28.3	27.3	26.5	25.6	24.8	24.0	23.3	22.6	21.9	21.3	20.7	20.1	19.5	19.0	18.5	18.0	17.5	17.0
66 (145)	30.3	29.3	28.3	27.4	26.5	25.7	24.9	24.1	23.4	22.7	22.0	21.4	20.8	20.2	19.7	19.1	18.6	18.1	17.7
68 (150)	31.4	30.3	29.3	28.3	27.4	26.6	25.7	25.0	24.2	23.5	22.8	22.2	21.5	20.9	20.3	19.8	19.3	18.7	18.3
70 (155)	32.4	31.3	30.3	29.3	28.4	27.5	26.6	25.8	25.0	24.3	23.6	22.9	22.2	21.6	21.0	20.4	19.9	19.4	18.9
73 (160)	33.4	32.3	31.2	30.2	29.3	28.3	27.5	26.6	25.8	25.1	24.3	23.6	23.0	22.3	21.7	21.1	20.5	20.0	19.5
75 (165)	34.5	33.3	32.2	31.2	30.2	29.2	28.3	27.5	26.6	25.8	25.1	24.4	23.7	23.0	22.4	21.8	21.2	20.6	20.1
77 (170)	35.5	34.3	33.2	32.1	31.1	30.1	29.2	28.3	27.4	26.6	25.8	25.1	24.4	23.7	23.1	22.4	21.8	21.2	20.7
79 (175)	36.6	35.3	34.2	33.1	32.0	31.0	30.0	29.1	28.2	27.4	26.6	25.8	25.1	24.4	23.7	23.1	22.5	21.9	21.3
82 (180)	37.6	36.4	35.2	34.0	32.9	31.9	30.9	30.0	29.1	28.2	27.4	26.6	25.8	25.1	24.4	23.7	23.1	22.5	21.9
84 (185)	38.7	37.4	36.1	35.0	33.8	32.8	31.8	30.8	29.9	29.0	28.1	27.3	26.5	25.8	25.1	24.4	23.8	23.1	22.5
86 (190)	39.7	38.4	37.1	35.9	34.8	33.7	32.6	31.6	30.7	29.8	28.9	28.1	27.3	26.5	25.8	25.1	24.4	23.7	23.1
88 (195)	40.8	39.4	38.1	36.8	35.7	34.5	33.5	32.4	31.5	30.5	29.6	28.8	28.0	27.2	26.4	25.7	25.0	24.4	23.7
91 (200)	41.8	40.4	39.1	37.8	36.6	35.4	34.3	33.3	32.3	31.3	30.4	29.5	28.7	27.9	27.1	26.4	25.7	25.0	24.3
93 (205)	42.8	41.4	40.0	38.7	37.5	36.3	35.2	34.1	33.1	32.1	31.2	30.3	29.4	28.6	27.8	27.0	26.3	25.6	25.0
95 (210)	43.9	42.4	41.1	39.7	38.4	37.2	36.0	34.9	33.9	32.9	31.9	31.0	30.1	29.3	28.5	27.7	27.0	26.2	25.6
98 (215)	44.9	43.4	42.0	40.6	39.3	38.1	36.9	35.8	34.7	33.7	32.7	31.8	30.8	30.0	29.2	28.4	27.6	26.9	26.2
100 (220)	46.0	44.4	43.0	41.6	40.2	39.0	37.8	36.6	35.5	34.5	33.5	32.5	31.6	30.7	29.8	29.0	28.2	27.5	26.8
102 (225)	47.0	45.4	43.9	42.5	41.2	39.9	38.6	37.4	36.3	35.2	34.2	33.2	32.3	31.4	30.5	29.7	28.9	28.1	27.4
104 (230)	48.1	46.5	44.9	43.5	42.1	40.7	39.5	38.3	37.1	36.0	35.0	34.0	33.0	32.1	31.2	30.3	29.5	28.7	28.0
107 (235)	49.1	47.5	45.9	44.4	43.0	41.6	40.3	39.1	37.9	36.8	35.7	34.7	33.7	32.8	31.9	31.0	30.2	29.4	28.6
109 (240)	50.2	48.5	46.9	45.3	43.9	42.5	41.2	39.9	38.7	37.6	36.5	35.4	34.4	33.5	32.6	31.7	30.8	30.0	29.2
111 (245)	51.2	49.5	47.8	46.3	44.8	43.4	42.1	40.8	39.5	38.4	37.3	36.2	35.2	34.2	33.2	32.3	31.5	30.6	29.8
113 (250)	52.3	50.5	48.8	47.2	45.7	44.3	42.9	41.6	40.4	39.2	38.0	36.9	35.9	34.9	33.9	33.0	32.1	31.2	30.4
116 (255)	53.3	51.5	49.8	48.2	46.6	45.2	43.8	42.4	41.2	39.9	38.8	37.7	36.6	35.6	34.6	33.6	32.7	31.9	31.0
118 (260)	54.3	52.5	50.8	49.1	47.6	46.1	44.6	43.3	42.0	40.7	39.5	38.4	37.3	36.3	35.3	34.3	33.4	32.5	31.6
120 (265)	55.4	53.5	51.8	50.1	48.5	46.9	45.5	44.1	42.8	41.5	40.3	39.1	38.0	37.0	35.9	35.0	34.0	33.1	32.3
122 (270)	56.4	54.5	52.7	51.0	49.4	47.8	46.3	44.9	43.6	42.3	41.1	39.9	38.7	37.7	36.6	35.6	34.7	33.7	32.9
125 (275)	57.5	55.5	53.7	52.0	50.3	48.7	47.2	45.8	44.4	43.1	41.8	40.6	39.5	38.4	37.3	36.3	35.3	34.4	33.5
136 (300)	62.7	60.6	58.6	56.7	54.9	53.1	51.5	49.9	48.4	47.0	45.6	44.3	43.0	41.8	40.7	39.6	38.5	37.5	36.5
159 (350)	73.2	70.7	68.4	66.1	64.0	62.0	60.1	58.2	56.5	54.8	53.2	51.7	50.2	48.8	47.5	46.2	44.9	43.7	42.6
181 (400)	83.6	80.8	78.1	75.6	73.2	70.9	68.7	66.6	64.6	62.6	60.8	59.1	57.4	55.8	54.3	52.8	51.4	50.0	48.7

☐ Underweight   ☐ Overweight
☐ Acceptable weight   ☐ Severe overweight
☐ Marginal overweight   ■ Morbid obesity

*Rowland ML: A nomogram for computing body mass index.
Dietetic Currents, vol 16, no. 2. Columbus, Ohio, Ross Laboratories, 1989, pp 5-12.

Figure 13-2 *(continued)*

Classification of Weight Status Based on BMI

	BMI	
	Men	*Women*
Overweight	27.8	27.3
(about 20% above desirable weight in Metropolitan Life Insurance tables)		
Severe obesity	31.1	32.3
(about 40% above desirable weight)		

From: Williamson, D. (1993) Descriptive epidemiology of body weight and weight change in US adults. Ann Intern Med, 119 (7 part 2) 646–649.

triglyceridemia, and low–high-density lipoprotein (HDL) cholesterol (Pi-Sunyer, 1993). Simple measurements of body fat appear in the display, Body Fat Check.

Waist:Hip Ratio

The **waist:hip ratio** is an easy method of determining upper body fatness: A high waist:hip ratio indicates a high distribution of abdominal fat and increased health risk. Waist:hip ratio can be obtained by dividing the waist measurement by the measurement of the hips taken at the widest point. Values should be less than 0.95 in men and less than 0.80 in women.

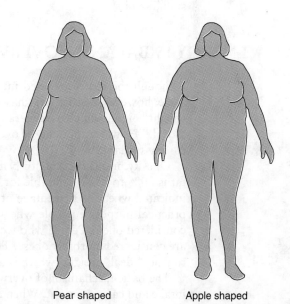

Figure 13-3

"Apple" shape vs. "pear" shape.

Pear shaped   Apple shaped

Body Fat Check

Mirror Test: Looking in the mirror can tell a great deal about body composition, without taking any kind of measurements.

Pinch Test: If you can pinch more than 1 inch of skin between the thumb and forefinger on the back of the upper arm, you're overfat.

Ruler Test: While lying on your back, place a 12-inch ruler on the stomach with the ends pointing toward the head and toes. If both ends of the ruler do not touch the body, you're overfat.

Skinfold Measurement

Skinfold measurements, which may be taken at the biceps, triceps, or subscapular or suprailiac region, provide an objective measurement of subcutaneous fat stores. Unfortunately, training and skill are required to obtain reliable measurements, and equipment is needed. See Chapter 9 for the procedure and interpretation of triceps skinfold measurements.

Laboratory Tests

Clinically impractical, objective measurements of body fatness can be obtained through the water displacement test: The percentage of body fat can be determined by measuring the amount of water that is displaced when a person is weighed underwater. Radioactive potassium counting, a procedure that has been used only for research purposes, measures lean body tissue by "counting" the radioactive potassium it emits.

ENERGY IMBALANCE: OVERWEIGHT AND OBESITY

Although the terms are used interchangeably, overweight and obesity are not the same; however, neither term has been precisely defined. **Overweight** refers to excess weight/height, which is generally considered as weight up to 20% higher than "ideal." However, one can be overweight without being overfat, particularly if muscle mass is large.

Obesity means the state of being overfat. For women, the desirable percent body fat is 20% to 25%; desirable for men is 15% to 18% body fat. Obesity (overfat) is indicated when the percentage of fat exceeds 30% in women and 25% in men. For practical purposes, people who weight 120% or more of their "ideal" weight are considered obese. People who weigh 100 pounds or more over their "ideal" weight are considered morbidly obese. The problem with all of these definitions is that they rely on "ideal" weight, which is also not precisely defined.

The basic mechanism of overweight and obesity is an imbalance between calorie intake and calorie output. When energy consumption exceeds energy expenditure, a positive energy balance results, leading to a weight gain over time. This can be caused by overeating, inactivity, or, most often, a combination of both. For instance, 1 pound of body fat equals 3500 calories; therefore, eating 500 extra cal/day for 7 days will produce a 1-lb weight gain. A person will gain 2 lb/week if daily intake exceeds expenditure by 1000 cal/day. Even a seemingly insignificant 1 extra glass of soft drink that supplies 145 calories will produce a 15-lb weight gain in a year if it is consumed daily and is not offset by an increase in activity.

$$145 \text{ cal} \times 365 \text{ days/year} = 52,925 \text{ extra cal/year}$$

$$\frac{52,925 \text{ cal/year}}{3500 \text{ cal/lb}} = 15 \text{ lb/year}$$

Although society in general assumes that obese people consume hoards of food, research has shown that many obese people actually eat less than their thin counterparts. The snowball effect of inactivity and increased weight perpetuates obesity—that is, inactivity can lead to increased weight, and weight gain can lead to social isolation and further reduction in activity (Fig. 13-4). Inactivity has been identified as a major cause of obesity among Americans.

Results from The National Health and Nutrition Examination Surveys (NHANES III) that were conducted from 1988 to 1991 reveal that for all racial and

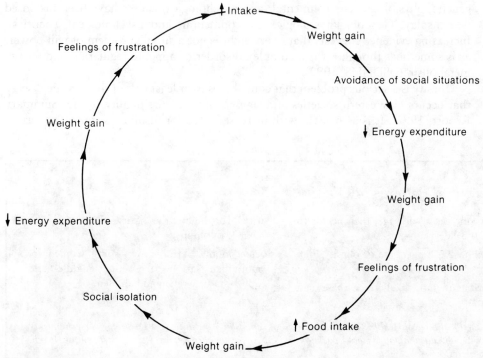

Figure 13-4
Perpetuating cycle of inactivity and weight gain.

ethnic groups in the United States combined, 31% of adult men and 35% of adult women are estimated to be overweight, with overweight defined as a BMI greater than or equal to 27.8 for men and greater than or equal to 27.3 for women (Kuczmarski et al, 1994). The incidence varies by race, ethnicity, sex, and age. This finding indicates a dramatic increase in the prevalence of overweight from the previous NHANES II study that was conducted from 1976 to 1980, during which 24% of both men and women for all racial and ethnic groups were overweight.

Despite the high incidence of overweight, the *perceived* incidence of overweight is even higher, especially among American women who are vulnerable to society's preoccupation with thinness. In 1990, 45% of Americans considered themselves overweight: 36.7% of men and 52% of women (Horm and Anderson, 1993). Reportedly, 25% of all men and 40% of all women in the United States are trying to lose weight at any given time (National Task Force on the Prevention and Treatment of Obesity, 1994). Although 58 million Americans are considered overweight, 65 million are dieting (Allred, 1995). Approximately 30% of people who are trying to lose weight are considered chronic dieters, who claim to be "dieting" for at least 1 year (Levy and Heaton, 1993).

The etiology of overweight and obesity is complex and multifactorial and differs among individuals. Sociocultural factors may be the most important influences on the prevalence of obesity (Summary Report, 1993) (see display, Sociocultural Patterns of Obesity). Black women have the highest prevalence of overweight at almost 49% of all those 20 years of age and older (Kuczmarski et al, 1994). Numerous genetic, physiologic, environmental, and psychological causes have been proposed (see display, Genetic, Physiologic, Environmental, and Psychological Theories). Increasing evidence suggests that overweight is not a simple problem of will power, as is sometimes thought; it is a complex disorder of appetite regulation and energy metabolism (USDHHS, 1992).

Obesity is a serious problem that contributes to at least half of the chronic disease that occurs in Western societies and significantly impairs quality of life (Summary Report, 1992). It is associated with increased risks for insulin resistance, hyperten-

Sociocultural Patterns of Obesity

Age: Obesity increases with age, then begins to decline in the elderly.

Sex: Females have a higher rate of obesity than males.

Race: Minorities are more likely to be obese than Caucasians.

Parity: The higher the parity, the greater the chance of obesity.

Socioeconomic Status: Lower-status women are more likely to be obese than middle- and upper-status women and all men.

From: National Institutes of Health, National Heart, Lung, and Blood Institute. (1992). Strategy Development Workshop for Public Education on Weight Education and Obesity: Summary Report. U.S. Department of Health and Human Services.

Genetic, Physiologic, Environmental, and Psychological Theories Related to the Etiology of Obesity

GENETIC THEORIES

Faulty ATP production: Obese people have lower levels of ATPase, an enzyme responsible for 15% to 40% of all the energy use not associated with physical activity. Because obese people have less ATPase than thin people, they use less energy performing metabolic activities.

Familial traits: The weight of natural children is highly correlated to that of their natural parents, whereas there is only a slight correlation between the weight of adopted children and their adoptive parents.

PHYSIOLOGIC THEORIES

Fat cell theory: People of normal weight have approximately 30 billion fat cells; morbidly obese people may have three to five times more. Although the biggest increase in the number of fat cells occurs from birth to age 5 and from 7 to 11, the number of fat cells can increase at any age. Once created, a fat cell exists for life. Fat cells can shrink in size when fat is broken down for energy, but the number of fat cells remains the same. Hence, obese people have extreme difficulty losing weight because of biologic pressures to keep the fat cells supplied with energy.

"Set point" theory: A center in the hypothalamus determines a "set point" or ideal biologic weight for the individual. When weight falls below what the body has determined as "ideal," metabolic rate is adjusted downward to reduce energy expenditure and conserve fat stores. Weight reduction becomes increasingly difficult below an individual's set point.

Brown fat: Obese people have less brown fat than people of normal weight, and therefore expend less energy producing heat through nonshivering or diet-induced thermogenesis.

Insulin response: Obese people respond more readily to external cues, such as the sight, sound, or smell of food, which stimulate the release of insulin. An increase in insulin → decrease blood glucose levels → the sensation of hunger and an increase in lipogenesis (fat formation).

Hormonal imbalances: An underactive thyroid gland → inadequate secretion of thyroid hormone → low BMR → weight gain.

ENVIRONMENTAL THEORIES

Food environment: An abundance of food may entice some people to overeat.

Family environment: A child with no obese parents has a 10% chance of becoming obese; with one obese parent, the chance increases to 40%; and if both parents are obese, children have a 80% chance of becoming obese, possibly related to familial eating patterns and attitudes regarding food and obesity.

Work environment: The mechanization of America has led to a decrease in energy expenditure. Likewise, even though work days and work weeks are generally shorter than at the turn of the century, people tend to spend their increased leisure time observing rather than participating in activities.

PSYCHOLOGICAL THEORIES

Obese people overeat

Because they have a compulsive behavioral disorder similar to alcoholics and drug abusers: Food controls the person's actions

As an emotional crutch

To compensate for a lack of affection, love, and companionship

To relieve boredom, tension, anxiety, and frustration

sion, hyperlipidemia, cardiovascular disease, non–insulin dependent diabetes, gallstones and cholecystitis, and respiratory dysfunction (Pi-Sunyer, 1993). Obese men have higher mortality rates for colorectal and prostate cancers, and overweight women have significantly higher rates of endometrial, gallbladder, cervical, ovarian, and breast cancers, although it is difficult to determine whether these effects are the result of obesity or of a high-fat, high-calorie diet. Obesity increases surgical risks, and it is associated with complications during pregnancy, labor, and delivery. Evidence suggests that obese people have a higher mortality and morbidity than their thin counterparts. However, it is important to remember that overweight does not automatically imply poor health (Cassell, 1995).

Obesity also presents psychological and social disadvantages. In a society that emphasizes thinness, obesity leads to feelings of low self-esteem, negative self-image, and hopelessness (Summary Report, 1992). Negative social consequences include stereotyping, prejudice, stigmatization, social isolation, and discrimination in social, educational, and employment settings.

Treatment

Because of its chronic nature and its complex, multifactorial origin, obesity is resistant to treatment and is rarely cured (Bray, 1993). In fact, there is no standard to even define successful treatment of obesity (Atkinson, 1993). For instance, moderate weight loss (10%–15% of body weight) decreases health risks and medical problems in 90% of obese people, even if "ideal" weight is not achieved (Robinson et al, 1995). Therefore, "success" is better measured by long-term improvements in health and improved quality of life, with or without weight loss (Robinson et al, 1995). Limiting "success" to weight loss alone inappropriately focuses on the symptom rather than the underlying problem. It may also create more problems than it solves by contributing to the increase in eating disorders (Robinson et al, 1995).

Unlike other chronic diseases such as diabetes and heart disease, obesity is usually treated without medical supervision (Blackburn, 1993). Americans spend $30–$50 billion annually on weight loss products and services (Robinson et al, 1993). Most commercial weight loss programs combine diet, exercise, and behavioral modification. Unfortunately, scientific studies on the effectiveness and safety of many of these programs are limited. In general, people tend to lose weight while they are enrolled in these programs, but they often regain weight after the program is completed. As such, conventional weight loss programs have been largely ineffective: Studies show that people who complete weight loss programs lose only 10% of their body weight and gain almost all of it back within 5 years (Committee to Develop Criteria . . . , 1995). Actual success rates vary with amount of initial weight, the length of the treatment period, the amount of weight loss desired, and the client's level of motivation (USDHHS, 1992).

Treatment programs vary according to the degree of overweightness, although there are key components that are common to all successful weight-control programs (Table 13-9). Approaches that focus on social support, a more active lifestyle, behavior modification, and, for moderately to morbidly obese patients, rapid weight loss diets, appear to be more effective than diet alone. Surgery and drug therapy are other options.

Table 13-9
Comparison of Treatment Components for Overweight and Obesity

	Degree of Overweightness	
Treatment Component	*Overweight →* **Mild Obesity**	*Moderate →* **Morbid Obesity**
Social support	X	X
Increased exercise	X	X
Behavior modification	X	X
Moderate calorie-restricted diet	X	
Very-low-calorie diet (VLCD)		X
Surgery		+
Drug therapy		+

"X" indicates appropriateness.
"+" indicates may be appropriate.

The problem with all obesity treatments is that weight slowly returns to baseline after the treatment ends (Foreyt and Goodrick, 1993). The repeated loss and regain of weight is known as **weight cycling**. It was once thought to be more harmful than static obesity; however, according to newer studies, there is no convincing evidence that weight cycling has adverse effects on body composition, energy expenditure, risk factors for cardiovascular disease, or the effectiveness of future weight loss attempts (National Task Force on the Prevention and Treatment of Obesity, 1994). They conclude that fears about weight cycling should not deter overweight people from trying to lose weight.

SOCIAL SUPPORT

Because social background and environment have a far greater and longer-lasting impact on an individual's food choices than information provided by a health professional, social support may be central to the success of any weight control program. Clearly, weight loss can be helped or hindered by family and friends. Some studies show that a disinterested or only marginally involved spouse may actually increase the likelihood of failure to lose weight (Parham, 1993). More common than couples programs are group programs, which provide social support through shared experiences, mutual understanding, and a sense of responsibility to each other. Group therapy is shown to be more effective than individualized therapy, even though actual contact with a health professional is less. Also, there is the potential for strong social support in the work setting, which results from the social relationships that develop and the close, almost daily interaction among workers. For children, parental involvement and school programs may be effective.

EXERCISE

In response to recommendations that have been made by leading health authorities, many Americans are adopting aerobic exercise activities for cardiovascular and weight-control benefits. Certainly, adding exercise to diet intervention produces more weight loss than can be attained by dieting alone: Exercise stimulates metabolic rate, thereby offsetting the compensatory decrease in REE that occurs within days when calorie intake is restricted. A sustained increase in REE that is induced by exercise prevails even after exercise ceases. Studies show that the body burns calories at a faster rate for 40 to 90 minutes post exercise: The increase appears to be greatest among beginning exercisers.

Although some people claim that the benefits of exercise are offset by an increase in appetite, research does not support this idea. In fact, animal and human studies indicate that exercise helps suppress appetite, and that even though vigorous exercisers do increase their food intake, the increase is not enough to prevent weight loss.

Exercise changes body composition by decreasing the percentage of fat and increasing the amount of lean body mass, which requires more calories to be maintained than fat. So, although initial weight loss may not be apparent because the weight of the lean body mass that develops offsets the weight of the fat that is lost, body dimensions improve and metabolic rate increases. Eventually the gain in lean body tissue is less than the weight of fat lost, and weight loss results. Exercise also reduces the waist:hip ratio, thus favorably altering the distribution of body fat (Blair, 1993).

Lowered blood pressure and serum glucose levels and an increase in HDL cholesterol are additional benefits of exercise, as is a subjective improvement in sense of well-being, reduced tension, increased agility, and improved alertness. However, exercise should be practiced with caution by people with back problems, hypertension, and insulin-dependent diabetes.

BEHAVIOR MODIFICATION

"Dieting" has negative connotations and is viewed by most people as a form of punishment or a short-term hurdle to be overcome. In order for a weight-control program to be successful and long-lasting, a permanent change in eating attitudes and behaviors must occur. Without a permanent lifestyle change, the perpetual cycle of weight loss followed by weight gain is inevitable.

Behavior modification, which is a conceptual approach to altering behavior, is widely used by many commercial programs and self-help groups such as Weight Watchers and TOPS (Take Off Pounds Sensibly). It involves 1) identifying eating and exercise behaviors that need improving, 2) setting specific behavioral goals, 3) modifying the "problem" behaviors, and 4) providing positive reinforcement of the desired behavior (USDHHS, 1992). Behavior modification can be practiced individually or in a group, alone or combined with other approaches.

Behavior modification is an essential component of any weight loss program because it offers techniques on "how to" and "how not to" change eating behaviors, rather than the standard list of "do's" and "don'ts" that is offered to most dieters (see display, Behavior Modification Techniques). Self-monitoring, such as recording food intake and the behaviors, thoughts, and feelings that occur before, during, and after eating and exercise, is a vital component of behavior modification (Foreyt and Goodrick, 1993). "Bad" eating behaviors are reprogrammed and "good" habits are reinforced. Positive reinforcement for achieving realistic goals is stressed.

Behavior Modification Techniques

THINK THIN

- Make a list of reasons why you want to lose weight before beginning a diet.
- Set long-term goals; avoid crash dieting based on getting into a particular dress or weighing a certain weight for an upcoming event or occasion.
- Give yourself a nonfood reward like new clothes or a night of entertainment for losing weight.
- Don't talk about food.
- Enlist the support of family and friends.
- Learn to distinguish hunger from cravings.

PLANNING

- Keep food only in the kitchen, not scattered around the house.
- Stay out of the kitchen except when preparing meals and cleaning up.
- Avoid tasting food while cooking; don't take extra portions in order to get rid of a food.
- Place the low-calorie foods in the front of the refrigerator; keep the high-calorie foods hidden.
- Remove temptation to better resist it; "out of sight, out of mind."
- Keep forbidden foods to a minimum.
- Plan meals, snacks, and grocery shopping to help eliminate hasty decisions and impulses that may sabotage dieting.

EATING

- Wait 10 minutes before eating when you feel the urge; hunger pangs may go away if you delay eating.
- Never skip meals.
- Eat only in one designated place and devote all your attention to eating. Activities like reading and watching television can be so distracting that you may not even realize you ate.

- Serve food directly from the stove to the plate instead of family style, which can lead to large portions and second helpings.
- Eat the low-calorie foods first.
- Use a small plate to give the appearance of eating a full plate.
- Chew food thoroughly and eat slowly.
- Put utensils down between mouthfuls.
- Leave some food on your plate to help you feel in control of food rather than having food control you.
- Eat before attending a social function that features food; while there, select low-calorie foods to nibble on.

SHOPPING

- Never shop while hungry.
- Shop only from a list; resist impulse buying.
- Buy food only in the quantity you need.
- Don't buy foods you find tempting.
- Buy low-calorie foods for when you need a snack.

LIFESTYLE CHANGES

- Keep busy with hobbies or projects that are incompatible with eating to take your mind off dieting and eating.
- Accept "diet" as it is really defined—a way of eating—not as a temporary reduction in calories that must be endured before "normal" eating habits can be resumed.
- Trim recipes of extra fat and sugar.
- Don't weigh yourself too often.
- If you eat something you shouldn't, accept it and go on with your plan. Don't let disappointment lure you into a real eating binge.
- Exercise.
- Get more sleep if fatigue triggers eating.

DIET INTERVENTION

Diet is the most frequently used approach to weight loss (USDHHS, 1992). Studies show that most people who are trying to lose weight seek weight loss information from friends, family, television, newspapers, or magazines, instead of from health professionals (Levy and Heaton, 1993).

Weight Loss Diets for the Overweight to Mildly Obese

For overweight to mildly obese clients, a nutritionally adequate diet that is mildly restricted in calories and allows for a 1- to 2-pound weight loss per week may be the safest and most effective method of achieving weight loss. Generally, calorie intake should not fall below 1200 calories for adult women and 1500 calories for adult men. Diets that provide less than 1200 calories may not provide adequate amounts of essential nutrients.

Individually, the number of calories needed for weight loss can be calculated by determining the number of calories needed to maintain ideal body weight and subtracting 500 to 1000 cal/day for a 1- to 2-lb weight loss per week, respectively. (500 cal/day $\times$ 7 days/week = 3500-calorie deficit/week, the equivalent of 1 lb of body weight; or 1000 cal/day $\times$ 7 days/week = 7000-calorie deficit/week, the equivalent of 2 lb of body weight.)

E X A M P L E
For the man and woman in the previous example to
Lose 1 lb/week:

Man	Woman
2418 cal − 500 cal = **1918 cal/d**	2176 cal − 500 cal = **1676 cal/d**

Lose 2 lb/week:

2418 cal − 1000 cal = **1418 cal/d**	2176 cal − 1000 cal = **1176 cal/d**

Remember it is generally recommended that men not consume fewer than 1500 calories/day, women not less than 1200 calories/day; neither may be getting adequate nutrition if they try to lose 2 pounds/week.

After desired weight loss has been achieved, the diet can be liberalized to provide enough calories for weight maintenance. However, because body mass is smaller, maintenance energy requirements are reduced after weight loss. As can be seen in Table 13-4, lighter people burn fewer calories than heavier people when doing the same activity.

There are numerous weight-loss diets available, and no one approach is ideal for all people. Important criteria for evaluating any weight-reduction diet are listed in the display, Criteria for Evaluating Weight-Reduction Diets. Low-calorie diets can be followed using the following methods.

Counting Calories

Unfortunately, counting calories does not ensure a nutritionally adequate diet. It is possible to lose weight on a diet that consists only of soft drinks and french fries, as long as the total calorie intake is less than total calorie expenditure. In addition, counting calories does not have long-term possibilities. Who would carry around a food composition table, paper, pencil, and calculator indefinitely?

Criteria for Evaluating Weight-Reduction Diets

A sound weight-reduction diet should

- Be realistic and flexible; that is, easily adaptable to your lifestyle and based on individual calorie requirements
- Suggest that a doctor be consulted
- Use food to meet nutritional requirements rather than vitamin or mineral supplements
- Encourage foods from each of the major food groups
- Meet the RDA for all nutrients
- Promote nutrition education
- Recommend exercise
- Promote a 1-lb to 2-lb weight loss/week

- Have long-term possibilities; diets recommended for only short periods of time obviously are not safe
- Be comprised of 50% to 55% carbohydrates, approximately 20% protein, and less than 30% fat
- Allow nutritious, low-calorie snacks
- Emphasize portion control
- Emphasize the need for behavior modification to attain and maintain weight loss
- Offer a maintenance plan after weight loss is achieved.

Counting Fat Grams

Because the body so efficiently processes fat, and because fat provides more than twice the calories contained in an equivalent amount of either carbohydrate or protein, low-fat diets seem effective at promoting weight loss, and even more effective at preventing the reaccumulation of fat after weight loss (Hill et al, 1993), if total calorie intake is less than total energy expended. It is recommended that fat should contribute less than 30% of total calories in all adult diets; "dieters" may benefit from limiting their fat intake to 20% to 25% of calories (see display, Fat Gram Guidelines).

Unfortunately, by focusing solely on fat content, the importance of nutrition and total calorie content may be overlooked. Indeed, many people believe that if a food is low in fat, they can have unlimited amounts without gaining weight (Allred, 1995).

Fat Gram Guidelines

	Grams of Total Fat Based on the Following Percentage of Total Calories		
Total Calories	20%	25%	30%
1200	27	33	40
1500	33	42	50
1600	36	44	53
1800	40	50	60
2000	44	56	67
2200	49	61	73

Data from NHANES III indicate that, although the percent of calories from fat in the diet has decreased over the last 45 years, the percentage of overweight Americans has increased. Obviously, losing weight is not as simple as limiting fat intake.

Eliminating Extras and Second Portions

This approach may produce a consistent, gradual weight loss for clients who do not have a lot of weight to lose. It may be particularly effective for children in that it enables them to "outgrow" their overweightness without actually losing weight and "dieting." For some adults, this approach may rely too much on willpower and self-control to be effective.

Using American Diabetic Association Exchange Lists for Meal Planning

The American Diabetic Association exchange lists and meal patterns, which are described in Chapter 18, allow flexibility in food choices. They are nutritionally adequate and consistent in calorie intake. A daily food allowance and sample menu for a 1500-calorie diet is shown in Table 13-10. For greatest client compliance, meal patterns should correlate as closely as possible with the individual's normal pattern of eating and likes and dislikes.

Self-help Groups Such as Weight Watchers and TOPS

Group weight-loss programs tend to be more successful than individual programs, even though the amount of individual time spent with a diet counselor is less. Although the cost of these programs may be a disadvantage to some, fee programs tend to have a smaller attrition rate than free programs, and deposit–refund programs are even more successful; requiring a fee or deposit tends to discourage unmotivated clients from entering and increases the motivation of those who do enroll.

Commercial Programs

Commercial programs, of which Weight Watchers, Jenny Craig, and NutriSystem are the most popular, provide diet and nutrition information, and may include behavior modification, exercise, psychotherapy, the provision of food, and group support (Brownell and Fairburn, 1995). The cost of these programs varies widely; programs that require the purchase of prepackaged food or supplements can cost thousands of dollars. Although these programs are widely used, their effectiveness is relatively unknown: Commercial groups are reluctant to share less than spectacular results for fear of damaging their profitability. Consumer surveys (which may or may not be reliable) indicate that participants tend to participate in the programs for about a year and lose 10% to 20% of their initial weight; but the average dieter gains back almost half that weight 6 months after ending the program (Consumer Reports, 1993). Within 2 years, most participants regain more than two thirds of their initial weight loss.

Other Techniques

Diet book, magazine, and tabloid publishers have given dieters in the United States what they want—a proliferation of quick-weight-loss schemes that add up to a multibillion dollar business each year. Fad diets may produce weight loss, especially diets that are high in protein and low in carbohydrates; however, they tend to be

Table 13-10
Sample Meal Plans and Menus for 1500-Calorie Diet Based on the American Diabetic Association Exchange Lists

Exchanges	Number of Exchanges (Servings)	Sample Menu
Breakfast:		
fruit	1	½ cup orange juice
starch	3	½ cup Shredded Wheat
		1 bagel
fat	1	2 Tbsp reduced fat cream cheese
milk, skim	1	1 cup skim milk
free foods	as desired	Coffee, tea
		2 tsp light jelly
Lunch:		
starch	2	1 hamburger bun
meat, lean	3	3 oz ground round hamburger
vegetable	1	1 cup salad made with greens, carrots, onions, mushrooms, and green peppers
fat	1	1 Tbsp regular salad dressing
fruit	1	1 small apple
free foods	as desired	1 Tbsp catsup
		mustard
		1 large dill pickle
		Coffee, tea
Dinner:		
meat, lean	3	3 oz grilled skinless chicken breast
starch	2	½ cup rice
		1 cup winter squash
vegetable	1	½ cup steamed broccoli
fruit	1	1¼ cup watermelon cubes
fat	1	1 tsp margarine
free foods	as desired	sugar-free gelatin
High-starch snack:		
milk, skim	1	1 cup skim milk
starch	1	3 cups microwave popcorn
fat	1	

Contains approximately 1482 calories: 54% CHO, 23% protein, 23% fat.

highly restrictive, which leads invariably not only to a decrease in intake and loss of weight but also to boredom and attrition. Besides their lack of long-term staying power, many of these diets are unbalanced, providing not enough of some nutrients and excessive amounts of others.

Other less frequently used weight-loss gimmicks include using weight-loss pills (appetite suppressants, diuretics, or thyroid pills), fasting for more than 24 hours, taking laxatives, using weight-loss devices such as body wraps, using fiber or protein supplements, and inducing vomiting after eating (Levy and Heaton, 1993). None of these practices are recommended and most are potentially harmful.

Weight Loss Diets for Moderately to Morbidly Obese Clients

As is indicated in Table 13-9, social support, increased exercise, and behavior modification are also appropriate approaches in the treatment of moderate to morbid obesity. However, for this population, moderately calorie-restricted diets may produce too slow a rate of weight loss, and therefore may not be the dietary treatment of choice. Very-low-calorie diets may be used under medical supervision when rapid weight loss is indicated. Total fasting is also an option, but it carries increased risk. Surgical intervention may be used when dietary intervention fails. Drug therapy is another option.

Very-Low-Calorie Diets

For moderately to morbidly obese clients, especially those with serious complications such as diabetes mellitus, hypertension, and sleep apnea, a more aggressive approach to traditional dieting is the use of a very-low-calorie diet (VLCD), otherwise known as a protein-sparing modified fast. It is designed for short-term, large, and rapid weight loss in patients whose health is so jeopardized by obesity that the risk of a modified fast is less than the risk of maintaining obesity.

Liquid protein modified fast formulas were introduced and became popular during the late 1970s. They were composed of an incomplete protein of low biologic value and lacked adequate vitamins, minerals, and electrolytes; no recommendations regarding the use of supplements were made. Diuresis and the extensive electrolyte losses that resulted from the use of these extremely low-calorie diets probably played a role in the numerous deaths that were attributed to the diet.

Today's VLCD bear little resemblance to their predecessors. Although they are virtually fasting diets, they furnish 400 to 800 calories/day, mostly from high–biologic value protein, which is provided at approximately twice the RDA for protein. The high protein content can be obtained either through small portions of meat, fish, or poultry, or as a powdered protein supplement mixed with water. This protein intake minimizes the loss of lean body tissue that occurs with complete fasting and promotes an average weekly weight loss of 1.5 to 2.0 kg in women and 2.0 to 2.5 kg in men (Wadden, 1993). Very-low-calorie diets also use critical amounts of supplemental vitamins and minerals based on laboratory data, especially serum electrolyte values. They contain small amounts of carbohydrates and little or no fat.

Studies show that today's VLCD are safe when they are provided for appropriate clients (ie, people who are 30% or more overweight) under close medical supervision. Average weight loss for 12 to 16 weeks of treatment is approximately 20 kg for women and 25 kg in men; these amounts are two to three times greater than amounts usually lost during the same length of treatment with conventional diets (Wadden, 1993). Other benefits include significant reductions in serum cholesterol and triglyceride levels, improved glucose tolerance, and improvements in hypertension, pulmonary problems, and surgical risks.

Unfortunately, loss of body protein and potassium remains a major concern with VLCD. Studies have shown that the degree of obesity is inversely related to the degree of protein depletion—lighter people tend to lose more protein than people with a higher percentage of body fat. Because of this, it is recommended that VLCD be used only in individuals who are at least 130% to 140% of ideal weight. Other contraindications include arrhythmias, unstable angina, protein-wasting diseases, major system failure, drug therapy causing protein wasting (eg, steroids), and pregnancy and lactation. Common side effects include moderate ketosis, decreased cold tolerance, hair loss, dry skin, fatigue, lightheadedness, nervousness, constipation or diarrhea, menstrual irregularities, and possibly an increased risk of gallstones (Wadden, 1993). In addition, the dropout rate is very high, and weight loss tends to be poorly maintained after the diet is discontinued. Some studies show that on the average participants regained 35% to 50% of their lost weight in the first year after cessation of treatment, even when they received lifestyle modification (Wadden, 1995). Studies suggest that the short-term effectiveness of VLCD may be related more to the fact that participants are provided with a choice-free menu of portion-controlled meals than to their severe caloric restriction.

Total Fasting

Because total fasting alters the normal physiology and biochemistry of the gastrointestinal tract, it should be used only under complete medical supervision. Potassium, sodium, bicarbonate, and multivitamin–mineral supplements are necessary. Although total fasting does produce weight loss, loss of lean body tissue is extensive and weight loss is poorly maintained. Other potential complications include dehydration, hyperuricemia, nausea, dizziness, hepatic and renal impairment, mineral depletion, acidosis, severe postural hypotension, and muscle wasting.

Surgical Procedures

Surgical intervention may be considered as a last resort for morbidly obese clients who fail to lose weight by nonsurgical means and who are at increased risk of morbidity and mortality because of their obesity. Surgery should be contemplated only when the risk of remaining obese is greater than the risk of surgery. Unfortunately, surgery cannot guarantee that weight loss will be maintained, especially if eating attitudes and habits do not change. Follow-up care and behavior modification are vital to the long-term success of any surgical weight-loss procedure.

The types of surgical procedures that may be performed include the following:

Gastric Restriction (gastroplasty), also known as "stomach stapling": A row of staples across the stomach limits the capacity of the stomach to 15 milliliters of solids and delays gastric emptying through the banded opening that has a diameter of 9 to 10 millimeters (Fig. 13-5). Unfortunately, limiting the stomach capacity does not automatically limit food intake. Over time, the pouch stretches to hold more food. Although the incidence of postsurgical complications is low, the staples may burst if too much food or liquid is consumed before the staple line heals. In addition, overindulgence can cause the pouch to accommodate more food, thereby reducing its effectiveness; obstruction can occur if food is improperly chewed. Nutritional complications that have been reported with this procedure include hypoalbuminemia and vitamin deficiencies, in addition to vomiting and nausea. Clients must understand the importance of eating small meals, eating slowly, chewing food thoroughly, and progressing the diet from liquids, to puréed foods, to soft foods gradually.

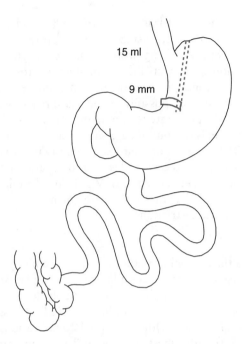

15 ml

9 mm

Figure 13-5
Vertical gastric stapling.

Intragastric Balloon Insertion: By endoscopy, a cylindrical implant is placed in the stomach and then inflated for the purpose of reducing stomach capacity. Diet therapy and behavior modification are included in the treatment program. Although standards were previously lower, the U.S. Food and Drug Administration (FDA) revised its criteria for eligibility to 100 pounds overweight in 1986 after complications of vomiting, ulcer, gastric perforation, and intestinal obstruction were reported. Few studies have been conducted on the dietary intake of balloon recipients. However, one study showed that weight loss ranged from 0% to 16% of original weight, which is comparable to weight loss achieved through diet and behavior modification alone. The effects of the balloon on long-term weight maintenance are not known. Some critics argue that the balloons have only marginal effects in reducing stomach capacity.

Combined Gastric Restriction and Malabsorption: This procedure combines gastric restriction with the bypass of more than 90% of the stomach, duodenum, and a portion of the jejunum of varying length, and produces greater weight loss than gastroplasty alone (Fig. 13-6). Rapid "dumping" of the stomach pouch contents into the small intestine produces a feeling of fullness or discomfort, and results in malabsorption, particularly of calcium, iron, and vitamin B_{12}. At 5 years after gastric bypass, the loss of excess weight is between 50% and 60% (Brownell and Fairburn, 1995).

Jaw Wiring: This is an approach that attempts to reduce intake by preventing the intake of solid foods. It is possible, however, to continue consuming a high-calorie

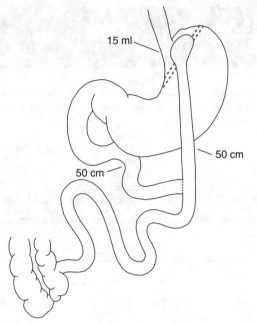

15 ml

50 cm

50 cm

Figure 13-6
Gastric bypass.

diet, depending on the client's choice of liquids. At best, jaw wiring is a temporary solution.

Fat Suctioning (Lipectomy): Fat cells are suctioned by a vacuum through a hollow tube that is inserted through an incision. This procedure is used primarily around the hips, abdomen, buttocks, and thighs, and is designed only for people under 40 with congenital fat bulges. It is not a cure for obesity because, at best, it addresses only the symptom of obesity rather than treating the underlying problem.

Drug Therapy

Historically, drug therapy has been used as a short-term intervention to initiate weight loss in clients with resistant obesity; after weight loss was achieved, drug therapy was discontinued. Newer views consider obesity a chronic disorder, like hypertension and diabetes, that requires continued intervention. Studies show that, when compared with patients using a placebo, people who are treated with active drugs tend to have greater weight loss (Bray, 1993). Unfortunately, drugs work only while they are being taken; the benefit stops when drug therapy stops. Drug therapy is usually reserved for clients who are unable to achieve weight loss through conventional methods alone. Amphetamines, a major category of appetite suppressants, are rarely used for obesity because of the high potential for abuse and the possibility of drug dependence (Brownell and Fairburn, 1995). The most frequently used appetite suppressants currently in use are listed in Table 13-11. Long-term benefits and complications must be evaluated.

Table 13-11
Appetite Suppressant Drugs Commonly Used for Obesity

Drug	Trade Name
Noradrenergic Drugs: Similar actions to amphetamines; however, they produce less CNS stimulation and have a much lower risk of abuse potential.	
Benzphetamine	Didrex
Phentermine	Fastin; Ionamin; Phentrol; Adipex-P; others
Diethylpropion	Tenuate; Tepanol
Mazindol	Mazanor; Sanorex
Phenylpropanolamine	Dexatrim (OTC)
Phendimetrazine	Anorex; Obalan; Phendiet; Wehless; others
Serotonineric Drugs: Serotonin-like properties that reduce physiological activity level, including a decrease in food intake.	
Fenfluramine	Pondimin

NURSING PROCESS

Before a plan of care can be devised, a thorough assessment is needed to determine who is likely to succeed in a weight-control program. Even though all obese clients have the potential to benefit from weight loss, not all obese clients are motivated to lose weight and to keep it off once lost. In addition, there are dangers if patients are selected indiscriminately for participation in a weight-loss program. For example:

- Failure can have devastating consequences that may preclude later attempts at dieting when the client may be more motivated and have a better chance at success.
- "Negative contagion" may spread to the rest of the participants in a group setting and hinder their progress.
- The health professional's morale may suffer.
- The health professional's time may be better spent on clients who are truly motivated to lose weight.

Assessment

Assess for the following factors:

Current weight, weight status: Compare actual weight to "ideal" standard.
Distribution and degree of body fatness, based on triceps skinfold measurements, waist:hip ratio, and measurements of bust/chest and thighs, if available.
Abnormal values, especially serum cholesterol, triglycerides, albumin, glucose, triiodothyronine (T_3), and thyroxine (T_4).
Signs or symptoms of malnutrition (see Chapter 9).

Usual 24-hour intake, including portion sizes, frequency and pattern of eating, method of food preparation, fat intake, and fiber intake.

The use of "diet" foods.

Eating behaviors and attitudes that can be improved. Early record keeping of the amounts and types of foods eaten, where the food was consumed, and the client's feelings about the meal or snack will help.

Previous history of dieting, especially "successes" that were followed by weight gain. Evaluate the types of diets followed, the length of dieting, and the reason for abandoning the diet to determine the client's level of motivation and determination.

Cultural, familial, religious, and ethnic influences on eating habits.

Emotional triggers that stimulate overeating, such as depression, boredom, anger, guilt, frustration, or self-hate. People who are identified as compulsive overeaters may benefit from Overeaters Anonymous, a self-help group that uses the 12-step program of Alcoholics Anonymous (see display, Overeaters Anonymous).

Nutritional knowledge, level of intelligence, and willingness to learn.

The duration of obesity, the age of onset, and whether a family history exists.

Presence of complications (eg, hypertension, diabetes, heart disease); determine their impact on nutritional status and whether dietary intervention is needed.

Usual activity patterns and the client's willingness to adopt an exercise program.

The client's sense of body image and self-esteem and the presence or lack of support systems.

Nursing Diagnosis

Altered Nutrition: More Than Body Requirements, related to excessive intake in relation to metabolic need.

Planning and Implementation

It is rarely effective to preach about the hazards of obesity and the virtues of being thin to someone who must lose weight. A positive, supportive approach is needed

---

Overeaters Anonymous

Overeaters Anonymous is founded on the belief that compulsive overeating is a physical, emotional, and spiritual disease. It is designed to complement medical and nutritional treatment of obesity; its focus is limited to the compulsive nature of overeating. There are no dues or fees, nor is there any weight requirement for entering the program. Like Alcoholics Anonymous, OA regards compulsive overeating as an addiction than can be arrested but not cured. A self-administered questionnaire that focuses on eating behaviors (such as eating in the absence of hunger, secret binge eating, feelings of guilt following overeating) may be used to help identify a compulsive eating disorder.

to establish rapport with the client and develop the an atmosphere that is conducive to weight control counseling. The more involved the patient is in developing personal eating and exercise plans, the greater the chance of achieving long-term weight control.

Set mutually agreeable realistic short- and long-term goals: Whereas a 100-lb weight loss in a year seems overwhelming and discouraging, a 6-lb weight loss per month may be within reach. For many, "ideal" weight may be unattainable and unnecessary; health benefits may be achieved with as little as 10% to 15% weight loss.

A balanced weight-reduction diet, like a normal diet, should provide approximately 20% of total calories from protein, less than 30% from fat, and the remainder from carbohydrate. Stress the importance of consuming a nutritionally adequate diet even though calorie intake is reduced. Include all major food groups in the diet; avoid items from the "Fats, Sweets, and Alcohol" group that provide mostly calories with few nutrients. Increase the intake of high-fiber foods: Fiber enhances a feeling of fullness and prolongs gastric emptying time.

Moderately restricted weight-loss diets usually do not provide less than 1200 calories for women and 1500 calories for men. Although extremely low-calorie diets can speed weight loss, they also make compliance more difficult and may be nutritionally inadequate. Multivitamins, and possibly mineral supplements, are indicated when intake falls below 1200 calories.

When a food is forbidden, it suddenly takes on mystical qualities and becomes all the more appealing. Keep forbidden foods to a minimum and emphasize portion control.

Weight-loss plateaus are to be expected because of a temporary increase in body water that results from the oxidation of fat tissue. Eventually, an increase in urine output rids the body of excess water and weight loss continues.

CLIENT GOALS

The client will

Increase physical activity.
Explain the relationship between diet, physical activity, and weight control.
Consume a nutritionally adequate, hypocaloric diet that contains less than 30% calories from fat.
Practice behavior modification techniques to avoid eating behaviors that lead to weight gain.
Not skip meals.
Lose 1 to 2 pounds/week until _____ pounds total weight loss is achieved.
Lessen health risks, as evidenced by a decrease in total cholesterol, low-density lipoprotein (LDL) cholesterol, and glucose; an increase in HDL cholesterol; and improved blood pressure, as appropriate.
Maintain weight loss.

NURSING INTERVENTIONS

Diet Management

- Decrease calorie intake by 500 to 1000 calories/day from calculated requirements to promote gradual weight loss.
- Individualize the diet as much as possible to correspond with the client's likes, dislikes, and eating pattern, because standard diets rarely fit into a person's lifestyle and eating habits.
- Limit fat intake to less than 30% of total calories/day; encourage an adequate protein intake and a liberal intake of complex carbohydrates.
- Increase fiber intake; fiber swells in the gut to provide a calorie-free feeling of fullness (fiber is not digested). Excellent sources of fiber include whole-grain breads and cereals, especially wheat bran, dried peas and beans, and fresh fruits and vegetables.

Client Teaching

Instruct the client

On the relationship between calorie intake, physical activity, and weight status.

That weight control can be achieved by reducing intake or increasing physical activity, but is most effectively and easily achieved by combining the two.

That permanent weight control can be achieved only through permanent lifestyle modification, not by "dieting."

That any amount and kind of exercise is better than no exercise at all. Encourage the client to participate in some kind of enjoyable activity; the intensity, duration, and frequency of exercise can be increased after the client gains confidence.

That food is used more efficiently when it is consumed in small quantities three to four times per day rather than at one large meal per day. Encourage the client to avoid meal skipping and hunger, which often leads to snacking and a higher calorie intake.

That occasional deviations from the diet should be expected. Encourage the client to accept these without feelings of failure and to resume "normal" dieting as soon as possible.

Not to get weighed too frequently; weight losses that are less than anticipated can be discouraging.

That fats in the diet provide the most concentrated source of calories—more than twice the calories in an equivalent amount of protein or carbohydrate. Calorie intake can be reduced drastically by limiting fat intake, such as fatty meats, whole-milk dairy products, fried foods, butter, margarine, salad dressings, oils, nuts and peanut butter, and rich desserts and pastries.

To keep a food record to increase awareness of amounts and types of foods eaten and precipitating factors.

To practice behavior modification techniques that are designed to change food attitudes and habits (see display, Behavior Modification Techniques). Successful weight control is possible when the attitude of "always being on a diet" changes to an acceptance of eating lighter and less as a way of life.

That a dieter's friends are as follows:

- A scale and measuring utensils to control portion sizes, at least during the early stages of "dieting"
- Baked, broiled, steamed, and boiled foods
- Fresh fruits and vegetables that have been prepared without added fat
- Lean meats, skinless poultry, and fish
- Starchy foods without added fat, such as bread, pasta, rice, potatoes, dried peas and beans, corn, peas, winter squash, and unsweetened cereals; whole-grain products and high-fiber foods are especially good at providing a feeling of fullness without a lot of excess calories
- Skim or low-fat milk and dairy products
- Herbs and spices, which impart flavor without any calories. The same is true of cooking with wine; as the food cooks, the calories evaporate, leaving only the flavor of wine

How to order from a menu while dining out:

- Estimate portion sizes of all foods. If the portion size is too big (eg, a 12-oz steak), eat half and take the rest home for the next day's meal. Consider ordering ala carte salad and appetizer for better portion control.
- Stick to plain foods rather than casseroles and stews. When in doubt, ask how the food is prepared; accommodating restaurants will prepare food without added fat, as requested.
- Choose tomato juice, unsweetened fruit juice, clear broth, bouillon, or consommé as an appetizer instead of sweetened juices, fried vegetables, seafood cocktail, or creamy or thick soups.
- Choose fresh vegetable salads, and use oil and vinegar or fresh lemon instead of regular salad dressings. If you use regular salad dressing, ask that the dressing be served separately and dip each forkful of salad into the dressing, rather than pouring the dressing on the salad. Avoid coleslaw and other salads with the dressing already added.
- Order plain roasted, baked, or broiled meat, fish, or poultry; avoid items that are au gratin, creamed, sauteed, or fried.
- Order steamed, boiled, or broiled vegetables.
- Choose plain baked, mashed, boiled, or steamed potatoes, rice, or noodles.
- Select fresh fruit for dessert. If you can't resist a high-fat dessert, order one and split it with a friend.
- At fast food restaurants, order the smallest size available; order burgers with lettuce, tomato, onions, pickles, mustard, relish, and ketchup if desired, but skip the cheese and special sauce.
- Order pizza with veggie toppings instead of pepperoni, sausage, other meats, and extra cheese.
- Request milk for coffee and tea, if desired, instead of cream.
- Most airlines will provide low-calorie meals if requested at the time that flight reservations are made.

- Be sure to "under"-eat for the rest of the day if you think you may overeat while you are out.

On food preparation:

- Food does not have to be prepared separately from the rest of the family's as long as extra sugar and fat are not added.
- Nonstick sprays are effective and virtually calorie free; you can also "saute" with a small amount of water or broth instead of margarine or oil.
- Trim all visible fat from meat after cooking, and remove the skin from poultry.
- Prepare soup stock a day ahead; refrigerate and remove the fat that hardens on the surface.
- Whenever possible, replace high-fat ingredients with low-fat substitutes (eg, replace whole and 2% milk with 1% and skim milk).
- When making casseroles or stews, halve the amount of meat called for and double the amount of rice, beans, pasta, or potatoes.
- Use low-calorie or diabetic cookbooks for variety.

On food purchasing and label reading:

- Avoid temptation by not buying problem foods.
- Stick to a shopping list.
- Do not shop while hungry.
- Buy only the amount needed.
- "Lite" or "Light" foods have 1/3 less calories or no more than 1/2 the fat of the higher-calorie, higher-fat versions.
- "Low-calorie" foods cannot have more than 40 cal/serving.
- "Calorie Free" items must have less than 5 calories/serving.
- "Sugar-free" and "dietetic" do not necessarily mean low-calorie.

Counsel overweight parents about the dangers of overfeeding infants and the inappropriate use of food to convey love, support, or acceptance. Advise parents to encourage their children to participate in regular physical activity.

Advise the client to consult his or her physician or dietitian if questions concerning the diet or weight loss arise.

Monitoring Progress

Monitor for the following signs or symptoms:

Compliance to diet, and the need for follow-up diet counseling
Effectiveness of the diet (ie, weight loss, improvement in serum lipids), and assess the need for further diet modification

Evaluation

Evaluation is ongoing. Provided the plan of care has not changed, the client will achieve the goals as stated above.

EATING DISORDERS: ANOREXIA NERVOSA
AND BULIMIA NERVOSA

Historically, the study of obesity and eating disorders has been separate: Obesity has been rooted in medicine, and eating disorders have been the focus of psychiatry and psychology. Yet there are commonalities between them, such as questions of appetite regulation, concerns with body image, and similar etiologic risk factors (Brownell and Fairburn, 1995).

Anorexia Nervosa

Anorexia nervosa is a condition of self-imposed fasting or severe self-imposed dieting that is characterized by dramatic weight loss or maintenance of weight that is at least 15% below the recommended weight for height (Krahn et al, 1993). Thinness is pursued compulsively, and self-perception of body weight is distorted. Clients with anorexia nervosa are intensely preoccupied with weight, and they see themselves as fat when they are emaciated (see display, Diagnostic Criteria for Anorexia Nervosa).

Although anorexia nervosa has been extensively studied, its basic causes remain unknown. It is now considered to be multifactorial in origin; risk factors include individual (biologic and psychological), familial, and cultural components. Some studies suggest that people with anorexia nervosa have disordered regulation of eating and mood related to alterations in the neurotransmitter serotonin (Garner, 1993). Certain personality traits, such as low self-esteem, perfectionism, and excessive compliance have been implicated as risk factors (Brownell and Fairburn, 1995). Studies strongly indicate a relationship between depression and eating disorders; many anorexics suffer from low mood, loss of interest, shortened attention span, disrupted sleep patterns, and suicidal tendencies. Studies suggest that alcohol and drug abuse may be four to five times higher in women with eating disorders than in the general population. Indeed, psychological and social factors, especially problems with family dynamics, are generally considered to be central to the problem. Major stressors, such as the onset of puberty, parents' divorce, death of a family member, broken relationships, and ridicule of being or becoming fat, are frequent precipitating factors. Eating disorders are most likely to occur immediately before or after the onset of puberty, and are almost always preceded by "dieting." Athletes, like dancers and gymnasts, may develop eating disorders to improve their performance.

Because the incidence of eating disorders is low, no studies have been conducted on their incidence in the general population (Brownell and Fairburn, 1995). Among mental health care facilities, the incidence rate for anorexia nervosa is about 5 per 100,000 of the total population (Brownell and Fairburn, 1995). Approximately 90% to 95% of cases of anorexia and bulimia occur in female patients, with a peak age of onset at 12 to 13 and 19 to 20 years of age. Anorexics typically are from white, middle- to upper-middle-class families that place heavy emphasis on high

Diagnostic Criteria For Anorexia Nervosa

For a definite diagnosis, all of the following are required:

(a) Body weight is maintained at least 15% below that expected (either lost or never achieved), or Quetelet's body-mass index is 17.5 or less. Prepubertal patients may show failure to make the expected weight gain during the period of growth.

(b) The weight loss is self-induced by avoidance of "fattening foods." One or more of the following may also be present: self-induced vomiting; self-induced purging; excessive exercise; use of appetite suppressants and/or diuretics.

(c) There is body-image distortion in the form of a specific psychopathology whereby a dread of fatness persists as an intrusive, overvalued idea and the patient imposes a low weight threshold on himself or herself.

(d) A widespread endocrine disorder involving the hypothalamic–pituitary–gonadal axis is manifest in women as amenorrhea and in men as a loss of sexual interest and potency. (An apparent exception is the persistence of vaginal bleeds in anorexic women who are receiving replacement hormonal therapy, most commonly taken as a contraceptive pill.) There may also be elevated levels of growth hormone, raised levels of cortisol, changes in the peripheral metabolism of the thyroid hormone, and abnormalities of insulin secretion.

(e) If onset is prepubertal, the sequence of pubertal events is delayed or even arrested (growth ceases; in girls the breasts do not develop and there is a primary amenorrhea; and in boys the genitals remain juvenile). With recovery, puberty is often completed normally, but the menarche is late.

Atypical Anorexia Nervosa: This term should be used for those individuals in whom one or more of the key features of anorexia nervosa, such as amenorrhoea or significant weight loss, is absent, but who otherwise present a fairly typical clinical picture. Such people are usually encountered in psychiatric liaison services in general hospitals or in primary care. Patients who have all the key symptoms but to only a mild degree may also be best described by this term. This term should not be used for eating disorders that resemble anorexia nervosa but that are due to known physical illness.

Note. From World Health Organization (1992). *The ICD-10 Classification of Mental and Behavioral Disorders: Clinical Descriptions and Diagnostic Guidelines* (pp. 176–181). Geneva: Author. Copyright 1992 by the World Health Organization. Reprinted by permission.

achievement, perfection, and physical appearance. Anorexics are often described as "model" children, although they tend to be immature, require parental approval, and lack independence.

Numerous physical and mental signs and symptoms may be observed in people with eating disorders (see display, Physical, Mental, and Behavioral Signs and Symptoms of Anorexia). Severe or chronic eating disorders may lead to fluid and electrolyte imbalances, erosion of tooth enamel, permanent brain damage, permanent sterility, chronic invalidism, damage to vital organs, and heart failure. Two long-term complications include Cushing's disease and osteoporosis. As many as one out of five to seven clients with chronic anorexia may die from complications.

Treatment seeks to restore normal eating behaviors and nutritional status through an oral diet; rarely are enteral or parenteral feedings necessary to stabilize the client medically. Because normalization of eating behaviors is the primary goal of nutri-

Physical, Mental, and Behavioral Signs and Symptoms of Anorexia

PHYSICAL SYMPTOMS

- Extreme weight loss and muscle wasting (weight loss ≥15% of original or expected weight)
- Arrested sexual development, amenorrhea
- Dry, yellow skin related to the release of carotenes as fat stores are burned for energy
- Loss of hair or change in hair texture
- Overgrowth of lanugo (fine, downy body hair)
- Pain on touch
- Hypotension, bradycardia
- Anemia
- Constipation
- Severe sleep disturbances, insomnia
- Dental caries and periodontal disease

MENTAL AND BEHAVIORAL SYMPTOMS

- Bizarre eating habits, refusal to eat
- Depressed mood, low self-esteem, social withdrawal
- Perfectionist, overachiever
- Preoccupation with food, dieting, and death
- Intense fear of becoming fat that does not lessen with weight loss
- Distorted body image and denial of eating disorder
- Frantic pursuit of exercise
- Frequent weighing
- Use of laxatives, diuretics, emetics, and diet pills
- Manipulative behavior

tion intervention, the use of commercial, nutrient-dense supplements should be limited or avoided. Step-by-step goals of diet intervention that have been designed to meet the client's physiologic and psychological needs are as follows:

1. Prevent further weight loss. Initially, 1500 calories or less may be recommended because larger amounts may not be well tolerated or accepted after prolonged semi-starvation (Beumont et al, 1993). The diet is advanced calorically only when the client is able to complete a full meal.
2. Improve nutritional status while low weight is maintained.
3. Gradually increase weight by reestablishing normal eating behaviors. Initially, patients may respond to nutritional therapy better if they are allowed to exclude high-risk binge foods from their diet. However, the binge foods should be reintroduced later so that the "feared food" (or trigger foods) idea is not promoted.
4. Maintain a set weight goal that has been agreed on by the health care team and the client. Sometimes a lower-than-ideal weight is selected as the initial weight goal (ie, enough weight to regain normal physiologic function and menstruation). When this has been achieved, the goals may be reevaluated. Many recovered clients have chronic problems with eating and weight.

The underlying problem of the eating disorder may be treated using a multidimensional approach, including nutrition counseling, behavior modification, individual psychotherapy, family counseling, and group therapy. Antidepressant drugs, such as serotonin reuptake inhibitors like fluoxetine, effectively reduce the frequency of, but do not eliminate, problematic eating behaviors. Depending on the severity of the eating disorder, clients may be treated on either an outpatient or an inpatient basis. All aspects of treatment (nutrition, behavior modification, psychotherapy) must be highly individualized; treatment is often time consuming and frustrating. Studies show that, on average, more than 40% of anorexics recover, one third improve, and 20% have a chronic course (Brownell and Fairburn, 1995).

NURSING PROCESS

Assessment

Assess for the following factors:

Abnormal eating behaviors, including undereating, refusal to eat high-calorie foods, cutting food into tiny pieces, choosing inappropriate utensils, eating extremely slowly, using excessive condiments, drinking too much or too little fluid, disposing of food secretly, counting calories, counting fat grams, and ritualistic eating behaviors

Food fears

The use of laxatives or diuretics; determine if self-induced vomiting is practiced

Weight, weight history, and current status; percent of weight loss and adequacy of growth, if appropriate

Overactivity, either in the form of actual physical activity or persistent restlessness

Fluid status; presence of edema

Abnormal laboratory values, especially electrolyte imbalances, and low hemoglobin, hematocrit, and albumin

Signs and symptoms of malnutrition, particularly the overgrowth of lanugo hair, alopecia, and dry, scaly skin

Amenorrhea, which may precede weight loss in some individuals

Nursing Diagnosis

Altered Nutrition: Less than Body Requirements, related to anorexia nervosa

Planning and Implementation

The optimal dietary intervention for promoting weight gain in clients with anorexia nervosa is unknown. Initially, a low-calorie diet (REE + 300–400 calories) that increases gradually to 3000 calories or more daily may be used. Central to all approaches is an individualized plan that promotes compliance and gains the client's trust.

Include the client in goal setting; link rewards to the quantity of calories consumed, not to weight gain. Initially, it may be beneficial to have the client record food intake and exercise activity.

Because gastrointestinal intolerance may exist, gassy and high-fat foods should be limited in the early stages of treatment.

Serve small, attractive meals based on individual food preferences. Foods that are nutritionally dense will help to minimize the volume of food needed. Finger foods that are served cold or at room temperature will help to minimize satiety sensations.

Never force the client to eat, and minimize the emphasis on food.

A high-fiber or low-sodium diet may be helpful in controlling symptoms of constipation and fluid retention, respectively. A multivitamin and mineral supplement may be prescribed. Because it is both a stimulant and a diuretic, caffeine should be avoided.

Tube feedings or parenteral nutrition should be used only if necessary to stabilize the client medically. Overly aggressive nutritional repletion carries medical risks of fluid retention and electrolyte changes; psychological risks may include a perceived loss of control, loss of identity, increased body distortion, and mistrust of the treatment team (ADA, 1994). Enteral support should never be used as punishment for difficult clients.

Prevention may be far more effective than the treatment of eating disorders. Encourage parents, teachers, and significant others

- To help children and adolescents establish a strong positive self-image and sense of worth regardless of their weight
- Not to expect perfection and to avoid putting pressure on children to excel beyond their capabilities
- To give adolescents an appropriate amount of independence, responsibility, and accountability for their own actions
- To recognize stresses in the child's life and provide support and encouragement
- To teach the basis of good nutrition and normal exercise
- To avoid putting pressure on young people to lose weight. If weight control is really indicated, a medically supervised plan of weight loss and weight maintenance should be followed. Discourage the use of fad diets and diet products.
- To recognize the signs and symptoms of eating disorders
- To seek professional help if eating disorders are suspected

CLIENT GOALS

The client will:

Change eating behaviors gradually until eating behaviors are normal.

Gain weight slowly (ie, 1–2 lbs/week) until reasonable weight goal is achieved, generally within a BMI range of 20 to 25. Achieve normal growth and development, if appropriate.

Achieve normal nutritional status, as evidenced by the lack of physical signs of malnutrition, the determination of normal laboratory values, and the resumption of menses.

Be free of other physical, mental, and behavioral signs and symptoms of anorexia (see display, Physical, Mental, and Behavioral Signs and Symptoms of Anorexia).

Maintain normal eating behaviors and healthy body weight.

NURSING INTERVENTIONS

Diet Management

Provide basal calorie requirements plus 300 to 400 calories initially; gradually increase to a high-calorie diet to promote weight gain.

Provide small frequent feedings to maximize intake and tolerance. Emphasize finger foods that are cold or at room temperature.

Limit fat intake initially, if gastrointestinal intolerance exists.

Limit sodium intake, if fluid retention is a problem.

Avoid caffeine, which acts as both a stimulant and a diuretic.

Client Teaching

The diet counselor should promote self-esteem in clients with eating disorders by using a positive approach, providing support and encouragement, fostering self–decision-making, and offering the client choices. Avoid preaching rules and reinforcing the client's preoccupation with food.

Instruct the client and family

On the principles of "healthy" weight, weight gain, and weight maintenance

On the importance of consuming small, frequent meals

On the characteristics of a healthy diet and the recommended servings from each food group. The Food Guide Pyramid may serve as a teaching aid (USDA, 1992).

On the dangers of dieting and of purging

On how to recognize signs of hunger

That the following volunteer organizations have information on treatment centers, hospitals, clinics, groups, and doctors who specialize in anorexia nervosa:

American Anorexia/Bulimia Association, Inc
133 Cedar Lane
Teaneck, NJ 07666

Anorexia Nervosa and Related Eating Disorders (ANRED)
PO Box 5102
Eugene, OR 97666

Monitoring Progress

Monitor for the following signs or symptoms:

Tolerance to fat (ie, absence of gastrointestinal upset, bloating) and sodium (ie, absence of fluid retention) in the diet

Compliance to the diet, and the need for follow-up diet counseling

Weight status, weight gain

Eating behaviors and attitudes about food, dieting, and weight

The effectiveness of the diet, and the need for further diet modifications

Evaluation

Evaluation is ongoing. Provided the plan of care has not changed, the client will achieve the goals as stated above.

Bulimia Nervosa

Bulimia nervosa, which was first defined in 1979, is a variant of anorexia nervosa with which it shares many clinical and background features (Brownell and Fairburn, 1995). Bulimia is characterized by recurrent episodes of gorging, that is, eating large amounts of food in a discrete period of time (eg, 2 hours) during which the client feels unable to stop or control the binge. Combined with the gorging is recurrent purging to prevent weight gain, such as self-induced vomiting; laxative, emetic, diuretic, or diet pill abuse; fasting; or vigorous exercise. Like anorexia, bulimia nervosa is usually preceded by prolonged "dieting." The binge and purge episodes must both occur at least twice a week, on average, for 3 months, according to the diagnostic criteria for bulimia nervosa (see display, Diagnostic Criteria for Bulimia Ner-

---

Diagnostic Criteria for Bulimia Nervosa

For a definite diagnosis, all of the following are required:

(a) There is a persistent preoccupation with eating, and an irresistible craving for food: the patient succumbs to episodes of overeating in which large amounts of food are consumed in short periods of time.

(b) The patient attempts to counteract the "fattening" effects of food by one or more of the following: self-induced vomiting; purgative abuse; alternating periods of starvation; use of drugs such as appetite suppressants, thyroid preparations, or diuretics. When bulimia occurs in diabetic patients they may choose to neglect their insulin treatment.

(c) The psychopathology consists of a morbid dread of fatness, and the patient sets herself or himself a sharply defined weight threshold, well below the premorbid weight that constitutes the optimum or healthy weight in the opinion of the physician. There is often, but not always, a history of an earlier episode of anorexia nervosa, the interval between the two disorders ranging from a few months to several years. This earlier episode may have been fully expressed, or may have assumed a minor cryptic form with a moderate loss of weight and/or a transient phase of amenorrhoea.

Atypical Bulimia Nervosa: This term should be used for those individuals in whom one or more of the key features listed for bulimia nervosa is absent but who otherwise present a fairly typical clinical picture. Most commonly this applies to people with normal or even excessive weight but with typical periods of overeating followed by vomiting or purging. Partial syndromes together with depressive symptoms are also not uncommon, but if the depressive symptoms justify a separate diagnosis of a depressive disorder, two diagnoses should be made.

Note. From World Health Organization (1992). *The ICD-10 Classification of Mental and Behavioral Disorders: Clinical Descriptions and Diagnostic Guidelines (pp. 176–181).* Geneva: Author. Copyright 1992 by the World Health Organization. Reprinted by permission.

vosa). Bulimics are preoccupied with body shape, weight, and food, and have an irrational fear of becoming fat (Brownell and Fairburn, 1995).

Initially, bulimics are secretive about their bingeing-purging episodes; the behaviors may go undetected by family members for years. Bulimics tend to have voracious appetites and may binge several times a day. Binges are frequently planned, with the client stockpiling food for a time when the binge can proceed uninterrupted. Binge foods are easy to swallow and regurgitate, and are usually the fatty, sweet, high-calorie foods that the client denies herself at other times. One single binge may involve the consumption of 1200 to 11,500 calories; usually the food is eaten rapidly over a period of minutes. Factors that may precipitate a binge include anxiety, tension, boredom, being reminded about food, drinking alcohol or smoking cannibus, and fatigue. Hunger is rarely cited as a reason for bingeing, even when the gorging follows a 24-hour fast (Brownell and Fairburn, 1995). Initially, bulimics may stick a finger down the throat to stimulate the gag reflex, but over time, many are able to vomit at will by contracting thoracic and abdominal muscles.

Like anorexia, the exact cause of bulimia is unknown, but it is considered multifactorial in origin. Although numerous psychological, physical, social, and cultural risk factors have been identified, it is not known how or why these factors interact to cause eating disorders. The variety of neuroendocrine and metabolic disorders that are often associated with eating disorders are more likely secondary, rather than primary, to the disorder (Brownell and Fairburn, 1995). Studies indicate that perhaps 30% of bulimics have a previous history of anorexia; however, bulimia in individuals of normal weight rarely develops into anorexia nervosa.

Bulimia nervosa is the most frequent eating disorder; some say it occurs at epidemic proportions among women in western countries (Brownell and Fairburn, 1995). Some surveys indicate that up to 19% of female students admit bulimic symptoms; approximately 85% of bulimics are college-educated females. Because of the secrecy that surrounds bulimia, the true incidence is not known.

Unlike anorexics, bulimics experience weight fluctuations and are of normal or slightly above normal weight. Bulimics are prone to depression, irritability, passivity, sadness, and suicidal tendencies, and may be at increased risk for alcohol and chemical abuse. Bulimics tend to have fewer serious medical complications than anorexics because the undernutrition is less severe. Frequent complaints include lethargy, fatigue, and "feeling bloated." Nausea, constipation, abdominal pain, tooth sensitivity, and irregular menses may also occur. Although results of a physical examination may be relatively normal, the client may appear to have puffy cheeks as a result of enlarged salivary glands, which occurs most often in the parotid glands. Calluses may be observed on the hand that is used to stimulate the gag reflex. Clients who have been vomiting for more than 4 years usually have destruction of tooth enamel. Edema may occur secondary to the abuse of laxatives or diuretics. Complications include electrolyte imbalances, particularly metabolic alkalosis, hypochloremia, and hypokalemia; esophagitis; esophageal erosion, perforation, and rupture; reflex constipation; dry skin; hypoglycemia; and other neuroendocrine abnormalities. Gastric dilation, with its risk of rupture, may be the most frequent cause of death among bulimics.

Most bulimics can be treated on an outpatient basis by a multidisciplinary team. Bulimia may be easier to treat than anorexia because bulimics know their behavior is abnormal and many are willing to cooperate with treatment. Psychotherapy, especially that involving cognitive-behavioral techniques, provides effective treatment for many bulimics. However, if psychotherapy fails, or the client is depressed, antidepressants may also be used. Nutritional intervention seeks to normalize eating behaviors, help the client gain control over eating, correct fluid and electrolyte imbalances, and promote long-term weight management.

NURSING PROCESS

Assessment

Assess for the following factors:

- Binge-eating behaviors, including eating large amounts of food when not physically hungry, eating rapidly, regurgitating (spitting out) food, eating in secrecy, and eating until feeling uncomfortably full
- Food fears, forbidden foods, binge foods
- Method of purging: self-induced vomiting; abuse of laxatives, diuretics, emetics, diet pills
- Weight, weight history, current weight status. Client's feelings about current weight and definition of "optimal" weight
- Overactivity, including both physical activity and restlessness
- Fluid status; presence of edema
- Abnormal laboratory values, especially hypochloremia and hypokalemia
- Signs, symptoms, and complications, including eroded tooth enamel, calluses on the hand, enlarged parotid glands, symptoms of esophagitis, irregular menses, weight fluctuations, and lethargy
- Use of alcohol, cannibus, and other drugs

Nursing Diagnosis

High Risk for Ineffective Management of Therapeutic Regimen, related to insufficient knowledge for self-care

Planning and Implementation

Initially, the diet for bulimia is structured and relatively inflexible to promote the client's sense of control. Meal patterns similar to those used for diabetics can be used to specify portion sizes, food groups to include with each meal and snack, and the frequency of eating.

To increase awareness of eating and satiety, meals should be eaten while sitting down, finger foods and cold or room temperature foods should be avoided, and the meal duration should be of appropriate length.

Eating strategies that may help to regulate intake include not skipping meals or snacks, using the appropriate-sized utensils, and not picking at food. Encourage clients to introduce forbidden binge foods into their diets.

Initially, the client may be required to eat no less than 1500 calories daily; having the client record intake before eating will promote a sense of control. The diet should provide adequate fat, which delays gastric emptying and contributes to satiety.

Nutritional counseling should focus on identifying and correcting food misinformation and fears. Bulimics must understand that gorging is only one aspect of a complex pattern of altered behavior; in fact, excessive dietary restriction is a major contributor to the disorder.

Expect minor relapses, especially after therapy is discontinued. When relapse occurs, the structured meal plan should be resumed immediately.

CLIENT GOALS

The client will

Eat regular meals and snacks of appropriate size, variety, and balance; client will not binge.

Not practice purging.

Maintain reasonable weight.

Be free of signs, symptoms, and complications of bulimia nervosa.

Maintain normal eating behaviors; client will not fear forbidden foods.

Nursing Interventions

DIET MANAGEMENT

- Provide a 1500-calorie diet in three balanced meals plus snacks, using a structured meal plan that provides adequate amounts of fat. Gradually increase calories as needed.
- Limit finger foods, avoid cold and room temperature foods, and advise the client to sit down for each meal and snack.

PATIENT AND FAMILY TEACHING

Instruct the patient and family

On the principles of healthy weight, weight gain, and weight maintenance

On the importance of adhering to the structured meal plan, at least initially

To record all meals and snacks prior to eating

On the dangers of bingeing and purging

How to recognize hunger

On the volunteer organizations that are available for clients with eating disorders (see anorexia nervosa)

That relapse is to be expected and should not be viewed as failure

MONITORING PROGRESS

Monitor for the following signs or symptoms:

Compliance to the diet; need for follow-up counseling
Weight; weight changes
Abnormal eating behaviors
The patient's attitude about food, dieting, and weight
Fluid and electrolyte balance

Evaluation

Evaluation is ongoing. Provided the plan of care has not changed, the client will achieve the goals as stated above.

KEY CONCEPTS

- Energy balance is determined by comparing calorie intake to calorie expenditure. A positive calorie balance, caused by eating too many calaories and/or expending too few calories, results in weight gain over time.
- For most Americans, the greatest proportion of their total calorie requirements are to support the involuntary activities of the body (resting energy expenditure).
- Ideal body weight and healthy body weight are imprecise terms that have not been universally defined. BMI may be the best method of evaluating weight status, but it does not account for how weight is distributed. "Apples" (people with upper body obesity) appear to have more health risks than "pears" (people with lower body obesity).
- Numerous physiologic and sociocultural theories about the etiology have been proposed; obesity appears to be multifactorial and is likely to have different causes in different people.
- Because of its multifactorial origin and chronic nature, obesity is resistant to treatment, when success is measured by weight loss alone. Rather than concentrating solely on weight loss to measure success, other health benefits, like lowered blood pressure and serum lipids, should also be considered.
- Exercise, behavior modification, and a hypocaloric diet are components of weight control for people who are mildly obese. Very-low-calorie diets, surgery, and drug therapy are also options for people who are moderately to morbidly obese.
- Obesity prevention is far more effective than "cure."
- Anorexia nervosa and bulimia nervosa are characterized by preoccupation with body weight and food and are usually preceded by prolonged dieting. Although their cause is unknown, they are considered to be multifactorial in origin.
- Anorexia nervosa is a condition of severe self-imposed starvation, which is often accompanied by a frantic pursuit of exercise. Although they appear severely underweight, anorexics have a distorted self-perception of weight and see themselves as overweight. They may have numerous physical and mental symptoms; anorexia can be fatal.

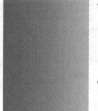

- Bulimia, which occurs more frequently than anorexia, is characterized by binge-ing (on large amounts of food in a short time) and purging (such as self-induced vomiting and laxative abuse). Bulimics usually appear to be of normal or slightly above normal weight and experience less severe physical symptoms than anorex-ics. Bulimia is rarely fatal.
- Eating disorders are best treated by a team approach, which includes nutrition intervention and counseling to restore normal eating behaviors and adequate nutritional status.

FOCUS ON **CRITICAL THINKING**

Mrs. Edwards is a sedentary 38-year-old who is 5'5" tall and weighs 160 pounds. Before the birth of her first child 10 years ago, Mrs. Edwards weighed 115 pounds; she has gained weight steadily since then. Mrs. Edwards wants to weigh 115 pounds by the end of 2 months, when her high school reunion is scheduled. She is deciding between starting a grapefruit and cottage cheese diet or joining Weight Watchers.

1. Calculate:
   a. her ideal weight and BMI
   b. her estimated calorie requirements
   c. the quantity of calories she should consume to lose 1 lb/wk; calories to lose 2 lb/wk
2. Discuss Mrs. Edwards weight loss goal, the time frame, and the reason she wants to lose weight.
3. What would you tell Mrs. Edwards about a grapefruit and cottage cheese diet? About Weight Watchers? What general guidelines would you suggest she look for in a weight-loss diet?
4. What strategies would you recommend Mrs. Edwards try to help promote weight loss?

REFERENCES

Allred, J. (1995). Too much of a good thing? JADA 95(4), 417–418.

American Dietetic Association (1994). Position of the American Dietetic Association: Nutri-tion intervention in the treatment of anorexia nervosa, bulimia nervosa, and binge eating. JADA, 94, 902–907.

Atkinson, R. (1993). Proposed standards for judging the success of the treatment of obesity. Ann Intern Med, 119(7 part 2), 677–680.

Beaumont, P., Russell, J., and Touyz, S. (1993). Treatment of anorexia nervosa. The Lancet, 341, 1635–1640.

Blackburn, G. (1993). Comparison of medically supervised and unsupervised approaches to weight loss and control. Ann Intern Med, 119(7 part 2),714–718.

Blair, S. (1993). Evidence for success of exercise in weight loss and control. Ann Intern Med, 119(7 part 2), 702–706.

Bray, G. (1992). Pathophysiology of obesity. Am J Clin Nutr 55(suppl), 488S–494S.

Bray, G. (1993). Use and abuse of appetite-suppressant drugs in the treatment of obesity. Ann Intern Med, 119(7 part 2), 707–713.

Brownell, K., and Fairburn, C. (editors)(1995). Eating Disorders and Obesity. A Comprehensive Handbook. New York: The Guilford Press.

Butterfield, G., and Gates, J. (1994). Fueling Activity: Current concepts. Topics in Nutrition and Food Safety, Fall 1994.

Callahan, M. (1991). The Healthy Weight. 2nd ed. Chicago: American Dietetic Association.

Cassell, J. (1995). Social anthropology and nutrition: A different look at obesity in America. JADA, 95(4), 424–427.

Committee to Develop Criteria for Evaluating the Outcomes of Approaches to Prevent and Treat Obesity, Food and Nutrition Board, Institute of Medicine, National Academy of Sciences. (1995). Summary: Weighing the options—Criteria for evaluating weight-management programs. JADA, 95, 96–105.

Consumer Reports. (1993). Losing weight. What works. What doesn't. Consumer Reports, 58(6), 353–357.

Foreyt, J., and Goodrick, G. (1993). Evidence for success of behavior modification in weight loss and control. Ann Intern Med, 119(7 part 2), 698–701.

Garner, D. (1993). Pathogenesis of anorexia nervosa. The Lancet, 341, 1631–1635.

Hill, J., Drougas, H. and Peters, J. (1993). Obesity treatment: Can diet composition play a role? Ann Intern Med, 119(7 part 2), 694–697.

Horm, J., and Anderson, K. (1993). Who in America is trying to lose weight? Ann Intern Med, 119(7 part 2), 672–676.

Krahn, D., Rock C., Dechert, R., et al. (1993). Changes in resting energy expenditure and body composition in anorexia nervosa patients during refeeding. JADA, 93, 434–438.

Kuczmarski, R., Flegal, K., Campbell, S., and Johnson, C. (1994). Increasing prevalence of overweight among US adults. The National Health and Nutrition Examination Surveys, 1960 to 1991. JAMA, 272(3), 205–211.

Levy, A., and Heaton, A. (1993). Weight control practices of US adults trying to lose weight. Ann Intern Med, 119(7 part 2), 661–666.

National Institutes of Health, National Heart, Lung, Blood Institute. (1992). Strategy Development Workshop for Public Education on Weight and Obesity. Sept. 22–25, Summary Report NIH Publication No 95-3314.

National Research Council (1989). Recommended Dietary Allowances. 10th ed. Washington, DC: National Academy Press.

National Task Force on the Prevention and Treatment of Obesity (1994). Weight cycling. JAMA, 272(15), 1196–1202.

Parham, E. (1993). Enhancing social support in weight loss management groups. JADA, 10, 1152–1156.

Pi-Sunyer, F. (1993). Medical hazards of obesity. Ann Intern Med, 119(7 part 2), 655–660.

Robinson, J., et al. (1993). Obesity, weight loss, and health. JADA, 93(4), 445–449.

Robinson, J., Hoerr, S., Petersmarck, K., and Anderson, J. (1995). Redefining success in obesity intervention: The new paradigm. JADA 95(4), 422–423.

U.S. Department of Agriculture, U.S. Department of Health and Human Services. (1995). Nutrition and Your Health: Dietary Guidelines for Americans, 4th ed. Home and Garden Bulletin No. 232.

U.S. Department of Agriculture. (1992). The Food Guide Pyramid. Home and Garden Bulletin No. 252.

U.S. Department of Health and Human Services, Public Health Service (1992). Methods for Voluntary Weight Loss and Control. National Institutes of Health Technology Assessment Conference Statement.

Wadden, T. (1993). Treatment of obesity by moderate and severe caloric restriction. Results of clinical trials. Ann Intern Med, 119(7 part 2), 688–693.

Williamson, D. (1993). Descriptive epidemiology of body weight and weight change in U.S. adults. Ann Intern Med, 119(7 part 2), 646–649.

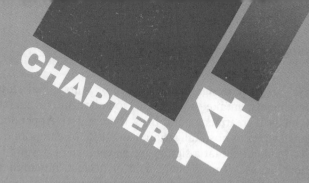

CHAPTER 14

Oral, Enteral, and Parenteral Nutrition

Chapter Outline

Key Terms

Bacterial translocation
Bolus feedings
Continuous drip
   method
Cracking
Cyclical TPN
Elemental formulas
Enteral nutrition
Esophagastomy
Gastrostomy
Hydrolyzed formulas

Intact protein/intact
   nutrient
Intermittent tube feedings
Isotonic
Jejunostomy
Modular
Osmolality
Ostomy tubes
Parenteral nutrition
Percutaneous endoscopic
   gastrostomy (PEG)

Peripheral parenteral
   nutrition (PPN)
Protein isolates
Specially defined formulas
Standard formulas
Total parenteral nutrition
   (TPN)
Total nutrient admixture
   (TNA)
Transnasal tubes

Illness can have a significant impact on nutritional status by altering nutrient requirements, intake, absorption, metabolism, or excretion. Diagnostic procedures, medical treatments, and drug therapy (see Appendix 5), combined with the emotional stress of hospitalization, can create or compound nutritional problems. It is well documented that a significant percentage of hospitalized clients develop malnutrition because of mismanagement or neglect. Impaired wound healing and susceptibility to infection are well-known consequences of malnutrition, both of which may prolong hospitalization and increase morbidity and mortality. Practices that are necessary to ensure optimal nutritional care appear in the display, Preventing Hospital Malnutrition.

"Hospital food," which may be a vital component of treatment, may be rejected for social, religious, or personal reasons. Frequently, appetite decreases as nutritional requirements increase (see display, Risk Factors for Poor Nutritional Status).

Nutritional support must not only provide adequate amounts of required nutrients—it must also deliver those nutrients in a form that the client will accept, use, and tolerate. Nutrients can be delivered orally, enterally, parenterally, or by a combination of those methods. Figure 14-1 illustrates the step-by-step decision-making process involved in selecting the appropriate type and method of feeding.

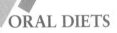

ORAL DIETS

Obviously, oral diets are the easiest, least expensive, least risky, and the preferred method of delivering nutrients, not only from a physiologic standpoint but also psy-

---

Preventing Hospital Malnutrition

To optimize nutritional care:

Record height and weight.

Provide consistent care despite staff rotation.

Assign accountability to nutritional care even if responsibility is diffused.

Discontinue IV glucose therapy as soon as possible.

Observe and record clients' food intake.

Assist clients who are unable to feed themselves.

Replace meals that are withheld for diagnostic tests.

Use tube feedings that are nutritionally adequate, consistent in composition, and prepared under sanitary conditions.

Know the composition of vitamin and nutritional products provided.

Recognize that illness and injury increase nutritional requirements.

Assess the nutritional status of clients who have or are at high risk for malnutrition.

Progress postsurgical diets as quickly as tolerated.

Realize the importance of nutrition in the prevention of, and recovery from, infection and to avoid unwarranted reliance on antibiotics.

Promote communication and interaction between the dietitian and physician.

Provide nutritional support to prevent malnutrition; once established, malnutrition may be difficult or impossible to reverse.

Use laboratory tests as part of nutritional assessment.

Risk Factors for Poor Nutritional Status

ANTHROPOMETRIC RISK FACTORS

Weight greater than 120% of ideal or less than 90% of ideal

Unintentional weight loss greater than 10% of weight within last 6 months

Arm muscle circumference or triceps skinfold <85% of standard

Inconsistent growth rates in children or abnormal weight for height

DIETARY RISK FACTORS

Inadequate food intake, fad dieting, numerous food intolerances or allergies

Use of inadequate modified diet (ie, clear liquid) for more than 3 days without adequate supplementation

NPO with simple IV therapy for longer than 3 days

Inadequate tube feedings

Difficulty chewing or swallowing

Changes in taste, smell, or appetite

MEDICAL–SOCIOECONOMIC RISK FACTORS

Medical conditions that alter intake or nutrient requirements: cancer, malabsorption, diarrhea, hyperthyroidism, severe infection, recent surgery, hemorrhage, physical or mental disabilities, multiple wounds or fractures, extensive burns

Persistent fever above 37°C for more than 2 days

Long-term use of drugs that affect nutritional status

Alcohol abuse

Inadequate food budget

BIOCHEMICAL RISK FACTORS

Low hematocrit and hemoglobin

Total lymphocyte count <1500/mm^3

Elevated or decreased serum cholesterol level

Serum albumin less than 3.5 g/dl

chologically (see display, Normal and Modified Diets). Normal diets are intended to maintain health by meeting the recommended dietary allowances (RDA) for the client's age and sex. No foods are excluded and portion sizes are not restricted on a normal diet.

Modified diets are used for clients who are unable to tolerate a normal diet or who have altered nutritional requirements. Modified diets can differ from normal diets in their consistency (ie, liquid or pureed), total calorie content (ie, high-calorie, low-calorie), concentration of macronutrients (ie, high-protein, low-fat), concentration of micronutrients (ie, low-sodium, low-potassium), or concentration of specific dietary components (ie, gluten free). Combinations of diet modifications may be necessary to meet a client's needs. All diets should be individualized as much as possible to ensure optimal tolerance and compliance.

When oral intake is resumed after acute illness, surgery, tube feedings, or total parenteral nutrition, clear liquids may be ordered and progressed to full liquids → soft diet → normal or modified diet (Table 14-1). Depending on the client's tolerance and condition, this routine progression may be accelerated by eliminating one or more of the transitional diets.

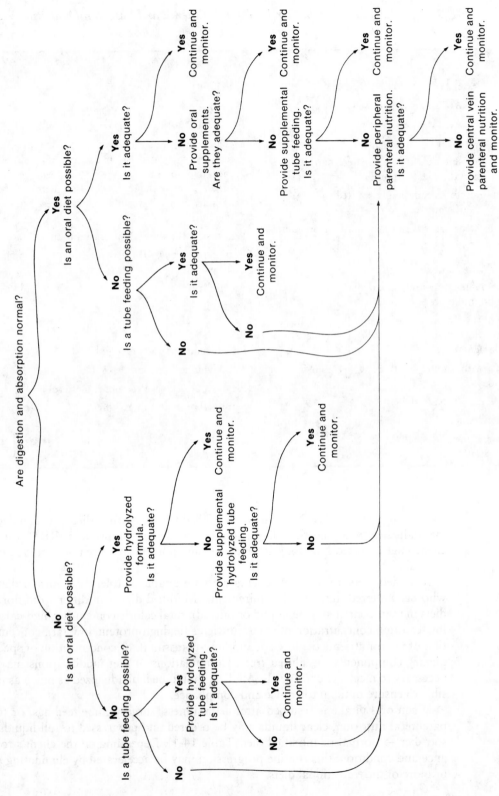

Figure 14-1

Selecting the appropriate type and method of feeding.

430

Normal and Modified Diets

"NORMAL" ("REGULAR" OR "HOUSE") DIETS FOR

Adults

Infants, children, and adolescents

Pregnancy and lactation

Vegetarians

DIETS MODIFIED IN CONSISTENCY AND TEXTURE

Clear liquid diet

Full liquid diet

Soft diet

Mechanical soft diet

Puréed diet

Tube feedings

Low-residue diet

High-fiber diet

Bland diet

CALORIE-MODIFIED DIETS

High-calorie diet

Low-calorie diet

Calorie-controlled diet (ie, diabetic diets)

MODIFIED NUTRIENT DIETS

High-CHO diet

Restricted CHO diet (ie, "anti-dumping" diets)

High-protein diet

Low-protein diet

Low-fat diet

Modified fat diet

Low-cholesterol diet

Low-potassium diet

High-potassium diet

Low-sodium diet

Low-calcium diet

Fluid-restricted diet

Force fluids

MODIFIED DIETS RESTRICTING OR ELIMINATING CERTAIN FOODS

Gluten-free diet

Low-lactose or lactose-free diet

Purine-restricted diet

Elimination diets for allergies

Tyramine-restricted diet

Phenylalanine-restricted diet

Various diagnostic tests that may be performed in the hospital setting require that specific diets be followed before the procedure. Although diet specifications vary among laboratories, examples of common "test" diets are outlined in Appendix 6.

Clients who are unable or unwilling to eat enough food to meet at least two thirds of their protein and calorie requirements may be given supplements orally or through a tube to augment their intake.

Oral Supplements

Oral supplements (homemade and commercial varieties) are frequently used to boost the protein and calorie intake of clients who are unable to meet their nutritional requirements through food alone. For example, oral supplements are frequently used in conjunction with full liquid diets, in clients with poor appetites, and when requirements are increased related to surgery or simple stress.

Milk shakes, instant breakfasts, eggnogs, and milk fortified with skim milk powder are high-protein, high-calorie "homemade" oral supplements that provide sig-

Table 14-1
Characteristics, Indications, and Contraindications for Liquid and Soft Diets

Diet Characteristics	Foods Allowed	Indications	Contraindications
CLEAR LIQUID			
A short-term, highly restrictive diet composed only of clear fluids or foods that are fluid at body temperature. It requires minimal digestion and leaves a minimum of residue. Although they provide some electrolyte and carbohydrates, clear liquid diets are inadequate in calories and all nutrients except vitamin C. Be sure to include bouillon in the diet if electrolyte replacement is needed; eliminate bouillon if the client requires a sodium restriction (one bouillon cube provides 424 mg of sodium).	Bouillon Fat-free broth Carbonated beverages Coffee, regular and decaf Fruit juices, strained and clear (apple, cranberry, grape) Gelatin Popsicles Tea Sugar, honey, hard candy	Initial feeding after surgery or parenteral nutrition; in preparation for surgery and various diagnostic tests of the bowel	Long-term use
FULL LIQUID DIET			
Composed of foods that are liquid or liquefy at body temperature. Full liquid diets can be carefully planned or supplemented to approximate the nutritional value of a regular or high-calorie–high-protein diet, making them suitable for long-term use. Full liquid diets may be inadequate in folic acid, iron, vitamin B_6, and fiber. If the diet is used longer than 2 to 3 days, the following modifications may be needed to increase calories and protein: Add sugar and syrups whenever possible. Use whole-fat milk unless the client has hypercholesterolemia. Melt butter or margarine on soup and cereal. Add glucose supplements to fruit juices, milk, and milk drinks. Add skim milk powder to milk, milk drinks, soup, custard, puddings, cereal. Add instant breakfast or commercial supplements (Appendix 7). Lactose-reduced milk is available for clients with lactose intolerance.	All the above plus: All milk and milk drinks, puddings, custards, desserts All vegetable juices All fruit juices Refined or strained cereals Eggs in custard Butter, margarine, cream	Used as a transitional diet between a clear liquid diet and a soft diet, and by clients who have difficulty chewing or swallowing	Severe lactose intolerance (diet relies heavily on milk and dairy products for protein and calories) Unless modified to decrease the cholesterol content, a liquid diet is not suitable for long-term use by clients with hypercholesterolemia

Table 14-1 *(Continued)* **Characteristics, Indications, and Contraindications for Liquid and Soft Diets**			
Diet Characteristics	**Foods Allowed**	**Indications**	**Contraindications**
May be adapted for clients with diabetes mellitus, renal disease, and other disorders. Low-sodium soups, eggnogs, and custard should be used by clients who require a sodium restriction. To avoid salmonella infection, raw eggs should not be used.			
SOFT DIET			
An adequate diet low in fiber, connective tissue, and fat. Restrictions vary considerably among institutions: Individual tolerances should determine the content of the diet.	All the above plus: Cooked vegetables as tolerated Lettuce in small amounts Cooked or canned fruit Avocado Banana Grapefruit and orange sections without membranes Whole-grain or enriched breads and cereals Potatoes Enriched rice, barley, pasta All lean, tender meats, fish, poultry Eggs, mild cheese, smooth peanut butter Butter, margarine, mild salad dressings	Used for clients who have difficulty chewing or swallowing. A mechanical soft diet is used primarily by clients who have difficulty chewing because they are endentulous or have ill-fitting dentures. A regular soft diet is used as a transition between liquids and a regular diet.	None

nificant amounts of protein and calories, are palatable, and are relatively inexpensive. However, these milk-based formulas are not appropriate for clients who (1) are lactose-intolerant (unable to tolerate milk sugar); (2) are unable to digest or absorb a normal diet; (3) need *complete* nutritional support in a liquid form; or (4) have metabolic disturbances that alter nutritional requirements.

Numerous commercial products, which vary in composition, taste, and cost, are available as alternatives to "homemade" supplements (see Appendix 7). As with use of homemade supplements, problems with taste fatigue arise with long-term use. To maximize acceptance, serve oral supplements cold, and experiment with different flavors.

Modular Products

Modular products are incomplete formulas that supply a single nutrient, either carbohydrate (eg, hydrolyzed cornstarch), protein (eg, whey protein), or fat (eg, MCT oil) (see display, Examples of Modular Products). They are not intended to be used as a sole source of nutrition but, rather, are used individually or in combination to alter the nutritional value of a food or enteral formula. For instance, a protein module may be added to a tube feeding to increase protein density without significantly affecting volume. Likewise, clients with chronic renal failure may receive carbohydrate-fortified mashed potatoes and juices to increase calorie intake without increasing protein content.

ENTERAL NUTRITION

Enteral nutrition is defined as the delivery of nutrients by mouth or tube into the gastrointestinal (GI) tract. In practice, the term enteral nutrition is used interchangeably with tube feeding. Tube feedings may be "homemade" blenderized diets or commercial formulas used as a total or supplemental feeding, and are often used as a transition between parenteral nutrition and an oral diet (see Appendix 7).

Compared to parenteral nutrition, enteral nutrition is safer and significantly less costly, and should be used whenever the GI tract is functional. Using the GI tract also helps prevent gut atrophy and helps reduce the risk of sepsis by preventing **bacterial translocation**, which is the movement of gut bacteria from the GI tract into lymph nodes and other internal organs. Criteria to consider when choosing a tube feeding appear in the display, "Ideal" Tube Feeding Characteristics. Clients who are unable to meet their nutritional requirements enterally may be candidates for supplemental parenteral nutrition.

Although tube feedings are useful for a variety of clinical conditions (see display, Common Indications for Tube Feedings), they are contraindicated when the GI tract is nonfunctional, as in the case of gastric or intestinal obstruction, paralytic ileus, intractable vomiting, and severe diarrhea (see Food for Thought: Terminal Illness . . . To Tube Or Not To Tube?).

Examples of Modular Products

Carbohydrate Modules

Moducal (Mead Johnson) (maltodextrins)

Polycose (Ross) (hydrolyzed cornstarch)

Protein Modules

Casec (Mead Johnson) (calcium caseinate)

ProMod (Ross) (D—whey protein concentrate)

Fat Modules

MCT oil (Mead Johnson) (coconut oil)

Nutrisource Lipid medium chain triglycerides (Sandoz Nutrition) (coconut oil)

Common Indications for Tube Feedings

NEUROLOGIC/PSYCHIATRIC

Post cerebrovascular accident

Neoplasms

Trauma

Inflammation

Demyelinating diseases

Severe depression, psychosis, other mental disorders

Anorexia nervosa

GASTROINTESTINAL

Severe dysphagia

Pancreatitis

Inflammatory bowel disease

Short bowel syndrome

Malabsorption

Low-output enterocutaneous fistula

OTHER

Thermal injury

Chemotherapy

Radiotherapy

Sepsis

Head and neck surgery, trauma, and cancer

Postoperative nutritional support

Ventilator-dependent clients

Protein–calorie malnutrition with inadequate oral intake

Types of Formulas

Complete tube-feeding formulas provide adequate amounts of all required nutrients, and, although they are intended for use as total feedings, they may also be given in smaller amounts to supplement an oral diet. The two major categories of commercial formulas are standard formulas and hydrolyzed formulas.

Standard formulas contain **intact proteins (or intact nutrients)** that are made from whole complete proteins (eg, milk, meat, and eggs), or **protein isolates** (semipurified, high-biologic-value proteins that have been extracted from milk, soybean, or eggs). Examples of standard formulas appear in the display, Examples of Standard Formulas. Most standard formulas provide approximately 1.0 cal/ml, although high-density formulas that supply 2.0 cal/ml also are available. Although variations exist, most standard formulas derive approximately 16% of total calories from protein, 54% from carbohydrate, and 30% from fat. Special standard formulas are available for clients with diabetes, renal insufficiency, and pulmonary disorders.

Many intact formulas are enriched with dietary fiber. Although high-fiber formulas have been promoted as preventing or controlling both constipation and diarrhea in tube-fed clients, definitive studies on fiber's efficacy are lacking. However, because of its role in maintaining gut mucosal integrity, fiber may be a desirable component of a standard tube-feeding regimen.

Because all intact formulas are made from complex molecules of protein, carbohydrate, and fat, they require normal digestion before they can be absorbed. They are more palatable, less costly, and lower in **osmolality** (see display, Osmolality) than hydrolyzed formulas.

Hydrolyzed formulas, which contain partially digested nutrients (ie, hydrolyzed peptides), are available for clients with impaired digestion or absorption (see the dis-

FOOD *for* THOUGHT

Terminal Illness . . . To Tube or Not to Tube? That Is the Question

Legal, ethical, and medical controversy surrounds the issue of tube feeding terminally ill adults. Although some argue that health care professionals have the responsibility to alleviate suffering and preserve the rights and dignity of all people, others contend that foregoing or discontinuing hydration and nutrition is inhumane and criminal. Central to any decision about whether to provide or withhold nutritional support are the wishes of the competent, informed client or his/her health care proxy. In addition, keep in mind that:

Each case is unique and must be decided individually.

The client's expressed wishes are the major determinant of the level of nutrition intervention.

The health care team must evaluate the potential risks and expected benefits of nonoral feedings and discuss these with the client. The client's physical and psychological comfort should be the focus of care.

Because the consequences of foregoing nutritional support may be irreversible within a period of days or weeks, the decision should be made with careful consideration.

The decision to forego "heroic" measures is not the same as withholding all nutrition support. "DNR" means "do not resuscitate," not "do not feed."

The decision whether to provide or forego nutrition support is documented in the medical record by the physician.

Defined, written guidelines for nutrition support protocol should be established and implemented in each institution with the help of an ethics committee, if available.

Source: American Dietetic Association (1992). Position of the American Dietetic Association: Issues in feeding the terminally ill adult. J Am Diet Assoc, 92(8), 996–1002.

Examples of Standard Formulas

Blenderized Formulas with Intact Protein

Compleat Regular (Sandoz Nutrition)

Vitaneed (Sherwood Medical)

Protein Isolate Formulas Containing Lactose

Mertitene (Sandoz Nutrition)

Sustagen (Mead Johnson)

Protein Isolate Formulas, Lactose-Free

Ensure (Ross)

Isocal (Mead Johnson)

Resource (Sandoz Nutrition)

Protein Isolate Formulas, Fiber-Enriched

Jevity (Ross)

Fibersource (Sandoz Nutrition)

Sustacal with Fiber (Mead Johnson)

Osmolality

Osmolality equals the number of particles (osmoles) per kg of water in solution.

The concentration of CHO, amino acid, and electrolytes determines osmolality of nutritional formulas. Generally, the more digested the protein, the greater the osmolality.

A solution that is *isotonic* has approximately the same osmolality as blood, about 300 mOsm.

The osmolality of a *hypertonic* or *hyperosmolar* solution is greater than that of blood (greater than 300 mOsm). If administered too rapidly or before the client has adapted to the high concentration of particles, hypertonic solutions can cause water to rush into the intestines to dilute particle concentrations, leading to cramping, nausea, and diarrhea ("dumping syndrome").

play, Examples of Hydrolyzed and Elemental Formulas). The osmolality of these products ranges from 300 to 810 mOsm/kg water. These formulas are often used as a transition diet between parenteral nutrition and a standard feeding. However, because most are hypertonic and relatively expensive, hydrolyzed formulas are contraindicated in patients who have a normally functioning GI tract.

Formulas that are made with crystalline amino acids, sometimes referred to as **elemental formulas**, are the simplest type of hydrolyzed protein formulas; they are made from free amino acids, simple sugar, and very little fat. Some elemental formulas are designed to be used for "stress"; they are high in branched-chain amino acids, which are metabolized primarily in the peripheral muscle tissue, and may be used preferentially for energy during stress. **Specially defined formulas** are designed for patients with specific metabolic disorders such as renal failure or hepatic failure.

Feeding Tubes

Large-bore feeding tubes made of rubber or polyvinyl chloride (PVC) were widely used in the past, even though they were extremely irritating to the nose and esophagus, needed to be replaced frequently because digestive juices caused them to stiffen,

Examples of Hydrolyzed and Elemental Formulas

Hydrolyzed Protein Formulas

Criticare HN (Mead Johnson)

Vital HN (Ross)

Reabilan (Elan Pharma Nutrition)

Elemental Formulas (Free Amino Acids)

Tolerex (Sandoz Nutrition)

Vivonex Plus (Sandoz Nutrition)

Specially Defined Formulas

Hepatic-Aid (McGaw) (hepatic failure)

Travasorb Renal (Clintec Nutrition) renal failure)

and interfered with normal cardiac sphincter function, which increased the risk of gastric reflux and aspiration.

These problems, especially severe irritation, have been greatly reduced by the introduction of soft, pliable, small-bore feeding tubes made of silicone, PVC, or polyurethane. Weighted tips of tungsten or molded plastic facilitate their passage into the intestines and help anchor them in position. The diameter of the tube that is used should be the smallest size possible that allows the formula to flow freely, generally size 12 French or less. Generally, the lower the residue content of a formula, the smaller the tube size needed. Small-bore tubes used for supplemental tube feedings allow the client to consume food orally while the tubes are left in place. Regardless of the type of tube used or its placement, proper care must be given to ensure that the tube does not clog, break, fall out, or fall "in."

FEEDING TUBE PLACEMENT

The placement of the feeding tube depends on the client's medical status and the anticipated length of time the tube feeding will be used. Generally, transnasal tubes, of which the nasogastric is the most common, are used for tube feedings of relatively short duration (ie, less than 6 weeks). Ostomies, or stomas, are surgically created openings made to deliver feedings directly into the stomach or intestines. They are the preferred method for permanent or long-term feedings because they eliminate irritation to the mucous membranes. Percutaneous endoscopic gastrostomy tube feedings are placed nonsurgically with the aid of an endoscope. The correct placement of any feeding tube should be determined by x-rays of the chest that are taken before the first feeding is initiated. Table 14-2 summarizes advantages and disadvantages of various feeding routes.

Transnasal Tubes

Transnasal tubes are inserted nonsurgically through the nose and extended into either the stomach (NG) or the intestine (NI). The client can participate actively in the procedure by swallowing small sips of water as the tube is passed, which minimizes discomfort and speeds its passage. The disadvantage with transnasal tubes is that they have the potential to irritate the nose and esophagus if they are used for prolonged periods or if the tube is too large. In addition, they can be easily removed by uncooperative or confused patients.

Tube Enterostomy

Ostomy tubes are inserted through a surgical opening in the stomach, esophagus, or jejunum, usually under general anesthesia. Compared to transnasal feedings, ostomy feedings may be more successful for long-term use and more acceptable to the client because they are hidden under clothing.

Esophagostomy, a surgical opening made in the esophagus through which a feeding tube is passed into the stomach, is commonly used for patients with head and neck cancer. Esophagostomy feedings are generally well tolerated because the stomach is used to hold and release food at a controlled rate, which prevents the "dump-

Table 14-2
Advantages and Disadvantages of Various Feeding Routes

Route	Indications	Advantages	Disadvantages
Nasogastric (NG)	Short-term feeding (less than 6 weeks) with functional GI tract	Uses stomach as reservoir Can use intermittent feedings "Dumping syndrome" less likely than with NI feedings	Contraindicated for clients at high risk for aspiration Not appropriate for long-term use Unaesthetic for client
Nasointestinal (NI)	Short-term feeding for clients with normal digestion and absorption	Less risk of aspiration, especially important for clients with impaired gag or cough reflex, decreased consciousness, who are ventilator-dependent, or who have a history of aspiration pneumonia	Increased risk of "dumping syndrome" Not appropriate for intermittent or bolus feedings Not appropriate for long-term use Unaesthetic for client
Gastrostomy	For long-term use in clients with a functional GI tract Frequently used for clients with impaired ability to swallow	Same advantages as NG, but more comfortable and aesthetic for client Confirmation of tube placement easier Can't be misplaced into trachea	PEG insertion contraindicated for clients who cannot have an endoscopy Risk of aspiration pneumonia in clients with gastro-esophageal reflux Risk of wound cellulitis
Jejunostomy	For long-term use in clients at high risk for aspiration pneumonia and for clients with altered GI integrity above the jejunum For short-term use after GI surgery	Low risk of aspiration No risk of misplacing tube into the trachea More comfortable and aesthetic for clients than transnasal tubes Can be used immediately after GI surgery	Small-diameter tubes become easily clogged Peritonitis can occur from tube dislodgment Cannot be used for intermittent or bolus feedings

ing syndrome." However, the risk of aspiration is high, and the danger of hemorrhagic injury to the thoracic duct exists.

A surgical **gastrostomy** is performed by inserting a tube directly into the stomach. Gastrostomy feedings are well tolerated because they take advantage of the stomach's role in digestion to hold and release food at a controlled rate, thereby avoiding the "dumping syndrome." A disadvantage is the high risk of aspiration. Also, if the gastric contents leak, the skin surrounding the exit site may become irritated and infected; the danger of peritonitis exists.

Percutaneous endoscopic gastrostomy (PEG) is a relatively new nonsurgical technique that is used for placing a feeding tube directly into the stomach. Although there are several different techniques, all methods use an endoscope with a light to determine placement. A flexible guidewire is inserted percutaneously into the stomach, and a tube is then inserted over the wire and secured by rubber "bumpers" or an inflated balloon catheter.

This procedure avoids laparotomy and usually can be performed under local anesthesia and intravenous sedation. As such, it is less costly and less risky than surgical gastrostomies, and feedings can be started sooner, usually within 24 hours after the procedure. Percutaneous endoscopic gastrostomy can also be used as a route of placement for a transpyloric feeding tube in patients with a contraindication for intragastric feedings. Percutaneous endoscopic gastrostomy feedings are contraindicated when an endoscopy cannot be performed, and in cases of active peptic ulcer disease or gastric outlet obstruction. Relative contraindications include previous gastric surgery, gastric or esophageal varices, ascites, severe gastroesophageal reflux, and gastroenteric fistulas. Because it makes the procedure more difficult, obesity may also be considered a contraindication. The most frequent complications of a PEG are accidental tube removal, wound cellulitis, aspiration pneumonia, and clogged tubes.

A **jejunostomy** is an opening in the jejunum that can be accomplished by way of a needle catheter placement, direct tube placement, or creation of a jejunal stoma that can be intermittently catheterized. Percutaneous endoscopic jejunostomy (PEJ), an extension of the percutaneous endoscopic gastrostomy procedure, is also performed. Jejunostomy feedings pose little risk of aspiration and have the advantage of using the GI tract for absorption even if digestion is impaired. Formula selection depends on where in the jejunum the tube is placed; intact formulas may be used if they are to be infused into the proximal jejunum, whereas hydrolyzed formulas are indicated for infusions into the mid- or distal jejunum and for needle catheter jejunostomies, because thicker formulas clog the small-bore tube. Jejunostomy feedings also require careful administration, that is, a slow, controlled, continuous drip by pump to avoid diarrhea.

Method of Delivery

The three methods of delivering tube-feeding formulas are bolus administration, intermittent infusion, and continuous drip. The rates may be regulated either by a pump or by gravity drip. The type of delivery method to be used depends on the type and location of the feeding tube, the type of formula being administered, and the patient's tolerance.

Bolus feedings can be used only when the tube is placed in the stomach. The feeding, which is poured into the barrel of a large syringe attached to a feeding tube, flows by gravity into the stomach. Generally, a 4- to 6-hour volume of formula is given four to six times per day. Intact formulas, either those prepared commercially or "homemade" versions, can be used. This method of feeding is most appropriate for patients who want to feed themselves and for disoriented patients who require observation throughout the feeding to ensure that the feeding actually is delivered. Unfortunately, rapid, uncontrolled bolus feedings of 300 to 400 ml of formula given four to six times per day are poorly tolerated and often cause the dumping syndrome: nausea, diarrhea, glucosuria, distention, cramps, vomiting, and increased risk of aspiration.

Intermittent tube feedings, administered in equal portions four to six times per day, have the advantage of resembling a more normal pattern of intake and allow the client more freedom of movement between feedings. Tolerance of intermittent feedings is optimized by infusing the formula by slow gravity drip or by pump over a 30- to 60-minute period. Generally, no more than 300 ml of formula should be given in a single feeding, unless the feeding is delivered very slowly. To decrease the risk of aspiration, gastric residuals should be checked before each feeding until tolerance is clearly established.

The **continuous drip method** of feeding is given over a 16- to 24-hour period to maximize tolerance and nutrient absorption; as such, it is the recommended method for feeding critically ill clients and for feedings delivered into the jejunum. It also is frequently used to begin a feeding into the stomach (ie, NG, gastrostomy, PEG), but may be replaced with intermittent feedings after 3 or 4 days without complications, to resemble more closely a normal intake. Because consistent flow rates are difficult to achieve by gravity drip, infusion pumps are recommended. Pumps have significantly reduced the incidence of diarrhea, and should always be used to prevent "dumping syndrome" when feedings are infused into the distal duodenum or jejunum. Feedings should be interrupted every 6 hours to infuse water into the line to clear the tubing and hydrate the client.

Table 14-3 summarizes appropriate formulas and delivery methods for enteral feeding based on feeding tube and GI function.

Administration

Before a tube feeding is initiated, tube placement must be verified, preferably by x-ray, and bowel sounds must be present. **Isotonic** feedings (approximately 300

Table 14-3
Appropriate Formulas and Delivery Methods for Enteral Feeding Based on Feeding Tube and GI Function

Tube (Caliber)		Gastrointestinal Function		Diet		Preferred Administration Schedule
Nasogastric (8–12 Fr)	→	Normal	→	Intact nutrient formula	→	Continuous or intermittent
		Abnormal	→	Elemental formula	→	Continuous
Esophagostomy/ pharyngostomy/ gastrostomy (>10 Fr)	→	Normal	→	Intact nutrient formula	→	Continuous or intermittent
		Abnormal	→	Elemental formula		
Jejunostomy (>6 Fr)	→	Normal	→	Intact nutrient formula	→	Continuous controlled by enteral pump
		Abnormal	→	Elemental formula		

mOsm/kg water) should be given full-strength at 25 to 50 ml/hr and advanced by 25 ml/hr every 12 to 24 hours until the desired rate is achieved. Initially, hypertonic feedings should be diluted to approximate isotonicity (ie, one-quarter to one-half strength) for clients who are malnourished (ie, serum albumin is less than 3.5 mg/dl). After tolerance is established, the rate is advanced by 25 ml/hr every 8 to 12 hours until the desired rate is achieved. The concentration is increased every 8 to 12 hours only after the desired rate is achieved, in gradations of one-half to three-quarters strength, as tolerated. Rate and concentration should never be advanced at the same time, and neither should be progressed until 8 to 12 hours after tolerance is established. When a fluid restriction is required, tube feedings can be started at 30 ml/hr.

Although feedings that are infused by continuous drip can be given chilled, intermittent and bolus feedings are better tolerated at room temperature. To reduce the risk of bacterial contamination, closed feeding systems are recommended. Other precautions include changing the extension tubing and bag daily, refrigerating prepared formulas until they are needed, never adding a new supply of formula to old formula, and hanging feeding solutions for less than 6 hours.

To prevent aspiration when feeding into the stomach, the head of the bed should be elevated at least 30° during the feeding and for 30 to 45 minutes afterward. Feedings should be held if gastric residuals are greater than 100 ml; aspirate should be replaced to reduce the loss of electrolytes and gastric juices. Some facilities color the feedings with food dye so that pulmonary secretions can be monitored for aspirated tube feedings. Although this practice may facilitate detection of aspirate, it does not protect against aspiration. In addition, blue food coloring causes a false-positive result in a Hematest for occult blood, and red or orange food coloring added to the formula makes the stool look bloody. A better approach for testing pulmonary secretions for aspiration is to use a glucose dipstick—unless they are bloody, pulmonary secretions normally do not contain glucose, whereas enteral formulas do.

To help ensure tube patency, intermittent and bolus feedings should be followed by an infusion of 40 to 50 ml of warm water, and continuous feeding tubes should be irrigated every shift with 40 to 50 ml of warm water. Likewise, every time the feeding is interrupted, the tube should be flushed with water.

Although many medications are frequently given through feeding tubes in patients who are unable to swallow, they should never be given while a feeding is infusing (Miller and Miller, 1995). Some drugs become ineffective if added directly to the enteral formula; also, adding drugs to the formula may result in a clogged tube. It is important to stop the feeding before administering drugs, making sure the tube is flushed with 15 to 30 cc of water before and after the drug is given. If more than one drug is given, flush the tube between doses. Drugs that are absorbed from the stomach should never be given through a nasointestinal tube. See Drug Alert for medications that should not be infused through an enteral tube.

Transition to Oral Diet

The goal of diet intervention during the transition period between enteral nutrition and an oral diet is to ensure an adequate nutritional intake while promoting an oral diet. To begin the transition process, the tube feeding should be stopped for 1 hour

DRUG
ALERT

Because they cannot be crushed and are not available in another oral form, substitutes should be requested when any of the following drugs are ordered for a tube-fed client who is unable to take oral medications:

Benzonatate (Tessalon)
Bisacodyl (Dulcolax)
Diclofenac (Voltaren)
Diltiazem (Cardizem SR)
Isotretinoin (Accutane)
Omeprazole (Prilosec)
Orphenadrine (Norflex)
Pentoxifylline (Trental)
Piroxicam (Feldene)

Source: Miller, D. and Miller, H. (1995). Giving meds through the tube. RN, 58(1), 44–46.

before each meal. Gradually increase meal frequency until six small oral feedings are accepted. Actual intake should be recorded and evaluated daily. When oral calorie intake consistently includes 500 to 750 calories/day, tube feedings may be given only during the night. When the client consistently consumes two thirds of protein and calorie needs orally for 3 to 5 days, the tube feeding may be totally discontinued.

NURSING PROCESS

Assessment

Initial and ongoing assessments are vital to evaluate the success of a tube feeding. Because the majority of patients who are receiving tube feedings have had feeding difficulties or medical problems that place them at increased risk, initial and periodic nutritional assessments should be performed. Although an in-depth nutritional assessment may be the dietitian's responsibility, the following screening data may be useful for the nurse.

Assess for the following factors:

Feeding route and the client's ability to digest and absorb nutrients (see Table 14-3); compare these to the form and source of nutrients provided in the formula. Be aware that clients with altered renal or liver function may require specialized metabolic formulas. Other considerations include the goals of therapy, the availability and cost of the formula, especially for home enteral nutrition, and "taste." Even though the client cannot truly taste a tube feeding, appearance and aroma may influence palatability and acceptance (see display, "Ideal" Tube Feeding Characteristics).

Weight status and any recent weight change.

Serum albumin and transferrin, if available, and evaluate any other abnormal laboratory values for their nutritional significance.

"Ideal" Tube Feeding Characteristics

Provides nutrients in a form the client can digest and absorb, is free from nutrients not tolerated by the client (e.g., lactose).

Nutritionally balanced and calorically adequate.

Provides 100% of the Recommended Dietary Allowances for vitamins and minerals in an acceptable volume of formula.

Well-tolerated: The client does not experience diarrhea, nausea, constipation, vomiting.

Easy to prepare and bacteriologically safe.

Convenient and easy to administer.

Of the proper viscosity to prevent clogging the tube.

Affordable and readily available.

Outward signs of malnutrition.

Hydration status.

Adequacy of intake before the initiation of tube feeding. Assess cultural, familial, religious, and ethnic influences on eating habits and how they may affect formula selection. Ask the client if there is a history of food intolerances or allergies (eg, lactose, gluten).

Past medical history and current problems, and evaluate the impact on intake and nutritional status. Assess GI and major organ function (renal, hepatic, cardiac).

For clients who are candidates for home enteral nutrition, assess the client's motivational level, social support system, and financial status. Evaluate the home environment to assess the availability of running water, electricity, refrigeration, and storage space.

Nursing Diagnosis

Altered Nutrition: Potential for more than or less than body requirements, related to tube feeding.

Planning and Implementation

Fluid, calorie, and protein requirements are individualized according to the client's nutritional assessment data.

The normal fluid requirement for adults is about 1.0 ml/cal. Patients who are experiencing a fever, draining fistulas or surgical tubes, diarrhea, hemorrhaging, extensive tissue breakdown, increased perspiration, or an inability to concentrate the urine (ie, characteristic of some renal diseases and the elderly) require more fluid. Patients with renal failure, liver failure, and heart disease may require less fluid. Generally, formulas that provide 1 cal/ml contain approximately 850 ml of water per liter of formula. Additional water given between feedings and the water used to clean the feeding tube also contribute to fluid intake.

Estimate calorie requirements. Use the Harris-Benedict equation (HBE) to estimate basal energy requirement (BEE); multiply BEE by an activity factor and an injury factor to estimate total calorie requirements (see display, Estimating Total Calorie Requirements).

Estimate the patient's protein requirement based on weight, laboratory data, and medical status. General guidelines are as follows:

0.8–1.0 g protein/kg for a normal, healthy adult
1.5–2.0 g/kg for fever, fracture, infection, protein depletion
2.0–2.5 g/kg for sepsis
1.5–3.0 g/kg for extensive burns

Be aware of the potential complications associated with tube feedings and nursing interventions to alleviate those problems (see display, Tube Feedings: Potential Problems, Rationale, and Nursing Interventions). In addition, clients who are receiving formula at a decreased volume or concentration may not be meeting their nutritional requirements and may need supplements.

Even though patients cannot taste tube feedings, the formula's appearance and aroma may influence its acceptance by the patient. For variety, add commercially available flavoring packets. If the formula's appearance is offensive, cover the feeding reservoir or remove it from the patient's field of vision, if possible.

(Text continues on page 450)

Estimating Total Calorie Requirements

1. Calculate BEE using the Harris-Benedict equation:
   for men: BEE (cal) = $66 + 13.7W + 5H - 6.8A$ W = weight in kg*
   for women: BEE (cal) = $655 + 9.6W + 1.7H - 4.7A$ H = height in cm
   A = age in years

2. Multiply BEE by activity and stress factors:
   Activity factor
   Confined to bed = 1.2
   Out of bed = 1.3
   Stress factor
   Mild starvation = 0.85–1.0   Severe infection or multiple trauma = 1.3–1.55
   Minor surgery = 1.2   Major sepsis = 1.6
   Long-bone fracture = 1.25–1.3 Severe burns = 2.1
   Skeletal trauma = 1.35

3. Total calorie requirement = BEE × activity factor × stress factor

Example: A person whose BEE is 1509 calories, confined to bed, with major sepsis would have total calorie requirements of 1509 × 1.2 × 1.6 = 2897 calories.

* *If actual body weight is greater than 125% of IBW, use adjusted body weight instead of actual weight. Adjusted body weight = (actual weight − IBW) × .25 + IBW (approximately 25% of body fat is metabolically active)*

Tube Feedings: Potential Problems, Rationale, and Nursing Interventions

POTENTIAL PROBLEM

Diarrhea

Although properly administered tube feedings do not cause diarrhea, diarrhea frequently develops in tube-fed clients. Clients fed low-residue formulas cannot be expected to have firm stools; rather, their stools are likely to be pasty or gruel-like. However, if it is established that the client is truly having diarrhea, the probable cause is investigated. If antidiarrheal medications are ordered by the physician, observe for constipation and signs of fecal impaction.

Rationale/Nursing Intervention and Considerations

1. Formula too cold

   Give canned formulas at room temperature; warm refrigerated formulas to room temperature in a basin of hot water.

2. Bacterially contaminated formula

   Handwashing and strict sanitation are required for formula preparation; equipment and utensils used in preparation should be washed in an automatic dishwasher or cleaned with hot, soapy water and rinsed thoroughly in boiling water; dry upside down.

   Administer formula promptly after opening; do not add newly opened formula to formula already in the feeding bag.

   Store unused formula in a tightly covered, dated container in the refrigerator; use within 24 hours or as recommended by the manufacturer.

   Rinse the equipment before each feeding with 30 to 50 ml of water.

   Replace the feeding bag and tubing every 24 hours.

   Be sure continuous drip feeding formulas do not hang at room temperature longer than 6 hours; do not hang "homemade" blenderized formulas longer than 4 hours.

3. Lactose intolerance

   Switch to a lactose-free formula.

4. Feeding rate too rapid

   Start initial feedings at 50 ml/hr and increase by 25 ml/hr every 12 hours depending on the client's tolerance.

   For existing feedings, decrease the rate of feeding to the level tolerated, increase by half the original increment.

5. Volume of formula too great

   Decrease the volume to a level tolerated by the client; gradually increase as tolerated.

   Feed smaller volumes of formula at more frequent intervals or switch to a continuous drip method of feeding.

6. Hypertonic formula (concentrated solution of sugars, amino acids, and electrolytes) delivered before adaptation has occurred.

   Give initial feedings at one-quarter to one-half strength for a minimum of 8 hours and gradually increase to allow the client time to adjust to a hypertonic solution (do not increase the rate and strength at the same time).

   Deliver by continuous drip method.

   Switch to an isotonic solution, if possible.

7. Nasogastric feeding misplaced into the duodenum → "dumping syndrome"

   Check the position of the tube before administering the formula.

8. Low serum albumin → decreased oncotic pressure → increased water within the bowel → diarrhea. A low serum albumin, which may indicate malnutrition, may also be accompanied by 1) a decrease in intestinal border enzymes (protein molecules); and/or 2) a decrease or flattening of the microvilli lining the intestinal tract, both of which lead to diarrhea.

   Dilute the formula and increase the concentration gradually, or switch to an isotonic formula and infuse at slow rates.

   Consider parenteral administration of albumin.

9. Secondary to antibiotics or other drugs. The overgrowth of certain strains of intestinal flora that are not affected by antibiotics is believed to cause diarrhea. These flora digest formula, producing excess gas and acid and resulting in diarrhea. Antibiotic-associated diarrhea may also be related to a superinfection with *Clostridium difficile* or *Staphylococcus aureus*. The use of undiluted, hypertonic oral electrolyte solutions and drugs, as well as sorbitol, has been implicated as a cause of diarrhea.

Determine if the client is receiving antibiotics or other medications that may produce diarrhea: antiarrhythmic drugs (quinidine propranolol), aminophylline, digitalis, potassium supplements, phosphorus supplements, cimetidine. Investigate possible alternatives; administer antidiarrheals as ordered.

POTENTIAL PROBLEM

Regurgitation of stomach contents → aspiration pneumonia

Rationale/Nursing Intervention and Considerations

1. Slowed gastric emptying time; that is, the gastric residual is greater than 100 ml
   Check gastric residual before each intermittent feeding and every 4 hours if continuous feeding is used. The physician should be notified and the feeding regimen should be evaluated if gastric emptying is consistently delayed.
   Switch to a continuous drip method of delivery.
2. Inhibited cough reflex related to debilitation, unconsciousness, or pulmonary complications
   Consider a nasoduodenal, nasojejunal, gastrostomy, or jejunostomy feeding.
3. Improper feeding position
   Elevate the head of the bed at least 30° during the feeding and for approximately 1 hour afterward.
4. Relaxed gastroesophageal sphincter related to a large-diameter feeding tube
   Switch to a pliable, small-diameter feeding tube.
5. High-fat content of formula (fat delays gastric emptying time)
   Switch to a low-fat formula.

POTENTIAL PROBLEM

Nausea
   Discontinue the feeding. Administer antiemetics if ordered by the physician.

Rationale/Nursing Intervention and Considerations

1. Malplacement of the tube
   Check the position of the tube.

2. Feeding rate too rapid
   Slow the rate of feeding; switch to a continuous drip method of delivery.
3. Volume of formula too great → delayed gastric emptying
   Check gastric residual and notify the physician if >100 ml.
   Reduce the volume and increase gradually.
   If distention is contributing to nausea, encourage ambulation.
4. Feeding too soon after intubation
   Allow approximately 1 hour between intubation and the first feeding.
5. Anxiety
   Explain the procedures to the client and encourage questions.
   Allow the client to verbalize his or her feelings; provide emotional support.
6. Intolerance to a specific formula, especially high-fat formulas
   Switch to a different formula.

POTENTIAL PROBLEMS

Distention and bloating

Rationale/Nursing Intervention and Considerations

1. High-fat content of the formula
   Switch to a low-fat formula.
2. Decrease in GI function, especially among critically ill clients
   Check for active bowel sounds; switch to a hydrolyzed formula if the bowel sounds are hypoactive.

POTENTIAL PROBLEM

Dehydration
   Monitor fluid intake and output. Provide fluid to balance urine output plus insensible water losses (approximately 500 ml/day in uncomplicated cases). Monitor serum BUN and sodium levels; elevated BUN and sodium levels indicate that the kidneys are unable to adequately excrete the nitrogenous wastes resulting from a high-protein intake combined with an inadequate intake of fluid. Monitor hematocrit and urine specific gravity, both of which increase as a result of dehydration.

(continued)

Tube Feedings: Potential Problems, Rationale, and Nursing Interventions *(Continued)*

Rationale/Nursing Intervention and Considerations

1. Diarrhea
   See above.
2. Excessive protein intake → increase in urea formation (end-products of protein metabolism) → compensatory increase in urine output
   Switch to a formula with less protein.
   Increase water intake, if possible.
3. Inadequate fluid intake
   Increase fluid intake.
4. Glycosuria
   Test for glucose in the urine; notify the physician of glucosuria of 3+ or 4+.
   Administer insulin if ordered by the physician.
   Switch to a continuous drip method to avoid giving a high-CHO load each feeding.

POTENTIAL PROBLEM

Fluid overload
   Monitor serum sodium, BUN, and hematocrit—all will decrease as a result of overhydration. Monitor intake and output.

Rationale/Nursing Intervention and Considerations

1. Excessive use of water to clean the tube after feedings
   Use only 30 to 50 ml of water to rinse the tube after each feeding.
2. Formula too dilute
   Check formula preparation for the proper dilution.

POTENTIAL PROBLEM

Constipation

Rationale/Nursing Intervention and Considerations

1. Low-residue content of the formula
   Increase residue content if appropriate (ie, change to a formula with added fiber or increase fruits and vegetables in a blenderized diet).
2. Decreased activity related to feeding apparatus
   Encourage ambulation as much as possible.
3. Dehydration
   Monitor intake and output. Add free water if intake is not greater than output by 500 to 1000 ml.
4. Obstruction
   Stop feeding and notify the physician.

POTENTIAL PROBLEM

Nose irritation

Rationale/Nursing Intervention and Considerations

1. Presence of an NG tube
   Remove dry mucous secretions with warm water or a water-soluble lubricant.
   Lubricate the tube regularly with water or a water-soluble lubricant.
   For persistent discomfort, withdraw the tube, clean, and reinsert.
   Notify the physician if irritation or bleeding is observed.
2. Too large an NG tube
   Switch to a smaller-diameter tube.

POTENTIAL PROBLEM

Skin irritation around the insertion site of a gastrostomy or jejunostomy tube

Rationale/Nursing Intervention and Considerations

1. Leakage of gastric or intestinal contents through the ostomy opening or tension from the tube
   Clean the skin around the catheter daily with warm water and mild soap to prevent skin irritation.
   Observe for drainage and signs of infection: edema, tenderness, or redness. If drainage is present, remove immediately, apply gauze around the tube, and notify the physician.

POTENTIAL PROBLEM

Gastric rupture

Rationale/Nursing Intervention and Considerations

1. Dangerous retention of feeding in the stomach related to gastric atony or obstruction

Check for residual before beginning each feeding.

Observe for signs of impending gastric rupture: distention, epigastric and upper quadrant pain, nausea, a large residual. If observed, discontinue feeding immediately and notify the physician.

POTENTIAL PROBLEM

Dry mouth

Rationale/Nursing Intervention and Considerations

1. NPO → irritation of the mucous membranes
   Apply petroleum jelly to the lips to prevent cracking.
   Allow ice chips, sugarless gum, and hard candies, if possible, to stimulate salivation
   Encourage good oral hygiene to alleviate soreness and dryness: mouthwash, warm water rinses, and regular brushing.
2. Breathing through the mouth
   Encourage the client to breathe through the nose as much as possible.

POTENTIAL PROBLEM

Clogged tube

Rationale/Nursing Intervention and Considerations

1. Feeding warmed formulas
   Do not heat formulas. Not only is the risk of clogging the tube increased, but water-soluble vitamins may be destroyed and the likelihood of bacterial contamination is increased.
2. Improper cleaning of the tube
   Replace the feeding tube and bag every 12 to 24 hours.
   Flush the tube before and after each infusion (regardless of the method) with 30 to 50 ml of water. If flushing fails to remove clog, the tube must be removed and replaced.
3. Formula too thick
   High-viscosity formulas (ie, blenderized tube feedings or commercial formulas that provide 1.5 cal/ml to 2 cal/ml) should be infused by pump and possibly through a large-bore feeding tube to prevent clogging.

If possible, consider switching to a less calorically dense formula.

Because it is desirable to use the smallest size tube, viscous formulas may be delivered by a pump to help prevent clogging.

POTENTIAL PROBLEM

Anxiety

Rationale/Nursing Intervention and Considerations

1. Deprivation of food → lack of sensory, social, and cultural satisfaction from eating
   Allow oral intake of food that the client requests, if possible. If oral intake is contraindicated, allow the client to chew his or her favorite food without swallowing.
   If possible, liquefy and add the client's favorite food to the tube feeding.
   Encourage the client to leave the room when others are eating and find other enjoyable activities.
   Encourage the client and family to view the tube feeding as another way of eating, rather than a form of treatment.
2. Altered body image
   Encourage the client to verbalize his or her feelings.
   Stress the positive aspects of the tube feeding.
3. Loss of control and fear
   Encourage the client to become involved in the preparation and administration of the formula, if possible.
   Inform the client of problems that may occur and how to prevent or cope with them.
   Encourage socialization with other well-adapted tube-fed clients.
4. Limited mobility
   Encourage normal activity.
   Control GI symptoms, such as diarrhea, nausea, vomiting, and constipation, that interfere with normal activity.
5. Discomfort related to the tube or formula
   Observe for intolerances; alleviate with appropriate interventions.
   Be sure to inspect and properly care for the tube exit site to avoid potential complications.

Before a patient is discharged on home tube feedings, a thorough evaluation of tolerance of the formula, ability and motivation to learn, manual dexterity, attitude toward the tube feeding, willingness to comply, and family support is necessary to determine the best formula and delivery system for the patient. In addition, the formula's cost and availability and the need for storage, electricity, running water, and refrigerator space must also be considered. Home health and community services can be used to provide additional support.

CLIENT GOALS

The client will:

Attain/maintain "healthy" body weight.

Receive _____ calories in _____ ml/day of _____ (product used), as ordered.

Be free of any signs and symptoms of tube-feeding intolerance (see display, Tube Feedings: Potential Problems, Rationale, and Nursing Interventions).

Prepare, administer, and monitor tube feeding as ordered for use at home, when home enteral nutrition is indicated.

Resume oral intake when and if possible.

Nursing Interventions

Diet Management

Select an appropriate formula based on calorie and protein requirements, tube placement, medical status, and diet therapy objectives.

Initially, dilute the formula to approximate isotonicity and administer slowly to give the client time to adapt to the tube feeding. The small intestine can tolerate changes in volume better than changes in concentration; therefore, the volume should be increased gradually to the optimal level before the concentration is increased. Isotonic formulas are given full strength.

Initiate continuous drip feeding at a rate of 25 ml/hour to 50 ml/hour for at least 8 hours. Increase the rate by 25 ml/hour every 8 to 12 hours as tolerated. If the client develops an intolerance (diarrhea, nausea, glucosuria), reduce the rate and then progress more slowly.

After the optimal volume is achieved, increase the concentration gradually, until full strength is achieved.

Flush tubing with water after every bolus or intermittent feeding, and every 3 to 6 hours with continuous feedings.

Encourage oral intake, if appropriate.

Client Teaching

Instruct the client

On the importance of tube feedings when oral intake is inadequate or impossible.

On the signs and symptoms of tube-feeding intolerance, and to alert the nurse if any problems arise.

To remain in an upright position or with the head elevated during and after the feeding to reduce the risk of aspiration.

Not to manipulate the flow rate unless otherwise instructed.

When home enteral nutrition is indicated, discharge teaching should encompass formula preparation, administration, and monitoring, as well as the rationale and interventions for tube-feeding complications (see display, Client Teaching for Home Enteral Nutrition).

Monitoring Progress

Ongoing assessment is necessary to evaluate the client's tolerance and response to the tube-feeding formula.

Evaluation

Evaluation is ongoing. Provided that the plan of care has not changed, the client will achieve the goals as stated above.

Time	Procedure
Before initiating a new or intermittent feeding	Check placement of an NG tube.
	Instill a small amount of water to make sure the tube is patent and to prevent the formula from sticking to it.
	Determine the amount of residual; if >150 ml, investigate reasons for delayed emptying.
Every ½ hour	Check gravity drip rates if applicable.
Every hour	Check pump drip rate if applicable.
Every 2 to 4 hours of continuous feeding	Check residual.
	After the first few days, residual should be checked at least once every 8 hours.
Every 4 hours	Check vital signs: blood pressure, temperature, pulse, and respiration.
	Check glucose and acetone in the urine.
	Discontinue nondiabetic monitoring if the client tests consistently negative for 48 hours. Monitor diabetic clients throughout the duration of the tube feeding.
	Refill feeding container.
Every 8 hours	Check intake and output and specific gravity of urine.
	Chart client's acceptance of and tolerance to the tube feeding.
Daily	Record the client's weight.
	Change feeding bag and tubing.
	Check serum electrolytes, BUN, and glucose until stabilized.
Every 3–4 days	Change irrigation set.
Every 7–10 days	Check all laboratory data.
	Reassess nutritional status.
PRN	Observe for intolerances: diarrhea, nausea, cramping, abdominal distention, vomiting, and glycosuria.
	Check NG tube placement, if appropriate.
	Check nitrogen balance and laboratory data.
	Perform delayed hypersensitivity skin testing.
	Clean feeding equipment.
	Chart significant information.

From Cataldo CB, Smith L: Tube Feedings: Clinical Applications. Reprinted with permission of Ross Laboratories, Columbus, OH. © Ross Laboratories

Client Teaching for Home Enteral Nutrition

Provide verbal and written instructions to the client and family on the following:

Formula preparation, including

- Handwashing techniques
- How to mix and prepare, if applicable
- How to store the formula and for how long

Enteral administration, including

- Proper procedure for intubation, if applicable
- How to check for proper tube position
- How to fill and hang the administration bag
- How to check for residuals
- The feeding schedule, with the volume and rate specified
- Correct body positioning during and after feedings
- Which medications to administer through the tube

Oral care, including

- Whether and what the client can eat by mouth
- Oral hygiene procedure

Insertion site care, including

- How the skin should look
- How to care for it

Tube care, including

- The name of the tube
- The measurement of the length of feeding tube outside the body

- How to flush the tube
- How to connect the feeding tube, how to cap/clamp the tube

Equipment care, including

- How to use an enteral pump, if indicated
- How to clean the pump
- Maintenance of alarms/batteries

Problem solving, including how to manage

- Cramps, diarrhea, bloating, constipation, nausea
- Tube malposition and breakage
- A clogged tube
- Mechanical problems with the pump

Data gathering for follow-up care, including

- Intake and output
- Weight
- Temperature and pulse
- Gastric residuals
- Urine glucose and acetone
- Signs and symptoms to report, such as increased breathing rate, fever, decreased urine output, altered level of consciousness, change in bowel function

Emergency phone numbers, including

- Home care agency/Nursing agency
- When to call the physician

How to dispose of equipment

PARENTERAL NUTRITION

Parenteral nutrition, such as simple intravenous (IV) solutions, peripheral parenteral nutrition (PPN), and total parenteral nutrition (TPN), delivers nutrients directly into the bloodstream, thereby bypassing the GI tract. Parenteral nutrition is used when a patient physically or psychologically cannot consume enough nutrients orally or enterally, or when alteration in GI function precludes oral and enteral feedings.

The usual fluid volume given to adults over a 24-hour period is 2 1/2 to 3 liters. Sterile water, dextrose (available in 5%, 10%, 20%, 30%, 50%, and 70% solutions), amino acids (available in 3.0%, 3.5%, 5.0%, 7.0%, 8.5%, and 10% solutions), lipid emulsions (10% or 20% solutions), electrolytes, multivitamins, minerals, and trace elements may all be given intravenously. The actual composition of the parenteral solution depends on the site of infusion and the patient's fluid and nutrient requirements.

Peripheral Nutrition

Solutions that are infused into peripheral veins must be isotonic (ie, must have low concentrations of dextrose and amino acids) to prevent phlebitis and increased risk of thrombus formation. Although lipid emulsions are isotonic and may be given for additional calories, the need to maintain isotonic concentrations of dextrose and amino acids while avoiding fluid overload limits the caloric value of peripheral solutions.

SIMPLE IV SOLUTIONS

The primary objective of a simple IV solution is to maintain or restore fluid and electrolyte balance on a short-term basis. They are used most frequently before and after surgery, after trauma, and during childbirth. Simple IV solutions contain water with dextrose (usually 5%, sometimes 10%), electrolytes, or both.

A liter of 5% dextrose in water (D_5W) provides 50 g of dextrose. When administered parenterally, one gram of dextrose provides 3.4 calories. Therefore, 1 liter of D_5W provides 170 calories (50 g dextrose x 3.4 cal/g = 170 calories). Usually no more than 3 liters of fluid is given daily; therefore, the maximum number of calories provided by a simple IV is 510 (170 cal/liter x 3 liters/day = 510 calories/day). Because simple IV solutions have little nutritional and caloric value, they should not be used longer than 1 to 2 days, or if nutritional requirements are high.

PERIPHERAL PARENTERAL NUTRITION

Peripheral parenteral nutrition (PPN) infuses a hypotonic or isotonic solution of dextrose (5% to 10%), amino acids (3% to 8.5%), vitamins, electrolytes, and trace elements into a peripheral vein. Because PPN is limited to 10% dextrose solutions, additional calories may be supplied in a lipid emulsion. Peripheral parenteral nutrition contains lesser concentrations of the same ingredients found in central vein TPN.

Peripheral parenteral nutrition provides temporary nutritional support to promote nitrogen balance and weight gain when oral intake is inadequate or is contraindicated. It may be used to supplement an oral diet or tube feeding, or as a transition from TPN to an enteral intake. Peripheral parenteral nutrition is used most effectively in patients who need short-term nutritional support (7 to 14 days) but do not require more than 2000 to 2500 cal/day. It may also be used in patients with a postsurgical ileus or an anastomotic leak, or in patients who require nutritional support but who are unable to use TPN because of limited accessibility to a central vein. Patients who receive peripheral parenteral nutrition should have normal kidney function and lipid metabolism. Peripheral parenteral nutrition is not adequate for patients who have increased nutritional requirements or who need more than 2000 to 2500 cal/day, and it is contraindicated in patients with abnormal lipid metabolism (ie, elevated serum triglycerides) or poor peripheral veins.

Central Vein Total Parenteral Nutrition

Total parenteral nutrition (TPN) is the infusion of a sterile, hypertonic solution through an indwelling central venous catheter (CVC), usually the superior vena cava, by way of the internal jugular or subclavian vein. Large-diameter veins with a high blood-flow rate are needed to dilute the solution quickly to isotonic.

TPN is used to provide complete nutritional support for patients who cannot or will not consume an adequate oral or enteral intake. Indications include the following conditions:

- Severe malnutrition; weight loss of 10% or more
- GI abnormalities: obstruction, peritonitis, impaired digestion and absorption, enterocutaneous fistulas, chronic vomiting, chronic diarrhea, prolonged paralytic ileus
- Anorexia nervosa, coma
- Severe malnutrition preoperatively
- Need for supplementation of inadequate oral intake in patients who are being treated aggressively for cancer
- After surgery or trauma, especially that involving extensive burns, multiple fractures, sepsis
- Acute liver and renal failure when amino acid requirements are altered

Because TPN is expensive, requires constant monitoring, and has potential infectious, metabolic, and mechanical complications (see display, Potential Complications of Total Parenteral Nutrition), it should be used only when an enteral intake is inadequate or contraindicated and when prolonged nutritional support is needed. Likewise, TPN should be discontinued as soon as possible. Gradual weaning to enteral nutrition or oral feedings is required to prevent metabolic complications and nutritional inadequacies. Total parenteral nutrition is never an emergency procedure and is always accompanied by potential risks.

COMPOSITION

The composition of TPN solutions is individualized according to the patient's nutritional requirements and medical condition. However, because there are standard concentrations of protein, carbohydrate, and fat in standard volumes, individualization is somewhat limited.

Monohydrous glucose, which provides 3.4 cal/g, is the most frequent source of carbohydrate in TPN solutions. Although initial glucose concentrations may range from 50% to 70%, final concentrations (after dilution with amino acids and water) are usually about 25%. Carbohydrates may be restricted in ventilator-dependent patients because the oxidation of glucose produces more carbon dioxide than does fat.

Protein is provided as a mixture of essential and nonessential crystalline amino acids that range in initial concentrations from 5% to 15% of the solution. After dilution (with water and dextrose), final concentrations are usually about 10%. The quantity of amino acids provided depends on the patient's estimated requirements

Potential Complications of Total Parenteral Nutrition

Infection and Sepsis Related to

Catheter contamination during insertion

Long-term indwelling catheter

Catheter seeding from blood-borne or distant infection

Contaminated solution

Metabolic Complications

Dehydration

Hyperglycemia

Rebound hypoglycemia

Hyperosmolar, hyperglycemic, nonketotic coma

Azotemia

Electrolyte disturbances

    Hypocalcemia

    Hypophosphatemia, hyperphosphatemia

    Hypokalemia

    Hypomagnesemia

High serum ammonia levels

Deficiencies of

    Essential fatty acid

    Trace elements

Altered acid–base balance

Elevated liver enzymes

Mechanical Complications Related to Catheterization

Catheter misplacement

Hemothorax (blood in the chest)

Pneumothorax (air or gas in the chest)

Hydrothorax (fluid in the chest)

Hemomediastinum (blood in the mediastinal spaces)

Subcutaneous emphysema

Hematoma

Arterial puncture

Myocardial perforation

Catheter embolism

Air embolism

Endocarditis

Nerve damage at the insertion site

Laceration of lymphatic duct

Chylothorax

Lymphatic fistula

Thrombosis

and hepatic and renal function. Generally, between 5% to 15% of total calories provided are from amino acids.

Lipid emulsions, made from safflower and soybean oil with egg phospholipid as an emulsifier, are isotonic, provide a significant source of calories, and can correct or prevent fatty acid deficiency. They are available in 10% and 20% concentrations, supply 1.1 and 2 cal/ml respectively, and come in 250- and 500-ml volumes. Lipid emulsions may be infused from a separate container and tubing that joins the glucose–amino acid mixture by way of a "Y" connector just before it enters the vein. They can also be added to compatible glucose–amino acid solutions to create a **total nutrient admixture (TNA)**. This eliminates the need for an extra peripheral IV line and reduces manipulation and potential contamination of the central line (Vaill, 1995). The usual dosage of fat is 0.5 to 1 g/kg/day to supply up to 30% of total calories.

The quantity of electrolytes provided is based on the patient's blood chemistry values and physical assessment findings. The electrolyte content can potentially be adjusted three times per day when a 1-liter bag is administered over 8 hours. However, TNA bags may hold a 24-hour quantity of TPN, which limits flexibility in changing the composition but reduces the risk of contamination.

A standard multivitamin preparation may be added to the TPN solution. Although it is now recognized that minerals and trace elements are a necessary component of TPN to prevent deficiency symptoms, exact parenteral requirements for zinc, selenium, chromium, manganese, iodine, copper, iron, and molybdenum are not known.

TPN-related medications may also be added to the TPN solution. Frequently, insulin may be ordered to help control serum glucose; this intervention is often necessary because of the high glucose concentration of the solution. Heparin may be added to reduce fibrin buildup on the catheter tip.

A sample calculation of a typical TPN order appears in the display, Calculating TPN.

CATHETER CONSIDERATIONS

The type of CVC used to deliver TPN depends on the patient's clinical status and the anticipated length of time that TPN will be used. For short-term use during hospitalization, a polyurethane catheter may be used; because it stiffens, thus increasing the risk of thrombophlebitis, it is appropriate only for short-term use. Polyurethane catheters are available with single, double, and triple lumens. In triple-lumen CVC, the middle port is usually used for TPN.

Patients who need TPN for up to 3 months may have a peripherally inserted central catheter (PICC), which is inserted in an arm vein and advanced until the tip rests in the superior vena cava. Another long-term option is an implanted port, which is often used for patients who are receiving chemotherapy and TPN; in using these

---

Calculating TPN

To determine the quantity of calories in a solution, the number of grams of dextrose and amino acids must first be calculated. A sample order may be 3 liters of 25% dextrose and 3.5% amino acids.

The percent of a nutrient in solution equals the grams of that nutrient in 100 ml of solution.

25% dextrose = 25 g dextrose/100 ml of solution, or 250 mg/liter of solution

3.5% amino acids = 3.5 g amino acids/100 ml or solution, or 35 g/liter

Determine the total amount given for the day if 3 liters are infused.

250 g dextrose/liter × 3 liters = 750 g dextrose/day

35 g amino acids/liter × 3 liters = 105 g amino acids/day

Calculate calories provided, knowing that IV dextrose provides 3.4 cal/g, amino acids 4.0 cal/g

750 g dextrose/day × 3.4 cal/g = 2550 dextrose calories

105 g amino acids/day × 4.0 cal/g = <u>420</u> amino acid calories

2970 total calories/day

If an additional 250 ml of a 20% lipid emulsion is added to the infusion:

250 ml lipid emulsion × 2.0 cal/ml = 500 calories from lipids

(500 fat calories divided by 9 calories/g = 55.5 g fat in 250 ml of lipid emulsion)

Total calorie intake: 2970 + 500 = 3470 calories

ports, a Silastic catheter, which is attached to a plastic or metal reservoir, is implanted subcutaneously, usually in the chest wall.

Catheter insertion is a surgical procedure that is performed under sterile conditions. The patient is given a local anesthetic and should be instructed to expect some pain. The placement must be confirmed by x-ray before the solution can be administered, and the catheter should be checked periodically for proper position, leaks, and obstructions. Although the site of insertion should be routinely cleaned, dressed, and checked for signs of infection, dressings or adhesives should not be removed for 48 hours after the catheter is inserted.

To prevent contamination, the central line should not be used to administer drugs (except insulin), measure central venous pressure, or withdraw blood. Equipment and solution containers should always be checked for leaks and cracks before use.

ADMINISTRATION

Initially, the infusion is started slowly (ie, 1 to 2 liters in the first 24 hours) to give the body time to adapt to the high concentration of glucose and the hyperosmolality of the solution. Continuous drip by pump infusion is needed to maintain a slow constant flow rate. After the first 24 hours, the rate of delivery is gradually increased by 1 liter/day until the optimal volume is achieved. If the rate falls behind or speeds up, the drip rate should be adjusted to the correct hourly infusion rate. Because of the dangers of hyperosmolar diuresis from an excessive glucose infusion, no attempts should be made to "catch up" to the ordered volume.

Cyclical TPN (10- to 16-hour infusion TPN) may be used if the patient is on home TPN, or if the client needs TPN only to support an inadequate oral intake. Cyclical TPN allows serum glucose and insulin levels to drop during the periods when TPN is not infused, thus promoting fat and glycogen mobilization and a more "normal" intake. When it is given during the night, cyclical TPN frees the patient to participate in normal activities during the day. When switching from continuous to cyclical TPN, the infusion time should be gradually decreased by several hours each day, as ordered, and assessment should be ongoing for signs of glucose intolerance and fluid overload (shortness of breath, crackles, pedal and sacral edema, more than 1 pound weight gain/day). To give the pancreas time to adjust to the decreasing glucose load, the infusion rate should be tapered near the end of each cycle (ie, reduce the rate by one-half during the last hour of infusion to prevent rebound hypoglycemia).

Patients must be weaned off TPN gradually to prevent rebound hypoglycemia. Enteral intake (either an oral diet or tube feeding) should increase as TPN decreases; enteral intake should be adequate before TPN is discontinued.

NURSING PROCESS

Assessment

Ongoing assessment of the patient's needs and tolerance to parenteral nutrition is necessary to ensure maximum benefit and prevent complications. Although an in-depth nutritional assessment may be the dietitian's responsibility, the following screening data may be useful for the nurse.

Assess for the following factors:

Weight status, any recent weight change.

Past medical history and current problems, and evaluate the impact on intake and nutritional status.

Food intolerances and allergies, especially an allergy to eggs, which is a contraindication to using lipid emulsions.

GI and major organ function (renal, hepatic, cardiac).

Serum albumin and transferrin, if available, and evaluate any other abnormal laboratory values for their nutritional significance.

Outward signs of malnutrition; assess hydration status.

For patients who are candidates for home parenteral nutrition, assess the patient's motivational level, social support system, financial status, and home environment.

Nursing Diagnosis

Altered Nutrition: Potential for more than or less than body requirements, related to total parenteral nutrition.

Planning and Implementation

Calculate parenteral calorie and protein requirements based on the patient's assessment data and medical status (Table 14-4). Approximately 30 to 50 ml of fluid/kg should be provided.

Inspect the solution for **"cracking,"** which appears as a layer of fat on the top or oily globules in the solution. This sometimes occurs in TNA mixtures if the calcium or phosphorus content is relatively high or if salt-poor albumin has been added (Vaill, 1995). A "cracked" solution cannot be infused; notify the pharmacy and physician, who may need to adjust the original TPN order to eliminate or reduce the offending component.

Because the exact requirements for vitamins, minerals, and trace elements given parenterally are not known, close monitoring of nutritional status is necessary to prevent the development of nutrient deficiencies or toxicities.

Table 14-4
Parenteral Calorie and Protein Requirements Based on Weight and Stress Level

	Calories/kg/day	Grams Protein/kg/day
Resting state (ie, medical clients)	20–30	0.8–1.0
Uncomplicated postoperative clients	25–35	1.0–1.3
Depleted clients	30–40	1.3–1.7
Hypermetabolic clients	35–45	1.5–2.0

Change the infusion equipment as needed to help prevent contamination. The infusion bottle should be changed every 12 hours, even if it still contains some solution. Change the infusion tubing from the bottle to the catheter hub once every 24 hours.

Monitor the flow rate to avoid complications and ensure adequate intake. Solutions that are infused too rapidly can cause hyperosmolar diuresis, leading to seizures, coma, and even death; solutions that are administered too slowly prevent an optimal nutritional intake.

Some patients may feel hungry while receiving TPN and should be allowed to eat, if possible. If an oral intake is contraindicated, give ice chips or allow the client to chew his or her favorite food without swallowing.

Begin weaning the client from TPN as soon as possible; enteral nutrition may be indicated until oral intake is adequate.

Patients who have permanently nonfunctional GI tracts may require TPN indefinitely. In order for home TPN to be successful, clients and their families must be physically and emotionally prepared. Intensive counseling should focus on the preparation and administration of the solution, catheter and equipment care, and assessment skills, as well as the psychological impact of permanent TPN.

CLIENT GOALS

The client will:

> Attain or maintain "healthy" body weight.
> Maintain or replenish body protein, as evidenced by normal serum protein levels (ie, albumin, transferrin).
> Receive _____ calories in _____ ml/day of _____ (mixture used), as ordered.
> Be free of any signs and symptoms of parenteral nutrition complications (see the display, Potential Complications of Total Parenteral Nutrition).
> Aseptically prepare, administer, and monitor TPN as ordered for use at home, if indicated.
> Resume enteral or oral intake when and if possible.

NURSING INTERVENTIONS

Diet Management

> Administer TPN as ordered.
> Notify the physician if an intolerance or complication develops.

Client Teaching

Instruct the client

> On the importance of TPN when oral or enteral intake is inadequate or impossible.
> To alert the nurse if any problems arise.
> Not to manipulate the flow rate unless otherwise instructed.

When home TPN is indicated, discharge teaching should encompass aseptic preparation and administration techniques, criteria to monitor signs and symptoms of system failure, when to call the doctor, when to call the dietitian, and when to call the pharmacist.

Encourage the client to discuss anxiety, anger, or adaptation to TPN and oral deprivation.

Monitoring Progress

Ongoing assessment is vital to the success of TPN.

Time	Procedure
Every 30 minutes	Check the flow rate.
Every 4–6 hours	Check urine glucose.
	Monitor vital signs.
	Check urine specific gravity.
Daily	Record the client's weight: A daily weight gain of ¼ lb to ½ lb is expected.
	Monitor intake (including any oral intake) and output.
2–3 times/week or daily	Check serum levels of glucose and electrolytes.
	Check BUN levels.
	Check hemoglobin.
Weekly	Check serum levels of protein, calcium, phosphorus and ammonia.
	Reassess nutritional status.
	Check liver function studies.
PRN	Check white blood cell count and differential count.
	Check cultures.
	Observe for intolerances and signs of complications.
	Chart significant information.

Evaluation

Evaluation is ongoing. Provided that the plan of care has not changed, the client will achieve the goals as stated above.

KEY CONCEPTS

- Oral diets may be modified in their consistency, or in their concentration of certain nutrients or dietary components, depending on the individual's need. Patients who are unable to consume enough food orally may need homemade or commercial supplements to augment thir intake. Tube feedings may also be used supplementally.

- Enteral nutrition commonly means tube feedings. Tube feedings are preferred over parenteral nutrition whenever the GI tract is functional. Tube feedings may be delivered through transnasal tubes, or through ostomy sites along the GI tract.

- The choice of tube feeding used depends on where the feeding is infused, the size of the feeding tube; and the patient's nutritional needs, GI function, present and past medical history, and tolerance.

- Standard tube feedings require normal digestion; they contain intact molecules of protein, carbohydrate, and fat. Hydrolyzed formulas are made from partially or totally predigested nutrients; they are higher in cost and osmolality. Specially defined formulas are available for specific metabolic disorders like renal failure and hepatic failure.

- Continuous drip infusion with a pump is the preferred method of delivering tube feedings to critically ill patients, and should be used whenever feedings are infused into the jejunum. Intermittent feedings may be preferable for long-term feedings and home enteral nutrition because they more closely resemble a normal intake and allow the client freedom between feedings. Bolus feedings are not recommended.

- Diarrhea is a frequent complication of tube feedings that may be caused by bacterial contamination, too rapid of a feeding rate, giving too much volume of formula, hyperosmolar formulas, misplacement of the feeding tube, hypoalbuminemia, or antibiotic therapy.

- Parenteral nutrition delivers nutrients by vein when the GI tract is nonfunctional or when oral/enteral intake is inadequate to meet the patient's needs. Amino acids, dextrose, lipid emulsions, electrolytes, multivitamins, minerals, and trace elements may be given by vein.

- Peripheral parenteral nutrition must be close to isotonic to avoid collapsing small-diameter veins. Central vein infusions are hypertonic, but they are quickly diluted by the rapid blood flow.

- Because parenteral nutrition has numerous potential metabolic, infectious, and mechanical complications, it should be used only when necessary and discontinued as soon as feasible.

 FOCUS ON **CRITICAL THINKING**

Mrs. Tanner is 5 foot tall, weighs 118 pounds, and is 72 years old. Four days ago, she suffered a stroke and subsequently has been unable to eat because of impaired swallowing. The doctor is hopeful she will regain her swallowing ability within the next couple of weeks. In the meantime, Mrs. Tanner will be fed via a tube feeding. She does not have a signficant medical history.

Calculate Mrs. Tanner's calorie requirements, using the Harris-Benedict equation, activity factor, and injury factor.

Presently, she appears to have an adequate protein status, based on a normal albumin level and adequate skin integrity. Estimate her protein requirement. What type of feeding tube placement would you recommend? Why?

The doctor has ordered full strengh Vital HN at 75 ml/hr. Is this adequate and appropriate? Why or why not? What product, strength, and method of feeding would you recommend?

Mrs. Tanner complains of nausea. What may be causing this and what actions could you take to help alleviate her nausea?

REFERENCES

American Dietetic Association. (1995). Position of The American Dietetic Association: Legal and ethical issues in feeding permanently unconscious patient. JADA 95(2), 231–234.

American Dietetic Association (1994). Position of The American Dietetic Association: Nutrition monitoring of the home parenteral and enteral patient. JADA 94(6), 664–666.

Bockus, S. (1993). When your patient needs tube feedings. Making the right decisions. Nursing 93, 23(7), 34–42.

Eisenberg, P. (1994). Nasoenteral tubes. RN, 57(10), 62–70.

Eisenberg, P. (1994). Gastrostomy and jejunostomy tubes. RN, 57(11), 54–59.

Eisenberg, P. (1994). Feeding formulas. RN, 57(12), 46–52.

McGinnis, C. and Matson, S. (1994). How to manage patient with a Roux-en-Y jejunostomy. AJN 94(2), 43–45.

Miller D. and Miller, H. (1995). Giving meds through the tube. RN, 58(1), 44–47.

Vaill, C. (1995a). Taking the mystery out of TPN. Part one. Nursing 95, 95(4), 34–41.

Vaill, C. (1995b). Taking the mystery out of TPN. Part two. Nursing 95, 95(5), 56–59.

Young, C. and White S. (1992). Preparing patients for tube feeding at home. AJN 92(4), 46–53.

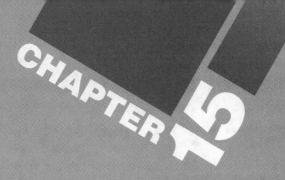

CHAPTER 15

Nutrition and Stress

Chapter Outline

Key Terms

Ebb phase
Flow phase

General adaptation syn-
    drome
Pathological stress

Physiological stress
Respiratory quotient (RQ)

Stress is any threat to an individual's emotional or physical well-being. **Physiolog-ical stress**, a normal part of everyday living, includes events like marriage, divorce, moving to a new house, and even going on a vacation; the amount of stress that is experienced varies among individuals and circumstances (see Food for Thought: Stressing Vitamins). **Pathological stress**, like trauma, surgery, burns, infec-tion, and fever, produces a more intense stress response; however, the same sequence of events occur as the body seeks to reestablish homeostasis.

FOOD *for* THOUGHT

Stressing Vitamins

Health food stores and pharmacies abound with "stress formula" vitamin and mineral preparations that claim to have the magic combination and concentration of nutrients needed to withstand the stress and strain of daily living. Most provide nutrients in "high-potency" or "super" concentrations, and many have ingredients that may not even be essential for humans. Naturally, such "protection" often comes at considerable cost. Unfortunately, manufacturers often rely on marketing, not scientific data, when developing new products.

Although it is true that increased metabolism and catabolism occur during severe or prolonged stress, the daily stress of living (eg, getting caught in traffic, worrying about an upcoming exam) does not produce the same intense and sustained physical response. Major stress does greatly increase calorie requirements, which are met by the body's stores of glycogen and then protein and fat tissue, if adequate calories are not consumed through the diet. By comparison, minor stresses come and go without any significant impact on nutrition.

The best nutritional insurance available to prepare for future major stress is to eat a varied diet that is adequate in all essential nutrients and to maximize glycogen storage through exercise. As for megavitamins and minerals, they just do not protect against future bouts of major stress. True, they are needed to metabolize energy, but they are not a source of energy. In addition, water-soluble vitamins that are taken in excess of need are generally excreted in the urine, whereas excesses of other vitamins and minerals taken over time can produce toxic effects.

For the stress of daily living, stress reduction techniques, rather than megadoses of vitamins and minerals, are your best bet.

THE STRESS RESPONSE

Hans Selye first described the **general adaptation syndrome** as the body's three-stage response to stress. Initially, an *alarm reaction* occurs as the body recognizes a threat; the secretion of hormones prepares the body for "fight or flight." Characteristically, heart rate increases, blood glucose rises, pupils dilate, and digestion slows. The *resistance* or *adaptive phase* follows, during which the body begins to reestablish balance as the acute stress symptoms diminish or disappear. Successful adaptation leads to recovery. If adaptation fails, the body eventually becomes unable to respond to the stress, resulting in *exhaustion* and possibly death.

The intensity of the stress response depends on the severity of the stress, the number of stressors, and the individual's ability to adapt to stress. The nutritional implications of various types of stress are outlined in Table 15-1. The stress of minor surgery in a well-nourished client may have little impact. Malnutrition is a stress that also requires adaptation. Patients who are burdened with malnutrition plus another form of stress (trauma, surgery, burns, infection, sepsis) may lack the nutrient reserves needed for adaptation to occur. The result may be multisystem organ failure and death.

Table 15-1
Nutritional Implications of Various Types of Stress

Stressor	Nutritional Objectives	Diet Management
Decubitus ulcer: a pressure sore caused by a lack of oxygen and nutrients to the affected area, usually at the bony or cartilaginous prominences of the hip, sacrum, elbow, or heels. Risk is highest among the elderly, bedridden and paralyzed clients, and people with protein–calorie malnutrition.	Attain normal protein status. Promote healing and prevent future sores.	Increase protein to 1.0–1.6 g/kg, depending on the "stage" of the ulcer. Increase nonprotein calories to promote healing. Supplements of zinc and vitamin C may be indicated. Provide small, frequent meals to maximize intake.
Fever: altered thermoregulation that may occur secondary to infections, neoplasms, connective tissue diseases, or unknown causes.	Meet increased calorie requirements related to the increase in REE: every 1°F increase in temperature above normal increases REE by 7%. Replenish nutrient losses, as needed: nitrogen, electrolytes, CHO stores. Correct and treat any concomitant GI symptoms.	Provide approximately 500 to 600 additional calories for each 1°F rise in temperature. Provide increased fluids: adults may need 10 to 15 cups/day. Modify the diet as needed to control GI symptoms. Small, frequent meals may be indicated. Provide a liquid diet if solids are not tolerated or accepted.
Infection: invasion and growth of pathogenic microorganisms.	Meet increased requirements related to hypermetabolism. Prevent or correct symptoms and complications. Replenish nutrient losses, as needed.	Provide high-calorie, high-protein diet. Provide adequate fluids. Small, frequent meals may be indicated.
Sepsis: infection that has spread to the bloodstream. Cause of 40% of all ICU deaths.	Same as infection, plus: Counteract nausea, vomiting, anorexia. Prevent/correct fluid imbalance. Prevent multiple system organ failure and death.	Increase protein to 1.6–2.5 g/kg. Provide 45 cal/kg. Impaired GI function (ileus) may necessitate the use of parenteral nutrition. However, sepsis may be worsened by bacterial translocation across the GI mucosa if the mucosa atrophies from nonuse.

TRAUMA AND SEVERE STRESS

Severe stress, such as that associated with trauma, produces a dramatic stress response. During the first 12 to 24 hours after trauma, the "ebb" or shock phase occurs, which parallels the alarm reaction. Increased levels of catecholamines and glucagon cause an increase in glycogen breakdown (glycogenolysis) and an increase in glucose production from amino acids (gluconeogenesis), resulting in hyperglycemia. Blood pressure, cardiac output, body temperature, and oxygen consumption are all decreased. Immediate goals are to restore tissue perfusion, maintain adequate oxygenation, and stop hemorrhage.

The "ebb" phase is followed by the acute, catabolic, or "flow" phase (ie, the adaptive phase). Increased levels of glucocorticoids, catecholamines, and glucagon, the "stress hormones," cause hypermetabolism (increased energy expenditure), accelerated nitrogen loss (protein catabolism), and persistent hyperglycemia despite normal or elevated serum insulin levels. Urinary losses of potassium and nitrogen increase, and sodium and fluid are retained. Decreased gastrointestinal (GI) motility can result in anorexia, distention, nausea, vomiting, or constipation. Often, loss of protein and fat tissue is significant, as the body breaks down its own reserves to meet increased energy needs. An adequate nutritional intake may help to minimize the effects of hypermetabolism and catabolism; however, symptoms may impair or preclude the ability to eat, necessitating the use of enteral or parenteral nutritional support. Hormonal and metabolic characteristics of "ebb" and "flow" phases are summarized in Table 15-2.

Within a few days after the initial stress response, catabolism peaks and the anabolic phase of recovery begins; this occurs only if adequate nutrients are available. As stress hormone levels subside, serum glucose levels decline and nitrogen balance is gradually achieved.

NURSING PROCESS

Assessment

Assess for the following factors:

- Extent of injuries and complications; significance of GI trauma, if appropriate
- Hemodynamic status; signs and symptoms of hemorrhaging
- Altered fluid and electrolyte balance, particularly sodium and fluid accumulation
- Altered neurologic status; ability to eat, ability to self-feed

Table 15-2
Metabolic and Hormonal Changes Characteristic of the Ebb and Flow Phases of Stress

Changes	Ebb Phase	Flow Phase
Hormonal	Decreased insulin	Normal or increased insulin
	Increased catecholamines	Increased catecholamines
	Increased glucagon	Increased glucagon
		Increased aldosterone
		Increased antidiuretic hormone
Metabolic	Hyperglycemia	Hyperglycemia, insulin insensitivity
	Decreased O_2 consumption	Hypermetabolism (increased O_2 consumption)
	Decreased blood pressure	Increased tissue catabolism
	Decreased cardiac output	Increased cardiac output
	Decreased body temperature	Increased body temperature
	Decreased renal output	Increased urinary nitrogen losses
		Muscle use of branched-chain amino acids for energy
		Sodium and fluid retention
		Increased fat oxidation

- Altered GI function, such as hypoactive bowel sounds, distention, complaints of nausea, anorexia
- Weight, weight changes
- Diminished renal output; measure intake and output (I & O)
- Serum albumin, glucose, and electrolyte levels
- Urinary urea nitrogen (UUN), if available; urine ketones
- Signs and symptoms of depression, anxiety

Nursing Diagnosis

Altered Nutrition, less than body requirements, related to inadequate intake secondary to hypermetabolism, hypercatabolism

Planning and Implementation

Major stress can have a profound impact on nutritional requirements; the greater the stress, the greater the impact on nutrition. Nutritional requirements should be determined on an individual basis.

Initially, trauma patients are treated with intravenous (IV) fluid, glucose, and potassium until they have stabilized. Life support and intensive monitoring may be required.

Nutritional intervention should begin when the flow phase begins, as indicated by a decrease in serum glucose, usually within 2 to 5 days post trauma. Providing aggressive support before the flow phase may be detrimental, because it increases metabolic demands on the body.

Oral and enteral nutrition are the preferred routes if the GI tract is functional. If the patient is able to tolerate oral feedings, supplements and small frequent feedings help to maximize intake. Calorically dense (ie, 2.0 cal/ml) formulas and specially formulated stress formulas may be used for patients who are receiving enteral nutritional support. Because of the increased risk of infectious, metabolic, and mechanical complications, parenteral nutrition is used only when necessary.

Adequate calories are essential to minimize weight loss and promote anabolism. Total calorie requirements can be estimated using Harris-Benedict equation and stress and activity factors. (See display, Estimating Total Calorie Requirements, p. 445.) Until stress is resolved, weight maintenance, not weight gain, should be the goal.

An adequate protein intake is essential to minimize or correct body protein catabolism and help maintain normal immune functioning. Because the body meets its energy requirements first, dietary protein is used for anabolism only if adequate nonprotein calories (carbohydrate and fat) are available to meet the body's calorie requirement. Generally, protein requirements range from 1.0 to 1.5 g/kg body weight for moderate stress, and from 1.5 to 3.0 g/kg body weight for severe stress. Arginine, normally a nonessential amino acid, may become conditionally essential during periods of stress. Whether the requirement for branched-chain amino acids increases during stress remains controversial.

During periods of stress, fluid requirements may be increased because of increased losses from exudates, hemorrhage, emesis, diuresis, and fever. To accurately assess fluid requirements and status, intake and output should be carefully monitored. Care should be taken to avoid overhydration; decreased renal output is a frequent complication of stress.

Vitamin, mineral, and electrolyte requirements during stress are unclear and undefined. Because of their role in tissue healing and immune function, supplements of the B complex vitamins, zinc, vitamin A, and vitamin C may be appropriate.

As patients enter the recovery phase, basal metabolic rate (BMR) returns to normal. Patients may be weaned from parenteral nutrition to enteral or oral diets; liquid or regular diets are usually tolerated.

CLIENT GOALS

The client will:

Consume adequate calories to maintain or restore pre-trauma weight
Consume adequate protein to achieve positive nitrogen balance and maintain or restore lean body mass
Maintain normal fluid and electrolyte balance
Experience adequate healing and recovery
Avoid complications, infection, respiratory failure, sepsis
Describe principles and rationale for post-trauma diet management, as appropriate, and implement the recommended dietary interventions

NURSING INTERVENTIONS

Diet Management

Initially, give IV fluid and electrolytes as ordered to maintain hydration until oral intake is resumed.

Progress oral intake, as tolerated, until a high-calorie, high-protein diet is achieved. Use small, frequent feedings to maximize intake. Clients who are unable or unwilling to consume an adequate oral intake may need total or supplemental enteral or parenteral nutrition.

Adjust fluid intake according to need, as based on I & O and physical findings.

Client Teaching

Instruct the client

On the importance of nutrition in promoting wound healing and recovery
How to increase calories and protein in the diet (see the display, Ways to Add Protein and Calories to the Diet)
To eat small, frequent meals if anorexia or nausea occurs

Monitoring Progress

Monitor for the following signs or symptoms:

Tolerance to the diet
Acceptance of the diet; adequacy of intake

> ## Ways to Add Protein and Calories to the Diet
>
> **For added protein and calories:**
> - Add skim milk powder to milk to make double-strength milk; chill well before serving.
> - Use double-strength milk on hot or cold cereals, and in scrambled eggs, soups, gravies, casseroles, milkshakes, milk-based desserts.
> - Substitute whole milk or evaporated milk for water in recipes.
> - Add grated cheese to soups, casseroles, vegetable dishes, rice, noodles.
> - Use peanut butter as a spread on slices of apple, banana, or pear, crackers, or waffles; use as a filling for celery.
> - Add finely chopped, hard-cooked eggs to sauces, soups, and casseroles.
> - Choose desserts made with eggs or milk, like sponge cake, angel food cake, custard, puddings.
> - Dip meat, poultry, and fish in eggs or milk and coat with bread or cereal crumbs before baking, broiling, or pan frying.
> - Use yogurt as a topping for fruit, plain cakes, or other desserts; use in gravies and dips.
>
> **For added calories:**
> - Mix cream cheese with butter and spread on hot bread and rolls.
> - Whenever possible, add butter to hot foods: breads, pancakes, waffles, soups, vegetables, potatoes, cooked cereal, rice, pasta.
> - Substitute mayonnaise for salad dressing in salads, eggs, casseroles, sandwiches.
> - Add dried fruit, nuts, or granola to desserts and cereal.
> - Use whipped cream on pies, fruit, pudding, gelatin, ice cream, and other desserts; to lighten coffee and tea; in hot chocolate.
> - Use marshmallows in hot chocolate, on fruit, and in desserts.
> - Top baked potatoes, vegetables, and fruits with sour cream.
> - Snack frequently on nuts; dried fruit, candy, buttered popcorn, cheese, granola, ice cream.
> - Use honey on toast, cereal, and fruits, and in coffee and tea.

Weight, weight changes.

Fluid balance. Rapid weight gain of more than 1 pound per day indicates fluid retention.

Laboratory values, especially serum glucose, albumin, electrolytes; UUN, if available; urine ketones

Evaluation

Evaluation is ongoing. Provided that the plan of care has not changed, the patient will achieve the goals as stated above.

SURGICAL NUTRITION

Ideally, patients should have an optimal nutritional status before surgery to enable them to withstand the stress of surgery and the short-term starvation that follows; the stress response may be mild to severe, depending on the extent and nature of the surgery and the development of complications. Good nutritional status can speed recovery time and shorten the period of hospitalization. Patients who are well nourished before surgery have a lower incidence of infections, complications, and postoperative mortality compared to malnourished patients.

Surgical patients are often malnourished. Disease-related symptoms that may be experienced before surgery, such as anorexia, nausea, vomiting, fever, malabsorption, and blood loss, may leave a patient nutritionally compromised. After surgery, nutrient requirements increase depending on the degree of hypermetabolism, hypercatabolism, and wound healing. Problems with ingestion, digestion, absorption, metabolism, or excretion resulting from surgery for cancer or disorders of the GI tract, pancreas, liver, or kidneys increase the risks for malnutrition and complications. To optimize the chance for a successful surgical outcome, malnourished patients and those at risk for malnutrition should be identified and given preoperative nutritional support (see the display, General Surgical Assessment Criteria).

NURSING PROCESS

Assessment

In addition to the general surgical assessment criteria, assess for the following factors:

Age status: Vulnerable age groups include infants, children, and the elderly because they have smaller reserves to sustain themselves through the stress of surgery and the postoperative period.

Nutritional status, based on nutritional screening criteria (see Fig. 9-1). If a nutritional problem is identified or suspected, a more in-depth nutritional assessment is indicated in order to develop appropriate diet therapy objectives and interventions to meet the patient's preoperative and postoperative nutritional needs.

ASSESSMENT CRITERIA

General Surgical Assessment Criteria

Presurgical history: symptoms of acute illness (ie, nausea, vomiting, diarrhea, anorexia) and existence of chronic illnesses (diabetes mellitus; pulmonary diseases; impaired cardiovascular, hepatic, or renal function; GI disorders; alcoholism)

Weight status; recent weight changes

Serum albumin, transferrin

Hydration status, electrolyte status

Blood pressure

Anemia

Nature and extent of anticipated surgery, especially GI surgery

Infections

Presurgical symptoms of illness or condition: onset, frequency, causative factors, severity, interventions attempted, and the results of interventions.

Dietary changes that have been made in response to symptoms—foods avoided, foods preferred. Determine which foods are best and least tolerated.

Weight status. Obesity increases the workload of the heart and increases the risks for infection, pulmonary complications, and delayed wound healing.

Past medical history.

Nursing Diagnosis

Altered Nutrition: Less than body requirements, related to increased requirements for healing secondary to surgery

Planning and Implementation

PREOPERATIVE NUTRITION

Although an optimal nutritional status before surgery can improve the outcome of surgery, IV fluid and electrolytes may be the only form of nutritional rehabilitation possible for patients who are undergoing emergency surgery.

Patients who are well nourished and who are scheduled for uncomplicated surgery do not need a special preoperative diet and can be maintained on their normal diet.

Deficiencies of vitamins, minerals, fluid, and electrolytes can be corrected quickly and easily, if detected. Adequate protein status and normal weight should be achieved, if time allows. However, it may not be possible to rehabilitate a patient nutritionally if emergency surgery is indicated or if the risks of delaying surgery are too great. Patients who are unable to consume an adequate oral intake may need enteral or parenteral nutritional support.

POSTOPERATIVE NUTRITION

Postoperative nutritional support varies with the location, extent, and type of surgery, as well as the occurrence of postsurgical complications and the patient's nutritional status and ability to eat. Minor surgery may have little effect on nutritional status and nutrient requirements. However, extensive surgery, surgery involving the GI tract, and the development of postoperative complications can increase nutritional requirements and influence the method of feeding.

Simple IV solutions are nutritionally and calorically inadequate and should be discontinued as soon as possible. Increased nutritional requirements combined with short-term starvation (NPO) or an inadequate diet may result in a weight loss of about 0.5 lb/day early in the postoperative period. A greater weight loss may be experienced by patients who have extensive surgery, postoperative complications, or other medical conditions. Weight loss may not be apparent if the patient has edema.

The following interventions may help to relieve discomfort, irritability, and the preoccupation with eating that can develop in patients who are NPO:

- Apply cold compresses or petroleum jelly to the lips to ease dryness.
- Encourage mouth-rinsing with cold water or a mouthwash.
- Divert the patient's attention away from eating by encouraging other activities, such as listening to the radio, watching television, talking with other patients, and so forth.

A needle-catheter jejunostomy tube may be inserted during surgery if the client is malnourished, hypermetabolic, or not expected to resume an oral intake within a few days after surgery. Unlike the stomach, which does not regain motility for 24 to 48 hours after surgery, the small intestine resumes peristalsis and the ability to absorb nutrients within several hours after surgery.

The postoperative diet varies according to the patient's previous nutritional status and the type and extent of surgery. Potential nutritional problems and diet interventions for various surgical procedures of the GI tract are listed in the display, Nursing Interventions and Considerations for Potential Nutritional Problems of Various Surgical Procedures of the GI Tract.

To maximize intake, especially in an anorexic client, solicit food preferences, individualize the diet, offer small, frequent meals, and allow food from home, if possible.

Encourage ambulation as soon as possible after surgery to prevent postoperative complications, to stimulate the appetite, and to prevent complications of immobility (eg, increased losses of protein and calcium).

CLIENT GOALS

The client will:

Attain or maintain "healthy" weight and optimal nutritional status before (if possible) and after surgery.
Avoid aspiration during anesthesia and recovery.
Maintain normal fluid and electrolyte balance.
Achieve nitrogen balance to promote wound healing.
Describe the principles and rationale for postoperative diet management, as appropriate, and implement the recommended dietary interventions.
Avoid GI complications, if appropriate.

NURSING INTERVENTIONS

Diet Management

Before Surgery

Provide a normal diet if patient is well nourished and scheduled for uncomplicated surgery; a high-calorie, high-protein diet may be indicated for malnourished patients or those facing extensive surgery.
Promote a liberal intake of nutrients that are important for wound healing (Table 15-3), especially vitamins C and K.

(text continues on page 476)

Nursing Interventions and Considerations for Potential Nutritional Problems of Various Surgical Procedures of the GI Tract

ESOPHAGEAL SURGERY

Surgical excision of diverticulum

Repair of gastroesophageal reflux disease (GERD): The Nissen, Belsy Mark IV, and Toupet partial fundoplication are three procedures that involve wrapping all or part of the fundus around the esophagus to reinforce lower esophageal sphincter (LES) pressure and to keep the fundus and cardia below the diaphragm.

Esophagogastrectomy: Partial removal of the esophagus and stomach (used as treatment for esophageal cancer), with remaining portions of each reattached. If so much tissue is removed that the structures cannot be reconnected directly, a colonic interposition (replacement of part of the esophagus with part of the colon) is performed. Gastrostomy or jejunostomy feedings are given for at least 1 week postoperatively, until swallowing is resumed.

Potential Problem/Rationale

Painful/difficult swallowing related to edema around the surgical site.

Nursing Interventions and Considerations

Provide liquid to soft diet, as tolerated.

Assure the client that swallowing ability should improve within 1 week.

Many clients undergoing esophageal surgery have a long history of difficulty swallowing; weight loss may be observed. Encourage a high-protein, high-calorie intake to facilitate healing and replenish losses.

Potential Problem/Rationale

Early satiety ("gas-bloat" syndrome) secondary to Nissen procedure for GERD related to fundus wrapped too tightly around the esophagus.

Nursing Interventions and Considerations

Encourage frequent ambulation to stimulate peristalsis.

Provide small, frequent meals; encourage the client to eat slowly.

Surgical intervention may be necessary.

GASTRIC SURGERY

Gastrectomy: Partial or total removal of the stomach or duodenum used in the treatment of gastric or duodenal ulcers, gastric cancer, gastric trauma.

Billroth I: Gastroduodenostomy. May cause *dumping syndrome,* anemia, malabsorption, weight loss.

Billroth II: Gastrojejunostomy; *dumping syndrome* and other problems are more common than with Billroth I.

Partial gastrectomy: Anastomosis between the remaining portion of the stomach and the jejunum.

Total gastrectomy: Radical removal of the stomach with anastomosis between the esophagus and jejunum.

Vagotomy: Partial or total severance of the vagus nerve; may cause *dumping syndrome,* diarrhea, increased feeling of fullness.

Potential Problems/Rationale

Diarrhea and the *dumping syndrome* related to a decrease in the holding capacity of the stomach; undigested food that is quickly "dumped" into the jejunum causes a rapid increase in the osmolarity of the intestinal contents. Extracellular fluid shifts from the circulating blood volume into the intestine to dilute the high particle concentration, resulting in distention, cramping, pain, and diarrhea, usually within 15 to 30 minutes after eating.

Because of a rapid transit time, fat may not be exposed to bile and pancreatic enzymes long enough to be thoroughly digested. As a result, steatorrhea and other symptoms of fat maldigestion may occur. The etiology of weight loss is

(continued)

Nursing Interventions and Considerations for Potential Nutritional Problems of Various Surgical Procedures of the GI Tract *(Continued)*

multifactorial: diarrhea, steatorrhea, a voluntary restriction of food intake, a restrictive diet, and so forth.

Nursing Interventions and Considerations

Instruct the client to follow the postgastrectomy (*antidumping*) diet (see display, Sample Postgastrectomy ["Antidumping"] Menu that includes the following modifications):

- Eat five to six or more small meals daily.
- Increase fat and protein intake; fat is isotonic and protein is hydrolyzed more slowly than CHO and therefore does not increase osmolarity as readily. Include some fat and protein in each feeding.
- Decrease CHO intake; avoid simple sugars that form a hyperosmolar solution in the jejunum.
- Avoid high-fiber foods that stimulate peristalsis.
- Adjust total calorie intake to attain and maintain weight.
- Avoid fluid with meals and 1 hour before and after eating.
- Eliminate individual intolerances.
- Lie down for 20 to 30 minutes after eating to delay gastric emptying time.

Clients with steatorrhea may need a low-fat diet, MCT oil, and water-soluble forms of the fat-soluble vitamins.

Lactose intolerance may develop, requiring a low-lactose or lactose-free diet (see Chap. 16).

Foods high in pectin (unripe bananas, raw apple, and white rice) may help prevent symptoms of the *dumping syndrome*.

Eventually the diet can be liberalized as the remaining portion of the stomach or duodenum hypertrophies to hold more food and allow for more normal digestion.

Potential Problem/Rationale

Reactive hypoglycemia (sweating, dizziness, and rapid heartbeat), which may occur as a sec-

ondary reaction 1 to 3 hours after eating, related to the rapid absorption of CHO from the duodenum → increase in blood glucose levels → oversecretion of insulin → rapid drop in blood glucose levels.

Nursing Interventions and Considerations

Advise the client to follow the modifications outlined above for the *antidumping* diet to avoid hypoglycemia.

Instruct the client to carry a source for concentrated sugar with him to treat reactive hypoglycemia when it occurs, such as hard candy, lumps of sugar, LifeSavers, and so forth.

Potential Problem/Rationale

Anemia may occur as a result of 1) chronic blood loss; 2) impaired iron absorption because of decreased exposure to HCl in the stomach or because the duodenal site of iron absorption is bypassed; or 3) vitamin B_{12} malabsorption related to inadequate secretion of intrinsic factor (IF) or because of bacterial overgrowth in a *blind loop*.

Nursing Interventions and Considerations

Observe for signs and symptoms of anemia (see Chap. 17). Adjust the diet and provide supplements accordingly.

Clients with pernicious anemia require intramuscular injections of vitamin B_{12}.

INTESTINAL SURGERIES

Intestinal bypass: Surgical removal of 50% or more of the small bowel because of inflammatory bowel disease, cancer, obstruction, and so forth.

Potential Problem/Rationale

Short bowel syndrome: Diarrhea, fluid and electrolyte imbalances, severe weight loss, muscle wasting, malabsorption, steatorrhea, anemia, and malnutrition resulting from a decrease in absorptive area of the intestine.

(continued)

Nursing Interventions and Considerations for Potential Nutritional Problems of Various Surgical Procedures of the GI Tract *(Continued)*

Nursing Interventions and Considerations

The client is usually maintained on total parenteral nutrition for 2 to 3 months after surgery. Oral intake resumes when fecal output is about 1 liter/day with clear liquids or a hydrolyzed (chemically defined) diet.

Monitor fluid and electrolyte balance and correct abnormalities. Antidiarrheals and potassium supplements may be needed for 5 or more months after surgery.

Low-residue foods are introduced as the client's tolerance improves.

Instruct the client

- To eat six to eight small, frequent meals
- To decrease fat intake; MCT oil may be used for additional calories
- To increase protein intake to replace losses
- To increase calorie intake to restore normal weight
- To take supplements as directed
- To avoid high-fiber foods.
- To avoid caffeine for at least the first year after surgery, because it stimulates GI motility.

Malabsorption of fat can result in deficiencies of the fat-soluble vitamins, calcium, and magnesium. Observe for signs and symptoms of deficiencies and provide supplements as needed.

Eventually the remaining small bowel can adapt by enlarging and by increasing its ability to absorb nutrients. However, depending on the extent of surgery, adaptation may not be possible and the client may need parenteral nutritional support indefinitely.

Ileostomy

An opening (stoma) in the abdominal wall into the ileum for continuous discharge of the liquid contents of the small intestine.

Colostomy

An opening (stoma) in the abdominal wall into the colon for defecation of liquid to formed stools after removal of the rectum and anus.

Either procedure may be used in the treatment of severe ulcerative colitis or inflammatory bowel disease, intestinal lesions, obstructions, or colonic cancer; ostomies may be temporary or permanent. Ileostomies are more likely to cause nutritional problems than colostomies.

Potential Problem/Rationale

Frequent, watery stools related to a decrease in absorptive surface (large amounts of water and electrolytes are normally absorbed in the colon).

Nursing Interventions and Considerations

Losses of fluid, sodium, and potassium may be considerable, depending on the location of the stoma and whether adaptation has occurred. Monitor fluid and electrolyte balance and correct abnormalities.

Initially, clear liquids are given and progressed to a low-residue diet to prevent irritation and slow GI transit time. As the client improves, gradually and individually add small amounts of foods containing fiber to the diet and assess the client's tolerance. Foods not tolerated initially can be reintroduced in a few months.

Encourage the client to drink a lot of fluid. Excess fluid intake does not contribute to diarrhea, but is excreted through the kidneys. It is important for ileostomy clients to maintain a normal urine output to minimize the risk of renal calculi.

Potential Problem/Rationale

Weight loss related to diarrhea or a fear of eating.

Nursing Interventions and Considerations

Provide a high-calorie, high-protein diet to replenish losses and restore normal weight.

Encourage the client to verbalize fears; counsel the client on the importance of eating to attain/maintain wellness.

(continued)

> ## Nursing Interventions and Considerations for Potential Nutritional Problems of Various Surgical Procedures of the GI Tract (Continued)
>
> **Potential Problem/Rationale**
>
> Anemia related to vitamin B_{12} malabsorption (vitamin B_{12} is normally absorbed in the distal ileum).
>
> **Nursing Interventions and Considerations**
>
> Clients with ileal resections require parenteral vitamin B_{12} injections for the rest of their lives.
>
> **Potential Problem/Rationale**
>
> Odor related to poor stomal hygiene or to the action of bacteria on food.
>
> **Nursing Interventions and Considerations**
>
> Encourage good stomal hygiene.
>
> Advise the client to eliminate foods that may produce odorous gas, such as beer and other alcoholic beverages, beans, onions, green pepper, broccoli, cabbage, asparagus, brussels sprouts, turnips, beets, corn, and spicy foods. Individual intolerances should also be eliminated.
>
> **Potential Problem/Rationale**
>
> Intestinal blockage related to improperly chewed food.
>
> **Nursing Interventions and Considerations**
>
> Advise the client to avoid high-fiber fruits and vegetables and to chew food thoroughly.
>
> **Potential Problem/Rationale**
>
> Depression and anxiety related to altered body image, altered body function, and dietary restrictions.
>
> **Nursing Interventions and Considerations**
>
> Provide emotional support and allow the client and family to verbalize their feelings.
>
> Advise the client that, with time, a more normal diet is possible as adaptation occurs. The stools usually become more firm and less frequent within 7 to 10 days after an ileostomy.

Withhold all food and liquids (NPO) for at least 8 hours before surgery to avoid aspiration related to anesthesia. To minimize fecal residue and postoperative distention after intestinal surgery, a low-residue, residue-free (see Chap. 16), or hydrolyzed formula diet may be used before surgery for 2 to 3 days (see Chap. 14).

After Surgery

Give IV fluid and electrolytes as ordered to maintain hydration until oral intake is resumed, usually with the return of bowel sounds 24 to 48 hours after surgery.

Progress oral intake from clear liquids to full liquids to a soft or regular diet as tolerated (see Chap. 14, Table 14-1).

Depending on the extent of surgery and the development of complications:

Increase protein intake to 1.5 g/kg body weight, or more, according to the extent of surgery and the patient's protein status. Protein is needed to promote wound healing and replace protein losses.

Increase caloric intake to meet increased energy requirements and to spare protein.

Encourage a liberal intake of those nutrients that are necessary for wound healing and recovery (see Table 15-3).

Table 15-3
Nutrients Important for Wound Healing and Recovery

Nutrient	Rationale for Increased Need	Possible Deficiency Outcome
Protein	To replace the lean body mass lost during the catabolic phase following stress To restore blood volume and plasma proteins lost during exudates, bleeding from the wound, and possible hemorrhage To replace losses resulting from immobility (increased excretion) To meet the increased needs for tissue repair and resistance to infection	Significant weight loss Impaired/delayed wound healing Shock related to decreased blood volume Edema related to decreased serum albumin Diarrhea related to decreased albumin Anemia Increased risk of infection related to decreased antibodies, impaired tissue integrity Decreased lipoprotein synthesis → fatty infiltration of the liver → liver damage Increased mortality
Calories	To replace losses related to NPO, hypermetabolism during catabolic phase following stress To spare protein To restore normal weight	Signs and symptoms of protein deficiency may develop when protein is used to meet energy requirements. Extensive weight loss
Water	To replace losses through vomiting, hemorrhage, exudates, fever, drainage, diuresis To maintain homeostasis	Signs, symptoms, and complications of dehydration such as poor skin turgor, dry mucous membranes, oliguria, anuria, weight loss, increased pulse rate, decreased central venous pressure (CVP)
Vitamin C	Important for capillary formation, tissue synthesis, and wound healing through collagen formation Needed for antibody formation	Impaired/delayed wound healing related to impaired collagen formation and increased capillary fragility and permeability Increased risk of infection related to decreased antibodies
Thiamine, niacin, riboflavin	Requirements based on metabolic rate: increased metabolic rate → increased requirements	Decreased enzymes available for energy metabolism
Folic acid, vitamin B_{12}	Needed for cell proliferation and therefore tissue synthesis Important for maturation of red blood cells Impaired folic acid synthesis related to some antibiotics; impaired vitamin B_{12} absorption related to some antibiotics	Decreased or arrested cell division Megaloblastic anemia
Vitamin A	Important for tissue synthesis, wound healing, and immune function Enhances resistance to infection	Impaired/delayed wound healing related to decreased collagen synthesis; impaired immune function Increased risk of infection
Vitamin K	Important for normal blood clotting Impaired intestinal synthesis related to antibiotics	Prolonged prothrombin time
Iron	To replace iron lost through blood loss	Signs, symptoms, and complications of iron deficiency anemia, such as fatigue, weakness, pallor, anorexia, dizziness, headaches, stomatitis, glossitis, cardiovascular and respiratory changes, possible cardiac failure
Zinc	Needed for protein synthesis and wound healing Needed for normal lymphocyte and phagocyte response	Impaired/delayed wound healing Impaired immune response

Modify the diet, as needed, to avoid potential nutritional problems related to GI surgery (see displays, Nursing Interventions and Considerations for Potential Nutritional Problems of Various Surgical Procedures of the GI Tract; and Sample Postgastrectomy ["Antidumping"] Menu).

Patients who are unable or unwilling to consume an adequate oral intake may require enteral or parenteral nutritional support. If the GI tract is functional, enteral nutrition is preferred over parenteral nutritional support.

Client Teaching

Instruct the client

On the importance of nutrition in recovery and wound healing

How to increase protein and calorie intake (see the display, Ways to Add Protein and Calories to the Diet)

On the principles and rationale of diet management of post-GI surgery, as appropriate

To eat small, frequent meals if anorexia or nausea exists

Monitoring Progress

Monitor for the following signs or symptoms:

Tolerance of oral diet (eg, absence of postprandial pain, nausea, vomiting, and distention)

Compliance with diet (as appropriate), and the need for follow-up diet counseling

Effectiveness of diet, and the need for further diet modification

Weight, weight changes

Healing, postsurgical course

Intake and output; observe for fluid and electrolyte imbalances

Bowel elimination; alterations in bowel function

Sample Postgastrectomy ("Antidumping") Menu

Breakfast
1 soft-cooked egg
1 slice white toast with butter
One Hour Later
1/2 cup milk

Midmorning Snack
Firm banana
Graham crackers

Lunch
1/2 cup cottage cheese with 2 canned peach halves
Dinner roll with butter
One Hour later
1/2 cup milk

Midafternoon Snack
1 oz cheddar cheese
4 saltine crackers

Dinner
2 oz baked chicken
1/2 cup white rice with butter
1/4 cup mashed butternut squash
One Hour Later
1/2 cup milk

Bedtime Snack
1/2 plain bagel with cream cheese

Evaluation

Evaluation is ongoing. Provided that the plan of care has not changed, the patient will achieve the goals as stated above.

BURNS

Burns are the third leading cause of accidental death in the United States. They may be caused by thermal, electrical, chemical, or radioactive insults. Burns are classified according to degree, based on the extent of damage. Burns over more than 20% of the body may be fatal.

Superficial partial-thickness (first-degree) burns destroy the epidermis. The area appears pink to red, with slight edema but no blisters. Pain may last up to 24 hours and is relieved by cooling. Healing occurs spontaneously within a week.

Deep partial-thickness (second-degree) burns may be superficial or deep. A superficial second-degree burn destroys the epidermis layer of the skin. The area appears red and blistered and is painful; however, healing occurs spontaneously if infection does not develop. Deep second-degree burns destroy all but the deep dermis layer of skin. The area appears mottled white and red; red, edematous areas blanch when touched. Healing takes several weeks; scarring may occur.

Full-thickness (third-degree) burns may appear red, white, black, or brown; burned areas do not blanch when touched. Third-degree burns destroy the epidermis and dermis layers of the skin and also the nerve endings; therefore, no pain is felt. Débridement and grafting are necessary; scarring and loss of skin function occur. Fourth-degree burns destroy skin, fat, muscles, and bone. Débridement, formation of granulation tissue, and grafting are necessary.

The patient's age and past medical history; the extent, depth, and cause of the burn; the presence of associated injuries; and the development of complications influence the patient's prognosis. Achieving nitrogen balance is imperative; weight loss of 40% to 50% may be fatal. Sepsis is the most common cause of death among burn victims, followed by pneumonia. Other complications include congestive heart failure, adrenal insufficiency, renal failure, hemorrhaging, and stress ulcers (Curling's ulcer) (see the display, Risk Factors for Complications in Burned Clients).

Treatment measures depend on the extent of the burn and the phase of recovery. The goals of treatment are to maintain fluid and electrolyte balance, relieve pain and anxiety, prevent complications and infection, promote healing, provide physical and emotional support, and meet increased nutritional requirements.

NURSING PROCESS

Assessment

Observe and assess:

The percentage of body surface area (BSA) burned
Thickness or degree of burn, and percentage of third-degree burn

Risk Factors for Complications in Burned Clients

Burn surface area greater than 20%

Poor nutritional status prior to burn

Preburn illness or disease

Morbid obesity

History of substance abuse

Associated injuries

Complications: pulmonary, circulatory, infectious, metabolic, GI

Weight loss of more than 10% or preburn weight while hospitalized

Low serum transferrin and anergy (impaired immunocompetence) are strongly correlated to a high risk of infectious complications.

Source: Jensen TG, Long JM, Dudrick SJ, et al (1985). Nutritional assessment indications of postburn complications. J Am Diet Assoc 85:68.

The type of burn: thermal, electrical, chemical, radioactive

The location of the burn; assess the client's ability to self-feed

The possibility of inhalation injury

Concomitant injuries

History of chronic illnesses and drug therapy

Prior nutritional status, especially usual/ideal preburn weight. Be aware that some nutritional assessment criteria may be difficult to obtain or invalid for burned patients. For instance, triceps skinfold and upper arm circumference measurements are contraindicated in patients with upper body burns, and massive fluid shifts make accurate weights impossible during the initial postburn period.

Nursing Diagnosis

Altered Nutrition: Less than body requirements, related to hypermetabolism secondary to thermal injury

Planning and Implementation

Extensive burns are the most severe form of stress that a person can experience. Because of hormonal responses and extensive evaporative water losses, metabolism may increase 100% above normal (hypermetabolism). Glycogen stores are quickly depleted, and the body uses its own lean body tissue for energy needs (hypercatabolism). Large quantities of fluid, electrolytes, protein, and other nutrients leach through the burned area. Nutritional support may be complicated by fluid and electrolyte imbalances, paralytic ileus, anorexia, pain, infection or other complications, emotional trauma, and medical–surgical procedures. Weight loss and malnutrition lead to increased morbidity and mortality unless aggressive nutritional support is initiated as soon as possible after fluid resuscitation.

Fluid replacement is the primary concern in the immediate postburn phase, also known as the "ebb" or shock phase. Individualized amounts and combinations of IV electrolytes, colloids (whole blood, plasma, or serum protein albumin), fluid, and dextrose may be given. Average fluid requirements range from 3 to 5 liters daily, although up to 10 liters/day may be needed for extensive burns. Generally, half of the calculated fluid volume that is needed for the first 24 hours is given in the first 8 hours when fluid loss is greatest; the remaining volume is given over the next 16 hours. Immediate use of IV fluids also helps to prevent gastric distention and paralytic ileus.

The high incidence of impaired immunocompetence and protein depletion among burned clients makes aggressive nutritional support vital in order to decrease the risk of infectious complications. Primary goals during the "flow" or recovery period that begins 48 to 72 hours post burn are to maintain fluid and electrolyte balance and to minimize the loss of lean body tissue and body weight. Oral intake should begin as soon as fluid resuscitation is completed and paralytic ileus is resolved, usually around the 3rd postburn day. If bowel sounds have not returned by the 4th postburn day, peripheral or central vein parenteral nutrition should be given. Although it is easier to meet calorie needs than protein needs, patients should be able to achieve neutral balances of both by the 7th postburn day. Goals of this secondary feeding period are to replace nutritional losses and promote wound healing.

The diet management recommendations listed below are guidelines. A starting level should be selected, and interventions should be implemented and evaluated for their effectiveness. Periodic diet adjustments should be made according to the patient's progress. Nutritional requirements are increased by the development of complications and are decreased as wound healing progresses.

Although it may be preferred, a regular diet with in-between meal supplements of high-calorie, high-protein liquids may not be adequate for some patients. Supplemental or complete enteral (nasogastric [NG] tube, gastrostomy, jejunostomy) or parenteral (central, jugular, femoral, or cut-down peripheral route) feedings may be necessary for patients with the following conditions:

- Extremely high calorie and protein requirements for those who cannot consume enough food orally to meet their needs
- Inability to swallow because of facial or neck burns
- Adynamic ileus
- Bleeding related to Curling's ulcer (need total parenteral nutrition [TPN])
- Anorexia related to fear, pain, altered body image, and frequent medical or surgical procedures; nutritional requirements are highest when appetite is poorest.

Total parenteral nutrition should be used with extreme caution because of the increased risks for infection and sepsis. Other considerations include the location of the burn and the compatibility of IV medications with the TPN solution.

There are no set guidelines for vitamin and mineral supplementation for burned patients. The need for some nutrients may increase directly to promote wound healing (eg, vitamin C, zinc) or indirectly because of the increased calorie intake (eg, requirements for thiamine, riboflavin, and niacin increase in proportion to the increase in calorie requirements) (see Table 15-3). Multivitamin and mineral supplements or megadoses of certain nutrients may be prescribed at the physician's discretion, depending on the patient's previous nutritional status.

Decreased weight-bearing during immobility results in increased bone resorption and a negative calcium imbalance, regardless of calcium intake. Encourage ambulation to minimize calcium and nitrogen excretion and to improve appetite and outlook. Once weight-bearing activity resumes, the calcium requirement increases to replace calcium that has been lost from bone.

As the patient enters the rehabilitation phase after wound healing, diet becomes less important. However, an adequate intake is needed to rebuild body stores and muscle tissue. Obesity is rare during the first 5 years after extensive burns.

CLIENT GOALS

The client will:

Attain or maintain fluid and electrolyte balance within 72 hours post burn
Avoid renal shutdown from decreased plasma volume and cardiac output
Have minimal catabolism of protein tissues to avoid protein–calorie malnutrition
Experience wound healing and retain grafts, as appropriate
Avoid weight loss greater than 10% preburn weight (if preburn weight was within the patient's "healthy" weight range)
Attain nitrogen balance
Avoid complications

NURSING INTERVENTIONS

Diet Management

After bowel sounds return, initiate an oral diet (ie, liquids) slowly and observe for signs of intolerance; progress the diet as tolerated. Hydrolyzed (elemental) tube feedings may decrease the incidence of GI bleeding and provide a higher and more consistent calorie intake than a mixed oral diet in the early secondary feeding period.

Increase protein intake to facilitate wound healing and to replace the loss of lean body mass. Depending on the severity of the burn, daily protein intake should be 1.5 to 3 g/kg, or approximately two to four times greater than the recommended dietary allowance (RDA).

Increase calorie intake to meet increased energy requirements related to hypermetabolism and spare protein for tissue repair. Daily calorie requirements may range from 40 to 60 cal/kg, a 30% to 100% increase above normal or may be calculated using the Harris-Benedict equation, accounting for activity and stress factors (see Example). Although metabolic rate peaks around the 10th postburn day, metabolism (and, therefore, the calorie requirement) remains high for several weeks or longer, depending on the extent of the burn. The distribution of calories should be approximately 25% protein, 50% carbohydrate, and 25% fat.

EXAMPLE

A 45-year-old man who is 5′9″ tall and weighs 165 lb has severe burns and is confined to bed.

Convert pounds and inches to metric:

$$165 \text{ lb} \div 2.2 \text{ lb/kg} = 75 \text{ kg}$$

$$5'9'' = 69'' \qquad 69'' \times 2.54 \text{ cm/in} = 175 \text{ cm}$$

1. Calculate BEE:

$$66 + 13.7(75) + 5(175) - 6.8(45) = \mathbf{1663}$$

2. Multiply BEE by activity factor:

$$1663 \times 1.2 = \mathbf{1996}$$

3. Multiply BEE/activity factor value by stress factor:

$$1996 \times 2.1 = \mathbf{4192 \text{ cal/day}}$$

Provide adequate fluid intake; water losses may be 10 to 12 times above normal in the first few postburn weeks. Encourage fruit juices high in potassium and vitamin C. Promote maximum intake:

- Work with the client and family to solicit food preferences. Young children may regress in their eating behaviors; adults may prefer foods that they associate with recovery as children (eg, chicken soup).
- Encourage the family to bring food from home.
- Discourage the intake of empty-calorie food and beverages.
- Provide small, frequent meals; assist as needed.
- Provide emotional support and allow the patient to verbalize feelings.
- If possible, schedule débridement and other medical and surgical procedures at a time when they are least likely to interfere with meals.
- Provide pain medication as needed before meals.

Client Teaching

Instruct the client

On the importance of nutrition in wound healing and avoiding complications.

On the rationale and principles of diet management for burns, and how to implement the appropriate dietary modifications, especially ways to add protein and calories to the diet (see the display).

That postburn weight loss is to be expected, but that weight eventually should be restored.

To take vitamins and minerals as ordered, to hasten recovery and wound healing.

Monitoring Progress

Monitor for the following signs or symptoms:

Fluid and electrolyte balance, and observe for signs of dehydration or overhydration

Progress and tolerance of the feeding regimen; progress or modify as indicated

The need for follow-up diet counseling and additional diet modifications

After fluid balance is restored and feedings have begun, record body weight and intake of protein and calories daily to assess diet adequacy. Suggested guidelines for weight gain (if complications do not develop) are as follows:

- <20% BSA burned: Regain weight in about 5 weeks.
- 20% to 30% BSA burned: Lose weight for the first 5 postburn weeks. Thereafter, the patient should gain weight slowly. Preburn weight may or may not be achieved before discharge.
- ≥40% BSA burned: May lose weight for about the first 8 postburn weeks. Thereafter, the patient should gain weight slowly.

Monitor laboratory studies (albumin, transferrin, total lymphocyte count, creatinine–height index) after the initial stress response and peak period of catabolism subside to assess nutritional status. Low serum transferrin and anergy are strongly correlated with the development of wound infection.

Monitor for signs and symptoms of sepsis: fever, abdominal distention, ileus, disorientation.

Evaluation

Evaluation is ongoing. Provided that the plan of care has not changed, the patient will achieve the goals as stated above.

RESPIRATORY STRESS: CHRONIC OBSTRUCTIVE PULMONARY DISEASE

Although they differ in pathologic progression, chronic bronchitis and emphysema are both characterized by chronic limited airflow and thus fall under the inclusive heading of chronic obstructive pulmonary disease (COPD).

Emphysema, the most severe form of COPD, is characterized by distention and destructive changes in the alveolar walls and air spaces. Although the exact cause is not known, emphysema appears to be the result of the body's inability to defend itself against the destructive effects of two enzymes that destroy the lung's connective tissue (elastin). The loss of elastin causes the lungs to become distended because they lose their ability to recoil. It also increases airway resistance, which results from the collapse or narrowing of small airways during expectoration. Air then becomes trapped in the distal spaces and contributes to distention. Increased pressure on the diaphragm eventually impairs the patient's ability to breathe effectively; accessory muscles are used to facilitate breathing. Initial symptoms include dyspnea, increased respiratory rate, prolonged expiratory phase, and pursed-lip breathing. Patients are often thin, because they experience poor appetites and increased calorie expenditure from labored breathing.

Chronic bronchitis is characterized by a productive cough that lasts for at least 3 months of the year for 2 consecutive years. Excess production of mucus and recurrent cough are related to hypertrophy and hyperplasia of the bronchial glands and an increased number of goblet cells. Chronic inflammatory changes cause narrowing of the small airways. Airway obstruction and air trapping occur from mucous plugging and inflammation, which pose a constant risk of infection. In addition to the productive cough, hypoxemia and hypercapnia may be noted. Later, accessory muscles assist with breathing.

Potentially life-threatening complications of both emphysema and chronic bronchitis include pneumonia, acute respiratory failure, and cor pulmonale. Although the course of chronic bronchitis may be variable, people with emphysema suffer progressive deterioration. COPD is the 6th leading cause of death in the United States.

COPD affects more than 23 million Americans, or roughly 10% of the population (Jess, 1992). Eighty to 90% of cases of COPD are attributed to cigarette smoking. Generally, it takes 30 to 35 years after the onset of smoking for symptoms of COPD to develop. Men over 45 years of age represent the greatest proportion of patients with COPD; however, since women started smoking in the 1930s and 1940s, the incidence of women with COPD has been increasing.

Treatment is intended to relieve symptoms, improve respiratory function, and prevent further lung damage. Drug therapy (bronchodilators, corticosteroids, expectorants, antibiotics), breathing exercises, and chest physiotherapy may be used.

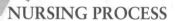

NURSING PROCESS

Assessment

In addition to the general pulmonary assessment criteria, assess for the following factors:

- The type and extent of respiratory disease; use of accessory muscles for breathing
- Symptoms that interfere with eating, such as shortness of breath, fatigue, nausea, vomiting, anorexia: Assess onset, duration, severity, interventions attempted, and results of interventions
- Dietary changes made in response to symptoms (ie, foods avoided, foods preferred). Determine which foods are best and least tolerated.

ASSESSMENT CRITERIA

General Pulmonary Assessment Criteria

Shortness of breath, exertional dyspnea	Rapid or altered respirations
Chronic cough, expectoration of mucus, dyspnea	Drowsiness, confusion, impaired judgment
Wheezing	Pallor, cyanosis, gray coloring; red, swollen nose
Recurrent respiratory tract infections	Distended neck veins during expiration
Fatigue, weakness, weight loss	

- Use of medications and their potential impact on nutritional status (see Drug Alert)
- Weight, recent weight changes
- Adequacy of usual intake, especially calories, protein, fat, and fluid
- Serum albumin; arterial blood gases; other abnormal laboratory values and their significance

Nursing Diagnosis: Altered Nutrition: Less than body requirement, related to anorexia, shortness of breath, and increased calorie expenditure secondary to labored breathing

Planning and Implementation

Weight loss and malnutrition in patients with COPD (especially emphysema) may be multifactorial and be characterized by the following: increased energy expenditure related to labored breathing; anorexia related to excess mucus, drug therapy, or decreased peristalsis and digestion secondary to inadequate oxygen to GI cells; and inadequate intake secondary to difficulty chewing and swallowing related to shortness of breath. A downhill spiral often occurs: A reduced respiratory rate reduces blood flow to the GI tract, thereby decreasing nutrient absorption and increasing the risk of malnutrition; conversely, malnutrition reduces respiratory rate and may exacerbate existing respiratory impairments.

Improving weight in underweight patients improves muscle strength, endurance, and exercise tolerance, even though it may not influence life expectancy (Whittaker et al, 1990). Calorie requirements may be estimated by multiplying BEE × 1.5. Overweight patients should be encouraged to lose weight to improve breathing. For depleted patients, provide 1.2 to 1.5 g protein/kg.

The metabolism of carbohydrates, protein, and fat yields carbon dioxide and water. **Respiratory quotient (RQ)** refers to the ratio of carbon dioxide produced to oxygen consumed; the more carbon dioxide is produced, the greater the burden on the lungs to exhale CO_2. Because the RQ is higher for carbohydrates than for either

DRUG ALERT

Drugs Commonly Used To Treat COPD

Theophylline (bronchodilator) commonly causes anorexia. A high-carbohydrate, low-protein diet slows the metabolism of theophylline, thereby increasing the risk of side effects, including dizziness, flushing, and headache. A sudden increase in protein intake may decrease the duration of theophylline action. Caffeine in any form also slows the rate of theophylline elimination; concurrent use of caffeine increases the risk for insomnia and cardiac arrhythmias.

Albuterol (bronchodilator) may cause hyperglycemia in diabetics.

Prednisone (antiinflammatory glucocorticoid) stimulates appetite and thus may cause weight gain. Hyperglycemia may occur in diabetics and nondiabetics. Promotes sodium retention, potassium excretion, loss of calcium from the bones, and GI upset.

protein or fat, it may be beneficial to limit carbohydrate intake in patients with hypercapnia or those on ventilator support. Instead of the normal calorie distribution of 50% to 60% carbohydrate, 20% to 30% fat, and 15% to 20% protein, it may be appropriate for them to limit carbohydrate intake to 25% to 30% of calories and increase fat intake to 50% to 55% of total calories. Low-carbohydrate, high-fat enteral products that are designed for use in patients with pulmonary disease are available. (See Appendix 7.)

A soft diet may be appropriate for patients who have difficulty chewing and swallowing related to shortness of breath. Fatigued patients may need assistance with cutting food, opening containers, and so forth. Breathing exercises should be avoided for at least 1 hour before and after eating.

Limiting "empty" liquids with meals (eg, coffee, tea, water, carbonated beverages) and providing small, frequent, nutritionally dense feedings help maximize intake and reduce gastric distention and pressure on the diaphragm. Gassy foods should be avoided, unless they are well tolerated. Consider "feedings" of high-calorie, high-protein eggnogs, shakes, and commercial supplements.

Unless it is contraindicated, a high fluid intake is needed to help thin mucus secretions; fever also increases fluid requirements. Generally, 1 cc/cal is adequate.

To avoid straining at stool, a high-fiber diet is indicated, which includes bran cereals, whole grains, prunes, fruits, and vegetables. Fiber intake should be increased gradually to avoid excessive gas, distention, and diarrhea.

Supplements of B-complex vitamins (for increased energy metabolism) and vitamins A and C (for healing and tissue repair) may be appropriate.

Additional diet modifications may be necessary, depending on the patient's drug therapy.

CLIENT GOALS

The client will:

Attain or maintain healthy weight and lean body mass
Avoid excessive CO_2 production, if hypercapnic
Maintain normal fluid and electrolyte balance
Avoid complications, such as respiratory infection and respiratory acidosis
Overcome symptoms (eg, anorexia, shortness of breath) to consume a nutritionally adequate diet
Avoid constipation and straining at stool

NURSING INTERVENTIONS

Diet Management

Provide calories for weight gain, if underweight; if patient is obese, decrease calories for weight loss to improve breathing. Limit carbohydrate and increase fat for patients who are hypercapnic.
Increase protein intake to 1.2 to 1.5 g/kg.

Modify food texture, as needed, to overcome problems with fatigue, chewing, and swallowing.

Allow 1 cc fluid/cal; modify as needed for overhydration or dehydration.

Provide small, frequent meals to lessen symptoms and maximize intake.

Increase fiber intake gradually.

Modify the diet, as needed, if the patient has side effects from medications.

Client Teaching

Instruct the client

On the principles and rationale of diet management for COPD

How to maximize intake (see the display, Ways to Add Protein and Calories to the Diet)

To rest before and after meals, and to avoid breathing treatments for at least 1 hour before and after eating

To eat slowly

To avoid extremely hot or cold foods, because they may precipitate coughing spells

Monitoring Progress

Monitor for the following signs or symptoms:

Compliance with the diet, and the need for follow-up diet counseling

Effectiveness of the diet (ie, "healthy" weight achieved, fluid balance maintained, constipation avoided) and evaluate the need for further diet modifications.

Tolerance to the diet (eg, avoids gastric distention, hypercapnia)

Evaluation

Evaluation is ongoing. Provided that the plan of care has not changed, the patient will achieve the goals as stated above.

KEY CONCEPTS

- The impact of stress on nutritional status and requirements depends on the severity of the stress, the number of stressors, and the individual's ability to adapt to stress.
- The release of stress hormones during the ebb phase following injury causes an increase in serum glucose, and decreases in oxygen consumption, blood pressure, cardiac output, body temperature, and renal output. Nutrition intervention during this period is usually contraindicated.
- Hypermetabolism and increased catabolism occur during the flow phase. Nutrition support begins when serum glucose levels fall, usually within 2 to 5 days posttrauma. Adequate calories are needed to minimize weight loss and promote anabolism; protein needs are also elevated.
- Patients who are well nourished before surgery have a lower incidence of infections and experience fewer complications than malnourished patients. If time allows, nutritional deficits should be corrected before surgery.

- The degree of stress associated with surgery depends on the location, extent, and type of surgery, and the development of postsurgical complications. Healing increases the requirements for calories, protein, vitamin C, and zinc.

- Extensive burns are the most severe form of stress that a person can experience. Calorie requirements may increase 100%, and protein needs may increase more than three times the normal RDA. Nutritional support may be complicated by paralaytic ileus, stress ulcers, anorexia, pain, and medical–surgical treatments.

- Patients with COPD are often underweight and malnourished. Shortness of breath can make eating difficult and decreased oxygenation of the GI cells can impair peristalsis and digestion. Conversely, poor nutrition can impair respiratory status.

- Nutrition-dense, easy-to-consume foods are preferred for patients with chronic respiratory disorders. Patients with hypercapnia or those on ventilator support may benefit from a restricted carbohydrate intake. Carbohydrates produce more CO_2 when metabolized than do either protein or fat, thus they create a greater burden on the lungs.

FOCUS ON **CRITICAL THINKING**

Mr. Stevens is 45 years old, 5'11" tall, weighs 160 pounds, and was brought to the emergency room after being struck by a car while jogging. It was quickly determined that Mr. Stevens suffered a ruptured spleen, broken femur, a broken jaw, and two cracked ribs. He underwent surgery to remove his spleen, set his leg, and wire his jaw; his course in the ICU was typical of post-trauma clients. By the third post-trauma day, Mr. Stevens still had a paralytic ileus, and parenteral nutrition was started.

Calculate Mr. Stevens' calorie and protein requirements. Why or why wasn't parenteral nutrition the best method of feeding to initiate? When would it be appropriate to discontinue parenteral nutrition? What method of feeding would you then recommend? When Mr. Stevens is able to tolerate oral feedings, what type of diet would you recommend? Devise an appropriate diet that would provide adequate calories and protein in a form Mr. Stevens could consume.

REFERENCES

Brown, K. (1994). Septic Shock: How to stop the deadly cascade. AJN 94(9), 20–26.

Brown, K. (1994). Critical interventions in septic shock. AJN 94(10), 20–25.

Escott-Stump, S. (1992). Nutrition and Diagnosis-Related Care. 3rd ed. Philadelphia: Lea & Febiger.

Jess, L. (1992). Chronic bronchitis and emphysema. Airing the differences. Nursing 92, 22(3), 34–41.

Lenaghan, N. (1992). After the trauma: Managing its effects down to the last letter. Nursing 92, 22(3), 45–48.

Roe, D. (1994). Handbook on Drug and Nutrient Interactions. 5th ed. Chicago: The American Dietetic Association.

Russell, S. (1994). Septic shock. Can you recognize the clues? Nursing 94, 24(4), 40–46.

Scherer, J. and Timby, B. (1995). Introductory Medical-Surgical Nursing. 6th ed. Philadelphia: JB Lippincott Company.

Shils, M., Olson, J. and Shike, M. (1994). Modern Nutrition in Health and Disease. 8th ed. Philadelphia: Lea & Febiger.

Weant, C. (1995). Easing the pain of esophageal surgery. RN, 58(8), 26–30.

Whittaker, J., et al (1990). The effects of refeeding on peripheral and respiratory muscle function in malnourished chronic obstructive pulmonary disease patients. Am Rev Respir Dis 142(2), 238–288.

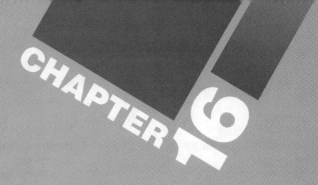

CHAPTER 16

Digestive System Disorders and the Role of Diet Therapy

Chapter Outline

(continued)

Chapter Outline (Continued)

Key Terms

BRAT Diet
Dysphagia
Dysphagia diets
Gluten-free diet
High-fiber diet
Lactose-restricted diet

Liberal bland diet
Low-fat diet
Low-residue diet
Lower esophageal sphincter
(LES)
Malabsorption syndrome

Medium-chain triglycerides
(MCT)
Progressive bland diet
Steatorrhea

The digestive system is composed of the alimentary canal (gastrointestinal tract) and the accessory organs (the liver, pancreas, and gallbladder). Alterations in GI function may be primary or secondary to other disorders. Nutrition intervention is often used to treat or control gastrointestinal (GI) disorders or to alleviate or prevent their symptoms. The reader will note that client goals are often to *lessen* symptoms rather than *eliminate* them; diet is not the sole cause or cure for most altered health states. Certain therapeutic diets have proved effective in the treatment of GI disorders. However, the validity of imposing rigid dietary restrictions on others is questionable. Because conservative diet therapy may be unnecessarily restrictive, the trend is toward more liberal dietary approaches. At the very least, diet intervention can help to correct nutritional deficiencies that are caused by GI disorders and their treatments.

Before the optimal diet intervention can be planned, a general assessment of GI status is indicated (see the display, General Gastrointestinal Assessment Criteria). Additional assessment criteria are provided, where applicable.

COMMON GASTROINTESTINAL PROBLEMS

Anorexia, nausea and vomiting, diarrhea, and constipation are common GI disorders that may occur as isolated incidents, as symptoms of underlying GI disorders, as a result of viral or bacterial infection, or secondary to drug therapy or medical treatment. Because they are common symptoms for a variety of disorders, they are dis-

ASSESSMENT CRITERIA

General Gastrointestinal Assessment Criteria

Appetite

Recent change in appetite

Ability to chew, swallow, and taste; oral and dental health

Activity: frequency, intensity

Feeding modality (oral, enteral, parenteral)

Signs or symptoms of altered GI function (reflux, indigestion, nausea, vomiting, diarrhea, constipation, bloating, cramping); onset, frequency, contributing factors, severity, interventions attempted and results

Weight status

Recent weight change: nature of change, onset, severity, contributing factors

Usual bowel habits: frequency; time of day; description of usual stool characteristics, including amount, consistency, shape, color, odor

Recent changes in bowel elimination

Use of elimination aids: fluids, particular foods, laxatives, stool softeners, enemas

Drug therapies: antacids, stool softeners, diuretics, laxatives, cimetidine, other

Psychological benefits or hazards of diet intervention

Client's attitude and willingness to modify diet

cussed here in depth. The nursing process for these disorders remains the same whether they are primary or secondary problems, and regardless of the underlying pathology.

Anorexia

Anorexia is defined as the lack of appetite, and differs from anorexia nervosa, a psychological condition that is characterized by the denial of appetite. In addition to the contributing factors listed above, anorexia may occur secondary to fear, anxiety, pain, and depression, or it may result from an impaired ability to smell and taste secondary to chronic rhinitis, olfactory and glossopharyngeal damage, laryngectomy, or certain drug therapies. The aim of diet management is to stimulate the appetite and attain or maintain adequate nutritional intake.

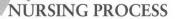

NURSING PROCESS

Assessment

In addition to the general GI assessment criteria, assess for the following factors:

Anorexia: onset, frequency, causative factors, severity, interventions attempted and the results.

Dietary changes made in response to anorexia (ie, foods avoided, foods preferred). Determine which foods are best and least tolerated.

Present intake, paying particular attention to meal frequency, food aversions, and fat intake—fat delays gastric emptying and provides a feeling of fullness, which inhibits appetite. Determine how much and how often high-fat foods are eaten: fried foods; fatty meats and luncheon meats; whole milk and milk products; butter, margarine, and oils; and rich desserts.

Intake and output; observe for signs of dehydration.

Weight. Compare actual weight to "healthy" weight. Assess amount and severity of any recent weight loss and observe for signs of malnutrition.

Activity patterns.

Nursing Diagnosis

Altered Nutrition: Less than body requirements, related to anorexia

Planning and Implementation

To enhance appetite, serve food attractively and season according to individual taste. If decreased ability to taste is contributing to anorexia, enhance food flavors with tart seasonings (orange juice, lemonade, vinegar, lemon juice) or strong seasonings (basil, oregano, rosemary, tarragon, mint).

If possible, schedule procedures and medications at a time when they are least likely to interfere with appetite. Also, control pain, nausea, or depression with medications, as ordered.

Liquid supplements that are provided as between-meal nourishments can significantly improve protein and calorie intake and generally are well accepted. In addition, liquids tend to leave the stomach quickly and are therefore less likely to interfere with meals.

CLIENT GOALS

The client will:

Experience less anorexia.

Consume adequate calories and protein to attain or maintain "healthy" weight.

Describe the principles and rationale for dietary management to relieve anorexia, and implement the appropriate dietary interventions.

Identify factors that contribute to anorexia, when known.

NURSING INTERVENTIONS

Diet Management

Provide small, frequent meals or between-meal supplements, as needed.

Limit fat intake, if fat is contributing to early satiety.

Solicit food preferences and allow food from home, if possible. Provide encouragement and a pleasant eating environment.

Client Teaching

Instruct the client

To stay calm, especially at mealtimes, and not to hurry through meals.
On the principles and rationale of diet management to relieve anorexia.
That small, frequent meals may be better tolerated than three large meals.
To eat a varied diet to stimulate appetite.
To avoid high-fat foods, if they are contributing to anorexia.
That an increase in activity, when possible, can help stimulate appetite.

Monitoring Progress

Monitor for the following signs or symptoms:

Compliance with the diet, and the need for follow-up diet counseling
Adequacy of intake
Effectiveness of diet interventions and the need for further modifications
Weight, weight changes

Evaluation

Evaluation is ongoing. Provided that the plan of care has not changed, the client will achieve the goals as stated above.

Nausea and Vomiting

Nausea is defined as the sensation of impending vomiting, which may or may not be followed by emesis. Nausea and vomiting may be related to a decrease in gastric acid secretion, a decrease in digestive enzyme activity, a decrease in GI motility, gastric irritation, or acidosis. Other causes include bacterial and viral infection; increased intracranial pressure; equilibrium imbalance; liver, pancreatic, and gallbladder disorders; and pyloric and intestinal obstruction. Drugs and certain medical treatments may also contribute to nausea. Prolonged nausea and vomiting can lead to weight loss; vomiting can cause metabolic alkalosis related to the loss of gastric hydrochloric acid.

NURSING PROCESS

Assessment

In addition to the general GI assessment criteria, assess for the following factors:

Nausea and vomiting: onset, frequency, causative factors, severity, interventions attempted, and results.
Dietary changes made in response to nausea and vomiting (ie, foods avoided, foods preferred). Determine which foods are best and least tolerated.

Fat intake: fat delays gastric emptying and provides a feeling of fullness, which inhibits appetite. Determine how much and how often high-fat foods are eaten: fried foods; fatty meats and luncheon meats; whole milk and milk products; butter, margarine, and oils; and rich desserts.

Fluid intake with meals: fluid can cause a full, bloated feeling.

Intake and output; observe for signs of dehydration.

Abnormal laboratory values, especially electrolyte imbalances (hyponatremia, hypochloremia).

Weight, and the severity of any recent weight loss; observe for signs of malnutrition.

Nursing Diagnosis

Fluid Volume Deficit, related to nausea and vomiting

Planning and Implementation

Solicit food preferences and observe individual food intolerances. Dry toast, crackers, or other carbohydrates eaten before the client gets out of bed in the morning may help avoid nausea.

Sodium and chloride are lost through emesis and may need to be replaced if vomiting is severe or prolonged.

CLIENT GOALS

The client will:

Experience less nausea and vomiting.

Maintain normal fluid and electrolyte balance.

Consume adequate calories and protein to attain or maintain "healthy" weight.

Describe the principles and rationale of diet management to relieve nausea and vomiting, and implement the appropriate dietary interventions.

Identify factors causing nausea and vomiting, when known.

NURSING INTERVENTIONS

Diet Management

Withhold food until nausea or vomiting subsides.

Progress oral feedings as the client's tolerance improves: clear liquids → full liquids → diet as tolerated. Small, frequent meals of readily digested carbohydrates (toast, crackers, plain rolls, pretzels, angel food cake, oatmeal, soft and bland fruit) are generally best tolerated.

Elevate the head of the bed.

Encourage the client to eat slowly.

Promote good oral hygiene with mouthwash and ice chips.

Limit liquids with meals because they can cause a full, bloated feeling; encourage a liberal fluid intake between meals.

Serve foods at room temperature or chilled; hot foods may contribute to nausea.

Client Teaching

Instruct the client

On the principles and rationale of diet management to relieve nausea and vomiting.

Not to eat when he or she feels nauseated.

To replace fluid and electrolytes with whatever liquids he or she can tolerate: clear soup and juice, gelatin, ginger ale, popsicles.

Monitoring Progress

Monitor for the following signs or symptoms:

Compliance with the diet, and the need for follow-up diet counseling

Adequacy of intake

Effectiveness of diet interventions and the need for further diet modifications

Weight, weight changes

Intake and output, and fluid balance (for vomiting)

Evaluation

Evaluation is ongoing. Provided that the plan of care has not changed, the client will achieve the goals as stated above.

Diarrhea

Diarrhea is characterized by the excretion of frequent, watery stools. It can cause large losses of potassium, sodium, and fluid, and also reduces the time that is available for the absorption of all other nutrients. Severe or prolonged diarrhea can quickly lead to nutritional complications, including weight loss, hypoproteinemia, and metabolic acidosis.

Emotional or physical stress, GI disorders and malabsorption syndromes, metabolic and endocrine disorders, surgical bowel intervention, certain drug therapies and medical treatments, and bacterial, viral, and parasitic infection are common causes of diarrhea (see the display, Drugs That Commonly Cause Diarrhea). Nutritionally, food allergies and the use of tube feedings are related to diarrhea. Also, coffee or caffeine stimulates peristalsis in some people, and an excessive intake of foods that are high in fiber or laxative properties can increase stool frequency.

NURSING PROCESS

Assessment

In addition to the general GI assessment criteria, assess for the following factors:

Diarrhea: onset, frequency, causative factors, severity, interventions attempted and results.

Drugs That Commonly Cause Diarrhea

Amphotericin B	Fluconazole
Azithromycin	Methotrexate
Cyclophosphamide	Misoprostol
Dactinomycin	Nitrofurantoin
Erythromycin	Olsalazine
Etretinate	Vincristine
5-Fluorouracil	

Source: Roe, D. (1994). Handbook on Drug and Nutrient Interactions. 5th ed. Chicago: American Dietetic Association.

Dietary changes made in response to diarrhea (ie, foods avoided, foods preferred). Determine which foods are best and least tolerated.

Intake of high-fiber foods that may be contributing to diarrhea: bran, whole-grain breads and cereals, raw vegetables, fresh fruits, and prunes or prune juice.

Milk intake and whether a relationship exists between milk consumption and diarrhea (ie, whether the client may have primary or secondary lactose intolerance).

Coffee or caffeine intake, and determine if a relationship exists between caffeine consumption and diarrhea.

Intake and output; observe for signs of dehydration and hypokalemia.

Abnormal laboratory values, especially potassium, sodium, and albumin.

If condition is chronic, client weight and signs of malnutrition.

Nursing Diagnosis

Diarrhea, related to _____ (causative factor)

Planning and Implementation

Because fluid and electrolyte balance is the principal concern when acute diarrhea occurs, a high fluid intake is the primary nutritional intervention.

Chronic diarrhea can cause not only fluid and electrolyte imbalances and metabolic acidosis, but also weight loss and nutrient inadequacies related to decreased transit time. Any foods that are suspected of causing or aggravating diarrhea (eg, milk, coffee, caffeine, high-fiber foods) should be eliminated. A **low-residue diet** (ie, foods low in fiber) reduces stool bulk and slows GI transit time. Sometimes a short-term diet called the **BRAT diet** is used (firm **B**ananas, white **R**ice, **A**pplesauce, **T**oast); it contains foods high in pectin to help firm stools. Clients who are not responding to traditional medical and dietary treatment (intractable diarrhea) may need bowel rest (total parenteral nutrition).

CLIENT GOALS

The client will:

Have fewer and less frequent stools.

Maintain normal fluid and electrolyte balance.

Consume adequate calories and protein to attain or maintain "healthy" weight.

Describe the principles and rationale of diet management to relieve diarrhea, and implement the appropriate dietary interventions.

Identify causative factors, if known.

NURSING INTERVENTIONS

Diet Management

Encourage clear fluids for acute diarrhea (usually subsides within 24 to 48 hours); no other diet intervention is necessary.

For chronic diarrhea, withhold food for 24 to 48 hours and provide intravenous fluid and electrolytes to maintain hydration.

Progress oral intake according to individual tolerance: clear liquids → full liquids → low-residue diet (see the display, Low-Residue Diet [Low-Fiber Diet]) until diarrhea has completely subsided.

Low-Residue Diet (Low-Fiber Diet)

CHARACTERISTICS

Restricts fiber and residue

Restrictions vary considerably among institutions and from mild to severe

OBJECTIVE

Reduce frequency and volume of fecal output and slow transit time

INDICATIONS FOR USE

Bowel inflammation, as seen in the acute stages of diverticulitis, ulcerative colitis, and regional enteritis

Esophageal and intestinal stenosis

Preparation for bowel surgery

CONTRAINDICATIONS

Irritable colon

Diverticulosis

FOODS ALLOWED

Meats: Eggs; ground or well-cooked tender meat, fish, and poultry

Dairy: Up to 2 cups of milk/day; mild cheeses

Fruits: Juices without pulp, except prune; canned fruit, and firm bananas

Vegetables: Vegetable juices without pulp; lettuce if tolerated, and most well-cooked vegetables without seeds

Breads and cereals: Only white bread and refined bread and cereal products; rolls, biscuits, muffins, pancakes, plain pastries; crackers, bagels; melba toast, waffles, refined cereals such as Cream of Wheat, Cream of Rice, and puffed rice

Miscellaneous: Plain desserts made with allowed foods such as fruit ices, plain cakes, puddings

(continued)

Low-Residue Diet (Low-Fiber Diet) (Continued)

(rice, bread, plain), cookies without nuts or coconut, sherbet, ice cream (no nuts or coconut); gelatin; candy such as butterscotch, jelly beans, marshmallows, plain hard candy; honey, molasses, sugar

FOODS NOT ALLOWED

Protein: Tough meats, dried peas and beans, lentils, peanut butter

Dairy: More than 2 cups of milk/day

Fruits: All other raw, cooked or dried fruits

Vegetables: Most raw vegetables and vegetables with seeds; sauerkraut, peas

Breads and cereals: Whole-grain breads and cereals, especially those made with bran or cracked wheat

Miscellaneous: Nuts, coconut, anything made with nuts or coconut, olives, pickles, seeds, popcorn

SAMPLE **MENU**

Low-Residue Diet

BREAKFAST

Strained orange juice
Cream of Rice
Poached egg
White toast with butter and jelly
1/2 cup milk
Coffee/tea
Salt/pepper/sugar

LUNCH

Tomato juice
Sandwich made with white bread, ham, and mayonnaise
Canned peach halves
Sponge cake
1/2 cup milk

Coffee/tea
Salt/pepper/sugar

DINNER

Roast chicken
White rice
Acorn squash
Italian bread with butter
Gelatin made with bananas
1/2 cup milk
Coffee/tea
Salt/pepper/sugar

SNACK

Saltine crackers
1/2 cup milk

POTENTIAL PROBLEM/RATIONALE

Nutrient deficiencies, especially of the following:

- Calcium, due to the limited amount of milk and dairy products allowed
- Iron, because many adults refuse to eat ground meats (meat is the richest source of iron in the diet). In addition, other sources

of iron, like dried fruits and many iron-fortified cereals, are prohibited
- Vitamins, because few kinds of vegetables are allowed on a low-residue diet; those that are allowed may be vitamin poor because processing techniques used to reduce the fiber content also remove vitamins

(continued)

Low-Residue Diet (Low-Fiber Diet) (Continued)

NURSING INTERVENTIONS AND CONSIDERATIONS

Monitor laboratory values and observe for signs of deficiencies. Provide supplements as needed.

Encourage as varied an intake as possible and liberalize the diet as soon as possible.

POTENTIAL PROBLEM/RATIONALE

Inadequate calorie intake related to the highly restrictive nature of the diet. Also, many adults refuse to eat strained food because it resembles baby food.

NURSING INTERVENTIONS AND CONSIDERATIONS

Honor special requests of allowed foods, if possible.

Liberalize the diet as soon as possible.

POTENTIAL PROBLEM/RATIONALE

Constipation related to the low fiber content of the diet: Insufficient fiber intake causes a decrease in stool bulk and slowing of intestinal transit time.

NURSING INTERVENTIONS AND CONSIDERATIONS

Liberalize the diet to allow more fiber.

POTENTIAL PROBLEM/RATIONALE

Persistent diarrhea related to poor tolerance to even the small amounts of fiber contained in a low-residue diet. Tolerance to fiber varies among clients and conditions.

NURSING INTERVENTIONS AND CONSIDERATIONS

Further reduce the residue content of the diet by eliminating all fruits and vegetables, except strained fruit juice.

LOW-RESIDUE DIET TEACHING

Instruct the client:

That fiber is a component of plants and, therefore, is found in fruits, vegetables, grains, and nuts.

That "Low Residue" means "low fiber," plus avoiding or limiting foods that increase residue and stool weight: prune juice, meat and shellfish with tough connective tissue, and milk/milk products (limit to 2c or less/day).

That reducing residue intake slows the passage of food through the bowel.

That the diet will probably be short-term.

On food preparation techniques to reduce residue:

- Skins, seeds, and membranes of fruits and vegetables are high in fiber and should be removed.
- Cook allowed vegetables until very tender.

Encourage the intake of foods that are high in pectin, which helps firm the stools: firm bananas, white rice, applesauce, dry toast. Increase protein, calorie, and potassium intake, as needed, to replenish losses.

Avoid very hot or cold food and beverages because they stimulate colonic activity. For that reason, caffeine should also be avoided: coffee, strong tea, some sodas, and chocolate.

Avoid milk and milk products until diarrhea has completely subsided, because lactose intolerance may be contributing to diarrhea.

Avoid carbonated beverages because their electrolyte content is low and osmolality is high, which can promote osmotic diarrhea.

Client Teaching

Instruct the client on the principles and rationale of diet management to relieve diarrhea, using these guidelines:

Follow a low-residue diet until diarrhea subsides.
Replace lost potassium with rich sources that the client can tolerate: bananas, canned apricots and peaches, apricot nectar, tomato juice, fish, potatoes, meat.
Eat small, frequent meals.
Avoid foods that may contribute to cramping: carbonated beverages, beer, gassy vegetables (such as broccoli, cauliflower, cabbage, brussels sprouts, onions, legumes, melons), spicy food, excessive sweets.
Drink plenty of liquids, but avoid milk and carbonated beverages until diarrhea subsides.
Eliminate coffee and caffeine for a trial period to see if any improvement occurs.

Monitoring Progress

Monitor for the following signs or symptoms:

Compliance with the diet, and the need for follow-up diet counseling
Effectiveness of diet interventions, and the need for further diet modification
Weight, weight changes
Intake and output, and fluid and electrolyte balance

Evaluation

Evaluation is ongoing. Provided that the plan of care has not changed, the client will achieve the goals as stated above.

Constipation

Constipation is marked by the difficult or infrequent passage of stools that may be hard and dry. Irregular bowel habits, psychogenic factors, lack of activity, chronic laxative use, inadequate intake of fluid and fiber, metabolic and endocrine disorders, and bowel abnormalities (tumors, hernias, strictures, diverticular disease, irritable colon) are causative factors. Likewise, constipation can occur secondary to certain drug therapies (see the display, Drugs That Commonly Cause Constipation).

NURSING PROCESS

Assessment

In addition to the general GI assessment criteria, assess for the following factors:

Constipation: onset, duration, causative factors, severity, interventions attempted and the results.

Drugs That Frequently Cause Constipation

Amantadine	Haloperidol
Benztropine	Morphine
Cholestyramine	Sulfalfate
Colestipol	Vincristine

Dietary changes made in response to constipation, (ie, foods avoided, foods preferred).

Usual fiber intake, especially foods high in insoluble fiber, which increases stool bulk and stimulates peristalsis (eg, wheat bran, whole-grain bread and cereals, raw vegetables, and fresh fruits). Assess client's ability to chew high-fiber foods, and his or her willingness to eat a high-fiber diet.

Adequacy of fluid intake: adults need 8 to 10 glasses of fluid a day.

Frequency and intensity of usual activity pattern.

Nursing Diagnosis

Constipation, related to an inadequate intake of fluid and fiber

Planning and Implementation

Elimination patterns vary with diet and activity. Daily bowel movements are not necessary, provided the stools are not hard and dry.

Generally, a high-fiber diet is used to alleviate constipation. Currently, American adults consume approximately 12 to 18 g fiber/day, about half the recommended intake of 20 to 35 g/d endorsed by leading health organizations (Anderson et al, 1994). A **high-fiber diet** is rich in both soluble and insoluble fiber, even though only insoluble fiber has been credited with increasing stool bulk and stimulating peristalsis. This diet must be initiated gradually to maximize tolerance, which varies among individuals (see Food for Thought: Defusing Gas). The major side effect of a high-fiber diet is increased intestinal gas production, which subsides with adaptation to the diet (Anderson et al, 1994). Regular aerobic exercise augments the health benefits of a high-fiber diet.

Discourage the use of mineral oil laxatives, which can cause malabsorption of the fat-soluble vitamins. Likewise, discourage the use of fiber "pills," which can cause constipation or even intestinal blockages, especially when taken in large amounts and with inadequate fluid.

In some cases of constipation, adding fat to the diet may have a laxative effect; fat stimulates bile secretion, which draws water into the GI tract (because of high salt content), to produce softer stools and stimulate peristalsis.

FOOD *for* THOUGHT

Defusing Gas

Leading health organizations recommend that American adults consume 20 to 35 g/fiber per day, or about double their current intake. Although the potential benefits abound (relief of constipation; decreased risk of numerous GI disorders, cardiovascular disease, and diabetes), the negatives (increased gas production) can intimidate people from adopting a more healthful diet.

Gas, or more precisely hydrogen, carbon dioxide, and in some people methane, is produced in the large intestine by the action of normal GI bacteria on undigested and unabsorbed sugars, starches, and fiber. Lactose is a frequent source of gas because of the high incidence of lactose intolerance. Other sources include soluble fibers like pectin in fruit and beta-glucans in oat bran, and even small amounts of starch from the incomplete digestion of wheat, oats, potatoes, and corn. Probably the most notorious sources of gas are indigestible oligosaccharides, called raffinose sugars, which are found in large quantities in dried pea and beans. Because humans lack the enzyme alpha-galactosidase, which is needed to break them down into digestible monosaccharides and sucrose, they enter the colon undigested, where gut bacteria feed on them, producing gas as a byproduct.

Alas, AkPharma manufactures a nonprescription hope on the horizon for gas-leary consumers. It is called Beano and it is actually alpha-galactosidase that is derived from the food-grade mold *Aspergillus niger*, which is classified by the USFDA as Generally Recognized As Safe (GRAS). Beano, when taken with an "offending" food, digests the raffinose sugars in the stomach so that digestible carbohydrates enter the small intestine, thereby depriving the GI flora of a feast. The manufacturer recommends 5 or more drops of liquid Beano or 2 to 3 tablets per ½ cup of food; more may be needed for larger servings.

Anedotal evidence indicates that Beano is effective in some people, but not in others. Results of a double-blind crossover study show that Beano prevents gas after ingestion of oligosaccharides, at least in some people; perhaps a larger dose would produce greater benefit (Ganiats et al, 1994). Because it is widely available, relatively inexpensive, and safe, people who are bothered by gas may want to hedge their bets and try Beano.

CLIENT GOALS

The client will:

Have soft bowel movements.
Consume an adequate fiber intake by substituting foods high in fiber for foods low in fiber.
Drink 8 to 10 glasses of fluid daily.
Describe the principles and rationale of diet management to relieve constipation, and implement the appropriate diet interventions.
Identify causative factors, if known.

NURSING INTERVENTIONS

Diet Management

Increase fiber intake gradually, until an effective, yet tolerable, level is achieved (see the display, High-Fiber Diet).

High-Fiber Diet

CHARACTERISTICS

Normal diet that substitutes high-fiber foods for foods low in fiber.

Unprocessed bran may be added as tolerated.

Fiber intake should come from eating a wide variety of plant foods, rather than fiber supplements.

At least eight 8-oz glasses of fluid are recommended daily.

OBJECTIVE

Insoluble fiber helps to increase fecal bulk and weight, increase GI motility, and decrease pressure within the bowel. Soluble fibers help lower serum cholesterol levels and improve glucose tolerance in diabetes.

INDICATIONS FOR USE

For the prevention or treatment of diverticular disease, constipation, irritable bowel disease, hypercholesterolemia, and diabetes mellitus

May aid weight reduction; may help protect against colon cancer

CONTRAINDICATIONS

Intestinal inflammation or stenosis

Guidelines to achieve high fiber diet

- Eat 6–11 servings from the bread and cereal group daily. Breads and cereals with adequate fiber provide 2–5 g fiber/svg. High-fiber cereals provide 7–11 g fiber/svg.
- Eat one serving dried peas or beans daily.
- Eat 2–4 servings of fruit/day. Apples, nectarines, oranges, peaches, bananas, pears, and berries are high in fiber.
- Eat 3–5 servings of vegetables/day. Cooked asparagus, green beans, broccoli, cabbage, carrots, cauliflower, greens, raw broccoli, tomatoes, celery, and zucchini are good choices.

SAMPLE **MENU**

High-Fiber Diet

BREAKFAST
Prune juice
Bran cereal
Milk
Whole-wheat toast with butter
Orange
Coffee/tea
Salt/pepper/sugar

LUNCH
Split pea soup
Julienne salad made with cheese, egg, lettuce, tomato, carrots, and other vegetables as desired
Salad dressing
Whole-wheat crackers
Apple
Milk

Coffee/tea
Salt/pepper/sugar

DINNER
Roast chicken
Brown rice
Buttered peas
Coleslaw
Bran muffin with butter
Fresh strawberries
Coffee/tea
Salt/pepper/sugar

SNACK
Oatmeal raisin cookies
Milk

(continued)

High-Fiber Diet *(Continued)*

POTENTIAL PROBLEM/RATIONALE

Flatus, distention, cramping, and osmotic diarrhea related to increasing the fiber content of the diet too much or too quickly.

NURSING INTERVENTIONS AND CONSIDERATIONS

Initiate a high-fiber diet slowly to develop the client's tolerance. If symptoms of intolerance persist, reduce the fiber content to the maximum amount tolerated by the client.

POTENTIAL PROBLEM/RATIONALE

Possible malabsorption of calcium, zinc, and iron, which may be related to the following situations:

- Increase in GI motility, which allows less time for absorption to occur
- Binding of fiber with nutrients to form compounds that the body cannot absorb
- Added bulk and water content of the intestines, which dilutes the concentration of nutrients

Actual fiber-induced deficiencies are unlikely, however, possibly because the body adapts to a high-fiber diet.

NURSING INTERVENTIONS AND CONSIDERATIONS

Monitor lab values and observe for signs of deficiencies. Provide supplements if needed.

Encourage the intake of foods rich in calcium, zinc, and iron.

HIGH-FIBER DIET TEACHING

Instruct the client:

That a high-fiber diet increases stool bulk and speeds the passage of food through the intestines.

On how to increase fiber intake by making subtle changes in eating and cooking habits, such as eating more fresh fruits and vegetables, especially with the skin on.

That switching to high-fiber bread and cereals can significantly increase fiber intake. The first ingredient on the label should be "whole wheat," not just "wheat."

To eat a variety of foods high in fiber; numerous forms of fiber exist and each performs a different action in the body (see Chap. 1).

To serve a meatless main dish made with legumes once a week.

To serve fresh or dried fruit for dessert or snack.

That although nuts and seeds are high in fiber, they are also high in fat and should be used sparingly.

That coarse unprocessed wheat bran is most effective as a laxative and generally is cheaper than fresh fruits and vegetables. It can be incorporated into the diet by the following methods:

- Mixing it with juice or milk
- Adding it to muffins, quick breads, casseroles, and meat loaves before baking
- Sprinkling it over cereal, applesauce, eggs, or other foods

To add bran to the diet slowly (up to 3 tablespoons/day) to decrease the likelihood of developing flatus and distention.

That (in addition to being high in fiber) certain foods have laxative effects: prunes and prune juice, figs, and dates.

To drink at least eight 8-oz glasses of fluid daily.

Promote adequate fluid intake. To help stimulate peristalsis, encourage the client to drink hot coffee, tea, or lemon water after waking.

Encourage the intake of prunes and prune juice, which have laxative effects.

Client Teaching

Instruct the client

On the principles and rationale of diet management to relieve constipation. Explain that diet can produce relief but does not cure constipation.

To establish a bowel elimination routine.

That physical activity promotes muscle tone and stimulates bowel activity. Encourage the client to exercise regularly.

To avoid the use of over-the-counter laxatives, stool softeners, and fiber "pills" unless recommended by the physician.

Monitoring Progress

Monitor for the following signs or symptoms:

Tolerance of increased fiber intake (ie, absence of excessive flatus, distention, diarrhea)

Compliance with the diet, and the need for follow-up diet counseling

Effectiveness of diet interventions (ie, relief of constipation) and the need for further diet modification

Evaluation

Evaluation is ongoing. Provided that the plan of care has not changed, the client will achieve the goals as stated above.

Impaired Ability to Swallow

Whether the cause is mechanical (ie, obstruction, inflammation, edema, surgery of the throat) or neurologic (ie, amyotrophic lateral sclerosis [ALS], myasthenia gravis, post cerebrovascular accident, traumatic brain injury, cerebral palsy, Parkinson's disease, multiple sclerosis), alterations in the ability to swallow (**dysphagia**) and chew can have a profound impact on intake and nutritional status, and greatly increase the risk of aspiration and its complications of bacterial pneumonia, bronchial obstruction, and chemical pneumonitis.

Swallowing is a complex series of events that is characterized by four distinct phases. The oral preparatory phase takes place in the mouth, where food (bolus) is chewed in preparation for swallowing. Obviously, liquids need little preparation compared to meat and raw vegetables. Clients who have difficulty with this phase may "pocket" food in the cheek, lose food from the lips, or be unable to move food toward the back of the mouth.

In the oral phase, the bolus is pushed steadily backward toward the pharynx, which opens to receive the bolus. Impairments in the tongue's muscles or nerves interfere with the oral phase and can cause coughing or choking before the client swallows. Liquids, because they are difficult to control, are especially problematic.

The pharyngeal phase follows; as the food reaches the opening of the pharynx, the swallowing reflex is triggered and the food moves toward and into the esophagus. Food remaining in the throat, prolonged chewing, nasal regurgitation, coughing, choking during or after swallowing, and hoarseness after swallowing are all signs of problems with this phase.

The process of swallowing is completed with the esophageal phase. Peristaltic movements carry the bolus through the esophagus into the stomach. Neurologically impaired clients have less difficulty with this phase than with the other phases. However, obstruction and reduced esophageal peristalsis are concerns. Unfortunately, problems with this phase are less amenable to intervention than problems with the other three phases.

NURSING PROCESS

Assessment

In addition to the general GI assessment criteria, assess for the following factors:

Swallowing dysfunction: observe for difficulty articulating words, facial drooping, drooling, a weak or hoarse cough, decreased gag reflex, impaired facial sensitivity, coughing and choking during or after meals, a gurgled voice, pocketing of food in the mouth. Assess causative factors, severity, and impact on intake.

Dietary changes made in response to impaired swallowing (ie, food avoided and foods preferred).

Foods and liquids that are easiest and hardest to swallow.

Weight. Compare actual weight to "healthy" weight; observe for signs of malnutrition.

Nursing Diagnosis

Altered Nutrition: Less than body requirements, related to impaired swallowing secondary to _____ (causative factor)

Planning and Implementation

Encourage dysphagic clients to rest before mealtime, and coordinate meals with peak drug action if the client's motor weakness is dose related. Give mouth care immediately before meals to enhance the sense of taste.

To stimulate salivation, instruct the client to think of a specific food. A lemon slice, lemon hard candy, or dill pickles may also help trigger salivation.

Reduce or eliminate distractions at mealtime so that the client can focus his attention on swallowing. Limit disruptions, if possible, and do not rush the client; allow at least 30 minutes for eating. Place the client in an upright or high Fowler's position. Suction equipment should be readily available.

Adaptive eating devices, like built-up utensils and mugs with spouts, may be indicated. Syringes should never be used to force liquids into the client's mouth because they may trigger choking or aspiration. Unless otherwise directed, do not allow the client to use a straw.

If the client has one-sided facial weakness, place the food on the other side of his/her mouth. Encourage small bites and thorough chewing.

Individualize texture, taste, and temperature of foods. Semisolid or medium-consistency foods like pudding, plain yogurt, and cooked cereals are usually safest for clients at risk of dysphagia. Cold foods may trigger the swallowing response; tepid foods that are difficult to locate in the mouth may be dangerous. The appropriate-consistency diet may be recommended by the speech pathologist (see Table 16-1, Dysphagia Diets). Progress the diet as the client's ability to swallow improves.

Provide nutritionally dense foods to maximize nutritional intake.

Consider tube feedings if the client is unable to consume an adequate oral diet.

Refer clients with actual or potential swallowing impairments to the speech pathology department for a thorough swallowing assessment.

Table 16-1
Dysphagia Diets

Based on results of a modified barium swallow, the speech pathologist and physician determine which of the following levels is most appropriate for the client:

Level	Description	Examples
I. Thick liquids	Blended or puréed liquids that are not solid, lumpy, or grainy. They must be able to run off a spoon slowly.	Applesauce; smooth, creamed soups; liquids thickened to pudding-like texture
II. Soft foods and thick liquids	May be gelatinous or sticky, but not crumbly	Pancakes soaked in syrup, plain custards, plain yogurts, mashed potatoes; smooth, cooked cereals; fruit nectars, eggnog, liquids thickened to pudding-like or nectar consistency
III. Semisolid foods, thick liquids, and carbonated beverages	Firm, but not tough	Soft fruit, poached eggs, pasta, puréed entree mixes, souffles, liquids thickened to nectar or honey consistency
IV. Solid foods and thick liquids	Can be firm, chewy, crispy, but not hard (eg, no raw vegetables)	Diced meat, soft-cooked vegetables, soft fruit, casseroles, toast, soft cookies, liquids thickened as necessary
V. Regular food and beverages		

CLIENT GOALS

The client will:

Swallow food and liquids without aspirating; return to a regular diet.
Consume adequate calories and protein to attain or maintain "healthy" weight.
Describe the principles and rationale for the dietary management of swallowing impairments, if appropriate, and implement the appropriate diet interventions.

NURSING INTERVENTIONS

Diet Management

Provide encouragement during meals.
Position the client in an upright position and tilt his or her head forward to facilitate swallowing. Postpone meals if the client is fatigued.
Individualize texture according to the client's tolerance; semisolid foods (pudding, custards, scrambled eggs, yogurt, cooked cereals, and thickened liquids) are easiest to swallow. See Table 16-1, Dysphagia Diets.
Serve food cold or at mildly warm temperature to stimulate swallowing and to avoid overreaction to extremely hot food.
Serve moderately flavored foods to stimulate salivation. Melted butter, gravy, and jelly help moisten foods.
Offer small, frequent meals to maximize intake.
Avoid sticky, mucus-forming foods: peanut butter, white bread, milk, chocolate, ice cream, bananas.

Client Teaching

Instruct the client

On the principles and rationale of diet management to promote swallowing, if appropriate.
To relax and eat slowly, and to avoid eating while fatigued.
To avoid alcohol, which interferes with effective swallowing and reduces cough and gag reflexes (Calianno, 1995).

Monitoring Progress

Monitor for the following factors:

Compliance with the diet, and the need for follow-up diet counseling or swallowing evaluation
Effectiveness of diet intervention and the need for further diet modification
Weight status, weight changes

Evaluation

Evaluation is ongoing. Provided that the plan of care has not changed, the client will achieve the goals as stated above.

Disorders of the Esophagus: Hiatal Hernia and Esophagitis

Hiatal hernia and esophagitis are two esophageal disorders whose symptoms can be greatly improved through appropriate diet interventions. Hiatal hernia, which is characterized by the protrusion of part of the stomach through the esophageal opening of the diaphragm, may be caused by a congenital or acquired weakness of the diaphragm or from increased intraabdominal pressure related to obesity, pregnancy, ascites, or physical exertion. Reflux esophagitis, commonly known as gastroesophageal reflux (GER), occurs when the backflow of acidic gastric juices causes irritation and inflammation of the lower esophageal mucosa. It may be caused by viral inflammation, ingestion of an irritant, or intubation. Recurrent GER is often related to hiatal hernia, recurrent vomiting, and reduced **lower esophageal sphincter (LES)** pressure, which means the sphincter fails to stay closed, thus allowing acidic gastric juice to splash into the esophagus. Hiatal hernia and esophagitis can lead to dysphagia and esophageal ulcerations and bleeding.

The presence of a hiatal hernia may not be apparent until the symptoms of reflux esophagitis develop: heartburn, which may radiate to the neck and throat; pain that worsens when the client lies down, bends over after eating, or wears tight-fitting clothing; regurgitation; and possible melena, hematemesis, and dysphagia.

Antacid therapy and diet intervention are the cornerstones of medical treatment for hiatal hernia and esophagitis. If reflux is not relieved by medical treatment, a vagotomy, or surgical repair, may be necessary.

NURSING PROCESS

Assessment

In addition to the general GI assessment criteria, assess for the following factors:

Symptoms: onset, frequency, relationship to eating, causative factors, severity, interventions attempted and the results

Dietary changes made in response to symptoms (ie, foods avoided, foods preferred). Determine which foods are best and least tolerated.

Usual intake of items known to decrease LES pressure, which contributes to "heartburn" (Table 16-2)

Intake of known gastric acid stimulants: coffee (regular and decaffeinated), caffeine (see Appendix 8), and pepper

---

Table 16-2
Factors That Decrease Lower Esophageal Sphincter (LES) Pressure

Alcohol	Fat
Caffeine	Peppermint and spearmint oils
Chocolate	Cigarette smoke

The frequency of eating, especially if a snack or meal is eaten immediately before bed

The client's use of tobacco, alcohol, caffeine, and drugs (See Drug Alert for Medications That Decrease LES)

Weight, weight status

Nursing Diagnosis

Altered Health Maintenance, related to the lack of knowledge of dietary management of _____ (causative factor).

Planning and Implementation

Low-residue and traditional bland diets were frequently used in the past to treat esophageal disorders, even though they are unnecessarily restrictive and not valid. The most effective interventions for GER are to lose weight, if overweight, and to avoid items that decrease LES pressure. Encourage a liberal intake of protein, because it increases LES pressure.

For optimal effectiveness, individualize the diet according to the client's tolerance. Common esophageal irritants include caffeine, cola, alcohol, red peppers, citrus juices, and tomato products.

Clients avoiding citrus juices because of their acidity should be encouraged to eat other sources of vitamin C: tomatoes, broccoli, brussels sprouts, strawberries, cantaloupe, greens, peppers, raw cabbage.

CLIENT GOALS

The client will:

Be free of symptoms of hiatal hernia or esophagitis.

Lose weight, if overweight.

Describe the principles and rationale for dietary management of hiatal hernia or esophagitis and implement the appropriate diet interventions.

Identify factors that contribute to hiatal hernia or esophagitis, when known.

NURSING INTERVENTIONS

Diet Management

Promote weight loss in overweight clients to decrease intraabdominal pressure. Eliminate factors that are known to decrease LES pressure (Table 16-2).

Encourage a liberal protein intake because protein increases LES pressure.

Provide small, frequent meals.

Avoid liquids immediately before and after meals to help prevent gastric distention.

Avoid items that stimulate gastric acid secretion: coffee (regular and decaffeinated), caffeine (see Appendix 8), alcohol, and pepper.

Eliminate foods that may irritate the esophagus, such as citrus juices, tomato products, and red pepper.

Client Teaching

Instruct the client

On the principles and rationale of diet management to relieve symptoms of esophageal disorders.

To avoid foods that decrease LES pressure to help reduce heartburn.

To eliminate any foods not tolerated.

To chew food thoroughly.

To avoid lying down, bending over, and rigorous exercise after eating.

To avoid tight-fitting clothing.

To sleep with the head of the bed elevated.

That small, frequent meals may be better tolerated than three large meals.

Monitoring Progress

Monitor for the following signs or symptoms:

Food intolerances; clients who severely limit their food choices and those who eliminate citrus fruits and vegetables may be at risk for vitamin and mineral deficiencies.

Compliance with the diet, and the need for follow-up diet counseling.

Effectiveness of diet intervention and the need for further diet modification.

Weight, if appropriate.

Evaluation

Evaluation is ongoing. Provided that the plan of care has not changed, the client will achieve the goals as stated above.

DRUG ALERT

Antacids

Interfere with iron absorption and may cause iron deficiency anemia.

Produce other side effects, depending on their composition:

Magnesium → diarrhea

Aluminum → constipation

Calcium → hypercalcemia

Sodium → fluid retention (sodium-containing antacids are contraindicated for clients who require low-sodium diets)

DRUG
ALERT   *Medications That Decrease LES*

Decreased LES and increased risk of GER may occur secondary to the following medications:

Anticholinergics (atropine, Bentyl, Librax)

Beta-blockers

Calcium channel blockers (Isoptin)

Prednisone

Valium (Diazepam)

Oral contraceptives

Theophylline

Disorders of the Stomach: Peptic Ulcers and Gastritis

Peptic ulcer, which is characterized by erosion of the mucosal layer of the stomach (gastric ulcer) or duodenum (duodenal ulcer), is caused by an excess secretion of, or decreased mucosal resistance to, hydrochloric acid. Recently, the *Helicobacter pylori* organism has been found to be present in 80% to 90% of clients with peptic ulcers; it appears to secrete an enzyme that may deplete gastric mucus, making it more susceptible to erosion.

Stress ulcers are a phenomenon that occurs secondary to severe stress, such as cardiac or respiratory arrest, severe burns, and trauma. The stress response causes decreased gastric blood flow and vasoconstriction, which impairs the mucosal cells' ability to secrete mucus. The mucosal lining becomes more vulnerable to erosion without adequate mucus to act as a protective barrier.

Approximately 5% to 15% of American adults develop ulcers, only half of which may be diagnosed. Duodenal ulcers occur 10 times more frequently than gastric ulcers, are 4 times more common in men than in women, and usually are diagnosed at about 50 years of age. Gastric ulcers occur twice as frequently among men than women and usually are diagnosed after age 45. They are more likely than duodenal ulcers to recur, and have a higher incidence of undergoing malignant changes (Scherer and Timby, 1995).

Typically, duodenal ulcers produce dull, burning, or piercing pain when the stomach is empty, usually 1 to 4 hours after eating; gastric ulcer pain may be worsened by intake of food (Chicago Dietetic Association, 1992). Heartburn, nausea, vomiting, and melena are possible. Scarring and obstruction can occur. The course of duodenal ulcers usually alternates between periods of exacerbation and remission, with occurrence more frequent in spring and fall. Cigarette smoking, genetics, and use of nonsteroidal antiinflammatory drugs have been identified as risk factors for ulcers; the effects of alcohol, caffeine, diet, and psychological stress are controversial.

Without proper treatment, ulcers can lead to hemorrhage, perforation, pyloric obstruction, and intractable ulcers. Various drug therapies (antacids, anticholinergics, H_2-receptor antagonists [cimetidine], antisecretory agents, antispasmodics, antimotility drugs, sedatives, tranquilizers, Bismuth and amoxicillin if *H. pylori* are present), bed rest (to reduce environmental stress), and diet intervention are used as treatment. Complications may be treated surgically if medical treatment fails.

Gastritis is an inflammation of the gastric mucosa. Acute gastritis is a temporary irritation, usually self-limiting, that is caused by the ingestion of corrosive or infectious substances, such as aspirin; food poisoning; acute alcoholism; and uremia. Symptoms vary with the source of the irritation and range from mild (heartburn) to severe (vomiting, bleeding, hematemesis). Chronic gastritis is marked by progressive and irreversible atrophy of the gastric mucosa, which can lead to achlorhydria and pernicious anemia. Symptoms include nausea, vomiting, stomach pain, malaise, anorexia, headache, hematemesis, and hiccupping. Perforation, hemorrhage, and pyloric obstruction related to scar tissue formation may occur. The exact cause of chronic gastritis is unknown, but it may be related to overeating, stress, coffee and alcohol consumption, cigarette smoking, or chronic uremia.

Gastritis is treated by eliminating the offender and controlling symptoms (ie, vomiting, pain, blood loss) through drugs and diet. Surgery may be needed to treat complications. The objectives of diet intervention for both peptic ulcer and gastritis are to decrease gastric acid secretion and eliminate gastric irritants.

NURSING PROCESS

Assessment

In addition to the general assessment criteria, assess for the following factors:

Symptoms: nature, onset, frequency, causative factors, severity, interventions attempted and the results. Determine if pain occurs when the stomach is empty or after eating.

Dietary changes made in response to symptoms (ie, food avoided, foods preferred). Determine which foods are best and least tolerated.

The client's use of tobacco, alcohol, drugs, and caffeine.

Weight, weight changes.

Abnormal laboratory values and their significance, especially hemoglobin and hematocrit.

Nursing Diagnosis

Altered Health Maintenance, related to the lack of knowledge of dietary management of _____ (causative factor)

Planning and Implementation

During an attack of acute gastritis, food is withheld and intravenous fluids are provided until symptoms subside. Thereafter, the diet is liberalized according to individual tolerance.

Traditionally, ulcers and gastritis have been treated with **progressive bland diets** in an attempt to eliminate foods that are chemically and mechanically irritating to the stomach. Bland diets were basically low-residue diets with the added restrictions of no fried foods, no spicy foods, no meat extracts, and no alcohol, caffeine, and pepper. Milk was used liberally to "soothe" the stomach. However, although the protein in milk effectively neutralizes stomach contents and provides immediate pain relief, protein and calcium act as powerful stimulants to acid secretion, and may cause irritation and the return of pain within 1 to 3 hours. Another drawback to the use of milk is the possibility of hypercalcemia, especially when milk therapy is used in combination with calcium antacids. Also, there is little agreement as to which foods are actually irritating to the GI mucosa, and there is no proof that a bland diet helps heal or prevent recurrent attacks of ulcer or gastritis. Bland diets have been replaced with a liberal bland diet (see the display, Liberal Bland Diet).

A **liberal bland diet** provides four to six small meals a day to help neutralize gastric contents, if pain is relieved by food. Pepper, chili powder, caffeine, and alcohol are eliminated because they are gastric acid stimulants. The only other recommendation is to eliminate any foods that are not tolerated by the person. Dietary restrictions should be kept to a minimum to help reduce stress in a client who may already be stressed.

Weight loss is experienced by many clients with ulcers or chronic gastritis. Encourage the client to attain and maintain "healthy" weight.

Iron deficiency anemia may result from blood loss and poor iron absorption related to antacid therapy or achlorhydria. Iron supplements may be indicated. Likewise, chronic gastritis can impair the secretion of intrinsic factor and result in pernicious anemia. Vitamin B_{12} status should be evaluated every several years.

Encourage protein and vitamin C intake to facilitate healing.

Discourage late evening snacks that can increase acid secretion and result in loss of sleep.

Be aware of the potential side effects and nutritional problems associated with antacid therapy (see section on Hiatal Hernias).

CLIENT GOALS

The client will:

Be free of symptoms of _____.
Consume adequate calories and protein to attain or maintain "healthy" weight.

Liberal Bland Diet

Eat four to six small meals/day.
Avoid individual intolerances.

Avoid
Pepper
Chili Powder
Regular and decaffeinated coffee
Caffeine
Alcohol

Avoid foods that are not tolerated.

Describe the principles and rationale of diet management in the treatment of gastric disorders, and implement the appropriate diet interventions.

Identify causative factors, if known.

NURSING INTERVENTIONS

Diet Management

Provide a well-balanced diet, with restrictions based on individual tolerance (see the display, Liberal Bland Diet).

Provide four to six small meals, if eating reduces pain.

Encourage adequate calories, protein, and vitamin C.

Client Teaching

Instruct the client

On the principles and rationale of a liberal bland diet to relieve symptoms.

To eat in a relaxed environment and chew food thoroughly.

To avoid rigorous activity immediately before and after eating.

To avoid cigarettes and alcohol. If the client refuses to give up alcohol, it should be consumed with meals or immediately after eating.

To avoid eating before going to bed to prevent acid stimulation during sleep.

Monitoring Progress

Monitor for the following signs or symptoms:

Compliance with the diet, and the need for follow-up diet counseling

Effectiveness of the diet and the need for further diet modification

Weight, weight changes

Evaluation

Evaluation is ongoing. Provided that the plan of care has not changed, the client will achieve the goals as stated above.

DRUG ALERT

Histamine H_2-blockers are commonly used in the treatment of peptic ulcers.

Cimetidine (Tagamet) decreases gastric secretion, which reduces the absorption of iron, folic acid, and vitamin B_{12}; hyperglycemia and diarrhea may occur.

Ranitidine (Zantac) generally produces fewer side effects and interactions than cimetidine, but may cause abdominal discomfort, constipation or diarrhea, and decreased absorption of vitamin B_{12} with long-term use.

The antisecretory drug omeprazole (Prilosec) can cause dry mouth and anorexia.

Disorders of the Intestines

Disorders of the intestines often cause altered bowel elimination; a primary objective of diet therapy is to promote normal bowel elimination by either increasing or decreasing transit time. Additional diet modifications are based on the underlying disease and the clinical manifestations.

DIVERTICULAR DISEASE

Diverticula are pouches that protrude outward from the muscular wall of the intestine, usually in the sigmoid colon, which characterize an asymptomatic condition known as diverticulosis. Diverticula are caused by increased pressure within the intestinal lumen, which may be related to chronic constipation and long-term low-fiber diets. Studies suggest that the incidence of symptomatic diverticular disease is increased by diets that are low in total dietary fiber and high in total fat or red meat (Aldoori et al, 1994).

Diverticulitis occurs when fecal matter gets trapped in the diverticula, causing inflammation and infection. Symptoms include cramping, alternating periods of diarrhea and constipation, flatus, abdominal distention, and low-grade fever. Complications include occult blood loss and acute rectal bleeding → iron deficiency anemia; abscesses; bowel perforation → peritonitis; fistula formation → bowel obstruction; and small bowel diverticula → bacterial overgrowth → fat and vitamin B_{12} malabsorption.

In the past, low-residue diets were believed to decrease the likelihood of diverticulitis, based on the idea that particles of fiber could get trapped in the diverticula and cause irritation and inflammation. Current thinking is that high-fiber diets can decrease the incidence of diverticular disease by producing soft, bulky stools that are easily passed, resulting in decreased pressure within the colon and shortened transit time. However, once the diverticula develop, a high-fiber diet cannot make them disappear. Foods with husks and seeds, like nuts, popcorn, cucumbers, raspberries, tomatoes, and corn, should be avoided because they can become trapped in diverticula and cause inflammation.

A high-fiber diet as tolerated (see the display, High-Fiber Diet) is recommended to prevent and treat diverticulosis. However, a low-residue diet may be used during an acute phase of diverticulitis, or when complications of intestinal bleeding, perforation, or abscess exist. Clients who are treated with a low-residue diet in the hospital may be reluctant to switch to a high-fiber diet upon discharge. Diet compliance depends on the patient's understanding of the rationale and benefits of a high-fiber diet for long-term prevention and treatment of diverticulosis and prevention of diverticulitis.

MALABSORPTION SYNDROME

A major clinical manifestation of many intestinal disorders is **malabsorption syndrome**, which is characterized by steatorrhea, diarrhea, weight loss, muscle wasting, abdominal cramps and distention, and numerous secondary nutrient deficiencies and metabolic disturbances (see the display, Secondary Nutrient Deficiencies and Metabolic Disturbances of Malabsorption Syndrome). Failure of the intestinal mucosa to adequately absorb nutrients can result in serious and sometimes life-threatening malnutrition and metabolic disturbances.

Malabsorption can result from maldigestion related to cystic fibrosis, pancreatitis, gallbladder disease, liver disease, and disaccharidase deficiencies, or from bacterial overgrowth related to blind loop syndrome. Alterations in bowel mucosa, as seen in regional enteritis, ulcerative colitis, celiac disease, radiation enteritis, and malignancy, also cause malabsorption. Other causes include short bowel syndrome related to intestinal surgery, and certain drug therapies.

Malabsorption is treated by correcting the underlying disorder and providing nutritional intervention aimed at reducing bowel stimulation, restoring optimal nutritional status, and promoting healing, where applicable. Diet intervention may also be necessary to control **steatorrhea**, or excess fat in the feces, related to fat maldigestion from impaired bile salt malabsorption. Selected digestive disorders that may cause malabsorption syndrome are highlighted in Table 16-3.

Secondary Nutrient Deficiencies and Metabolic Disturbances of Malabsorption Syndrome

POTENTIAL PROBLEMS/RATIONALE

Muscle weakness related to hypokalemia

Hypoalbuminemia → edema related to the following problems:

- Protein malabsorption
- Decreased albumin synthesis
- Leakage of albumin into the gut (protein-losing enteropathy)

Iron deficiency anemia related to iron malabsorption and/or blood loss

Folic acid deficiency anemia related to folic acid malabsorption

Vitamin B_{12} deficiency anemia related to vitamin B_{12} malabsorption

Purpura and easy bleeding related to vitamin K malabsorption

Roughening of the skin and impaired night vision related to vitamin A malabsorption

Osteomalacia → bone pain related to calcium, magnesium, and vitamin D malabsorption

Tetany related to hypocalcemia, hypomagnesemia

Stomatitis, cheilosis, glossitis, and dermatitis related to malabsorption of the B-complex vitamins

Lactose intolerance → cramping, distention, flatus, and diarrhea after milk ingestion related to lactase deficiency resulting from intestinal mucosa damage

Kidney stone formation related to increased oxalate absorption (normally, most dietary oxalate binds with calcium in the intestine and is excreted in the feces; calcium malabsorption leads to a secondary increase in oxalate absorption)

Cholesterol gallstone formation related to bile salt malabsorption: bile salt malabsorption → cholesterol-saturated bile → precipitation of cholesterol from bile into gallstones

Table 16-3
Selected Malabsorption Disorders: Description, Symptoms, Diet Management

Disorder	Symptoms	Diet Management for Malabsorption PLUS
Lactose intolerance: Maldigestion of lactose (milk sugar) caused by a deficiency of the digestive enzyme lactase, which is normally found in the intestinal villi. May be congenital or acquired, or occur secondary to bowel disorders, malnutrition, GI surgery, or radiotherapy.	Distention, cramps, flatus, and diarrhea occurring 15 to 30 minutes after lactose ingestion and usually subsiding within 2 hours; undigested lactose increases the osmolality of the intestinal contents and results in a large fluid shift into the intestines to dilute the particle concentration. Individual tolerance to lactose varies considerably.	Reduce lactose to the maximum amount tolerated by the individual (see display, Lactose-Restricted Diet).
Regional enteritis (Crohn's disease): Chronic, progressive, inflammatory disease involving the entire thickness of the bowel wall. Commonly affects the terminal ileum, but it can occur anywhere along the entire GI tract.	Diarrhea with possible melena, weight loss, crampy abdominal pain, fever, fatigue, anorexia, alternating periods of exacerbation and remission. Complications include fistulas and abscesses, hemorrhage, bowel perforations, intestinal obstructions, anemia, malnutrition.	Low lactose. During remission, encourage a well-balanced diet based on individual tolerance.
Ulcerative colitis: Chronic, inflammatory disease involving the mucosal and sometimes submucosal layer of the colon and rectum.	Anorexia, nausea, vomiting, frequent passage of hard or liquid stools containing blood, pus, or mucus; abdominal pain and distention; weight loss, fever, dehydration, alternating periods of exacerbation and remission. Complications include anal fissures, abscesses, bowel perforations, intestinal stenosis from scar tissue, iron deficiency anemia, bleeding tendency re: vitamin K deficiency, malnutrition, colon cancer.	Low lactose. Encourage a well-balanced diet based on individual tolerance during remission.
Celiac disease (gluten-induced enteropathy, nontropical sprue): Sensitivity to gliadin (the protein component of gluten) causes flattened, atrophied intestinal villi, a decreased absorptive surface with a loss of disaccharidases, leading to malabsorption syndrome. Gluten is found in wheat, oats, rye, and barley.	Steatorrhea, malabsorption, weight loss, muscle wasting, disaccharide intolerance, weakness, malnutrition, fatigue.	Gluten-free diet (see display, Gluten-Free Diet). Complete and permanent elimination of gluten causes the villi to return toward normal, usually within a few weeks. Complete regeneration may never occur. A low-lactose diet may be needed temporarily or permanently.
Pancreatitis: Inflammation of the pancreas. Retention of pancreatic enzymes within the pancreas leads to autodigestion. Chronic pancreatitis is characterized by scarring and tissue calcification.	Severe abdominal pain, nausea and vomiting, fever, jaundice. Chronic pancreatitis can lead to hyperglycemia, steatorrhea, weight loss, and malnutrition.	Low-fat diet (ie, 25–50 g), as tolerated. Eliminate gastric acid stimulants: regular and decaf, coffee, tea, alcohol, and pepper. A CHO-controlled diet may be needed if symptoms of diabetes mellitus develop.

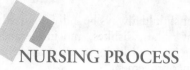

NURSING PROCESS

Assessment

In addition to the general GI assessment criteria, assess for the following factors:

Symptoms: onset, frequency, causative factors, severity, interventions attempted and the results.

Dietary changes made in response to malabsorption symptoms (ie, foods avoided, foods preferred). Determine which foods are best and least tolerated.

Fat intake, which can aggravate existing steatorrhea.

Intake and output; observe for signs of dehydration and electrolyte imbalance, especially hypokalemia and hypernatremia.

Abnormal laboratory values, especially hemoglobin, hematocrit, sodium, potassium, albumin, and glucose.

Weight status; observe for signs of malnutrition and nutrient deficiencies (see the display, Secondary Nutrient Deficiencies and Metabolic Disturbances of Malabsorption Syndrome).

Nursing Diagnosis

Altered Nutrition: Less than body requirements, related to malabsorption secondary to _____ (causative factor)

Planning and Implementation

Many factors contribute to the malnutrition that characterizes malabsorptive disorders: diarrhea, loss of nutrients through the stool, possible blood loss, drug therapy, and sometimes surgical intervention. Decreased food intake, which may be related to restrictive diets, decreased appetite, fear of eating, decreased pleasure from eating, or depression, is an important factor in weight loss (Riguad et al, 1994). The task of restoring nutritional status without aggravating the bowel in an anorexic client is difficult and frustrating for both the health care team and the client.

Some malabsorptive disorders, such as Crohn's disease, may require complete bowel rest (ie, total parenteral nutrition) to facilitate healing. Although elemental (predigested) formulas are frequently used for enteral support of Crohn's disease clients, they may not offer any advantages over standard formulas (Griffiths et al, 1995). Likewise, during an acute attack of celiac disease, the client may be ordered NPO (nothing by mouth) and given intravenous fluid and electrolytes to rest the bowel temporarily. Bowel rest has been less effective in treating ulcerative colitis. Food is also withheld initially during an acute attack of pancreatitis. If the client is malnourished, nasojejunal tube feeding of a hydrolyzed formula diet or total parenteral nutrition may be used until oral intake is resumed (see Chap. 14). Oral intake should progress to a nutrient-rich diet as soon as possible.

Regardless of the underlying disorder, the diet should always be individualized as much as possible to correspond with the client's likes, dislikes, and intolerances. Small, frequent meals are indicated to maximize intake. Clients who are apprehensive about eating need emotional support and encouragement.

Fat intake is limited whenever steatorrhea is present, such as when the ileum is inflamed. Because the enzyme activity of lactase may be temporarily impaired during malabsorption syndromes, it is prudent to restrict dietary lactose (milk sugar) even when a lactase deficiency has not been objectively diagnosed. Lactase activity may return to normal after malabsorption has been resolved.

Malabsorption can lead to numerous nutrient deficiencies: protein, calcium, magnesium, zinc, iron, vitamin B_{12}, folic acid, vitamin C, potassium, and the fat-soluble vitamins. Multivitamin and mineral supplements and water-soluble supplements of the fat-soluble vitamins are needed not only to replenish losses, but also for the metabolism of a high-calorie, high-protein diet and to facilitate healing.

It is difficult to meet protein and calorie needs with a low-residue diet, especially if the client is lactose-intolerant. If commercial formulas are used to supplement intake,* the following should be taken into consideration:

- Osmolality: hypertonic formulas may need to be diluted and administered gradually to prevent diarrhea
- Residue content
- Lactose content
- Client acceptance: To improve palatability, formulas may be served over ice, enhanced with commercial flavor packets, or incorporated into appropriate recipes

The length of time the diet should be followed depends on the underlying disorder and the client's medical status. For instance, during remission of regional enteritis and ulcerative colitis, a well-balanced diet based on individual tolerance is recommended; lactose and fiber tolerance varies among individuals. Clients with celiac disease must follow a **gluten-free diet** (see the display, Gluten-Free Diet) permanently, but they may regain their ability to tolerate lactose.

CLIENT GOALS

The client will:

Experience fewer or no symptoms.
Attain or maintain normal fluid and electrolyte balance.
Consume adequate calories and protein to attain or maintain "healthy" weight.
Be free of symptoms of nutrient deficiencies (see display, Secondary Nutrient Deficiencies and Metabolic Disturbances of Malabsorption Syndrome).
Describe the principles and rationale of diet management for malabsorption syndrome and its symptoms, and implement the appropriate diet interventions.
Identify causative factors, if known.

---

* Use of commercial supplements is covered in Chapter 14; supplements are outlined in Appendix 7.

Gluten-Free Diet

CHARACTERISTICS

Eliminates gliadin, a protein fraction of gluten found in wheat, rye, oats, and barley

OBJECTIVE

Prevent intestinal villi changes, steatorrhea, and other symptoms characteristic of celiac disease

INDICATIONS FOR USE

Gluten-induced enteropathy (nontropical sprue, celiac sprue, celiac disease)

Dermatitis herpetiformis

CONTRAINDICATIONS

None

FOODS ALLOWED

Beverages: Carbonated drinks, cocoa, coffee, tea, fruit juice, milk, decaffeinated coffee containing no wheat flour

Breads and cereals: Products made with arrowroot, cornstarch, cornmeal, potato, rice, soybean, and gluten-free wheat starch flours; pure rice, sago, and tapioca; gluten-free macaroni products; cornbread, muffins, and pone made without wheat flour; corn or rice cereals such as cornflakes, Cream of Rice, hominy, puffed rice, rice flakes, Rice Krispies; rice cakes; grits; popcorn

Desserts: Cakes, cookies, pastries, and other baked products made with allowed flours; custard, gelatin, homemade cornstarch, tapioca, and rice puddings; ice cream and sherbet prepared without gluten stabilizers

Fats: Butter, corn oil, French dressing, pure mayonnaise and olive oil, margarine, other pure animal and vegetable fats and oils

Soups: Broth, bouillon, clear soups, cream soups thickened with allowed flours

Miscellaneous: Pepper, pickles, popcorn, potato chips, sugars and syrups, vinegar, molasses

Plain meats, fruits, and vegetables, or those prepared with allowed foods

FOODS NOT ALLOWED

Beverages: Ale, beer, instant coffee containing wheat, Postum, Ovaltine and other cereal beverages, malted milk

Breads and cereals: All products made from wheat, rye, oats, barley, buckwheat, durum, or graham, including the following items:

- All commercial yeast and quick bread mixes
- All-purpose flour
- Baking powder biscuits
- Bran
- Bread crumbs
- Bread flour
- Bulgur
- Crackers and cracker crumbs
- Farina
- Graham flour
- Kasha
- Macaroni
- Malt and malt flavoring
- Matzoh
- Millet
- Noodles
- Pancakes
- Pastry flour
- Pretzels
- Quinoa
- Rye flour
- Self-rising flour
- Semolina
- Spelt
- Teff
- Vermicelli
- Waffles
- Whole- or cracked-wheat flours
- Wheat germ
- Zwieback

Cooked or ready-to-eat cereals containing malt, bran, rye, wheat, oats, barley, or wheat germ

Desserts: Cakes, cookies, pastries, and other baked products made with flours not allowed; prepared mixes, prepared pudding thickened with wheat flour

(continued)

Gluten-Free Diet *(Continued)*

Fats: Commercial salad dressings that contain gluten stabilizers or homemade salad dressings thickened with flour

Soups: All soups thickened with wheat products or containing barley, noodles, or other wheat, rye, and oat products in any form

Meats prepared with wheat, rye, oats, or barley, or gluten stabilizers or fillers

Any thickened or prepared fruits; some pie fillings

Any creamed or breaded vegetables, unless allowed ingredients are used; canned baked beans; commercially prepared vegetables with cream sauce or cheese sauce

Miscellaneous: Because the following ingredients may contain gluten, check with the manufacturer before using products containing the following ingredients:

- Emulsifiers
- Flavorings
- Hydrolyzed vegetable protein (HVP)
- Modified starch and modified food starch
- Stabilizers
- Soy sauce, soy sauce solids
- Vegetable gum
- Vegetable protein or textured vegetable protein (TVP)

ADDITIONAL CONSIDERATIONS

Clients may be discouraged and overwhelmed when faced with a lifelong restricted diet. Provide support, encouragement, and thorough diet instructions.

The client may be temporarily or permanently lactose-intolerant and may require a lactose-restricted diet.

A celiac crisis may be precipitated by emotional stress.

POTENTIAL PROBLEM/RATIONALE

Difficulty obtaining a variety of allowed foods from grocery stores related to the highly restrictive nature of the diet.

NURSING INTERVENTIONS AND CONSIDERATIONS

Encourage the client to use as many "normal" items as possible, such as corn cereals, cornmeal, grits, rice, and rice cereals. Not only are they easily obtained from any grocery store, but they are also less expensive than special products.

Encourage the client to shop in health food or specialty stores to obtain hard-to-find items such as potato and soybean flours.

GLUTEN-FREE DIET TEACHING

Instruct the client:

On the importance of adhering to the diet, even when no symptoms are present.

That "cheating" on the diet will cause the return of symptoms, which will disappear after resumption of the diet.

To eliminate all wheat, oat, rye, and barley flours and products permanently.

To eat an otherwise normal, well-balanced diet adequate in nutrients and calories.

To read labels to identify less obvious sources of wheat, rye, oats, and barley used as extenders and fillers. Clients should check with the manufacturer *before* using products of questionable composition.

To use corn, potato, rice, arrowroot, and soybean flours and their products.

To use the following as thickening agents: arrowroot starch, cornstarch, tapioca starch, rice starch, sweet rice flour

That weight gain may be slowly achieved.

To avoid milk and other sources of lactose if not tolerated.

Provide the client with the following aids:

- A detailed list of foods allowed and not allowed
- Information regarding support groups, such as the American Celiac Society, the Gluten Intolerance Group, and the Midwestern Celiac Sprue Association
- Gluten-free recipes

NURSING INTERVENTIONS

Diet Management

At the very least, clients with malabsorption require a diet that is low in residue to reduce bowel stimulation. Other diet modifications for malabsorptive disorders depend on the actual underlying disorder and the presenting symptoms. For instance, clients with significant weight loss need a high-calorie, high-protein diet; only clients with celiac disease require a gluten-free diet (see the display, Gluten-Free Diet).

General diet interventions for malabsorption are as follows:

Limit residue and fiber to slow transit time and reduce bowel stimulation. With the control of symptoms, fiber intake may be increased, as tolerated.

Reduce fat intake to 50 g or less for clients with steatorrhea (see the display, Low-Fat Diet). If necessary, use medium-chain triglycerides to increase calorie intake (see Chapter 4).

(text continues on page 528)

Low-Fat Diet (50 g)

CHARACTERISTICS

Limits the total amount of fat, regardless of the type.

Foods are baked, broiled, or boiled instead of fried or prepared with added fat.

Visible fat on meats is trimmed and poultry skin removed, preferably before cooking.

Allowed fats can be used as seasonings or in cooking.

OBJECTIVE

Reduce the symptoms of steatorrhea and pain in clients intolerant of fat

INDICATIONS FOR USE

Chronic pancreatitis

Malabsorption syndromes: celiac disease, cystic fibrosis, radiation enteritis, short bowel syndrome, tropical sprue

Some cases of gallbladder disease

Type I hyperlipoproteinemia (25 to 35 mg fat)

CONTRAINDICATIONS

None

FOODS ALLOWED

Meats: Up to 6 oz of lean meat, fish, and skinless poultry daily; up to three egg yolks/week; egg whites and low-fat egg substitutes as desired

Dairy products: Two or more servings/day of skim milk; skim-milk cheeses, yogurt, and puddings

Fruits and vegetables: A total of six servings/day or more of any fruit and vegetable prepared without added fat, except avocado

Bread and cereals: Four or more servings/day of plain cereals, pasta, macaroni, rice, whole-grain or enriched breads

Miscellaneous: Sherbet, fruit ices, gelatin, angel food cake, fat-free or skim-milk soups, soft drinks, honey, sugar, seasonings as desired

Fats: Three to five servings of fat daily. Each of the following constitutes one serving:

- 1 teaspoon butter, margarine, shortening, oil, or mayonnaise
- 1 tablespoon diet margarine or diet mayonnaise
- 1 strip crisp bacon

(continued)

Low-Fat Diet (50 g) *(Continued)*

- 1 tablespoon heavy cream, Italian or French dressing
- ⅛ avocado
- 2 teaspoons peanut butter
- 2 tablespoons light cream
- 6 small nuts
- 5 small olives

FOODS NOT ALLOWED

Meats: Fried, fatty, or heavily marbled meats; sausage, lunch meat, spare ribs, frankfurters, salt pork, tuna and salmon packed in oil

Dairy products: Whole milk; whole-milk cheeses and yogurt, ice cream

Fruits and vegetables: Any buttered, au gratin, creamed, or fried vegetables

Breads and cereals: Products made with added fat such as biscuits, muffins, pancakes, doughnuts, waffles, and sweet rolls; breads made with eggs, cheese, or added fat; buttered popcorn; granola-type cereals; popovers; snack crackers with added fat; snack chips; stuffing

Miscellaneous: Cream sauces, gravy; desserts, candy, and anything made with chocolate or nuts

SAMPLE **MENU**

Low-Fat Diet

BREAKFAST

Orange juice
Toast with 1 tsp margarine and jelly
Oatmeal
Skim milk
Coffee/tea
Salt/pepper/sugar

LUNCH

Sandwich made with whole-wheat bread, 2 oz skinless chicken breast, lettuce, and 1 tbsp mayonnaise
Tossed salad with fat-free dressing
Fruit cocktail
Skim milk
Coffee/tea
Salt/pepper/sugar

DINNER

3 oz broiled fish
Baked potato with fat-free sour cream
Steamed broccoli
Carrot and celery sticks
Dinner roll with 1 tsp butter
Sherbet
Fresh strawberries
Skim milk
Coffee/tea
Salt/pepper/sugar

SNACK

Unbuttered popcorn
Fruit juice

POTENTIAL PROBLEM/RATIONALE

Noncompliance related to decreased palatability and satiety from the reduction in fat intake.

NURSING INTERVENTIONS AND CONSIDERATIONS

Encourage the client to eat a variety of the foods allowed. Allow fat exchanges to be substituted

(continued)

Low-Fat Diet (50 g) (Continued)

for meat and dairy products of a higher fat content than is normally allowed (eg, decrease the fat allowance by one serving to allow 1 cup of 2% milk instead of skim milk).

Encourage the client to try low-fat or fat-free substitutes of high-fat items, such as fat-free mayonnaise, salad dressings, and frozen desserts.

Encourage the client to use low-calorie butter seasonings to flavor hot vegetables and potatoes. Butter-flavor vegetable sprays can add flavor to unbuttered popcorn.

POTENTIAL PROBLEM/RATIONALE

Persistent symptoms of steatorrhea or pain after eating related to fat intolerance. Fat tolerance varies considerably among clients and conditions.

NURSING INTERVENTIONS AND CONSIDERATIONS

Decrease the fat content of the diet by reducing or eliminating fat exchanges and limiting the amount of low-fat meat allowed. A 25-g-fat diet is achieved by limiting lean meat intake to 5 oz/day and eliminating all fat exchanges.

POTENTIAL PROBLEM/RATIONALE

Inadequate intake of iron related to the limited allowance of meat (red meat is the best source of iron in the diet)

NURSING INTERVENTIONS AND CONSIDERATIONS

Monitor laboratory values and observe for signs of iron deficiency. Provide supplements as needed.

Encourage a liberal intake of low-fat, high-iron foods, such as dried fruits, fortified cereals and grains, green leafy vegetables, and dried peas and beans. Instruct the client to eat a good source of vitamin C at each meal to enhance iron absorption from plant sources.

LOW-FAT DIET TEACHING

Instruct the client:

That the total amount of dietary fat is reduced, regardless of the source.

That the sources of fat may be visible (butter, margarine, shortening, fat on meat, and salad dressings) or invisible (marbled meat, whole milk and whole-milk products, egg yolks, and nuts).

That substitutions can be made to individualize the diet.

That oil-packed tuna and salmon may be used if thoroughly rinsed.

That fat-free salad dressings may be used as desired.

How to order off a menu while dining out:

- Choose juice instead of soup as an appetizer.
- Use lemon, vinegar, low-calorie dressing (if available) or fresh ground pepper on salad, or request that the dressing be brought on the side.
- Order plain baked or broiled foods.
- Avoid warm bread and rolls that absorb more butter than those at room temperature.
- Order fresh fruit, gelatin, or sherbet for dessert.
- Request milk for coffee or tea in place of cream and nondairy creamers.

On food preparation techniques to reduce fat content.

- Trim fat from meat and remove skin from chicken before cooking.
- Place meats to be baked or roasted on a rack to allow the fat to drain.
- Bake, broil, steam, or sauté foods in vegetable cooking spray or allowed fats.
- Cook with bouillon, lemon, vinegar, wine, herbs, and spices instead of adding fat.
- Make fat-free soup stock by preparing the stock a day ahead and refrigerating it overnight. The fat will harden and can be easily removed from the surface. Make fat-free gravies by this method also.

To purchase "select" grade meats because they are lower in fat than "choice" and "prime" grades.

Increase protein and carbohydrate intake to restore weight that has been lost. Clients with increased requirements for healing (eg, regional enteritis, ulcerative colitis) may need 2000 to 3500 calories/day, and 1.0 to 1.5 g protein/kg.

Provide small, frequent feedings to maximize intake, if appropriate.

Increase fluid intake to compensate for increased fluid output (eg, diarrhea, fistula drainage, blood loss).

Modify the diet as needed to alleviate any secondary nutrient deficiencies and metabolic disturbances that develop (see display, Secondary Nutrient Deficiencies and Metabolic Disturbances of Malabsorption Syndrome). Reduce lactose to the maximum amount tolerated by the individual (see the display, Lactose-Restricted Diet), as indicated.

Additional diet interventions for selected malabsorptive disorders are summarized in Table 16-3.

Lactose-Restricted Diet

CHARACTERISTICS

Limits lactose (milk sugar) to the level tolerated by the individual

INDICATIONS FOR USE

Primary, secondary, and acquired lactose intolerance

CONTRAINDICATIONS

None

FOODS HIGH IN LACTOSE

Milk: whole, 2%, 1%, skim, evaporated, nonfat dry milk, milk solids

Cream; sour cream

All cheese, except aged natural cheeses

Creamed soup and sauces

Specialty-flavored instant coffee blends made with creamer

Cocoa and most chocolate beverages

Ice cream, sherbet, ice milk, custard, puddings, commercial desserts and mixes

FOOD WITH LESS LACTOSE

Liver, sweetbreads

Products that have milk, butter, margarine, dry milk solids, or whey listed as ingredients, including the following foods:

- Breads and cereals, such as Total, Special K, and Cocoa Krispies
- Cookies, cakes, pastries, commercial fruit pie fillings, sherbet
- Cold cuts and hot dogs
- Creamed or breaded meats and vegetables
- Gravy, dried soups, dips, salad dressings
- Commercial french fries, instant potatoes, mashed potatoes
- Butterscotch, caramels, chocolate candy, molasses, peppermints, toffee, chewing gum
- Cordials and liqueurs
- Maraschino cherries
- Powdered soft drinks, powdered coffee creamer
- Some dietetic and diabetic foods
- Sugar substitutes (Sweet 'n Low and Equal tablets)
- Monosodium glutamate (MSG)
- Some vitamin and mineral preparations

POTENTIAL PROBLEM/RATIONALE

Calcium deficiency related to the reduction or elimination of milk and dairy products from the diet.

(continued)

Lactose-Restricted Diet *(Continued)*

NURSING INTERVENTIONS AND CONSIDERATIONS

Encourage the client to drink small amounts of milk as tolerated; tolerance may be greatly improved when milk is consumed with solids. Some clients may tolerate yogurt, milk with acidophilus added, or milk treated with Lactaid. Sometimes chocolate milk is better tolerated because of its higher sucrose content and slower emptying rate from the stomach.

Encourage the intake of calcium from nondairy sources, such as green leafy vegetables, dates, prunes, canned sardines and salmon with bones, egg yolks, whole grains, nuts, dried peas and beans, and calcium-fortified orange juice.

Provide calcium supplements as needed.

LOW-LACTOSE DIET TEACHING

Instruct the client:

On the sources of lactose.

To include nondairy sources of calcium in the diet and to take calcium supplements if needed.

To read labels to identify sources of lactose. Lactate, lactalbumin, and calcium compounds are lactic acid salts and are lactose-free. Kosher foods labeled *pareve* are made without milk.

That some amount of milk may be tolerated by those with acquired lactose intolerance, especially if consumed slowly, at room temperature, and with food.

That nondairy creamer is lactose-free and may be used in beverages, on cereal, and in cooking, if desired.

That acidophilus milk or Lactaid milk may be tolerated. The lactose in Lactaid has been converted into other absorbable sugars. Lactaid is available in supermarkets and can be used as a beverage or in cooking.

Client Teaching

Instruct the client

On the principles and rationale of diet management to relieve malabsorption syndrome symptoms, as indicated (see Table 16-3, and the appropriate displays for specific diet modifications).

On the relationship between eating and recovery.

To eat small, frequent meals to maximize intake. Advise the client to eat slowly and chew food thoroughly.

To avoid extremely hot or cold food and beverages because they can stimulate peristalsis.

Monitoring Progress

Monitor for the following signs or symptoms:

Tolerance of fat intake (ie, decrease or absence of steatorrhea and pain after eating)

Compliance with the diet, and the need for follow-up diet counseling

Effectiveness of the diet, and the need for further diet modification

Intake and output; fluid and electrolyte balance
Weight, weight changes
Clinical signs of malnutrition

Evaluation

Evaluation is ongoing. Provided that the plan of care has not changed, the client will achieve the goals as stated above.

DRUG
ALERT   *Corticosteroids and Sulfasalazine*

CORTICOSTEROIDS

Can cause calcium and potassium depletion, sodium retention, and glucose intolerance.

ACTIONS

Monitor potassium and sodium status. Encourage intake of potassium-rich and calcium-rich foods. Limit sodium if edema or hypertension develops. Monitor serum glucose; long-term use of corticosteroids may necessitate the use of a diabetic diet.

SULFASALAZINE

Interferes with the metabolism and physiologic function of folic acid, leading to folic acid deficiency anemia. May also lead to crystalluria and renal stone formation. Other common side effects include anorexia, nausea, and GI upset.

ACTIONS

Provide folic acid supplements as needed. Encourage a high fluid intake to prevent renal stones. Give with food or milk.

Disorders of the Liver

The liver is a highly active organ that is involved in the metabolism of almost all nutrients. After absorption, almost all nutrients are transported to the liver, where they are "processed" before being distributed to other tissues. The liver synthesizes plasma proteins, blood clotting factors, and nonessential amino acids, and forms urea from the nitrogenous wastes of protein. Triglycerides, phospholipids, and cholesterol are synthesized in the liver. Glucose is formed (gluconeogenesis), and glycogen is formed, stored, and broken down, as needed. Vitamins and minerals are metabolized and many are stored in the liver. Finally, the liver is vital for detoxifying drugs, alcohol, ammonia, and other poisonous substances.

Liver damage can have profound and devastating effects on the metabolism of almost all nutrients. Liver damage can range from mild and reversible (eg, fatty liver) to severe and terminal (eg, hepatic coma).

HEPATITIS AND CIRRHOSIS

Hepatitis is an inflammation of the liver. It can be caused by viral infections (type A, type B, type C, type D, and type E), alcohol abuse, and hepatotoxic chemicals such as chloroform and carbon tetrachloride. Early symptoms include anorexia, nausea and vomiting, fever, fatigue, headache, and weight loss. Later, dark-colored urine, jaundice, liver tenderness, and possibly liver enlargement may develop. Liver cell damage that occurs from hepatitis is reversible with proper rest and nutrition.

Cirrhosis encompasses all forms of end-stage liver disease that are characterized by extensive loss of liver cells, fibrosis, and fatty infiltration of the liver. Liver function is seriously impaired as liver cells are replaced by functionless scar tissue; normal blood circulation through the liver also is disrupted. During the early stages of cirrhosis, fever, anorexia, weight loss, and fatigue may be evident. Impaired glucose tolerance is common. Later, portal hypertension, dyspepsia, diarrhea or constipation, jaundice, esophageal varices, hemorrhoids, ascites, edema, bleeding tendencies, anemia, hepatomegaly, and splenomegaly may develop. Cirrhosis can progress to terminal hepatic coma.

The major cause of cirrhosis is alcoholism, with a 10% to 12% incidence rate among alcoholics. Other causes include chronic viral hepatitis, repeated exposure to toxic chemicals, chronic biliary obstruction, malignancies, and malnutrition.

The objectives of diet intervention for hepatitis and cirrhosis are to avoid or minimize permanent liver damage, promote liver cell regeneration, restore optimal nutritional status, and alleviate symptoms. For clients with cirrhosis, diet intervention may help avoid complications of ascites, esophageal varices, and hepatic coma; however, depending on the extent of liver damage, regeneration may not be possible.

NURSING PROCESS

Assessment

In addition to the general GI assessment criteria, assess for the following factors:

Symptoms: onset, frequency, causative factors, severity, interventions attempted and the results

Dietary changes made in response to symptoms (ie, foods avoided, foods preferred). Determine which foods are best and least tolerated.

Protein intake: meat, fish, poultry, milk and milk products, dried peas and beans, grain products

Fat intake, and determine if the client is experiencing any symptoms of fat intolerance, such as distention, indigestion, or early satiety

Intake and output; observe for edema, ascites; measure abdominal girth

Abnormal laboratory values, especially low white blood cell, red blood cell, and platelet counts; high serum bilirubin and ammonia; elevated liver enzymes; low albumin, sodium, potassium, serum transferrin, and BUN; prolonged clotting times; occult blood

Weight, weight changes: rapid weight gain signals fluid retention

Nursing Diagnosis

Altered Nutrition: Less than body requirements, related to faulty metabolism secondary to altered liver function

Planning and Implementation

The importance of optimal nutrition in the management of liver disorders cannot be overestimated. Adequate protein and calories are of paramount importance—protein is needed for liver cell regeneration; calories are used to spare protein. However, depending on the extent of liver cell damage and regenerative capacity, high protein intakes may overburden the liver and precipitate a hepatic coma. In the later stages of cirrhosis, there is a fine line between enough protein and too much protein. Likewise, it may be difficult to provide adequate calories if the client experiences steatorrhea or an intolerance to fat.

Alcohol must be eliminated.

Malnourished, anorexic clients have difficulty consuming an adequate diet, and nausea may worsen as the day progresses. High-calorie, high-protein liquid nourishments may be better tolerated than traditional meals. Solicit individual food preferences and work closely with the family.

A texture-modified diet (ie, soft, low-residue, or full liquids) may be needed if a regular diet irritates esophageal mucosa. Withhold food if esophageal varices bleed.

For unknown reasons, clients with cirrhosis cannot handle a normal sodium load. If ascites is present, restrict sodium intake to 2 g/day or less. Unfortunately, high-protein foods are also relatively high in sodium. Low-sodium milk is an option; however, it is unpalatable and most clients find its taste offensive.

If sodium restriction alone is not effective, fluid intake also may need to be limited to as few as 1000 ml. However, a high fluid intake may be needed to replace losses caused by fever and vomiting. Fluid needs must be assessed on an individual basis.

Clients with severe anorexia, nausea, or vomiting may need enteral or parenteral nutritional support.

Multivitamin and mineral supplements, especially iron, B vitamins, vitamin C, and vitamin K, may be necessary to compensate for alterations in metabolism.

CLIENT GOALS

The client will:

Experience fewer and less severe symptoms of _____.
Consume adequate calories and protein to attain or maintain "healthy" weight and regenerate liver cells, if possible.
Describe the principles and rationale of diet management of hepatic disorders, and implement the appropriate diet interventions.
Identify causative factors, if known.

NURSING INTERVENTIONS

Diet Management

Provide 1.0 to 2.0 g protein/kg, emphasizing high-biologic-value sources: milk, meat, and eggs. If hepatic coma is impending, decrease protein to the maximum amount tolerated by the individual.

Increase calories to 2000–3000/day to spare protein and meet energy needs, allowing a liberal carbohydrate intake of 300 to 400 g, but moderate amounts of fat. Restrict fat intake if steatorrhea develops.

Provide small, frequent meals and encourage the client to eat all meals and snacks. Offer nutrient-rich morning meals if nausea worsens as the day progresses.

Limit sodium and fluid for clients with ascites. Allowances are determined by the accumulation of fluid as measured by sudden weight gain. Sodium allowance ranges from 1000 to 2000 mg (see Chapter 17); fluid allowance ranges from 1000 to 2000 ml/day; amounts are liberalized as liver function improves.

Client Teaching

Instruct the client

On the importance of eating an adequate diet and taking vitamins and minerals as prescribed.

On the principles and rationale of diet management to relieve symptoms of hepatic disorders, and how to implement necessary changes.

To avoid spices, pepper, caffeine, and coarse foods that may irritate esophageal varices.

To chew food thoroughly.

Monitoring Progress

Monitor for the following signs or symptoms:

Tolerance to protein intake (eg, absence of central nervous system manifestations, controlled/decreased serum ammonia levels)

Compliance with the diet, and the need for follow-up diet counseling

Effectiveness of the diet, and the need for further diet modification

Weight, weight status

Intake and output, and fluid balance

Evaluation

Evaluation is ongoing. Provided that the plan of care has not changed, the client will achieve the goals as stated above.

Hepatic Systemic Encephalopathy

Hepatic systemic encephalopathy refers to the central nervous system (CNS) manifestations of cirrhosis, and is characterized by mental disturbance or loss of consciousness. Impaired memory and concentration, slow response time, drowsiness, irritability, flapping tremor, and fecal odor to breath may progress to a terminal coma.

The exact cause of hepatic encephalopathy is not known; however, increased serum ammonia levels may be at least partially responsible. Ammonia is a CNS toxin that is produced by the action of GI flora on protein (dietary sources, products of muscle catabolism, and protein from GI blood loss). Because the malfunctioning liver cannot convert ammonia to urea, serum ammonia levels increase. Another possible cause is the formation of false neurotransmitters, which is related to an alteration in serum amino acid patterns that characterizes altered liver function.

The primary objective of treatment for hepatic encephalopathy is to decrease intestinal ammonia by controlling dietary protein, controlling GI bleeding, alleviating constipation, and reducing GI flora. Additional goals include correcting fluid and electrolyte imbalances and treating or preventing infection.

NURSING PROCESS

Assessment

In addition to the general GI assessment criteria, assess for the following factors:

Symptoms: onset, frequency, causative factors, severity, interventions attempted and the results.

Dietary changes made in response to symptoms (ie, foods avoided, foods preferred). Determine which foods are best and least tolerated.

Protein intake and adequacy of calorie intake.

Serum ammonia levels, and clinical signs of impending coma.

Intake and output; observe for signs of fluid and electrolyte imbalance.

Weight and weight changes.

Nursing Diagnosis

Fluid Volume Excess, related to ascites secondary to liver disease

Planning and Implementation

Sodium intake is restricted to alleviate the fluid accumulation of ascites. Restrictions may be severe, allowing only 250 mg/day, which makes compliance extremely difficult.

Manipulation of dietary protein is critical. Providing protein in excess of what the liver can handle increases serum ammonia levels and worsens CNS symptoms. The same results occur from too little protein; a protein intake that is inadequate to meet the body's needs stimulates body protein catabolism, which, in effect, is like eating too much protein. In fact, some studies suggest that low protein intake may be independently associated with worsening of hepatic encephalopathy (Morgan et al, 1995). Optimal protein allowance is derived by observation of clinical symptoms and serum ammonia levels. Protein intake may need to be adjusted daily, or even more frequently, depending on the course of the disease.

To prevent tissue breakdown, a high calorie intake is indicated.

Texture modification may be necessary to prevent damage to esophageal varices. A soft, puréed, or liquid diet may facilitate swallowing.

Specially defined commercial tube-feeding formulas that comprise altered amino acid patterns may be used to supplement the diet of clients with liver failure (see Appendix 7).

CLIENT GOALS

The client will:

Avoid hepatic coma.

Experience a decrease in ascites, avoid complications of esophageal varices.

Consume adequate calories and an optimal amount of protein, based on his or her clinical symptoms.

NURSING INTERVENTIONS

Diet Management

Limit sodium and fluid for clients with ascites. Sodium allowance ranges from 250 to 2000 mg/day; fluid allowance ranges from 1500 to 2000 ml/day.

Reduce protein to 20 to 40 g/day and increase by 10 to 15 g/day as the client improves. Adjust the protein content of the diet according to mental symptoms, and eliminate all protein if the client is comatose. Restrict foods that are sources of preformed ammonia or that contain amino acids that convert readily to ammonia: cheese, chicken, ground beef, ham, salami, buttermilk, gelatin, Idaho potatoes, onions, and peanut butter.

Supply at least 2000 cal/day to prevent tissue breakdown. To increase calorie intake without increasing protein, use the following supplements:
- Butter or margarine on potatoes, bread, vegetables, rice, cereal
- Honey, sugar, glucose in coffee or fruit juice, on toast or cereal
- Hard candy and jelly
- Modular carbohydrate supplements (see Appendix 7)

Client Teaching

Client teaching is not indicated, because of the severity of the condition. Clients who respond to treatment will be maintained on the diet as indicated for cirrhosis; however, protein allowance may be less.

Monitoring Progress

Monitor for the following signs or symptoms:

Effectiveness of diet and the need for further diet modification

Intake and output; ascites

Serum ammonia levels

CNS symptoms

Evaluation

Evaluation is ongoing. Provided that the plan of care has not changed, the client will achieve the goals as stated above.

DRUG
ALERT   *Neomycin*

Neomycin kills intestinal bacteria → decreased vitamin K synthesis → vitamin K deficiency → easy bleeding and diarrhea.

Pancreatic Disorders: Pancreatitis

Inflammation of the pancreas, known as pancreatitis, causes the retention of pancreatic enzymes, leading to autodigestion of the pancreas. Symptoms of both acute and chronic pancreatitis include severe abdominal pain, nausea, vomiting, distention, fever, and jaundice. Hyperglycemia, steatorrhea, weight loss, and malnutrition may develop as chronic manifestations.

Acute pancreatitis may develop from unknown causes, alcoholism, biliary tract disease, pancreatic cancer, post gastric or biliary tract surgery, or secondary to mumps or a bacterial infection. Chronic pancreatitis, characterized by scarring and tissue calcification, is most often caused by alcohol abuse, although it is also associated with gallstones, hyperparathyroidism, and hyperlipidemia.

Acute pancreatitis is treated by reducing pancreatic stimulation; the client is ordered NPO, and a nasogastric tube is inserted to suction gastric contents. Appropriate measures are taken to correct fluid and electrolyte imbalance, to control pain, and to treat or prevent symptoms. The treatment of chronic pancreatitis focuses on pancreatic enzyme replacement to control maldigestion, and diet therapy to reduce steatorrhea, to minimize pain, and to avoid acute attacks. Surgical intervention may be necessary if medical treatment fails.

NURSING PROCESS

Assessment

In addition to the general GI assessment criteria, assess for the following factors:

Symptoms: onset, duration, causative factors, severity, interventions attempted and the results.

Dietary changes made in response to symptoms (ie, foods avoided, foods preferred). Determine which foods are best and least tolerated.

Fat intake and its relationship to the onset of symptoms.

Alcohol intake; the intake of other gastric acid stimulants, such as regular and decaffeinated coffee, tea, and pepper.

Signs and symptoms of hyperglycemia.

Weight, weight changes.

Abnormal laboratory values, especially high serum glucose, lipase, amylase, triglycerides; decreased serum calcium, magnesium, sodium, chloride, potassium, albumin.

Symptoms of malnutrition (see the display, Secondary Nutrient Deficiencies and Metabolic Disturbances of Malabsorption Syndrome).

Nursing Diagnosis

Altered Nutrition: Less than body requirements, related to faulty digestion secondary to pancreatitis

Planning and Implementation

Food is withheld initially during an acute attack of pancreatitis. If the client is malnourished, nasojejunal tube feeding of an elemental diet or total parenteral nutrition may be used until oral intake is resumed (see Chapter 14). As bowel sounds return, serum amylase levels fall, and pain subsides, clear liquids are given and progressed to a low-fat diet as tolerated (see the display, Low-Fat Diet).

A low-fat diet is used to alleviate steatorrhea. **Medium-chain triglycerides**, which do not require digestion by pancreatic lipase before being absorbed, may be used for calories. However, medium-chain triglycerides do not provide essential fatty acids and are unpalatable.

Liberal quantities of protein and carbohydrates are recommended to replace calorie and nutrient losses. However, a carbohydrate-controlled diet may be necessary if signs and symptoms of hyperglycemia develop.

Small, frequent meals may help reduce the amount of pancreatic stimulation at each meal. Known gastric stimulants, such as alcohol, caffeine, coffee, and pepper, should be prohibited.

Steatorrhea may necessitate the use of vitamin C and B-complex vitamin supplements, water-soluble supplements of the fat-soluble vitamins, and vitamin B_{12} injections.

CLIENT GOALS

The client will:

Avoid or experience alleviation of symptoms of pancreatitis and chronic complications (eg, hyperglycemia, steatorrhea, malnutrition).

Describe the principles and rationale of dietary management of pancreatitis, and implement the appropriate dietary changes.

Identify and avoid gastric stimulants.

NURSING INTERVENTIONS

Diet Management (for Chronic Pancreatitis)

Limit fat to the maximum amount that the client can tolerate without causing steatorrhea or pain, usually 50 to 70 g/day. Encourage a liberal intake of protein and carbohydrates.

Eliminate individual intolerances and gastric acid stimulants: alcohol, regular and decaffeinated coffee, tea, and pepper.

Provide a carbohydrate-controlled diet if signs or symptoms of hyperglycemia develop (see Chapter 18).

Provide six small meals per day.

Client Teaching

Instruct the client

On the principles and rationale of diet management of pancreatitis, and how to implement the appropriate dietary changes.

To eliminate individual intolerances and gastric acid stimulants.

That if pancreatic replacements are prescribed, they must be taken with every meal and snack.

Monitoring Progress

Monitor for the following signs or symptoms:

Tolerance to fat intake (ie, absence of steatorrhea and pain after eating)

Compliance with the diet, and the need for follow-up diet counseling

Effectiveness of the diet and the need for further diet modification

Weight, weight changes

Signs of malnutrition related to malabsorption (see the display, Secondary Nutrient Deficiencies and Metabolic Disturbances of Malabsorption Syndrome)

Signs of hyperglycemia

Evaluation

Evaluation is ongoing. Provided that the plan of care has not changed, the client will achieve the goals as stated above.

Gallbladder Disorders: Cholelithiasis and Cholecystitis

Abdominal pain, nausea and vomiting, jaundice, fever, fat intolerance, and flatulence are symptoms of cholecystitis, an inflammation of the gallbladder. Cholecystitis may be caused by gallstones (cholelithiasis) obstructing the cystic duct, trauma, or previous surgery. It occurs mostly in women, especially those who are obese, older than age 40, and multiparous. Cystic duct obstruction can lead to abscess, necrosis, perforation, and peritonitis.

NURSING PROCESS

Assessment

In addition to the general GI assessment criteria, assess for the following factors:

Symptoms: onset, frequency, causative factors, severity, interventions attempted and results.

Dietary changes made in response to symptoms (ie, foods avoided, foods preferred). Determine which foods are best and least tolerated.

Fat intake and its relationship to the onset of symptoms.

Weight.

Nursing Diagnosis

Altered Health Maintenance, related to the lack of knowledge of dietary management of cholelithiasis/cholecystitis.

Planning and Implementation

The role of diet intervention in the treatment of cholecystitis is to minimize gallbladder stimulation. During an acute attack of cholecystitis, food is withheld and the client is maintained on intravenous fluid and electrolytes. After 12 to 24 hours, a clear liquid diet may be offered and progressed to a regular diet as tolerated.

Low-fat diets (varying from 20 to 60 g/day of fat) are frequently used in the management of gallbladder disease, based on the rationale that limiting fat intake reduces stimulation to the gallbladder and minimizes pain. Although some clients are aggravated by fat, some studies indicate that fat intolerance is no more common among clients with gallbladder disease than it is among the general population. Diet modification, therefore, should be based on individual tolerance.

Coffee, both regular and decaffeinated, has been shown to induce significant increases in plasma cholecystokinin, the hormone released in the upper small bowel that stimulates gallbladder contraction. It is recommended that clients with symptomatic gallstones avoid coffee.

Fat-soluble vitamin deficiencies may develop as a result of impaired bile secretion, making water-soluble forms of vitamins A, D, E, and K necessary.

After gallbladder surgery, some physicians recommend a low-fat diet for 4 to 6 weeks; others believe no diet modification is necessary.

CLIENT GOALS

The client will:

Lose weight, if overweight, to reduce intraabdominal pressure.
Describe the principles and rationale of diet management for cholecystitis, and implement the appropriate diet interventions.
Identify and avoid foods that produce symptoms.

NURSING INTERVENTIONS

Diet Management

Promote weight loss, if indicated.
Eliminate individual foods that are not tolerated.
Some clients may benefit physically or psychologically from a low-fat diet (see display, Low-Fat Diet); otherwise, provide diet as tolerated.

Client Teaching

Instruct the client

To lose weight, if overweight.
To avoid any foods not tolerated. Some clients are bothered by highly seasoned food, coffee, eggs, and certain fruits and vegetables such as broccoli, cauliflower, brussels sprouts, cabbage, onions, legumes, and melons.
To limit fat intake, if fat appears to produce symptoms.

Monitoring Progress

Monitor for the following signs or symptoms:

Compliance with the diet, and the need for follow-up diet counseling
Effectiveness of the diet, and the need for further diet modification
Weight, if overweight

Evaluation

Evaluation is ongoing. Provided that the plan of care has not changed, the client will achieve the goals as stated above.

KEY CONCEPTS

- Diet intervention for GI disorders is usually aimed at minimizing or preventing symptoms; for some disorders, diet intervention may be the primary treatment.
- The trend is toward liberalizing diet restrictions; diet intervention should always be individualized according to the client's tolerance.
- Small, frequent meals may help maximize intake in clients who are anorexic, and avoiding high-fat foods may lessen the feeling of fullness.

- After nausea and vomiting subside, progress oral feedings based on the client's tolerance. Carbohydrates that are low in fat, such as crackers, toast, oatmeal, and bland fruit, are usually well tolerated. A high fluid intake may be indicated to replenish losses, but fluids should not be given to meals because they can promote the feeling of fullness.

- A low-residue diet is similar to a low-fiber diet; its purpose is to reduce the frequency and volume of fecal output and slow transit time. It may be used on a short-term basis for diarrhea, diverticulitis, malabsorption syndromes, and in preparation for bowel surgery.

- A high-fiber diet is high in both soluble and insoluble fiber. Soluble fiber has been credited with lowering serum cholesterol and promoting glucose control in diabetics. Insoluble fiber increases stool bulk and stimulates peristalsis, and thus is effective against constipation. The average American consumes about half the recommended quantity of fiber recommended daily.

- Semisolid foods, like pudding, yogurt, and cooked cereals, are usually the easiest and safest foods for people with dysphagia. Thin liquids and sticky foods should be avoided.

- A liberal bland diet eliminates any foods the individual cannot tolerate plus pepper, chili powder, alcohol, caffeine, and all coffee. This diet may be used to treat hiatal hernia, esophageal reflux, gastritis, and ulcers.

- Depending on the severity and chronicity, malabsorption syndromes can cause numerous nutritional problems. When steatorrhea occurs, a low-fat diet is indicated; MCT oil may be used to increase calorie intake when fat digestion is impaired.

- A gluten-free diet prevents intestinal villi changes, steatorrhea, and other symptoms in clients with celiac disease. All forms and sources of wheat, oats, rye, and barley must be permanently eliminated from the diet. Secondary lactose intolerance may be permanent or temporary.

- In people with hepatitis, liver cell regeneration can occur if adequate calories and protein are provided, and the underlying cause is treated.

- With increasing liver damage, the cells' regenerative capacity diminishes. The diet is modified according to the client's symptoms, such as soft foods or liquids for esophageal varices, and low sodium for ascites. Although a high-protein diet may be indicated to promote liver regeneration, protein can overburden the liver in advanced stages of cirrhosis and precipitate a hepatic coma.

- Chronic pancreatitis is treated with a low-fat diet. A liberal bland diet may also be recommended, and a diabetic diet may be necessary for clients with glucose intolerance.

- Although low-fat diets are frequently used in the treatment of gallbladder disease, fat intolerance may be no more common among clients with gallbladder disease than it is among the general population. Clients with symptomatic gallstones should avoid coffee (regular and decaffeinated) and eliminate individual intolerance. Weight loss, if overweight, reduces intraabdominal pressure.

FOCUS ON **CRITICAL THINKING**

Mrs. Templeton is 45 years old, weighs 153 pounds, and is 5'1" tall. Recently, she has been complaining about heartburn that radiates to her throat and regurgitation. She notes that the pain is particularly bothersome when she eats before going to bed. Her doctor has diagnosed hiatal hernia with GER. She avoids all citrus products because they are "too acidic," but has not made any other dietary changes related to her diagnosis.

In questioning Mrs. Templeton about her usual dietary habits, on which foods would you specifically focus? Why is it important to find out how frequently and at what times Mrs. Templeton eats? What would be the most effective dietary intervention for her? What other advice would you give Mrs. Templeton to help relieve her symptoms? What nutrient may be deficient in her diet because she avoids all citrus products? What foods would you recommend she consume to avoid a deficiency of that nutrient?

REFERENCES

Aldoori, W., Giovannucci, E., Rimm, E., Wing, A., Trichopoulos, D., and Willett, W. (1994). A prospective study of diet and the risk of symptomatic diverticular disease in men. Am J Clin Nutr, 60, 757–764.

Anderson, J., Smith, B., and Gustafson, H. (1994). Health benefits and practical aspects of high-fiber diets. Am J Clin Nutr, 59(suppl), 1242S–1247S.

Butler, R. (1994). Managing the complications of cirrhosis. AJN, 94(3), 46–49.

Calianno, C. (1995). Guarding against aspiration complications. Nursing 95, 25(6), 52–53.

Chicago Dietetic Association and the South Suburban Dietetic Association (1992). Manual of Clinical Dietetics. 4th ed. Chicago: The American Dietetic Association.

Cole-Arvin, C, Notich, L., and Underhill, A. (1994). Identifying and managing dysphagia. Nursing 94, 24(1), 48–49.

Dehkordi, N. and Warren, A. (1995). Lactose malabsorption as influenced by chocolate milk, skim milk, sucrose, whole milk, and lactic cultures. J Am Diet Assoc, 95(4), 484–486.

Escott-Stump, S. (1992). Nutrition and Diagnosis-Related Care. 3rd ed. Philadelphia: Lea & Febiger.

Ganiats, T., Norcross, W., Halverson, A., Burford, P., and Palinkas, L. (1994). Does Beano prevent gas? A double-blind crossover study of oral alpha-galactosidase to treat dietary oligosaccharide intolerance. J Fam Pract, 39(5), 441–445.

Griffiths, A., Ohlsson, A., Sherman, P., and Sutherland, L. (1995). Meta-analysis of enteral nutrition as a primary treatment of active Crohn's disease. Gastroenterology, 108, 1056–1067.

Leibman, B. (1991). Out of gas? Nutrition Action Health Letter, 18(2), 1, 6–7.

Meissner, J. (1994a). Caring for patients with ulcerative colitis. Nursing 94, 24(7), 54–55.

Meissner, J. (1994b). Caring for patients with cirrhosis. Nursing 94, 24(9), 44–45.

Morgan, R., Moritz, T., Mendenhall, C., Haas, R., and VA Cooperative Study Group #275 (1995). Protein consumption and hepatic encephalopathy in alcoholic hepatitis. J Am Coll Nutr, 14, 152–158.

Riguad, D., Angel, L., Cerf, M., Carduner, M., Melchior, C., Sautier, C., Rene, E., Apfel-baum, M., and Mignon, M. (1994). Mechanisms of decreased food intake during weight loss in adult Crohn's disease patients without obvious malabsorption. Am J Clin Nutr, 60, 775–781.

Scherer, J. and Timby, B. (1995). Introductory Medical-Surgical Nursing. 6th ed. Philadel-phia: JB Lippincott.

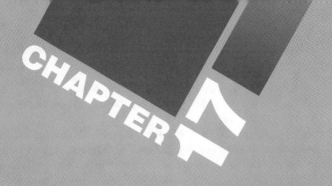

CHAPTER 7

Cardiovascular Disorders and Nutritional Anemias

Chapter Outline

Key Terms

Arteriosclerosis	Low-density lipoproteins	Step Two diet
Atherosclerosis	(LDL-cholesterol)	*Trans* fatty acids
Cardiac cachexia	Nonheme iron	Very-low-density lipopro-
Heme iron	Omega-3 fatty acids	teins (VLDL-cholesterol)
High-density lipoproteins	Plaque	
(HDL-cholesterol)	Step One diet	

THE CARDIOVASCULAR SYSTEM

The cardiovascular system is composed of the heart, arteries, capillaries, and veins. The muscle action of the heart pumps oxygen-depleted blood through veins to the lungs, where carbon dioxide is removed and oxygen is replenished. Arteries carry oxygen-rich blood away from the heart to the capillaries. Oxygen and nutrients are freely exchanged between the blood and body cells through the capillary walls.

Diseases of the heart are the leading cause of death in the United States in people older than 35 years of age, and 90% of those deaths are attributed to atherosclerosis and hypertension. Approximately 1,250,000 Americans have heart attacks each year, and more than 500,000 die annually from coronary heart disease (CHD) (NCEP, 1993a). Substantial evidence that has accumulated over the past 2 decades indicates that diet can play a significant role in reducing the risk of heart disease. Studies show that, although making healthful food choices may not prevent heart disease in all *individuals*, Americans in general can reduce their risk of heart disease by lowering serum cholesterol levels through diet modification.

CARDIAC DISORDERS

Atherosclerotic Heart Disease and Coronary Heart Disease

Arteriosclerosis is a poorly defined general condition that is characterized by thickening and hardening of the arterial walls; to some degree, it occurs in all people as they age (Leibman and Hurley, 1993). **Atherosclerosis**, a more common and severe form of arteriosclerosis, is caused by the formation of plaques along the smooth inner walls of arteries, which results in progressive narrowing. It is estimated that 70% of adult Americans have some atherosclerotic narrowing of their coronary arteries (NCEP, 1993a).

The process of atherosclerosis begins asymptomatically with the development of fatty streaks on the lining of the arterial wall; exactly why fatty streaks form is not known. A complex and dynamic interplay between many factors (monocytes, platelets, abnormal blood clotting, damaged endothelial cells, dysfunctional macrophages and smooth muscle cells, oxidized low-density lipoproteins [LDL-cholesterol]) causes the streaks to enlarge and harden, forming **plaques** (NCEP, 1993b).

Plaques, which are composed mostly of fats, cholesterol, calcium, other blood components, and connective tissue, eventually cause artery walls to lose their elasticity and become narrowed, resulting in restricted blood flow and increased blood pressure. When blood flow is impaired, damage to organs and tissues that are "serviced" by those arteries can occur secondary to the decreased availability of oxygen. The increase in blood pressure further damages artery walls, making them more susceptible to plaque formation. Thus, the progression of atherosclerosis is self-perpetuating (Fig. 17-1).

The three sites most often affected by atherosclerosis are the legs (peripheral vascular disease and increased risk of gangrene), the brain (cerebral vascular accident [CVA]), and the coronary arteries (CHD). Although angina may be a symptom of blocked coronary arteries, most people are asymptomatic until three fourths of a coronary artery is occluded (Leibman and Hurley, 1993).

Complications of atherosclerosis can occur in several ways. In rare instances, plaques can grow to fully occlude an artery. Another possibility is that arteries can weaken and balloon out from the increased pressure, forming an aneurysm. A ruptured aneurysm in a major artery can lead to massive bleeding and death.

Perhaps the most likely complication from atherosclerosis arises from clot formation. Platelets interpret plaque formation as an injury and respond in normal fashion by stimulating clot formation. Once they have been formed, clots may enlarge and remain stationary (thrombus) until they completely block off the blood supply to tissues fed by that artery (thrombosis). Slow tissue death occurs and scar tissue forms. Thrombosis can occur in coronary arteries (coronary thrombosis) or in arteries that nourish the brain (cerebral thrombosis). A clot can break off from the thrombus (embolus) and travel until it gets stuck in a narrowed artery (embolism). The surrounding tissue is then deprived of oxygen and suddenly dies; this occurs in the death of heart tissue (heart attack) or brain tissue (stroke).

RISK FACTORS

Although the exact cause of CHD is unknown, epidemiologic studies show a direct relationship between the level of LDL-cholesterol (and total cholesterol) and the rate of CHD (NCEP, 1993b). Table 17-1 outlines risk based on levels of total serum cho-

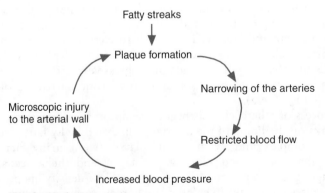

Figure 17-1
Perpetuating progression of atherosclerosis.

Table 17-1
Classification of Total Serum and LDL Cholesterol

Classification	Total Serum Cholesterol	LDL Cholesterol
Desirable	<200 mg/dl	<130 mg/dl
Borderline–high risk	200–239 mg/dl	130–159 mg/dl
High	≥240 mg/dl	≥160 mg/dl

Source: Public Health Service, United States Department of Health and Human Services, National Institutes of Health: National Cholesterol Education Program: Second Report of the Expert Panel on Detection, Evaluation, and Treatment of High Blood Cholesterol in Adults. NIH Publication No. 93-3095. Washington, DC: Government Printing Office, 1993.

lesterol and LDL-cholesterol. A low serum high-density lipoprotein (HDL)–cholesterol (35 mg/dl or less) also increases the risk of CHD, whereas levels of 60 mg/dl or above are associated with decreased risk of CHD. Other nonlipid risk factors appear in the display, Nonlipid CHD Risk Factors.

Although it is well documented that saturated fats raise serum cholesterol, plaque development is complex and is more than simply the result of excess serum cholesterol. The belief that a high-fat diet raises serum cholesterol, and thus causes atherosclerosis and CHD, is an oversimplified but frequently held view. Opponents to this hypothesis raise several thought-provoking questions:

Why is it that people who eat high-fat diets do not always have elevated cholesterol levels?

Why do many people with low or normal serum cholesterol levels have CHD, but a majority of those with elevated serum cholesterol levels do not have CHD? (Nelson, 1995)

Nonlipid CHD Risk Factors

Modifiable Risk Factors	Nonmodifiable Risk Factors
Cigarette smoking	Age:
Hypertension (140/90 or higher or on antihypertensive therapy)	Males: 45 years and older Females: 55 years or older, or premature
Physical inactivity	menopause without estrogen replacement therapy
Diabetes mellitus	Male sex
Obesity (BMI >27), especially visceral obesity	Family history of premature CHD (definite myocardial infarction or sudden death before 55 years of age for father or other male first-degree relative; or before 65 years of age for mother or other female first-degree relative)

> Why does death from cardiovascular disease occur in clients with minimal atherosclerosis? Conversely, why do so many people with extensive atherosclerosis exhibit no apparent clinical problems? (Nelson, 1995)

Clearly, questions remain about whether a low–saturated fat diet can reduce the risk of heart disease. Debate also continues on whether diet intervention should be reserved for "high-risk" clients only, or whether it is appropriate for "population health," as promoted by the Healthy People 2000 campaign (Posner et al, 1993). Beyond the issue of fat, there are other dietary substances that may affect risk, such as omega-3 fatty acids, soluble fibers, folic acid, and antioxidant vitamins (Fraser, 1994) (see Food for Thought, Beyond Fat). Risk reduction may require preventing

---

FOOD for THOUGHT

Beyond Fat

Although the focus of diet intervention for reducing the risk of CHD has been on reducing saturated fat and cholesterol intake to reduce serum LDL-cholesterol levels, it may be that there are other dietary factors that impact on CHD risk without directly affecting serum concentrations of LDL-cholesterol. Consider:

Folic acid. Results from more than 20 studies indicate that people with high levels of the amino acid homocysteine in their blood are more likely to have an MI or CVA than their counterparts with normal homocysteine levels. Although the mechanism isn't known, it may be that high homocysteine levels damage arteries, setting the stage for plaque development. Although vitamins B_6, B_{12}, and folic acid are all required for normal homocysteine metabolism, it appears that a deficiency of folic acid is more likely to cause elevated homocysteine levels than deficiencies of either of the other two B vitamins. Researchers speculate that some people have high homocysteine levels because they are born with an inefficient form of an enzyme that normally enables folic acid to interact with homocysteine (Leibman, 1995). Years of additional study may be needed before the role of folic acid in CHD is understood. Until then, it may be a good idea to be sure to get 400 micrograms of folic acid daily, preferably through diet, but with the aid of supplements if necessary. Sources of folic acid include fortified cereals, brewer's yeast, lentils, dried peas and beans, spinach, asparagus, orange juice, wheat germ, brussels sprouts, and peas.

Vitamin E. Evidence linking vitamin E to a decreased risk of heart disease is growing. Many studies indicate that vitamin E, as well as other antioxidants, delays and reduces the oxidation of LDL, which may be a vital step in the development of plaque. It appears that LDL-cholesterol that has been oxidized by endothelial cells damages tissues, which triggers macrophages to defend the body by engulfing the oxidized LDL molecules. Researchers believe that macrophages are able to handle only a limited amount of oxidized LDL-cholesterol; diets that are high in fat may overwhelm macrophages, especially if they are high in PUFA, which are easily oxidized. On the other hand, studies show that vitamin E may be able to stop LDL from being oxidized. People who take as little as 100 IU of vitamin E daily seem to have a lower risk of heart disease. The NCEP claims that there is not enough evidence to recommend that people take vitamin E supplements, but it is impossible to get 100 IU of vitamin E through diet alone. Until all the results are in, it may be prudent, safe, inexpensive, easy, and effective to take 100 IU of vitamin E daily. The only potential drawback is that large doses of vitamin E (>400 IU/day) may increase the risk of hemorrhagic stroke.

the oxidation of LDL-cholesterol, decreasing the propensity of blood to clot, or altering platelet aggregation. In the meantime, the consensus of the American Heart Association and the National Cholesterol Education Program (NCEP) is to lower total fat, saturated fat, and cholesterol.

CHOLESTEROL AND LIPOPROTEINS

Cholesterol, a fatlike substance, is found in all animal cell membranes and is a precursor of bile acids and sex hormones. Because it is insoluble in water (blood), all serum cholesterol is attached to protein in lipoprotein molecules when it is transported through the blood. High-density lipoproteins (HDL), low-density lipoproteins (LDL), and very-low-density lipoproteins (VLDL) are the three main types of lipoproteins that are found in fasting blood. Table 17-2 outlines their composition and function. **Hyperlipoproteinemia or hyperlipidemia** is characterized by elevated levels of one or more of the lipoprotein types. Table 17-3 summarizes various types of lipid abnormalities and the nutritional implications of each.

Total serum cholesterol is influenced by many variables, including genetics, diet, various diseases, activity, certain drugs, and age. It is a measure of all cholesterol (HDL-cholesterol + LDL-cholesterol + VLDL-cholesterol) and does not distinguish between the "good" and "bad" cholesterol.

HDL-cholesterol is the "good" cholesterol that acts as a scavenger to take cholesterol out of the serum and transport it to the liver, where it is either recycled or excreted in the bile. HDL are composed mainly of protein and make up about 20% to 30% of total serum cholesterol. Their levels are inversely correlated with the risk of CHD: The higher the HDL levels, the lower the risk of heart disease. Exercise, smoking cessation, weight loss if overweight, and moderate alcohol consumption can increase HDL-cholesterol levels.

LDL-cholesterol is the major atherogenic class of lipoproteins and is thus labeled "bad." LDL, which make up 60% to 70% of total serum cholesterol, transport cholesterol out of the liver to the cells. Numerous clinical, epidemiologic, metabolic, and animal studies strongly indicate that high levels of total and LDL cholesterol increase

Table 17-2
Fasting Lipoproteins: Types, Composition, and Functions

Type	Composition	Function
Very-low-density lipoproteins (VLDL)	Mainly endogenously produced triglycerides with a small amount of cholesterol	Transport cholesterol from the liver to the cells. Precursor of LDL. Role in CHD is unclear.
Low-density lipoproteins (LDL)	Mainly cholesterol	Transport cholesterol out of the liver to the cells. Strong positive association between elevated LDL and CHD.
High-density lipoproteins (HDL)	Mainly protein with some cholesterol	Transport cholesterol from the cells to the liver. Elevated HDL are protective against CHD.

Table 17-3
Various Lipid Abnormalities and Their Nutritional Implications

Abnormality	Nutritional Implications
Familial hypercholesterolemia (FH): caused by a defective gene. People with one defective gene usually have cholesterol levels that reach 350–500 mg/dl. Two defective genes rarely occur and are characterized by cholesterol levels of 700–1200 mg/dl. Severe and often fatal heart disease frequently develops in adolescent years.	Diet intervention rarely is effective as the sole mode of treatment. Step Two Diet is recommended to potentiate the action of cholesterol lowering drugs.
Familial combined hyperlipidemia (FCHL): characterized by high cholesterol, high triglycerides, or both. Problem may be due to over-production of VLDL by the liver, but other metabolic defects also may be present. Associated with premature CHD.	Treatment includes weight reduction and control of diabetes, if present. A low-saturated fat, low-cholesterol diet may further reduce LDL levels. Drug therapy may be needed to completely or adequately control serum lipoproteins.
Familial dysbetalipoproteinemia (type 3 hyperlipoproteinemia): relatively uncommon condition characterized by a high total cholesterol related to an increase in VLDL. Cholesterol and triglycerides usually are increased to nearly equal levels. Increased risk of premature CHD and peripheral vascular disease; obesity, glucose intolerance, hyperuricemia, and hypothyroidism accentuates hyperlipidemia.	Calorie restriction is indicated for overweight clients. Low-saturated fat, low-cholesterol diet often helpful; however, drug therapy may be needed.
Reduced HDL cholesterol: characterized by HDL levels <35 mg/dl and classified as a major risk factor for CHD. Common causes of reduced HDL include cigarette smoking, obesity, lack of exercise, use of androgenic steroids, use of beta-adrenergic blocking agents, hypertriglyceridemia, and genetic factors.	Calorie restriction is indicated for obese clients. Smoking cessation in cigarette smokers and increased activity in sedentary people are emphasized.
Diabetic dyslipidemia: abnormal lipid and lipoprotein levels are often observed in diabetics, especially hypertriglyceridemia and low HDL levels.	Improved glucose control can reduce serum triglycerides. Low-saturated fat, low-cholesterol diet may improve lipid levels.
Severe polygenic hypercholesterolemia: characterized by LDL-cholesterol levels >220 mg/dl. No unique genetic defect is responsible; appears related to complex interaction of environmental and genetic factors. Associated with increased risk for premature CHD.	Low-saturated fat, low-cholesterol diet recommended; drug therapy often necessary.

Source: Public Health Service, United States Department of Health and Human Services, National Institutes of Health: National Cholesterol Education Program: Second Report of the Expert Panel on Detection, Evaluation, and Treatment of High Blood Cholesterol in Adults. NIH Publication No. 93-3095. Washington, DC: Government Printing Office, 1993.

the risk of CHD: high levels are associated with obesity and excessive intakes of saturated fat, total fat, and dietary cholesterol. Conversely, lowering total and LDL cholesterol levels reduces CHD risk, and may even help prevent recurrent myocardial infarction and death in clients who have already had a heart attack (NCEP, 1993b).

VLDL-cholesterol makes up 10% to 15% of the total serum cholesterol, and VLDL are precursors of LDL. VLDL are composed mostly of triglycerides; the significance of hypertriglyceridemia is debated (see display, Hypertriglyceridemia). VLDL remnants appear to be atherogenic (NCEP, 1993b).

Hypertriglyceridemia (High Serum Triglycerides)

- Relationship between triglycerides (TG) and CHD is complex.

- Uncertainty exists over whether risk is from TG-rich lipoproteins (small VLDL and VLDL remnants) or from the consequences of high TG (low HDL-cholesterol, small LDL particles, and/or enhanced thrombogenesis).

- Not all forms of hypertriglyceridemia impart the same risk for CHD; high triglycerides that are accompanied by familial combined hyperlipidemia, familial dysbetalipoproteinemia, diabetes mellitus, central visceral obesity, and family history of premature CHD appear more closely associated with early-onset CHD than when high TG is present with primary lipoprotein lipase deficiency and some familial hypertriglyceridemias.

- Definitions of hypertriglyceridemia are as follows:

Normal	TG <200 mg/dl
Borderline-high	TG = 200–400 mg/dl
High	TG = 400–1000 mg/dl. Clinical significance uncertain; some develop premature CHD, others do not.
Very high	TG > 1000 mg/dl. Increased risk of pancreatitis.

- Weight control, elimination of alcohol, and a low-fat, low-saturated fat diet are recommended.

Source: Public Health Service, United States Department of Health and Human Services, National Institutes of Health: National Cholesterol Education Program: Second Report of the Expert Panel on the Detection, Evaluation, and Treatment of High Blood Cholesterol in Adults. NIH Publication No. 93-3095. Washington, DC: Government Printing Office, 1993.

DEFINING RISK AND INTERVENTION STRATEGIES

The National Cholesterol Education Program recommends that total serum cholesterol be measured at least every 5 years in all adults 20 years of age and older, preferably as part of a total physical examination so that other risks can be identified (NCEP, 1993a). Total serum cholesterol and HDL-cholesterol can be used to screen adults who have no symptoms of CHD. Both measurements can be obtained any time of day in the nonfasting state because they change little after eating.

Figure 17-2 depicts intervention strategies based on total cholesterol and HDL-cholesterol. Because the level of LDL-cholesterol more accurately reflects CHD risk than does total cholesterol, a lipoprotein analysis is recommended to estimate LDL-cholesterol for anyone with the following: total cholesterol more than 240 mg/dl; total cholesterol 200 to 239 mg/dl with two or more risk factors for CHD; and HDL levels of 35 mg/dl or less.

A lipoprotein analysis obtains fasting levels of total cholesterol, total triglycerides, and HDL-cholesterol. If the total triglyceride value is less than 400 mg/dl, then triglycerides divided by 5 is an accurate estimate of VLDL-cholesterol. The following formula can be used to estimate LDL-cholesterol:

$$\text{LDL-cholesterol} = \text{total cholesterol} - \text{HDL-cholesterol} - (\text{triglycerides}/5)$$

Accurate LDL-cholesterol cannot be estimated when triglyceride values exceed 400 mg/dl; in that case, ultracentrifugation is needed for accurate lipoprotein determination.

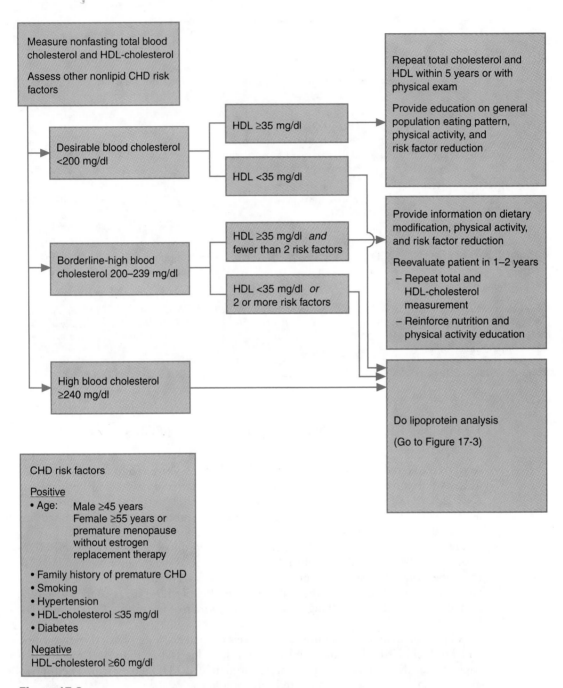

Figure 17-2

Primary prevention in adults without evidence of CHD: Initial classification based on total cholesterol and HDL-cholesterol. (Source: National Cholesterol Education Program (1993). Second Report of the Expert Panel on Detection, Evaluation, and Treatment of High Blood Cholesterol in Adults (Adult Treatment Panel II). Bethesda: USDHHS, Public Health Service, National Institutes of Health, NIH Publication No. 93-3095.)

Treatment recommendations and goals based on LDL-cholesterol values appear in Figure 17-3. Diet therapy is the cornerstone of treatment; drug therapy may be added for clients at high risk for development of CHD (Table 17-4).

DIET THERAPY

Although the term "diet" is used to describe the nutritional recommendations put forth by the NCEP to treat hypercholesterolemia, diet really is a misnomer. Permanent lifestyle changes among both the well population and those with high cholesterol levels are urged for the prevention and treatment of hypercholesterolemia.

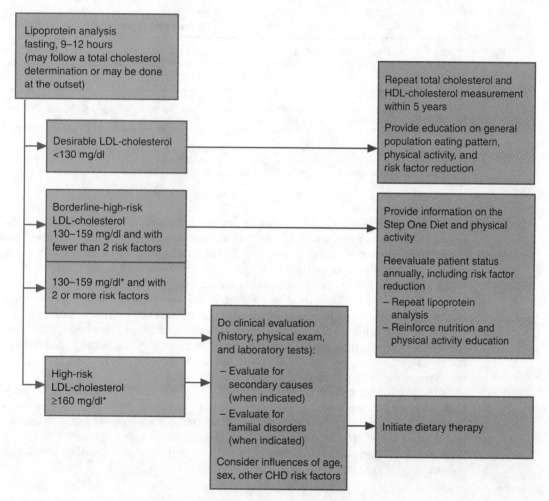

* On the basis of the average of two determinations. If the first two LDL-cholesterol tests differ by more than 30 mg/dL, a third test should be obtained within 1–8 weeks and the average value of three tests used.

Figure 17-3

Primary prevention in adults without evidence of CHD: Subsequent classification based on LDL-cholesterol. (Source: National Cholesterol Education Program (1993). Second Report of the Expert Panel on Detection, Evaluation, and Treatment of High Blood Cholesterol in Adults (Adult Treatment Panel II). Bethesda: USDHHS, Public Health Service, National Institutes of Health, NIH Publication No. 93-3095.)

Table 17-4
Treatment Decisions Based on LDL-Cholesterol

	Dietary Therapy	
	Initiation Level	*LDL Goal*
Without CHD and with fewer than 2 risk factors	≥160 mg/dl	<160 mg/dl
Without CHD and with 2 or more risk factors	≥130 mg/dl	<130 mg/dl
With CHD	>100 mg/dl	≥100 mg/dl
	Drug Treatment	
	Consideration Level	*LDL Goal*
Without CHD and with fewer than 2 risk factors	≥190 mg/dl*	<160 mg/dl
Without CHD and with 2 or more risk factors	≥160 mg/dl	<130 mg/dl
With CHD	≥130 mg/dl†	≤100 mg/dl

* In men under 35 years of age and premenopausal women with LDL-cholesterol levels 190–219 mg/dl, drug therapy should be delayed, except in high-risk patients such as those with diabetes.

† In CHD patients with LDL-cholesterol levels 100–129 mg/dl, the physician should exercise clinical judgment in deciding whether to initiate drug treatment.

Source: Public Health Service, United States Department of Health and Human Services, National Institutes of Health: National Cholesterol Education Program: Second Report of the Expert Panel on Detection, Evaluation, and Treatment of High Blood Cholesterol in Adults. NIH Publication No. 93-3095. Washington, DC: Government Printing Office, 1993.

Generally, the diet to lower serum cholesterol is limited in saturated fat and cholesterol, with calories adjusted to attain healthy weight, if overweight. A varied and nutritious diet that is rich in fruits, vegetables, grains, and fish supplies other substances that may protect against CHD. A high fiber intake, especially soluble fiber, is recommended for its effect in lowering serum cholesterol levels.

The NCEP has outlined the low–saturated fat, low-cholesterol diet in two steps (Table 17-5). The **Step One Diet,** which is similar to the eating pattern recommended for the general public, limits the major and obvious sources of saturated fat and cholesterol, like whole milk and high-fat meats. The Step One Diet is the initial therapy for clients who have not yet modified their diets. Many clients can comply with this diet by making only moderate changes in their dietary habits.

If the goals of the Step One Diet are not accomplished after 3 months of good compliance, the client may need to progress to the **Step Two Diet,** which more severely limits intake of saturated fat and cholesterol. Examples of foods to include and avoid for both the Step One and Step Two Diets appear in Table 17-6. Clients who are unable to achieve acceptable lipid levels through diet modification may require drug therapy.

NURSING PROCESS

Assessment

In addition to the general cardiovascular assessment criteria, assess for the following factors:

Table 17-5
Characteristics of the Step One and Step Two Diets

Nutrient	Recommended Intake	
	Step One Diet	**Step Two Diet**
Total fat	30% or less of total calories	
Saturated fatty acids	8%–10% of total calories	Less than 7% of total calories
Polyunsaturated fatty acids	Up to 10% of total calories	
Monounsaturated fatty acids	Up to 15% of total calories	
Carbohydrates	55% or more of total calories	
Protein	Approximately 15% of total calories	
Cholesterol	Less than 300 mg/day	Less than 200 mg/day
Total calories	To achieve and maintain desirable weight	

Source: Public Health Service, United States Department of Health and Human Services, National Institutes of Health: National Cholesterol Education Program: Second Report of the Expert Panel on Detection, Evaluation, and Treatment of High Blood Cholesterol in Adults. NIH Publication No. 93-3095. Washington, DC: Government Printing Office, 1993.

Table 17-6
Examples of Foods To Choose or Decrease for the Step One and Step Two Diets*

Food Group	Choose	Decrease
Lean Meat, Poultry, and Fish ≤5–6 oz per day	Beef, pork, lamb—lean cuts well trimmed before cooking	Beef, pork, lamb—regular ground beef, fatty cuts, spare ribs, organ meats
	Poultry without skin	Poultry with skin, fried chicken
	Fish, shellfish	Fried fish, fried shellfish
	Processed meat—prepared from lean meat (eg, lean ham, lean frankfurters, lean meat with soy protein or carrageenan)	Regular luncheon meat (eg, bologna, salami, sausage, frankfurters)
Eggs ≤4 yolks per week, Step I ≤2 yolks per week, Step II	Egg whites (two whites can be substituted for one whole egg in recipes), cholesterol-free egg substitute	Egg yolks (if more than four per week on Step One or if more than two per week on Step Two); includes eggs used in cooking and baking
Low-Fat Dairy Products 2–3 servings per day	Milk—skim, 1/2% or 1% fat (fluid, powdered, evaporated), buttermilk	Whole milk (fluid, evaporated, condensed), 2% fat milk (low-fat milk), imitation milk
	Yogurt—nonfat or low-fat yogurt or yogurt beverages	Whole-milk yogurt, whole-milk yogurt beverages
	Cheese—low-fat natural or processed cheese	Regular cheeses (American, bleu, Brie, cheddar, Colby, Edam, Monterey Jack, whole-milk mozzarella, Parmesan, Swiss), cream cheese, Neufchatel cheese
	Low-fat or nonfat varieties (eg, cottage cheese—low-fat, nonfat, or dry curd [0 to 2% fat])	Cottage cheese (4% fat)
	Frozen dairy dessert—ice milk, frozen yogurt (low fat or nonfat)	Ice cream
	Low-fat coffee creamer Low-fat or nonfat sour cream	Cream, half & half, whipping cream, nondairy creamer, whipped topping, sour cream

(continued)

Table 17-6
Examples of Foods To Choose or Decrease for the Step One and Step Two Diets* *(Continued)*

Food Group	Choose	Decrease
Fats and Oils ≤6–8 teaspoons per day	Unsaturated oils—safflower, sunflower, corn, soybean, cottonseed, canola, olive, peanut	Coconut oil, palm kernel oil, palm oil
	Margarine—made from unsaturated oils listed above, light or diet margarine, especially soft or liquid forms	Butter, lard, shortening, bacon fat, hard margarine
	Salad dressings—made with unsaturated oils listed above, low fat or fat free	Dressings made with egg yolk, cheese, sour cream, whole milk
	Seeds and nuts—peanut butter, other nut butters	Coconut
	Cocoa powder	Milk chocolate
Breads and Cereals 6 or more servings per day	Breads—whole-grain bread, English muffins, bagels, buns, corn or flour tortilla	Bread in which eggs, fat, and/or butter is a major ingredient; croissants
	Cereals—oat, wheat, corn, multigrain	Most granolas
	Pasta	
	Rice	
	Dry beans and peas	
	Crackers, low-fat—animal-type, graham, soda crackers, breadsticks, melba toast	High-fat crackers
	Homemade baked goods using unsaturated oil, skim or 1% milk, and egg substitute—quickbreads, biscuits, cornbread muffins, bran muffins, pancakes, waffles	Commercial baked pastries, muffins, biscuits
Soups	Reduced- or low-fat reduced-sodium varieties (eg, chicken or beef noodle, minestrone, tomato, vegetable, potato, reduced-fat soups made with skim milk)	Soup containing whole milk, cream, meat fat, poultry fat, or poultry skin
Vegetables 3–5 servings per day	Fresh, frozen, or canned, without added fat or sauce	Vegetables fried or prepared with butter, cheese, or cream sauce
Fruits 2–4 servings per day	Fruit—fresh, frozen, canned, or dried	Fried fruit or fruit served with butter or cream sauce
	Fruit juice—fresh, frozen, or canned	
Sweets and Modified Fat Desserts	Beverages—fruit-flavored drinks, lemonade, fruit punch	
	Sweets—sugar, syrup, honey, jam, preserves, candy made without fat (candy corn, gumdrops, hard candy), fruit-flavored gelatin	Candy made with milk chocolate, coconut oil, palm kernel oil, palm oil
	Frozen desserts—low-fat and nonfat yogurt, ice milk, sherbet, sorbet, fruit ice, popsicles	Ice cream and frozen treats made with ice cream
	Cookies, cake, pie, pudding—prepared with egg whites, egg substitute, skim milk or 1% milk, and unsaturated oil or margarine; ginger snaps; fig and other fruit bar cookies, fat-free cookies; angel food cake	Commercial baked pies, cakes, doughnuts, high-fat cookies, cream pies

*Careful selection of processed foods is necessary to stay within the sodium <2400 mg guideline.
Source: Public Health Service, United States Department of Health and Human Services, National Institutes of Health: National Cholesterol Education Program: Second Report of the Expert Panel on Detection, Evaluation, and Treatment of High Blood Cholesterol in Adults, NIH Publication No. 93-3095. Washington, DC: Government Printing Office, 1993.

ASSESSMENT CRITERIA

General Cardiovascular Assessment Criteria

Age, especially over age 40

Sex

Presence of obesity, especially visceral (upper body) obesity

Blood pressure

Serum cholesterol

Lipid profiles

Other laboratory results: electrolyte imbalances, LDH and CPK levels

Results of other diagnostic procedures: angiograms, ECG

Ascites, edema

Chest pain

Xanthomas

Diet high in fat, cholesterol, and calories

Use of alcohol, tobacco

Positive family history of heart disease

Other medical conditions, such as diabetes mellitus, hypertension, hypothyroidism, nephrotic syndrome, and obstructive liver disease

Medications used

Type A personality, stressful lifestyle

Meal timing and frequency: Determine when the client's largest meal is eaten.

Total fat, saturated fat, and cholesterol intake: Determine how much, how often, and what types of meats, eggs, dairy products, fried foods, baked goods, convenience foods, table fats, and snacks are consumed. Figure 17-4 is a dietary assessment questionnaire that can be used to evaluate a client's usual intake according to Step One and Step Two Diet recommendations.

Fiber intake, especially foods high in soluble fiber: oatmeal, oat bran, dried peas and beans, citrus fruits, apples, and certain vegetables.

Likes and dislikes: Determine which foods the client cannot live without, and which foods can be easily forfeited.

The impact of lifestyle and work schedule on eating (ie, are most meals eaten at home, at a restaurant, in a cafeteria?).

Cultural, familial, religious, and ethnic influences on eating habits.

The client's medical history and any possible effects on intake or nutritional status, especially such risk factors as diabetes, hypertension, and obesity.

The client's use of alcohol, drugs, and tobacco.

Weight, weight status.

Dietary changes made in response to diagnosis of atherosclerosis or CHD, if appropriate.

The client's willingness to make dietary changes.

The client's educational level, social status, and previous counseling experiences.

Frequency and intensity of exercise.

Nursing Diagnosis

Health Seeking Behaviors, as evidenced by the lack of knowledge of a heart-healthy diet and a desire to learn

Name _____ Date _____

MEDFICTS: Dietary Assessment Questionaire

(**M**eats, **E**ggs, **D**airy, **F**ried foods, **I**n baked goods, **C**onvenience foods, **T**able fats, **S**nacks)

Directions: For each food category for both Group 1 and Group 2 listings: Please check a box in the "Weekly Consumption" column and in the "Serving Size" column. If patient rarely or never eats the food listed, please check only the "Weekly Consumption" box.

FOOD CATEGORY			WEEKLY CONSUMPTION			SERVING SIZE			SCORE
			Rarely/ Never	3 or less serv/wk	4 or more serv/wk	Small	Average	Large	For office use

M Meats

- Average amount per day: 6 oz (equal in size to 2 decks of playing cards)
- Base your estimate on the food you consume the most of

Group 1

Beef	Processed meats	Pork & others
Ribs	Regular Hamburger	Pork shoulder
Steak	Fast food hamburger	Pork chops, roast
Chuck blade	Bacon	Pork ribs
Brisket	Lunchmeat	Ground pork
Ground beef	Sausage	Regular ham
Meatloaf	Hot dogs	Lamb steaks, ribs, chops
Corned beef	Knockwurst	Organ meats
		Poultry with skin

Weekly Consumption: □ Rarely/Never, ■ 3 or less serv/wk (3 pts), ■ 4 or more serv/wk (7 pts) × Serving Size: ■ Small (1 pts), ■ Average (2 pts), ■ Large (3 pts) =

Group 2

Lean Cuts of Beef	Low-fat Processed Meats	Poultry, Fish, Meat
Sirloin tip	Low-fat lunchmeat	Poultry without skin
Flank steak	Low-fat hot dogs	Fish, seafood
Round steak	Canadian bacon	Lamb flank, leg-shank, sirloin, roast
Rump roast		Lean ham cured and fresh
Chuck arm roast		Pork loin chops, tenderloin
		Veal chops, cutlets, roast
		Venison

Weekly Consumption: □ Rarely/Never, □ 3 or less serv/wk, □ 4 or more serv/wk × Serving Size: □ Small, □ Average, ■ Large + (6 pts) =

E Eggs

- Weekly consumption is expressed as times/week

Group 1
Whole eggs, yolks

How many eggs do you eat each time?

Weekly Consumption: □ Rarely/Never, ■ 3 or less serv/wk (3 pts), ■ 4 or more serv/wk (7 pts) × ≤1 (1 pts) 2 (2 pts) ≥3 (3 pts) =

Group 2
Egg whites, egg substitutes (½ cup = 2 eggs)

Weekly Consumption: □ Rarely/Never, □ 3 or less serv/wk, □ 4 or more serv/wk × ≤1 2 ≥3 =

D Dairy

Milk • Average serving: 1 cup

Group 1
Whole milk, 2% milk, 2% buttermilk, yogurt (whole milk)

Weekly Consumption: □ Rarely/Never, ■ 3 or less serv/wk (3 pts), ■ 4 or more serv/wk (7 pts) × ■ Small (1 pts), ■ Average (3 pts), ■ Large (3 pts) =

Group 2
Skim milk, 1% milk, skim milk-buttermilk
Yogurt (nonfat & low-fat)

Weekly Consumption: □ Rarely/Never, □ 3 or less serv/wk, □ 4 or more serv/wk × □ Small □ Average □ Large =

Cheese • Average serving: 1 oz.

Group 1
Cream cheese, cheddar, Monterey jack, Colby, Swiss, American processed, blue cheese
Regular cottage cheese and ricotta (½ cup)

Weekly Consumption: □ Rarely/Never, ■ 3 or less serv/wk (3 pts), ■ 4 or more serv/wk (7 pts) × ■ Small (1 pts), ■ Average (2 pts), ■ Large (3 pts) =

Group 2
Low-fat & fat-free cheeses, skim-mild mozzarella
String cheese
Low-fat & fat-free cottage cheese, and skim-milk ricotta (½ C)

Weekly Consumption: □ Rarely/Never, □ 3 or less serv/wk, □ 4 or more serv/wk × □ Small □ Average □ Large =

Frozen Desserts • Average serving: ½ cup

Group 1
Ice cream, milk shakes

Weekly Consumption: □ Rarely/Never, ■ 3 or less serv/wk (3 pts), ■ 4 or more serv/wk (7 pts) × ■ Small (1 pts), ■ Average (2 pts), ■ Large (3 pts) =

Group 2
Ice milk, frozen yogurt

Weekly Consumption: □ Rarely/Never, □ 3 or less serv/wk, □ 4 or more serv/wk × □ Small □ Average □ Large =

+ Score 6 points if this box is checked

Comments: _____ Total _____

Figure 17-4

Medficts: Dietary Assessment Questionnaire. (Source: National Cholesterol Education Program (1993). Second Report of the Expert Panel on Detection, Evaluation, and Treatment of High Blood Cholesterol in Adults (Adult Treatment Panel II). Bethesda: USDHHS, Public Health Service, National Institutes of Health, NIH Publication No. 93-3095.)

FOOD CATEGORY	WEEKLY CONSUMPTION			SERVING SIZE			SCORE
	Rarely/ Never	3 or less serv/wk	4 or more serv/wk	Small	Average	Large	For office use

F Fried Foods • Average serving: see below

Group 1
French fries, fried vegetables: (½ cup)
*Fried chicken, fish, and meat: (3 oz.)
  *check meat category also

3 pts   7 pts   × 1 pts   2 pts   3 pts =

Group 2
Vegetables, - not deep fried
Meat, poultry, or fish - prepared by baking, broiling, grilling,
  poaching, roasting, stewing

I In Baked Goods • Average serving: 1 serving

Group 1
Doughnuts, biscuits, butter rolls, muffins, croissants, sweet rolls, danish,
cakes, pies, coffee cakes, cookies

3 pts   7 pts   × 1 pts   2 pts   3 pts =

Group 2
Fruit bars, low-fat cookies/cakes/pastries, angel food cake, homemade
baked goods with vegetable oils

C Convenience Foods • Average serving: see below

Group 1
Canned, packaged, or frozen dinners; e.g., pizza (1 slice),
Macaroni & cheese (about 1 cup), pot pie (1), cream soups (1 cup)

3 pts   7 pts   × 1 pts   2 pts   3 pts =

Group 2
Diet/reduced calorie or reduced-fat dinners (1 dinner)

T Table Fats • Average serving: see below

Group 1
Butter, stick margarine: 1 pat
Regular salad dressing or mayonnaise, sour cream: 1–2 Tbsp

3 pts   7 pts   × 1 pts   2 pts   3 pts =

Group 2
Diet and tub margarine, low-fat & fat-free salad dressings
Low-fat & fat-free mayonnaise

S Snacks • Average serving: see below

Group 1
Chips (potato, corn, taco), cheese puffs, snack mix, nuts,
Regular crackers, regular popcorn,
Candy (milk chocolate, caramel, coconut)

3 pts   7 pts   × 1 pts   2 pts   3 pts =

Group 2
Air-popped or low-fat popcorn, low-fat crackers, hard candy, licorice,
fruit rolls, bread sticks, pretzels, fat-free chips, fruit

Directions for scoring:
Multiply weekly consumption points (3 or 7) by serving size points (1, 2, 3)
for Group 1 foods only except for a large serving of Group 2 meats

Example:

3 pts   7 pts   1 pts   2 pts   3 pts
3 × 7 = 21 points
Add score on page 1 and page 2 to get Final Score

Key
40 - 70   -Step I Diet
less than 40   -Step II diet

= Foods high in fat, saturated
  fat, and/or cholesterol

Total _____

Score from
page 1   + _____

Final Score _____

Comments: _____
        (Note frequent use of foods high in fat or saturated fat, e.g. coffee creamer, whipped toping)

Figure 17-4 *(Continued)*

Planning and Implementation

The goal of diet therapy is to provide a nutritionally adequate, palatable diet, while reducing serum cholesterol levels; for every 1% drop in serum cholesterol, the risk of CHD decreases by 2%. Diet may also be used to control other medical risk factors that are responsive to diet modification, such as hypertension, obesity, and diabetes mellitus.

Although diet intervention is considered the first line of treatment for clients with elevated cholesterol levels, "diet" should be viewed as a lifestyle change that is consistent with good health. All people, regardless of cholesterol level, should be educated about diet and risk reduction for the possible prevention of CHD. It has been suggested that it may take 2 to 10 years to make drastic changes in eating habits. Compliance may improve when dietary changes are individualized and are instituted gradually. LDL-cholesterol levels should begin to decrease within 3 to 4 weeks from when the diet is initiated.

Because saturated fats raise LDL-cholesterol levels, foods that are high in saturated fat are limited. To implement the Step One Diet, average Americans must reduce their usual intake of saturated fat by 1/3, and by about 1/2 for the Step Two Diet (NCEP, 1993b). Animal fats, from both butterfat (butter, cheese, ice cream, cream, whole and 2% milk) and meats, usually provide 2/3 of the saturated fat in the typical American diet. Lean cuts of meat should be chosen and visible fat removed. Skinless chicken and fish should frequently be used in place of red meats, and meatless meals should be served occasionally. Egg yolks should be limited to four or fewer per week, and organ meats used sparingly. Coconut oil, palm oil, and palm kernel oil are high in saturated fat, but their overall contribution to the diet is relatively small.

Hydrogenation is a process that converts a vegetable oil to a more solid fat by adding hydrogen molecules. The resultant product has more saturated fat than the original vegetable oil and also contains *trans fatty acids*; *trans* refers to the type of configuration around the fatty acid's double bond (Fig. 17-5). Although small quantities of *trans* fatty acids occur naturally in meat and dairy products, the majority of double bonds in food fats are in the *cis* configuration (Lichtenstein, 1995). Studies show that *trans* fatty acids raise LDL-cholesterol, possibly to the same levels as saturated fats do. At high intakes, they may also lower HDL-cholesterol. Today, most *trans* fatty acids in the American diet are obtained from the intake of partially hydrogenated fats. These are used in commercially prepared baked goods and fried foods, both of which are restricted in Step One and Two Diets. Margarine also contributes a significant number of *trans* fatty acids. Recent controversy surrounding the effects of *trans* fatty acids on serum cholesterol led to claims that butter is healthier than margarine. However, butter is higher in saturated fat than the highest *trans* fatty acid margarine, and also contains cholesterol, unlike vegetable oil margarines. To lower *trans* fatty acid intake, clients should be advised to select the softest margarine available: The softer the margarine, the less hydrogenated the product.

Polyunsaturated fats (corn oil, sunflower oil, safflower oil, soybean oil) currently provide about 7% of total calories in the average American diet, which is an acceptable level (NCEP, 1993). At one time, Americans were advised to increase their

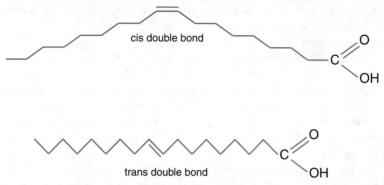

Figure 17-5
Structure of *cis* and *trans* fatty acids.

intake of PUFA (polyunsaturated fatty acids) to help lower LDL-cholesterol; however, concerns about long-term safety and evidence that PUFA lower HDL-cholesterol as well have led to the recommendation that PUFA intake remain at its current level, and that intake not exceed 10% of total calories.

Omega-3 fatty acids, which are most abundant in fish oils, are a type of PUFA that have been shown to lower serum triglycerides; their effect on LDL-cholesterol levels is variable (Chicago Dietetic Association, 1992). They may also decrease platelet aggregation and slow the proliferation of smooth muscle cells in the artery wall. Limited epidemiologic studies indicate that frequent consumption of fish, especially fatty fish, is related to a lower incidence of heart disease. Although increased consumption of fatty fish appears prudent, the use of fish oil capsules has not been proven effective or safe; their use should be discouraged.

Monounsaturated fats, including those predominant in olive oil, canola oil, and peanut oil, tend to lower LDL-cholesterol without adversely affecting HDL-cholesterol. Up to 15% of total calorie intake should comprise monounsaturated fats.

Dietary cholesterol may augment the serum cholesterol–raising effect of saturated fat (NCEP, 1993). Cholesterol is found only in animal products, especially those that are high in saturated fat. Because cholesterol is found in both animal fat and muscle, a low-fat diet is not necessarily low in cholesterol.

Carbohydrates (CHO) should provide up to 55% of total calories for both the Step One and Step Two Diets (see Table 17-5). Because complex carbohydrates are generally low in fat and rich in fiber, vitamins, and minerals, a liberal intake is recommended. High-CHO, low-fat diets tend to lower HDL-cholesterol and raise VLDL; the significance of these changes is debatable.

Obesity often raises LDL-cholesterol, VLDL-cholesterol, and triglycerides, and lowers HDL-cholesterol. It also increases the risks for hypertension and diabetes mellitus. Clients with upper body obesity are at greater health risk than those with lower body obesity. Consuming a low-calorie diet and increasing activity promote weight loss and lower CHD risk.

High-fiber diets, especially those rich in soluble fiber, lower serum cholesterol without lowering HDL-cholesterol (Fraser, 1994). Oatmeal, oat bran, dried peas and beans, citrus fruits, apples, and some vegetables are rich sources of soluble fiber. Clients should be encouraged to eat at least five servings of fruits and vegetables, and at least six servings of whole-grain breads and cereals.

Moderate alcohol consumption has been shown to increase HDL-cholesterol. Unfortunately, alcohol can also raise blood pressure and triglyceride levels, and impede weight loss. Because the potential adverse effects are great, it is not recommended that people who don't drink start, or that people who do drink increase their intake. The Dietary Guidelines for Americans recommends that if clients choose to drink, their daily intake should not exceed 2 drinks for men and 1 drink for women.

The role of vitamins in reducing CHD risk is currently being investigated (see Food for Thought: Beyond Fat). The consumption of fruits and vegetables should be encouraged not only for their low fat content, but also because they are rich sources of fiber, vitamins, minerals, and other substances that may eventually be determined to lower CHD risk.

Garlic oil can significantly lower both serum triglyceride and cholesterol levels and raise HDL levels. The amount of garlic needed, however, is so large that its use is not practical, and the effectiveness of odorless garlic pills is questionable.

Even though dietary changes can lower serum cholesterol levels, it is not known whether atherosclerosis can be prevented through diet modification, or if all Americans should alter their current eating habits. Most experts agree that the majority of Americans older than 2 years of age have the potential to benefit from a low-fat, low–saturated fat, low-cholesterol diet with calorie intake appropriate for "healthy" weight. Possible exceptions include high-risk elderly clients and pregnant women.

Although the Step One and Step Two Diets refer to "percentage of total calories" and "milligrams" of cholesterol, these terms are meaningless to the general public (see Table 17-5). Overall, emphasizing portion sizes and portions/day is much more effective and less intimidating than discussing specific caloric breakdown of the diet.

It is helpful to instruct clients to record their total intake for one or more days. This activity increases their awareness of eating and food choices, and the written account provides the clinician with a tool for identifying areas that need improvement.

Sample menus for the Step One and Step Two Diets of traditional American cuisine appear in the display, Sample Step One and Step Two Diet Menus. Be aware of the potential problems associated with a Step One Diet, and the corresponding nursing interventions and considerations.

CLIENT GOALS

The client will:

Experience a decrease in serum cholesterol/LDL-cholesterol to the desired level or below (see Table 17-4); clients with desirable serum cholesterol levels will maintain those levels.

Explain the principles and rationale of diet management for hypercholesterolemia, implement the appropriate dietary changes, and incorporate these changes into his or her lifestyle.

Step One and Step Two Diet Menus

Traditional American Cuisine: Males 25–49 Years

Step One Sample Menus

BREAKFAST

Bagel, plain (1 medium)
  Cream Cheese, low-fat (2 tsp)
Cereal, shredded wheat (1½ cups)
Banana (1 small)
Milk, **1%** (1 cup)
Orange juice (¾ cup)
Coffee (1 cup)
  Milk, **1%** (1 oz)

LUNCH

Minestrone soup, canned, low sodium (1 cup)
Roast beef sandwich
  Whole wheat bread (2 slices)
  *Lean roast beef, unseasoned (**3 oz**)
  American cheese, low fat and low sodium
    (¾ oz)
  Lettuce (1 leaf)
  Tomato (3 slices)
  Mayonnaise, low fat and low sodium (2 tsp)
Fruit and cottage cheese salad
  Cottage cheese, **2%** and low sodium (½ cup)
  Peaches, canned in juice (½ cup)
Apple juice, unsweetened (1 cup)

DINNER

***Salmon** (3 oz)
  Vegetable oil (1 tsp)
Baked potato (1 medium)
  Margarine (2 tsp)
*Green beans (½ cup), seasoned with margarine
  (½ tsp)
*Carrots (½ cup), seasoned with margarine
  (½ tsp)
White dinner rolls (1 medium)
  Margarine (1 tsp)
Ice milk (1 cup)
Iced tea, unsweetened (1 cup)

Step Two Sample Menus

BREAKFAST

Bagel, plain (1 medium)
  Margarine (2 tsp)
  Jelly (2 tsp)
Cereal, shredded wheat (1½ cups)
Banana (1 small)
Milk, **skim** (1 cup)
Orange juice (¾ cup)
Coffee (1 cup)
  Milk, **skim** (1 oz)

LUNCH

Minestrone soup, canned, low sodium (1½ cups)
Roast beef sandwich
  Whole wheat bread (2 slices)
  *Lean roast beef, unseasoned (**2 oz**)
  American cheese, low-fat and low sodium
    (¾ oz)
  Lettuce (1 leaf)
  Tomato (3 slices)
  Margarine (2 tsp)
Fruit and cottage cheese salad
  Cottage cheese, **1%** and low sodium (½ cup)
  Peaches, canned in juice (½ cup)
Apple juice, unsweetened (1 cup)

DINNER

***Flounder** (3 oz)
  Vegetable oil (1 tsp)
*Baked potato (1 medium)
  Margarine (2 tsp)
Green beans (½ cup), seasoned with margarine
  (½ tsp)
Carrots (½ cup), seasoned with margarine
  (½ tsp)
White dinner roll (1 medium)
  Margarine (1 tsp)
Frozen yogurt (1 cup)
Iced tea, unsweetened (1 cup)

(continued)

Boldface food items represent differences between the Step One and Step Two Diets. See companion menu.
*No salt is added in recipe preparation or as seasoning. All margarine is low sodium.

Step One and Step Two Diet Menus *(Continued)*

SAMPLE **MENUS**

Traditional American Cuisine: Males 25–49 Years

Step One Sample Menus *(Continued)*

SNACK

Popcorn (3 cups)
  Margarine (1 T)

Calories	2518
Total fat, % kcals:	29
SFA, % kcals:	8.6
Cholesterol, mg:	181
Protein, % kcals:	18
Total carb, % kcals:	53
Simple carb, % carb:	36
Complex carb, % carb:	64
*Sodium, mg:	1821

100% RDA met for all nutrients except:
  Zinc 90%

Step Two Sample Menus *(Continued)*

SNACK

*Popcorn (3 cups)
  Margarine (1 T)

Calories	2533
Total fat, % kcals:	28
SFA, % kcals:	6.6
Cholesterol, mg:	150
Protein, % kcals:	17
Total carb, % kcals:	55
Simple carb, % carb:	36
Complex carb, % carb:	64
*Sodium, mg:	1803

100% RDA met for all nutrients except:
  Zinc 90%

POTENTIAL PROBLEM/RATIONALE

Inadequate iron intake related to the restriction on the amount of red meat allowed. Red meats are the richest source of iron in the diet.

NURSING INTERVENTIONS AND CONSIDERATIONS

Assess iron status periodically and provide supplements as needed.

Encourage the client to eat other foods high in iron, such as dried fruits, fortified cereals and grains, green leafy vegetables, and dried peas and beans. Instruct the client to consume a good source of vitamin C at each meal to enhance iron absorption from plant sources.

POTENTIAL PROBLEM/RATIONALE

Increased sodium intake related to the use of specially prepared low-cholesterol products, such as imitation cheese, bacon, and eggs.

NURSING INTERVENTIONS AND CONSIDERATIONS

If the client also is following a low-sodium diet, calculate the amount of sodium being consumed from these products. If possible, revise the low-sodium diet to include as many of these products as desired. If necessary, encourage only limited use of high-sodium, cholesterol-free imitation foods.

POTENTIAL PROBLEM/RATIONALE

Difficulty buying a variety of specialty foods related to increased cost. Polyunsaturated margarines, egg substitutes, and other imitation foods often cost more than the items they are intended to replace.

NURSING INTERVENTIONS AND CONSIDERATIONS

Advise the client that polyunsaturated margarines must be used if the diet is to be followed

(continued)

Step One and Step Two Diet Menus *(Continued)*

successfully; for economy, they can be purchased in quantity while on sale and kept frozen until ready to use. Although other imitation products add variety to the diet, they are not essential and need not be used.

POTENTIAL PROBLEM/RATIONALE

Boredom related to the restrictive nature of the diet.

NURSING INTERVENTIONS AND CONSIDERATIONS

Provide a variety of recipes using allowed foods.

Refer the client to the local American Heart Association for additional resources.

Consume a varied and nutritious diet.

Name foods that are high in saturated fats, polyunsaturated fats, monounsaturated fats, and cholesterol.

Lose weight, if overweight.

NURSING INTERVENTIONS

Diet Management

Reduce total fat, saturated fat, and cholesterol to levels recommended in the Step One Diet (see Tables 17-5 and 17-6).

Adjust calorie intake to attain or maintain healthy weight.

Increase intake of carbohydrates, especially complex carbohydrates and soluble fiber.

Allow moderate use of alcohol, if appropriate.

Client Teaching

Instruct the client:

That the three most effective dietary modifications for lowering serum cholesterol are 1) to decrease saturated fat; 2) to limit dietary cholesterol; and 3) to lose weight, if overweight.

That fat in food is usually a mixture of all three types of fats: saturated, polyunsaturated, and monounsaturated. A food is considered a saturated fat or a polyunsaturated fat based on which type of fat is included in the food in the largest concentration (see Table 3-4).

On the role of saturated fat. Saturated fats raise LDL-cholesterol levels and are found mostly in animal fats: meats, cheese, lard, butter, suet, salt pork, and bacon drippings. Saturated fat intake should decrease. Coconut oil, palm oil, and palm kernel oil, which are economical tropical oils used in food processing, are also highly saturated but contribute far fewer calories to the diet than animal fats.

On the role of cholesterol. Dietary cholesterol tends to raise serum cholesterol, although the impact is less than that of saturated fat. Cholesterol is produced by the body, so that dietary intake is not essential. Cholesterol is found only in animal products, both in the muscle and the fat; therefore, a low-fat animal product is not necessarily low in cholesterol (eg, shrimp). The richest sources of cholesterol are organ meats and egg yolks (see Table 3-5); organ meats should be avoided, and egg yolks limited to four or fewer per week, including those used in food preparation. Fruits, vegetables, grains, cereals, nuts, and legumes contain no cholesterol. Egg whites are also cholesterol-free and may be used as desired.

On the role of polyunsaturated fats. Polyunsaturated fats, which are found in highest concentrations in vegetable oils, tend to lower both the "good" and the "bad" cholesterol. The average American does not need to alter his or her current intake of PUFA.

On the role of monounsaturated fats. Monounsaturated fats, which are found in highest concentrations in peanut oil, olive oil, and canola oil, tend to lower the "bad" cholesterol without having an adverse effect on the "good" cholesterol. They should provide more calories in the diet than either saturated or polyunsaturated fats.

That the fats in fatty fish, like herring, salmon, mackerel, and trout, may help prevent heart disease. If the client likes fatty fish, encourage its consumption. Caution the client against using fish oil supplements.

On the sources of "hidden" fats in the diet: baked goods, cheese, processed meats.

That soluble fiber, which is abundant in oatmeal, oat bran, dried peas and beans, citrus fruits, apples, and certain vegetables, helps to lower serum cholesterol. Encourage the client to gradually increase fiber intake so that the risk of unpleasant side effects (gas, bloating, and diarrhea) is reduced.

On general diet guidelines:
- Limit egg yolks to four or fewer per week for the Step One Diet, and two or fewer for the Step Two Diet, including those used in food preparation.
- Limit meat intake to 5 to 6 oz/day, using mostly skinless poultry; lean, well-trimmed cuts of beef, pork, and lamb; and fish, shellfish, and processed meats made from lean meat.
- Avoid organ meats, regular processed meats, poultry with skin, fatty cuts of meat; and fried fish, shellfish, or poultry.
- Use canola, olive, peanut, corn, and other polyunsaturated oils; use soft or liquid margarine made from those oils. Avoid butter, solid margarine, shortening, and lard.
- Substitute skim milk and skim-milk products for whole milk and whole-milk products.
- Eat more fruits, vegetables, and whole grains, which are naturally low in fat and are cholesterol-free.
- Choose low-fat desserts, like low-fat and nonfat yogurt, ice milk, sherbet, sorbet, fruit ice, popsicles, angel food cake, fig bars, ginger snaps, and other low-fat cakes and cookies.

On food preparation techniques and meal planning ideas to reduce saturated fat content:
- Eat occasional meatless meals.

- Trim fat from meat before cooking; chicken can be cooked with the skin on, but the skin should be removed before eating.
- Tender cuts of meat—sirloin and rib—are higher in fat and calories than less tender cuts such as round, loin, and flank.
- Use meat more as a condiment than as the main entree. For example, when preparing casseroles, reduce the meat by half and double the complex CHO (rice, potato, pasta).
- Place meats to be baked or roasted on a rack to allow the fat to drain.
- Bake, broil, steam, or saute foods in vegetable cooking spray or allowed oils.
- Prepare foods from "scratch" instead of purchasing convenience foods and mixes, which tend to be high in saturated fat.
- Use allowed oils to season cooked vegetables and in the preparation of salad dressings, marinades, pie crusts, barbecue sauces, and skim-milk cream sauces.
- Reduce fat by one half or more in casserole and quickbread recipes.
- Substitute low-fat items for high-fat items whenever possible (see the display, Low-Fat Cooking).
- Make fat-free soup stock by preparing the stock a day ahead and refrigerating it overnight. The fat will harden and can be removed easily from the surface. Also, make fat-free gravies, thickened with cornstarch, by this method.
- Use herbs and spices, lemon juice, and flavored vinegars to flavor foods without fat.
- Use these low-fat snack ideas: low-fat yogurt, fresh fruits and vegetables, dried fruit, unbuttered popcorn, unsalted pretzels, bread sticks, melba toast, frozen juice bars, low-fat crackers.

On how to interpret descriptive terms about calories, fat, saturated fat, and cholesterol on labels (see display, Descriptive Labeling Terms).

On how to order from a menu while dining out (see display, Ordering Out With Fat in Mind).

Provide the client with appropriate teaching materials, recipes, and information on additional resources.

Monitoring Progress

Monitor for the following signs or symptoms:

Compliance with the diet, and the need for follow-up diet counseling.

Effectiveness of the diet: LDL-cholesterol should begin to decline 3 to 4 weeks after the diet is initiated; if the client fails to achieve the desired goal after 3 months of good compliance, progress to the Step Two Diet.

Weight, weight changes.

Other risk factors, if appropriate (eg, hypertension, diabetes, smoking).

Evaluation

Evaluation is ongoing. Provided that the plan of care has not changed, the client will achieve the goals as stated above.

Low-Fat Cooking

High-Fat Food	Low-Fat Alternatives	Grams of Fat "Saved"
1 oz hard cheese	1 oz low-fat cheese	4
	1 oz low-fat processed cheese	7
	2 tbsp grated parmesan cheese	6
1 whole egg	¼ cup egg substitute	6
	2 egg whites	6
1 cup whole milk	1 cup 2% milk	5
	1 cup 1% milk	7
	1 cup skim milk	10
1 cup sour cream	1 cup reduced-fat sour cream	32
	1 cup low-fat cottage cheese (puréed)	44
	1 cup plain nonfat yogurt	48
1 cup regular mayonnaise	1 cup reduced-fat mayonnaise	111
	1 cup nonfat mayonnaise	175
1 cup whole-milk ricotta cheese	1 cup part-skim ricotta	12
	1 cup regular cottage cheese	22
	1 cup low-fat cottage cheese	28
1 cup heavy cream, liquid	1 cup half-and-half	61
	1 cup evaporated whole milk	69
	1 cup evaporated skim milk	87
1 cup regular ice cream	1 cup ice milk	8
	1 cup frozen yogurt	10
	1 cup nonfat frozen dessert	14
1 oz cream cheese	1 oz reduced-fat cream cheese	5
	2 tbsp puréed low-fat cream cheese	9.5
1 cup white sauce	1 cup paste-method white sauce made with:	
	2% milk	63
	1% milk	65
	skim milk	67
1 tbsp regular Italian dressing	1 cup low-calorie Italian	8

DRUG ALERT *Cholesterol-Lowering Drugs*

Bile acid sequestrants (cholestyramine, colestipol) are used to lower LDL-cholesterol. They are both powders that must be mixed with water or fruit juice, and are usually taken once or twice a day with meals. Because they are not absorbed from the gastrointestinal (GI) tract, they do not produce systemic toxicity. Decreased absorption of the fat-soluble vitamins and folic acid has been reported with prolonged high doses (NCEP, 1993). GI symptoms may include constipation, bloating, epigastric fullness, nausea, and flatulence.

Nicotinic acid lowers serum total and LDL-cholesterol levels and triglyceride levels, and raises HDL-cholesterol levels. Nicotinamide, which is also frequently referred to as niacin, has no effect on serum lipids and cannot be used as a substitute for nicotinic acid. Nicotinic acid has frequent side effects, including flushing, which may be mini-

Descriptive Labeling Terms

Term	What It Means
FAT	
Fat-free	Less than 0.5 g of fat per serving
Saturated fat-free	Less than 0.5 g per serving and the level of *trans* fatty acids does not exceed 1% of total fat
Low-fat	3 g or less per serving. If the serving is 30 g or less or 2 tablespoons or less, must be 3 g or less per 50 g of the food
Low-saturated fat	1 g or less per serving and not more than 15% of calories from saturated fatty acids
Reduced or less fat	At least 25% less per serving than reference food
Reduced or less saturated fat	At least 25% less per serving than reference food
CHOLESTEROL	
Cholesterol-free	Less than 2 mg of cholesterol and 2 g or less of saturated fat per serving
Low-cholesterol	20 mg cholesterol or less and 2 g or less saturated fat per serving. If the serving is 30 g or less or 2 tablespoons or less, must be 20 mg cholesterol or less and 2 g or less of saturated fat per 50 g of the food.
Reduced or less cholesterol	At least 25% less and 2 g or less of saturated fat per serving than reference food
SODIUM	
Sodium-free	Less than 5 mg per serving
Low-sodium	140 mg or less per serving. If the serving is 30 g or less or 2 tablespoons or less, must be 140 mg or less sodium per 50 g of the food.
Very-low-sodium	35 mg or less per serving. If the serving is 30 g or less or 2 tablespoons or less, must be 35 mg or less per 50 g of the food.
Reduced or less sodium	At least 25% less per serving than reference food

Source: FDA (1993). Focus on Food Labeling. Read the label, set a healthy table. Rockville, MD: FDA, US Public Health Service, Department of Health and Human Services. DHHS Publication No. (FDA) 93-2262.

mized by gradually increasing the dose, taking the drug during or after meals, and taking an aspirin 30 minutes before the drug. Nausea, dyspepsia, flatulence, vomiting, diarrhea, and activation of peptic ulcer may also occur (NCEP, 1993).

Hydroxymethylglutaryl coenzyme A (HMG CoA) reductase inhibitors (statins—lovastatin, pravastatin, simvastatin) lower LDL-cholesterol. Because they are more effective at lowering LDL-cholesterol when taken in the evening than in the morning, the U.S. Food and Drug Administration (FDA) recommends that lovastatin be taken with the evening meal, pravastatin at bedtime, and simvastatin in the evening (NCEP, 1993). Side effects are most often gastrointestinal: dyspepsia, flatus, constipation, abdominal pain or cramps.

Myocardial Infarction

A myocardial infarction (MI) involves the destruction of heart tissue in areas of the heart that are deprived of blood and oxygen. An MI can occur as a result of athero-

Ordering Out With Fat in Mind

	Instead of Ordering:	Request:
Appetizers	Cream soups	Clear broth, vegetable soup
	Clams casino	Shrimp cocktail
	Stuffed mushrooms	Fresh vegetable tray
Salads	Caesar, potato, taco, or pasta	Fruit salad without whipped cream or mayonnaise
	Tossed salad with dressing	Ask that dressing be served "on the side," then dip the fork in the dressing before loading the greens on the fork
Entrees	Anything fried, breaded, creamed, braised, or in a butter sauce	Broiled, baked, grilled, or stir-fried. Ask for sauces and gravies "on the side"
	King or Queen cuts	No more than 6 oz of meat, or ask for a doggie bag and save half for another meal
Side dishes	Hash browns, fried potatoes	Baked potato with margarine "on the side"
	Coleslaw	Vegetables without sauces or breading
Desserts	Pie, cake, other rich desserts	Angel food cake with fresh fruit or gelatin
		Or indulge, but split the serving with a companion. Another alternative: gourmet coffee, but watch for cream and alcohol
	Ice cream	Ice milk, frozen yogurt, sorbet, fruit ice
Breakfast	Regular eggs	Scrambled egg substitutes
	Toast, English muffin, bagel	Good choices, but ask that they be served dry, with margarine "on the side"
Sandwiches	Traditional sandwiches and burgers with mayonnaise or "special sauce"	Ask that they be served plain and add mustard or ketchup. Lettuce, tomato, onions, sprouts, and green pepper add texture and interest
	Super size	Regular size
	Fried chicken or fish	Broiled or baked chicken or fish
Pizza		Load up on vegetables
	Pepperoni, sausage, and other meat	Pat the pizza surface with a paper napkin to absorb grease before eating

sclerosis, arterial occlusion from embolus or thrombus, or myocardial hypertrophy caused by congestive heart failure and hypertension, or secondary to a temporary reduction in blood flow to the heart related to shock, GI bleeding, severe dehydration, or hypotension. MI are the most frequent cause of death in North America; 15% to 20% of white Americans die from MI, with a slightly lower incidence among blacks.

Symptoms of an impending or actual MI include spontaneous, constrictive, prolonged chest pain, which is not relieved by rest or nitrates; the pain may radiate to one or both arms, the neck, and the back. Symptoms of shock, such as hypotension, gray facial color, cold diaphoresis, tachycardia or bradycardia, and weak, irregular pulse, may be observed. The client may experience nausea, vomiting, shortness of breath, physical or mental fatigue, dizziness, anxiety, and apprehension. However, half of all acute MI victims have none of the typical symptoms (Hicks, 1994).

"Silent" MI, although it is not diagnosed at the time of an impending heart attack, can be as deadly as a symptomatic MI and just as likely to cause complications.

Myocardial infarctions that do not result in sudden death can cause severe and life-threatening complications: arrhythmias, shock, congestive heart failure (CHF), rupture of the heart, pulmonary embolism, and recurrent heart attacks.

Treatment of an acute MI seeks to alleviate symptoms and prevent further damage with continual assessment and monitoring, complete rest, sedation, narcotics, oxygen, and intravenous fluids. The diet is modified to prevent diet-induced arrhythmias and to reduce cardiac workload. After the acute phase has passed, treatment focuses on rehabilitation and education of the client and the family. Diet modification is aimed at reducing the diet-responsive risk factors, such as hypercholesterolemia, obesity, diabetes mellitus, and hypertension.

NURSING PROCESS

Assessment

In addition to the general cardiovascular assessment criteria (see display, General Cardiovascular Assessment Criteria), assess for the following factors:

State of recovery: acute, subacute, or rehabilitative

The presence of symptoms that interfere with eating, such as shortness of breath, fatigue, anorexia, nausea, or apprehension

Other medical conditions that require diet intervention, such as hypertension, diabetes mellitus, or obesity

The use of medications that produce nutritional side effects, such as potassium-depleting diuretics

Nursing Diagnosis

Health Seeking Behaviors, as evidenced by a lack of knowledge of dietary management of heart disease and a desire to learn

Planning and Implementation

Initially, clients who experience an MI are ordered nothing by mouth (NPO) and are given intravenous fluids; a clear to full liquid diet may resume within 24 to 48 hours post MI. In an attempt to reduce cardiac workload, total calories and meal size are often restricted. When the diet is progressed, soft, bland foods that are easily digested may be given in 4 to 6 meals daily. Gassy foods are avoided, but fiber intake should be adequate to prevent constipation. Because they may produce cardiac arrhythmias and slow the heart rate, food and liquid served at extreme temperatures are avoided. Caffeine is a stimulant and therefore should be eliminated.

When the client enters the rehabilitative phase, usually 5 to 10 days post MI, the diet is individualized according to the client's weight, serum lipid levels, and medical condition. A Step One or Step Two Diet (see Table 17-6) may be indicated, and calories are adjusted for healthy weight. A sodium-restricted diet is usually prescribed to treat or prevent hypertension, edema, or CHF. Ongoing client education is extremely important to maximize diet compliance. Dietary changes should be initiated gradually and sequentially.

CLIENT GOALS

Acute Phase
   The client will:

   Avoid diet-induced arrhythmias and cardiac stimulants
   Avoid food and liquids that increase cardiac workload; avoid gastric distention, flatulence, and constipation
   Begin healing and convalescence

Rehabilitative Phase (begins 5 to 10 days post MI)
   The client will:

   Reduce serum lipid levels and control medical risk factors, if appropriate
   Consume a nutritionally adequate diet with calories for healthy weight

NURSING INTERVENTIONS

Diet Management

Initial Diet (begins 24 to 48 hours post MI until the rehabilitative phase begins):

   Limit calories and provide small, frequent meals to avoid abdominal distention that could exert pressure on the heart. Calorie intake is increased as the client improves.
   Provide liquids or soft, bland foods that are easy to digest; eliminate gassy foods and individual intolerances.
   Avoid foods and liquids served at temperature extremes, which may produce cardiac arrhythmias.
   Eliminate caffeinated beverages that may stimulate heart rate.
   Provide complete or partial assistance with eating, depending on the client's strength.

Rehabilitative Phase (begins 5 to 10 days post MI):

   Advance the diet as tolerated to three meals per day; however, small, frequent meals are recommended for clients with persistent angina.
   Individualize the diet according to the client's weight, serum lipid levels, and medical conditions. A Step One or Step Two Diet may be indicated (see Table 17-6).
   Restrict intake of sodium to prevent or treat hypertension, edema, or CHF.

Client Teaching

Client teaching is not indicated during the acute and subacute phases. During the rehabilitative phase, the client may be instructed on the Step One or Step Two Diet (see Table 17-6) and be advised to limit sodium; additional instructions may be necessary to control other diet-responsive risk factors, such as obesity, diabetes mellitus, and hypertension.

Monitoring Progress

Monitor for the following signs or symptoms:

Tolerance of the diet (ie, absence of postprandial cardiac changes such as arrhythmias and increased heart rate)
The client's ability to self-feed; as the client moves into the rehabilitative phase, monitor the presence of other risk factors and the need for diet counseling.

Evaluation

Evaluation is ongoing. Provided that the plan of care has not changed, the client will achieve the goals as stated above.

Congestive Heart Failure

Congestive heart failure (CHF) is a syndrome that is characterized by the inability of the heart to maintain adequate blood flow through the circulatory system, which leads to decreased blood flow to the kidneys, excessive sodium and fluid retention, peripheral and pulmonary edema, and finally, an overworked and enlarged heart. The severity of CHF can vary from mild to severe. Although the heart and its circulatory efficiency are principally affected initially, the entire circulation eventually is altered.

CHF develops in 50% to 60% of all cases of organic heart disease that weaken the muscle action of the heart: MI, hypertension, congenital heart disease, cardiomyopathies, valve disorders, and arrhythmias. CHF also may occur secondary to circulatory overload related to excessive intravenous fluids or renal failure. Circulatory deficits such as hemorrhage and dehydration, as well as pulmonary diseases such as chronic lung disease and pulmonary embolism, may also lead to CHF. In addition, any condition that increases metabolic demands can result in CHF (eg, hyperthyroidism, pregnancy, anemia, fever, infection, and obesity). Frequently, CHF arises from a combination of factors.

Initially, CHF may be classified as left-sided or right-sided failure; eventually, symptoms of both occur. Symptoms of left-sided heart failure, such as dyspnea, orthopnea, paroxysmal nocturnal dyspnea, pleural effusion, and pulmonary edema, are caused by inefficient oxygenation of the blood related to lung congestion. Right-sided heart failure most often causes dependent edema (especially of the feet and ankles), pitting edema, ascites, sudden weight gain related to fluid retention, upper abdominal pain related to liver congestion, anorexia and nausea, nocturia, weakness, and distended neck veins. Almost all clients with CHF are at risk for sudden death from frequent, complex tachyarrhythmias; chronic CHF may also lead to pneumonia and pulmonary embolism (Lewandowski, 1995).

The treatment of CHF involves treatment of the underlying cause. Physical and mental rest help to decrease cardiac workload. Digitalis may be used to slow the heart rate and strengthen its beat. Diuretic therapy is used to help rid the body of excess fluid. Oxygen therapy may be necessary. Diet intervention is used to reduce sodium and fluid retention and to minimize cardiac workload.

NURSING PROCESS

Assessment

In addition to the general cardiovascular assessment criteria (see display, Cardiovascular Assessment), assess for the following factors:

Edema: areas affected, severity, interventions attempted and the results.

The presence of symptoms that may affect intake (eg, nausea, anorexia, dyspnea, upper abdominal pain, weakness).

Dietary changes made in response to symptoms (ie, foods avoided, foods preferred). Determine which foods are best and least tolerated.

Weight, recent weight changes. Note that sudden weight gain is a symptom of fluid retention.

Usual intake of sodium, which is abundant in table salt, canned soups, meats, vegetables, processed meats, convenience foods, many condiments, and traditional snack foods (see display, Sources of Sodium and Potassium).

Intake of foods high in potassium, such as fresh and dried fruits, fruit juices, many fresh and frozen vegetables, dairy products, whole grains, meats, fish, and poultry.

Intake and output.

Abnormal laboratory values and their significance, especially blood urea nitrogen (BUN), creatinine, albumin, glucose, sodium, potassium, chloride, and lipids.

The use of diuretics; determine whether they are potassium-sparing or potassium-wasting.

Nursing Diagnosis

Fluid Volume Excess, related to CHF

Planning and Implementation

Edema related to CHF can be relieved by reducing sodium intake, as extracellular fluid retention does not occur in the absence of sodium. Permitted sodium intake may vary from 250 to 2000 mg, depending on the severity of CHF.

In most cases, sodium restriction, used alone or in combination with diuretics (low-sodium diets enhance the sodium-excreting effects of diuretics), effectively reduces fluid volume without the need for fluid restriction. However, fluid restriction may be necessary if edema persists despite a low-sodium diet.

A diet that is low in calories but otherwise nutritionally adequate is indicated for overweight clients. Attaining ideal or slightly under ideal weight reduces the cardiac workload.

Sources of Sodium and Potassium

SODIUM SOURCES

The rule of 6 S's:

Soups

Canned, freeze-dried soup mixes, broth, bouillon (unless salt-free)

Sauces

Canned gravy, spaghetti sauce, and other cooking sauces; packaged sauce mixes and convenience mixes

Snacks

Processed varieties like chips, popcorn, pretzels, snack crackers, and salted nuts

Smoked meats or fish

Like bacon, chipped beef, corned beef, cold cuts, ham, hot dogs, sausage

Sauerkraut

And other foods preserved in brine, like pickles, pickled beets, pickled sausage, pickled herring, pickled eggs

Seasonings

Horseradish, soy sauce, Worcestershire sauce, ketchup, mustard, meat tenderizer, monosodium glutamate

POTASSIUM SOURCES

Fruit

Especially bananas, citrus fruits and their juices, melon, raisins, dried dates, apricots, avocados

Vegetables

Sweet and white potatoes, tomatoes and tomato products, dried peas and beans, green leafy vegetables, carrots, corn, spinach, winter squash

Whole grains, especially those containing bran

Fresh meat

Milk, yogurt, ice cream, pudding

Potassium-containing salt substitutes

NoSalt, Seasoned NoSalt, Morton Salt Substitute, Morton Lite Salt Mixture, Adolph's Salt Substitute, Adolph's Seasoned Salt, Diamond Crystal, Co-Salt

The diet should be individualized according to the client's tolerance. Emphasize easy-to-digest foods, such as carbohydrates, rather than protein, fat, and gas-forming foods.

It should be noted that malnutrition resulting from poor nutritional intake and long-term medication use may not be apparent in clients with edema. **Cardiac cachexia** is characterized by anorexia and muscle wasting that is not readily apparent because of edema.

CLIENT GOALS

The client will:

Attain or maintain normal fluid balance.
Consume adequate calories to attain or maintain healthy body weight; correct any nutritional deficits.

Describe the principles and rationale of diet management for CHF and implement the appropriate dietary changes.

Avoid potassium imbalance by consuming the appropriate potassium intake, based on the type of diuretic used.

Avoid agents that act as cardiac stimulants.

Avoid agents that induce gastric distention and increase pressure on the heart.

NURSING INTERVENTIONS

Diet Management

Limit sodium intake (acceptable range: 250 mg to 2000 mg; see display, Sodium-Restricted Diets). Initial allowance may be progressed as edema subsides. Some clients may tolerate 4 to 6 g of sodium after their condition has stabilized.

(text continues on page 581)

Sodium-Restricted Diets

The objective of low-sodium diets is to rid the body of excess sodium and fluid accumulation associated with certain disorders, such as liver disease characterized by edema and ascites, congestive heart failure, renal disease characterized by edema and hypertension, and adrenocortical therapy. Low-sodium diets also are used in the treatment, and possible prevention, of hypertension.

Low-sodium diets are contraindicated for sodium-wasting renal diseases, such as pyelonephritis, polycystic renal disease, and bilateral hydronephrosis; pregnancy; clients with ileostomies; and myxedema.

The characteristics of low-sodium diets vary according to the level of restriction; 500-mg and 250-mg sodium diets are unpalatable, are extremely difficult to follow, and are likely to be inadequate in some nutrients. To promote compliance and to allow greater flexibility, exchange lists featuring the sodium content of high- and low-sodium foods may be used.

LEVELS OF RESTRICTION

3000 mg sodium (130 mEq)

Up to ¼ teaspoon of salt allowed daily
Eliminate high-sodium processed foods and beverages

2000 mg (87 mEq)

Eliminate processed and prepared foods and beverages high in sodium
No salt is allowed in cooking or at the table
Limit milk and milk products to 16 oz/day

1000 mg (45 mEq)

Follow 2000-mg sodium restrictions plus:
Omit regular margarines and salad dressings
Limit regular breads to 2 servings per day.

500 mg (22 mEq)

Follow 1000-mg sodium restrictions plus:
Eliminate vegetables naturally high in sodium: beets, beet greens, carrots, kale, spinach, celery, white turnips, rutabagas, mustard greens, chard, peas, and dandelion greens
Use only low-sodium bread in place of regular bread
Use distilled water for cooking and drinking
Eliminate sherbet and flavored gelatin
Limit meat to 6 oz/day; one egg may be substituted daily for 1 oz of meat
Limit milk and milk products to 8 oz daily

250 mg (11 mEq)

Follow 500-mg sodium restrictions plus:
Use low-sodium milk in place of regular milk
(continued)

Sodium-Restricted Diets *(Continued)*

FOODS HIGH IN SODIUM

Food Group	Foods High in Added Sodium	Foods Naturally High in Sodium	Foods Lower in Sodium
Meats	Real and imitation bacon, cold cuts, chipped or corned beef, frankfurters, smoked meats, sausage, salt pork, canned meats, codfish, canned, salted or smoked fish, kosher meats, frozen and powder egg substitutes, regular peanut butter	Brain, kidney, clams, crab, lobster, oysters, scallops, shrimp, and other shellfish	Fresh, frozen, or canned low-sodium meat and poultry; eggs; low-sodium cheeses and peanut butter; fresh bass, bluefish, catfish, cod, eel, flounder, halibut, rockfish, salmon, sole, trout, tuna; canned low-sodium tuna and salmon
Dairy products	Buttermilk, regular cheeses and cottage cheese; commercial milk products such as ice cream, malted milk, milk mixes, milk shakes, sherbet		Skim, 2%, whole, evaporated, and low-sodium milk; low-sodium cheeses, low-sodium cottage cheese
Fruits and vegetables	Crystallized or glazed fruit, maraschino cherries, dried fruit with sodium preservatives added; canned vegetables and vegetable juices unless low sodium, sauerkraut, frozen vegetables with added salt	Spinach, celery, beets and beet greens, carrots, artichokes, white turnips, Swiss chard, dandelion greens, kale, mustard greens	Fresh, frozen without salt, and low-sodium canned vegetables, except those listed Fresh, frozen, canned or dried fruits without added sodium
Breads and cereals	Commercial mixes, bread and rolls made from frozen bread dough, graham and all other crackers except low-sodium crackers, instant rice and pasta mixes, commercial casserole mixes, commercial stuffing, instant and quick-cooking cereals, most dry cereals (except puffed rice, puffed wheat, and shredded wheat), self-rising flour, self-rising cornmeal, waffles, quick breads, and other baked products containing salt, baking soda, baking powder, or egg white		Low-sodium breads, crackers, cereals, and cereal products; baked products made without salt, baking powder containing sodium, and baking soda; low-sodium mixes; unsalted cooked cereals, puffed rice, puffed wheat, shredded wheat, barley, cornmeal, cornstarch, unsalted matzo; unsalted macaroni, and rice

(continued)

Sodium-Restricted Diets (Continued)

FOODS HIGH IN SODIUM

Food Group	Foods High in Added Sodium	Foods Naturally High in Sodium	Foods Lower in Sodium
Fats	Salted butter and margarine, regular commercial salad dressings and mayonnaise		Unsalted butter, margarine, salad dressings, and mayonnaise; cooking oils and shortening
Miscellaneous	Regular canned or frozen soups; soup mixes; salted popcorn, nuts, potato chips, and snack foods; instant cocoa mixes; powdered drink mixes, canned fruit drinks; pastries; commercial candies, cakes, cookies, and gelatin desserts		Alcohol; coffee and coffee substitutes, lemonade, tea, salt-free or low-sodium candy, unflavored gelatin, jam, jelly, maple syrup, honey; unsalted nuts and popcorn
Seasonings and condiments	Sea salt, rock salt, and kosher salt; barbecue sauce, bouillon cubes, catsup, celery salt, seed, and leaves; chili sauce; tartar sauce; garlic salt; horseradish made with salt; meat extracts, sauces, and tenderizers; Kitchen Bouquet, gravy, and sauce mixes; monosodium glutamate; prepared mustard, olives, onion salt, pickles, relishes, saccharin, soy sauce, teriyaki sauce, sugar substitutes containing sodium, Worcestershire sauce		Allspice, almond extract, anise seed, basil, bay leaf, low-sodium bouillon, caraway seed, cardamon, low-sodium catsup, chili powder, chives, cinnamon, cloves, cocoa (1 to 2 teaspoons), coconut, cumin, curry, dill, fennel, garlic and garlic powder, ginger, horseradish made without salt, juniper, lemon juice, mace, maple extract, marjoram, low-sodium meat extracts, low-sodium meat tenderizers, mint, mustard (dry and seeds), nutmeg, orange extract, oregano, paprika, parsley, pepper, peppermint extract, poppy seed, poultry seasoning, purslane, rosemary, saffron, sage, salt substitutes (if approved by a physician), savory, sesame seeds, sorrel, sugar, tarragon, thyme, turmeric, vanilla, vinegar, walnut extract, wine

(continued)

Sodium-Restricted Diets (Continued)

2000-MG SODIUM DIET	250-MG SODIUM DIET
BREAKFAST	**BREAKFAST**

2000-MG SODIUM DIET

BREAKFAST

½ cup orange juice
¾ cup shredded wheat
2 slices toast
2 tsp margarine
1 tbsp strawberry jam
1 cup 1% milk
Sugar
Coffee/tea
Pepper

LUNCH

2 oz sliced chicken breast on 2 slices whole-
  wheat bread with 2 tsp mayonnaise, tomato,
  and lettuce
Tossed salad with oil-and-vinegar dressing
Fresh fruit
4 vanilla wafers
1 cup 1% milk
Coffee/tea
Sugar/pepper

DINNER

4 oz broiled halibut
Baked potato
2 tsp margarine
½ cup broccoli
Coleslaw made with oil-and-vinegar dressing
1 dinner roll
½ cup sherbet
Coffee/tea
Sugar/pepper

SNACK

1 cup unsalted popcorn
Apple juice

POTENTIAL PROBLEM/RATIONALE

   Hyponatremia (nausea, malaise, possible confusion, seizures, and coma) related to a sodium
intake that is too low, especially when combined
with the use of diuretics. For most people, the

250-MG SODIUM DIET

BREAKFAST

½ c orange juice
¾ c shredded wheat
2 slices low-sodium toast
2 tsp unsalted margarine
1 tbsp strawberry jam
1 cup low-sodium milk
Sugar
Coffee/tea
Pepper

LUNCH

2 oz sliced chicken breast on 2 slices low-sodium
  bread with 2 tsp low-sodium mayonnaise,
  tomato, lettuce
Tossed salad with oil and vinegar dressing
Fresh fruit
Fruit ice
Sugar/pepper
Coffee/tea
Apricot nectar

DINNER

4 oz broiled beef patty
Baked potato
2 tsp unsalted margarine
½ cup broccoli
1 slice low-sodium bread
Fresh strawberries
Coffee/tea
Sugar/pepper

SNACK

1 cup plain popcorn
Apple juice

risk of hyponatremia is insignificant. However,
clients with renal disease and the elderly may not
be able adequately to reabsorb enough sodium
while following a low-sodium diet

(continued)

Sodium-Restricted Diets (Continued)

NURSING INTERVENTIONS AND CONSIDERATIONS

To allow homeostatic mechanisms time to adapt in the elderly and clients with renal disease, initiate a low-sodium diet gradually. Observe for signs of sodium deficiency and liberalize the diet if necessary.

POTENTIAL PROBLEM/RATIONALE

Noncompliance, which may be related to the following situations:

Pervasiveness of sodium in the diet. Not all high-sodium foods taste salty.

Preference of salt taste

Ethnic or religious customs. For instance, Chinese cooking relies heavily on soy sauce and MSG for seasoning. Kosher meats are bathed in a brine solution for 1 hour after slaughter. Although rinsing does remove some of the salt, kosher meats remain high in sodium.

Reliance on convenience products and canned foods, which are high in sodium. This is especially common among the elderly and people living alone.

NURSING INTERVENTIONS AND CONSIDERATIONS

Assure the client that with time, the taste for salt lessens, and it becomes easier to follow the diet.

Advise the client that label-reading is essential. Foods that supply >480 mg sodium/serving (ie, 20% DV) are high-sodium foods and should be avoided.

Provide thorough and periodic instructions on how to incorporate the diet into the client's lifestyle and budget, information on sources of sodium in food and drugs, and lists of sodium alternatives.

If expense and convenience are a problem, allow the client to continue using regular canned meats and vegetables, if possible. Rinsing canned foods under running water for at least 1 minute removes much of the sodium content.

Encourage support from the client's family and urge them to follow the diet if possible.

LOW-SODIUM DIET TEACHING

(Be more or less specific depending on the level of sodium allowed.) Instruct the client

That reducing sodium intake will help the body rid itself of excess fluid and help lower high blood pressure.

That the body may need only about 200–250 mg of sodium a day (less than one tenth of a teaspoon of salt), although most Americans consume 2500 to 5000 mg/day and can tolerate intakes much higher than this.

That sodium appears in the diet in the form of salt (40% sodium) and to some degree in almost all food and beverages. Most unprocessed, unsalted food generally is low in sodium.

That approximately 15% of our sodium intake comes from salt added during cooking and at the table, 75% from processed foods, and 10% from food and water naturally high in sodium.

That sodium compounds are used extensively as preservatives (sodium propionate, sodium sulfite, and sodium benzoate), leavening agents (sodium bicarbonate, baking soda, and baking powder), and flavor enhancers (salt, MSG), and are found in foods that may not taste salty.

That many nonprescription drugs (such as aspirin, cough medicines, laxatives, and antacids), toothpastes, toothpowders, and mouthwashes contain large amounts of sodium and should not be used without a physician's approval.

That salt substitutes replace sodium with potassium or other minerals. "Low-sodium" salt substitutes are not sodium-free and may contain half as much sodium as regular table salt. Use neither type without a physician's approval.

That preference for salt taste eventually will decrease.

(continued)

Sodium-Restricted Diets *(Continued)*

If he or she "cheats" by eating a high-sodium meal or snack, to compensate by eating less sodium than normally allowed for the rest of the day.

How to order off a menu while dining out:

- Request that food not be salted, if possible.
- Choose fruit juice instead of soup for an appetizer.
- Use oil and vinegar or fresh lemon instead of regular salad dressing.
- Order plain meat and vegetables without gravy or sauce.
- Choose plain baked potatoes and season sparingly with sour cream, butter, or just with pepper.
- Select fresh fruit for dessert. If the client is going to splurge, ice cream or sherbet are better choices than pie, cake, cookies, and other desserts.
- Avoid fast-food restaurant meals, which generally are high in sodium.

On food preparation techniques to minimize sodium intake:

- Foods made from "scratch" generally have less sodium than processed foods and mixes.
- Experiment with sodium-free seasoning, such as herbs, spices, lemon juice, vinegar, and wine. Fresh ingredients are more flavorful than dried.
- Commercial "salt alternatives" are sodium-free blends of herbs and spices not intended to taste like salt but to be used as flavor enhancers.
- If permitted by a physician, salt substitutes may be used, although they taste bitter to some people.
- A variety of low-sodium cookbooks are available.

On how to read labels:

- Salt, monosodium glutamate, baking soda, and baking powder contain significant amounts of sodium. Other sodium compounds such as sodium nitrite, benzoate of soda, sodium saccharin, and sodium propionate add less sodium to the diet.
- "Sodium free," "low sodium," "very low sodium," and "reduced" or "less sodium" are defined terms (see display, Descriptive Labeling Terms).
- Numerous low- and reduced-sodium products are available: milk, bread and bread products, cereal, crackers, cakes, cookies, pastries, soups and bouillon, canned vegetables, tomato products, meats, entrées, processed meats, hard and soft cheeses, condiments, nuts and peanut butter, butter, margarine, salad dressings, baking powder, and snack foods.
- The difference in taste between some low-sodium products and their high-sodium counterparts is barely noticeable; others taste flat and may need to have herbs or spices added.

Provide adequate potassium, based on the type of diuretic prescribed. A high-potassium diet may be indicated for clients who are taking thiazide diuretics (potassium-wasting) and digitalis. Spironolactone and triamterene are potassium-sparing diuretics that do not warrant the intake or use of additional potassium.

Provide calories for "healthy" body weight. Decrease calories for weight loss, if overweight, to lessen cardiac workload.

Provide 5 to 6 small meals per day of nonirritating and non–gas-forming foods to limit gastric distention and pressure on the heart. Fluid may be limited to 2 liters per day or less, depending on the client's response to the sodium restriction.

Initially, eliminate caffeine. After the client's condition has stabilized, coffee intake may be liberalized to 4 to 5 cups/day as tolerated.

Client Teaching

Instruct the client:

On the principles and rationale of diet management for CHF.

On how to implement the changes that are necessary to ensure compliance with a low-sodium diet (see Low-Sodium Diet Teaching section in the display, Sodium-Restricted Diets).

To weigh himself or herself daily without clothes before breakfast. Weight gain that exceeds 2 pounds should be reported.

Monitoring Progress

Monitor for the following signs or symptoms:

Compliance with the diet, and the need for follow-up diet counseling.

Effectiveness of the diet (ie, reduction in edema, weight loss), and evaluate the need for further diet modifications.

Serum potassium; observe for signs of hypokalemia and hyperkalemia.

Evaluation

Evaluation is ongoing. Provided that the plan of care has not changed, the client will achieve the goals as stated above.

VASCULAR DISORDERS

Hypertension

Hypertension is a symptom, not a disease, that is arbitrarily defined as sustained elevated blood pressure greater than or equal to 140/90 mm Hg. It is estimated that hypertension affects one of every four Americans, although only one third of these may actually be diagnosed.

Fewer than 5% of cases of hypertension occur secondary to renal disease, stenosis of the aorta, endocrine imbalance, sodium retention during pregnancy, increased intracranial pressure related to brain tumors, or advanced collagen disease. Eliminating the underlying disorder cures secondary hypertension.

The remaining 95% or more of cases of hypertension occur from unknown causes and are classified as essential, primary, or idiopathic hypertension. Essential hypertension is more common among blacks than whites, and occurs more frequently among men than women until late middle age. In the United States and other developed countries, the prevalence of hypertension rises progressively with aging (National High Blood Pressure Education Program Working Group, 1993). However, animal, clinical, and population studies show that age-related increases in blood pressure cannot be blamed only on biologic changes. Age-related increases in blood pressure appear to be related as well to certain environmental factors: high salt intake, obesity, physical inactivity, excessive alcohol consumption, and an inadequate intake of potassium (National High Blood Pressure Education Program Working Group, 1993). Essential hypertension cannot be cured but may be prevented in large numbers of people through lifestyle changes. Health authorities in the United States and in fourteen other countries advocate reducing salt intake as one way of preventing hypertension (Adams et al, 1995).

Most hypertensive clients are asymptomatic. However, because the blood pressure–cardiovascular disease risk relationship is continuous and progressive (even within the "normal" blood pressure range), blood pressure–related vascular complications can occur even before a client is definitively diagnosed with hypertension (National High Blood Pressure Education Program Working Group, 1993). Damage to the small and large vessels throughout the body can affect the heart, brain, eyes, or kidneys. The client may experience angina, intermittent claudication, retinal hemorrhage, severe headache, polyuria, nocturia, dyspnea on exertion, and edema of the extremities. Prolonged hypertension accelerates coronary atherosclerosis. If left untreated, hypertension can lead to peripheral vascular disease, MI, CHF, renal insufficiency, renal failure, CVA, and blindness.

Diet management that is designed to reduce cardiac workload, alleviate sodium retention, and help maintain potassium balance may effectively control essential hypertension in a significant number of clients and preclude the use of drug therapy. Because it has the potential to be completely effective and has no adverse side effects, diet management should be the initial treatment of choice. If the client fails to achieve desired goals, drug therapy (eg, diuretics, vasodilators, adrenergic blocking agents) may be added to diet therapy.

NURSING PROCESS

Assessment

In addition to the general cardiovascular assessment criteria, assess for the following factors (see the display, General Cardiovascular Assessment Criteria):

Lifestyle risk factors: high salt intake, excess weight, physical inactivity, ingestion of more than 1 oz of ethanol/day, low potassium intake, smoking, or a high–saturated fat, high-cholesterol intake (see display, Sources of Sodium and Potassium).

The use of diuretics; identify whether they are potassium-sparing or potassium-wasting.

Coexisting medical conditions that may require diet modification: diabetes, renal insufficiency, atherosclerosis.

Abnormal laboratory values and their significance, especially sodium, potassium, serum lipids, glucose, and BUN.

Nursing Diagnosis

Noncompliance, related to poor understanding of the dietary management of hypertension

Planning and Implementation

The role of diet in the treatment of hypertension has been widely debated since 1904, when the Kempner "rice diet" was found to effectively lower blood pressure. The diet was drastically low in sodium (200 mg) and consisted only of rice, fruit, and sugar. Because the diet was unpalatable, nutritionally inadequate, and difficult to follow, diet therapy was discounted as a practical means of treating hypertension. Studies now show that high blood pressure can be effectively lowered or prevented by reducing sodium intake, losing weight, increasing physical activity, reducing alcohol consumption, and possibly increasing potassium intake.

Observational and experimental studies show that reducing sodium intake lowers blood pressure; even a mild sodium restriction can modestly lower blood pressure in hypertensive clients. Although adults only need 200 to 250 mg of sodium daily, the average American consumes 2500 to 5000 mg of sodium. The National High Blood Pressure Education Program Working Group (1993) recommends that Americans moderate their salt intake and that 2400 mg of sodium per day be established as a national dietary goal.

A gradual reduction in intake may be better accepted and easier to comply with than an abrupt withdrawal of sodium. Because the preference for salt gradually diminishes when intake is limited, following a low-sodium diet tends to get easier with time. Clients who are diagnosed with hypertension are advised to follow a low-sodium diet indefinitely.

Losing weight without reducing sodium intake also lowers blood pressure, even if ideal weight is not attained and regardless of the degree of overweight. In the Trials of Hypertension Prevention, people who lost an average of 8 pounds through dieting and exercise cut their risk of hypertension in half (Leibman, 1995b). Weight loss may also reduce or eliminate the need for medication and thus the potential for toxicity and unpleasant side effects associated with drug therapy. Because weight control has the potential to control hypertension effectively for a large number of people, it is recommended that weight reduction be used as the initial step in treating overweight clients with mild to moderate hypertension.

Studies show that increasing activity, either alone or as part of a weight loss program, lowers blood pressure. It appears that 30 to 45 minutes of moderate-intensity aerobic exercise may actually be better than a more intense workout (Leibman, 1995b). It is recommended that individuals participate in activities such as walking, cycling, dancing, and gardening three to five times per week.

Consistent and powerful evidence links alcohol consumption (3 or more drinks/day) with hypertension. Clients who drink habitually should be advised to limit their consumption to 2 drinks/day or less (1 oz of ethanol or less).

Numerous studies show an inverse relationship between potassium intake and blood pressure: The higher the intake of potassium, the lower the blood pressure.

Some researchers believe that the ratio of potassium to sodium may be equally important. Although adding potassium to an already high intake may not produce much effect, switching from a low-potassium to a high-potassium diet may lower blood pressure. In animals, potassium has been shown to protect against strokes caused by a high salt intake (Leibman, 1995b).

Although a low-fat, low-cholesterol diet does not have a direct effect on blood pressure, a Step One or Step Two Diet (see Table 17-5) is advised because of the synergistic relationship between atherosclerosis and high blood pressure.

Other nutritional factors that are being investigated for their potential effect on blood pressure include calcium, magnesium, and fish oil. Until all the evidence is in, researchers are urging clients to eat a healthy diet, rather than rely on supplements.

Be aware of the potential side effects of antihypertensive and diuretic therapies.

CLIENT GOALS

The client will:

Control blood pressure to avoid complications such as CHF, stroke, and renal disease.

Consume adequate calories to attain or maintain healthy weight.

Maintain normal fluid and electrolyte balance.

Describe the principles and rationale of diet management for the treatment of hypertension, and implement the appropriate dietary changes.

NURSING INTERVENTIONS

Diet Management

Decrease calories for weight loss, if more than 10% overweight.

Reduce sodium intake, usually to between 2 and 4 g/day (see display, Sodium-Restricted Diets). To promote a rapid drop in blood pressure, initial sodium allowance may be severely restricted to 200 to 250 mg/day. At this level, the diet is unpalatable and extremely difficult to follow; it is appropriate only for temporary use in an acute care setting.

Provide Step One or Step Two Diet (see Table 17-6).

Adjust potassium intake, depending on drug therapy.

Restrict or eliminate alcohol consumption.

Client Teaching

Instruct the client:

That weight loss in overweight people may effectively control blood pressure without any other dietary or drug therapy.

That a low-sodium diet may help prevent hypertension, and is almost always used in the treatment of hypertension (see Low-Sodium Diet Teaching section in display, Sodium-Restricted Diets).

On the principles and rationale of diet management for hypertension, and how to implement the appropriate dietary changes.

That salt substitutes may contain potassium in place of sodium or may be a combination of sodium and potassium chloride. Neither type should be used without a physician's permission.

That it is important to consume adequate amounts of potassium in the diet, especially when potassium-wasting diuretics are used. Often, clients who require an increased potassium intake are told to "eat a banana and drink orange juice every day," without any further explanation. Explain the rationale of this oversimplified advice and instruct the client on the many other sources of potassium, especially those that are low in sodium (see display, Sources of Sodium and Potassium).

To get 30 to 45 minutes of regular aerobic exercise, such as walking, bicycling, dancing, or gardening, three to five times each week.

Monitoring Progress

Monitor for the following signs or symptoms:

Compliance with the diet and the need for follow-up diet counseling.
Effectiveness of the diet (ie, lowered blood pressure, weight loss if indicated), and evaluate the need for further diet modifications.
Fluid and electrolyte balance, if diuretics are used.

Evaluation

Evaluation is ongoing. Provided that the plan of care has not changed, the client will achieve the goals as stated above.

DRUG ALERT   *Antihypertensive Drugs*

Potassium-wasting diuretics (thiazide and related agents, loop diuretics) can cause constipation, diarrhea, nausea, vomiting, GI upset, dry mouth, increased thirst, anorexia, and fluid and electrolyte imbalances. Modify the diet to alleviate unpleasant GI side effects, if possible. Monitor for signs of potassium deficiency, and encourage the intake of potassium-rich foods (see display, Source of Sodium and Potassium). Advise the client to avoid natural licorice, which tends to cause potassium depletion and sodium retention.

Potassium supplements can lead to nausea, vomiting, GI discomfort, and diarrhea, and can produce hyperkalemia when used with salt substitutes that contain potassium. Monitor serum potassium levels and observe for signs of hyperkalemia. Advise against the use of potassium-containing salt substitutes.

Because the absorption of beta-adrenergic blocking agents (propranolol, metoprolol, atenolol) is enhanced by food, clients should be advised to take them with food.

Elderly patients who are receiving high doses of captopril may experience loss of taste.

Some calcium channel blockers (eg, diltiazem [Cardizem, Dilacor]) should be taken on an empty stomach because foods that contain fat may decrease their absorption.

NUTRITIONAL ANEMIAS

Anemia is a syndrome that is characterized by a deficiency in the oxygen-carrying capacity of the blood; this deficiency is related to a decrease in hemoglobin, red blood cell volume, and red blood cell number.

Nutritional anemias occur when one or more of the nutrients that are necessary for red blood cell production are deficient. Shortages of iron, vitamin B_{12}, and folic acid are the most common causes of nutritional anemias. Table 17-7 outlines the roles of various nutrients in the production of red blood cells (RBC). For hematologic assessment criteria, see the display, General Hematologic Assessment Criteria.

Iron Deficiency Anemia

Iron deficiency anemia occurs when total iron stores become depleted, leading to a decrease in hemoglobin. It is classified as microcytic (small blood cells) and hypochromic (pale red blood cells related to the decrease in hemoglobin pigment).

Iron deficiency anemia is the most common nutritional deficiency disorder in the United States. The incidence rate among high-risk populations may be as high as 10% to 50%. Groups who are most vulnerable include infants under 2 years of age, menstruating women, the elderly, minorities, and people in low-income groups.

Iron deficiency anemia can result from an inadequate iron intake, such as that found among low-income groups and vegetarians, or from inadequate absorption secondary to chronic diarrhea, malabsorption syndrome, partial or total gastrectomy, pica, or poor bioavailability of the iron consumed. Chronic blood loss related to bleeding ulcers, gastritis, malignancy, parasites, excessive menstrual losses, or closely spaced pregnancies, may also lead to anemia. Finally, iron deficiency may occur secondary to an increased need for iron due to accelerated growth during pregnancy, infancy, and puberty.

Table 17-7
Role of Various Nutrients in RBC Formation

Nutrient	Role in RBC Formation
Vitamin C	Enhances the absorption of iron and folic acid
Vitamin B_6	Coenzyme in hemoglobin formation
Copper*	Mobilizes iron from storage to plasma
Protein	Necessary for the formation of hemoglobin and enzymes involved in the production of RBC
Vitamin E*	Exact function is unclear; premature infants deficient in vitamin E develop hemolytic anemia
Vitamin A	Exact function is unclear; may aid in the mobilization of iron from the liver

* Rare incidence of dietary deficiency.

ASSESSMENT CRITERIA

General Hematologic Assessment Criteria

Hemoglobin, hematocrit, transferrin

Clinical signs of deficiency: beefy red tongue, anorexia, fatigue

General dietary intake

Use of alcohol or tobacco

Concurrent illness, medical history

Recent surgery; history of GI surgery

Infection, sepsis

Family history of anemia

Use of prescription and over-the-counter medications

Signs and symptoms of anemia vary with the degree of severity and chronicity: Mild anemia may be asymptomatic. Possible symptoms include fatigue, weakness, pallor, sensitivity to cold, anorexia, dizziness and headaches, stomatitis, glossitis, and thin, spoon-shaped fingernails. Some people with iron deficiency anemia practice pica (ingestion of nonfood substances such as dirt, clay, or laundry starch). Complications of iron deficiency anemia include cardiovascular and respiratory changes that may result in cardiac failure.

The treatment of iron deficiency anemia begins with correcting the underlying disorder, when appropriate. Iron supplements are used; parenteral iron may be given if oral supplements fail or are not tolerated. Although diet therapy is not effective in curing anemia once it is established, it is used adjunctively to increase iron intake and absorption, and to alleviate symptoms, if indicated.

NURSING PROCESS

Assessment

In addition to the general hematologic assessment criteria, assess for the following factors:

Symptoms that may affect intake (eg, fatigue, anorexia, stomatitis, glossitis); assess onset, severity, interventions attempted and the results.

Dietary changes made in response to symptoms (ie, foods avoided, foods preferred). Determine which foods are best and least tolerated.

Usual intake of foods high in iron (Table 17-8).

Vitamin C intake when plant sources of iron (eg, fortified, enriched, and whole-grain breads and cereals) are consumed. Rich sources of vitamin C include citrus fruits and juices, tomatoes, broccoli, cabbage, baked potatoes, and strawberries.

The intake of tea and coffee when plant sources of iron are consumed; tea and coffee inhibit the absorption of iron.

Table 17-8
Selected Sources of Iron

Heme Iron	Nonheme Iron
Beef: muscle meats, heart, kidney, liver, and tongue	Bran flakes
Chicken, especially dark meat	Brewer's yeast
Egg yolk	Brown rice
Lamb	Chocolate, cocoa
Liver sausage	Enriched and whole grain breads, cereals, and flours
Oysters	Fortified cereals
Pork	Dried beans, peas, and soybeans
Shellfish	Dried fruit: apricots, currants, dates, figs, peaches, prunes, raisins
Shrimp	Green peas
Tuna	Greens: beet, dandelion, kale, spinach, Swiss chard, turnip
Turkey, especially dark meat	Lentils
Veal	Molasses
	Nuts: almonds, brazil nuts, cashews, hazelnuts, pecans, peanuts, walnuts
	Oatmeal
	Sauerkraut
	Sweet potatoes

The quantity and quality of protein usually consumed; determine if the client is a vegetarian.

Pica. If the client practices pica, determine what items are eaten and how frequently they are consumed.

Nursing Diagnosis

Altered Nutrition: Less than body requirements, related to poor bioavailability of iron consumed

Planning and Implementation

There are several reasons why inadequate intake is a frequent cause of iron deficiency anemia. First, the typical American diet provides 10 to 20 mg/day. Men, who typically consume more food than women, can easily meet their Recommended Dietary Allowance (RDA) for iron (10 mg). Women tend to eat less iron (mean intake of 12.4 mg/day for women 12 to 49 years of age, according to advanced data of the National Health and Nutritional Examination Survey [NHANES] II data) (CDC, 1994), but require more iron (RDA of 15 mg). Also, on the average, only 10% of the iron that is consumed is absorbed. The actual rate of iron absorption varies with both need (the rate of absorption increases in response to need) and the form of iron consumed (heme iron or nonheme iron).

Heme iron (organic iron) is the most abundant form of iron in animal sources, such as meat, fish, and poultry; however, it accounts for only 5% to 10% of total iron consumed. The average absorption rate of heme iron, which is influenced only by body need, is about 15% (Herbert, 1992). Heme iron promotes the absorption of nonheme iron from other foods when it is eaten at the same time.

Nonheme iron (inorganic iron) is the most abundant form of iron in plant sources: grains, vegetables, legumes, and nuts. It is the most prevalent form of iron in the diet, yet on average, only about 3% of nonheme iron is absorbed. Like heme iron, its rate of absorption is influenced by body need; however, it also is significantly affected by the presence of other dietary factors (Table 17-9). Nonheme iron absorption is enhanced by Vitamin C, certain animal proteins, and gastric acidity. Nonheme iron absorption is sharply reduced by many natural substances, including tannic acid (found in tea), calcium phosphate (found in dairy products), phytates

Table 17-9
Factors That Influence Nonheme Iron Absorption

	Comments
NONHEME IRON ENHANCERS	
Vitamin C	The most potent iron enhancer known; it reduces and binds iron to form a readily absorbable compound. Its enhancing effect is proportional to the amount of vitamin C consumed. To be effective, vitamin C must be eaten at the same time as the iron.
Certain animal proteins	Meat, fish, and poultry enhance nonheme iron absorption when consumed at the same time as nonheme iron.
Gastric acidity	Increases the solubility and availability of iron.
NONHEME IRON INHIBITORS	
Tea	Contains tannin, which combines with nonheme iron to form insoluble complexes that cannot be absorbed.
	Can reduce iron absorption by as much as 87% when consumed with meals.
Coffee	Exact mechanism is unclear; appears to render iron unabsorbable by changing it from the ferrous to the ferric state.
	When consumed with meals or up to 1 hour later, can reduce iron absorption by 39%. Does not interfere with iron absorption when consumed 1 hour before eating.
	Inhibitory effect is dose related: absorption decreases as the strength of the coffee increases.
Binding agents	Various compounds combine with iron to form insoluble complexes the body cannot absorb. Common binding agents include bran (whole grains), phosphates (dairy products, whole grains, legumes), oxalates (certain fruits and vegetables, soybean products), and phytates (oatmeal, whole grains).
Alkalinity	Antacids decrease iron solubility by increasing gastric pH.
Increased GI motility; steatorrhea	Diarrhea reduces the time available for absorption.
THE FORM OF ELEMENTAL IRON IN SUPPLEMENTS AND ENRICHED PRODUCTS	
Well absorbed	Ferrous sulfate, lactate, fumarate, succinate, glycinesulfate, glutamate
Poorly absorbed	Ferrous citrate, tartrate, pyrophosphate

(found in many cereals), bran, oxalates, and antacids. Increased GI motility also impairs iron absorption.

Anorexia may necessitate the intake of small, frequent meals. Acidic and salty foods, strong spices, coarse breads, raw vegetables, and hot foods and beverages should be eliminated if the oral mucosa is inflamed.

Iron stores are replenished slowly; iron therapy may be needed for up to 1 year after anemia is diagnosed.

Because iron deficiency and iron overload produce many common symptoms (eg, fatigue, headache, irritability, palpitations) and anemia, a definitive diagnosis of iron deficiency should be made before iron and vitamin C supplements are used (Herbert, 1992).

Be aware of the potential side effects of iron supplementation (see Drug Alert).

CLIENT GOALS

The client will:

Experience alleviation of anemia; be free of signs and symptoms.
Replace poor sources of iron in the diet with rich sources of iron (eg, consume iron-fortified cereals, organ meats).
Include a source of vitamin C at every meal to enhance nonheme iron absorption.
Modify the diet as needed, to alleviate symptoms that may interfere with eating (anorexia, inflamed oral mucosa)
Avoid foods or beverages that are known to inhibit iron absorption.
Describe the principles and rationale of diet management for iron deficiency anemia.
Modify the diet, as needed, to alleviate anemia symptoms or side effects of iron therapy.

NURSING INTERVENTIONS

Diet Management

Increase iron intake (see Table 17-8), especially of heme iron and preferably at every meal.
Include a source of vitamin C at every meal to enhance nonheme iron absorption; avoid foods that are known to inhibit nonheme iron absorption.

Client Teaching

Instruct the client:

* On ways to increase the iron content of the diet:
  Add dried fruit to cereals and baked goods.
  Use crushed, iron-fortified cereal as a breading for meat, fish, poultry, and vegetables; mix with butter or margarine for a casserole topping; use as a meat extender in meatloaf, meatballs, and burgers; sprinkle on ice cream; add to yogurt and pudding for extra crunch.

Substitute whole-grain products for refined products; brown rice for white rice.
Cook in iron pots whenever possible, especially acidic foods (eg, dishes made with tomatoes).
- On ways to increase the iron availability of the diet:
Eat meat at every meal, if possible.
Consume a rich source of vitamin C at every meal: citrus fruits and their juices, brussels sprouts, strawberries, broccoli, greens, cabbage, cantaloupe, tomatoes.
Avoid coffee and tea both with and after meals.

Monitoring Progress

Monitor for the following signs or symptoms:

Tolerance to oral feedings (ie, absence of mouth pain), if oral mucosa is inflamed.
Compliance with the diet, and the need for follow-up diet counseling.
Effectiveness of the diet, and the need for further diet modifications.
Hemoglobin and hematocrit.

Evaluation

Evaluation is ongoing. Provided that the plan of care has not changed, the client will achieve the goals as stated above.

DRUG
ALERT   *Iron Supplements*

Oral iron supplements:

Are better absorbed if taken between meals; antacids and food in the stomach inhibit absorption.

Commonly cause GI upset, nausea, heartburn, diarrhea or constipation, and black stools, which are dose-related. Administering a smaller dose, several times a day, for a longer period of treatment or taking the supplements with meals may be necessary to alleviate side effects.

Can be toxic when taken in excessive amounts. Keep these and all medications out of the reach of children.

Vitamin B_{12} Deficiency Anemia

A lack of vitamin B_{12} leads to decreased deoxyribonucleic acid (DNA) synthesis, which can result in megaloblastic anemia (red blood cells with delayed and abnormal nuclear maturation). Vitamin B_{12} is absorbed in the ileum and requires intrinsic factor, which is produced and secreted in the stomach. Vitamin B_{12} is found only in animal products.

Vitamin B_{12} deficiency related to an inadequate intake occurs rarely and usually is seen only in strict vegetarians who consume no animal products and do not take vitamin B_{12} supplements. The most frequent cause of vitamin B_{12} deficiency is impaired absorption, which can result from numerous factors.

Pernicious anemia is vitamin B_{12} deficiency anemia that is caused by the lack of intrinsic factor production in the stomach, which renders vitamin B_{12} incapable of being absorbed. Pernicious anemia occurs in only 0.1% of the population, most often in people over 50 years of age, and may be related to a genetic defect, chronic iron deficiency, an autoimmune disorder, or total, and sometimes subtotal, gastrectomy.

Absorption of vitamin B_{12} also may be impaired secondary to disorders of the ileum and pancreas, malabsorption syndrome, bacterial overgrowth related to intestinal stasis, or fish tapeworm.

Because normal body stores of vitamin B_{12} are extensive, the onset of deficiency symptoms may be delayed for 5 to 10 years. Symptoms related to anemia include pallor, dyspnea or orthopnea, weakness, fatigue, and palpitations. GI changes may occur: sore mouth with a smooth, red, "beefy" tongue, anorexia, indigestion, recurring diarrhea or constipation, and weight loss. Neurologic changes that may be observed include paresthesia of the hands and feet, decreased sense of position, poor muscle coordination, poor memory, irritability, depression, paranoia, delirium, and hallucinations. Prolonged pernicious anemia can lead to permanent neurologic damage; untreated pernicious anemia can result in death. Pernicious anemia also is associated with an increased incidence of benign gastric polyps and gastric carcinoma. Thirty-three percent of people with vitamin B_{12} deficiency also have iron deficiency (Herbert, 1992).

The treatment of pernicious anemia requires lifelong parenteral vitamin B_{12} injections. Vitamin B_{12} deficiency anemia that occurs secondary to GI disorders is treated by correcting the underlying problem and administering vitamin B_{12} as needed. Strict vegetarians who become vitamin B_{12} deficient because of an inadequate intake can be treated with oral vitamin B_{12} supplements, and should be encouraged to increase their dietary intake, if possible (ie, through use of fortified soybean milk, or inclusion of some animal products). Adjunctive diet therapy may be used to provide nutrients that are essential for RBC production, to help correct any existing nutritional deficiencies, and to minimize GI symptoms.

NURSING PROCESS

Assessment

In addition to the general hematologic assessment criteria, assess for the following factors:

Symptoms that may affect eating (eg, sore mouth, anorexia, indigestion, diarrhea, constipation); assess onset, frequency, severity, interventions attempted and the results.

Dietary changes made in response to symptoms (ie, foods avoided, foods preferred). Determine which foods are best and least tolerated.

Usual intake of vitamin B_{12}; vitamin B_{12} is found only in animal products.

Past and present medical history, especially GI history, to determine if there are any conditions contributing to anemia.

Nursing Diagnosis

Altered Oral Mucous Membranes, related to vitamin B_{12} deficiency as manifested by stomatitis

Planning and Implementation

A liquid or soft diet may be necessary if glossitis and oral inflammation interfere with eating. Likewise, other dietary changes may be necessary to alleviate anorexia, diarrhea, or constipation (see Chapter 16).

Fat may not be tolerated by clients with achlorhydria because of delayed gastric emptying and decreased rate of digestion.

Iron deficiency may occur as a result of achlorhydria or may develop secondary to treatment. If iron supplements are prescribed, be aware of the potential side effects (see Drug Alert section under Iron Deficiency Anemia).

Folic acid deficiency can also cause megaloblastic anemia and the same GI symptoms as pernicious anemia. Folic acid that is given to clients with pernicious anemia reverses the anemia and GI symptoms without affecting the neurologic disturbances, which can be irreversible if left untreated. It is imperative that the correct cause of megaloblastic anemia be ascertained before treatment is begun.

CLIENT GOALS

The client will

Experience alleviation of anemia, if possible.

Modify the diet, as needed, to alleviate symptoms.

Describe the principles and rationale of diet management for vitamin B_{12} deficiency anemia and implement the appropriate dietary changes.

NURSING INTERVENTIONS

Diet Management

Increase vitamin B_{12}, protein, iron, and folic acid intake by providing more meat (especially liver, beef, and pork), eggs, green leafy vegetables, milk, and milk products.

Provide liquid or soft foods if oral mucosa is inflamed. Modify the diet as needed for other GI symptoms (see Chapter 16).

Client Teaching

Instruct the client:

> On the principles and rationale of diet management for vitamin B_{12} deficiency anemia, and how to implement the appropriate dietary changes.

Monitoring Progress

Monitor for the following signs or symptoms:

> Tolerance to oral feedings (ie, absence of pain), if oral mucosa is inflamed.
> Compliance with the diet, and the need for follow-up diet counseling.
> Effectiveness of the diet, and the need for additional diet modifications.
> Anemia and symptoms.

Evaluation

> Evaluation is ongoing. Provided that the plan of care has not changed, the client will meet the goals as stated above.

Folic Acid Deficiency Anemia

> A lack of folic acid leads to decreased DNA synthesis, which can result in megaloblastic anemia. Folic acid deficiency may occur because of inadequate intake, as in the elderly and alcoholics, or may occur secondary to increased requirements related to growth, such as during pregnancy and infancy. Malabsorption syndromes can also cause folic acid deficiency, as can the use of certain medications, such as anticonvulsants, antimetabolites, and oral contraceptives.
>
> Normal body stores of folate usually become depleted in 2 to 4 months on a folate-deficient diet. Symptoms related to anemia include pallor, dyspnea or orthopnea, weakness, fatigue, and palpitations. GI changes that may be observed include sore mouth with a smooth, red, "beefy" tongue, anorexia, indigestion, recurring diarrhea or constipation, and weight loss. Unlike pernicious anemia, no neurologic changes occur.
>
> Folic acid deficiency is treated by correcting the underlying disorder, if appropriate. Oral folate supplements are used; however, intramuscular injections may be necessary in patients with malabsorption. Diet therapy may help to promote RBC production.

NURSING PROCESS

Assessment

> In addition to the general hematologic assessment criteria, assess for the following factors:

Symptoms that may affect intake (eg, sore mouth, anorexia, indigestion, diarrhea, constipation, weight loss); assess onset, frequency, severity, interventions attempted and the results.

Dietary changes made in response to symptoms (ie, foods avoided, foods preferred). Determine which foods are best and least tolerated.

Usual intake of foods rich in folic acid, such as liver, organ meats, broccoli, green leafy vegetables, asparagus, milk, eggs, orange juice, wheat bran, wheat germ, whole wheat bread, brewer's yeast, dried peas and beans.

Usual intake of vitamin C: Vitamin C converts folic acid from its inactive to its active form.

Nursing Diagnosis

Altered Oral Mucous Membrane, related to folic acid deficiency anemia as manifested by stomatitis

Planning and Implementation

A liquid or soft diet may be necessary if glossitis and oral inflammation interfere with eating. Likewise, other dietary changes may be needed to alleviate anorexia, diarrhea, or constipation (see Chapter 16).

Encourage the intake of both vitamin C and folic acid at every meal; folic acid supplements may be required.

Because heat destroys folic acid, fruits and vegetables should be eaten raw or cooked minimally.

About 60% of clients with folate deficiency also have iron deficiency (Herbert, 1992); iron deficiency leads to RBC hemolysis and therefore an increased need for folate to replenish RBC. Observe for signs of iron deficiency and provide supplements as ordered.

CLIENT GOALS

The client will:

Experience alleviation of anemia, if possible.

Modify the diet, as needed, to alleviate symptoms (ie, stomatitis, anorexia, diarrhea, constipation, weight loss).

Describe the principles and rationale of diet management for folic acid deficiency anemia and implement the appropriate dietary changes.

NURSING INTERVENTIONS

Diet Management

Increase folic acid intake by eating more foods that are high in folic acid: liver, organ meats, broccoli, green leafy vegetables, asparagus, milk, eggs, orange juice, wheat germ, whole-wheat bread, brewer's yeast, dried peas and beans.

Provide a rich source of vitamin C with every meal to enhance absorption.

Modify the diet, as needed, to alleviate GI symptoms (see Chapter 16).

Client Teaching

Instruct the client:

> On the principles and rationale of diet management for folic acid deficiency anemia and how to implement the appropriate dietary changes.
> To modify the diet, as needed, to alleviate GI symptoms.

Monitoring Progress

Monitor for the following signs or symptoms:

> Tolerance to oral feedings (ie, absence of pain), if oral mucosa is inflamed
> Compliance with the diet, and the need for follow-up diet counseling
> Effectiveness of the diet, and the need for further diet modification

Evaluation

Evaluation is ongoing. Provided that the plan of care has not changed, the client will meet the goals as stated above.

KEY CONCEPTS

- Although diet intervention may not prevent heart disease in individuals, it can reduce the risk of heart disease in Americans.
- HDL-cholesterol takes cholesterol out of the serum and delivers it back to the liver, where it can be recycled or excreted in bile. It is commonly known as the "good" cholesterol: the greater the HDL, the lower the risk for heart disease.
- HDL-cholesterol is not significantly influenced by diet. The three main factors that have been shown to increse HDL-cholesterol are exercise, weight loss, if overweight, and smoking cessation. Moderate alcohol consumption appears to raise HDL levels.
- LDL-cholesterol is the "bad" cholesterol. A variety of studies strongly indicate that the higher the LDL-cholesterol, the higher the risk of heart disease.
- Excessive intakes of saturated fats, total fat, and dietary cholesterol, and excessive body weight increase LDL-cholesterol.
- Diet intervention should always be used for the treatment of hypercholesterolemia; drug therapy may be added for clients who fail to achieve goals through diet alone and who are at high risk for CHD.
- The Step One Diet is lower in saturated fat, total fat, and cholesterol than the current typical American diet. Calories should be adjusted for healthy weight. The majority of calories should be from carbohydrates–grains, vegetables, and fruit. Many experts believe all Americans 2 years of age and older should follow a Step One Diet.
- The Step Two Diet is recommended when the goals of the Stop One diet are not achieved after 3 months of good compliance because it more severely limits saturated fat and cholesterol.
- Changing eating patterns is a lifestyle modification that should be made gradually and sequentially for the greatest chance of long-term success.

- Sources of saturated fat include animal fats (butterfat, meat) and coconut oil, palm oil, and palm kernel oil.
- Cholesterol is found only in animal products; it is in both fat and lean tissue; therefore, low-fat meats are not necessarily low in cholesterol.
- When intake resumes after an MI, small frequent meals of easily digested soft foods are recommended. Temperature extremes and caffeine are avoided.
- Usually a low-sodium diet, used with or without diuretics, effectively controls fluid balance in clients with CHF, without the need for a fluid restriction.
- High blood pressure is linked to high salt intake, obesity, physical inactivity, excessive alcohol consumption, and an inadequate intake of potassium. Diet intervention should be the initial treatment of choice because it has the potential to effectively control blood pressure without the risk of side effects.
- Nonheme iron absorption is influenced by numerous dietary components. Vitamin C and certain animal proteins promote its absorption; coffee, tea, phytates, bran, calcium phosphate, and oxalates impair its absorption. To promote maximum absorption, coffee and tea should not be consumed with meals, and a rich source of vitamin C should be consumed at every meal.
- Pernicious anemia is vitamin B_{12}-deficiency anemia caused by a lack of intrinsic factor; it occurs rarely. Vitamin B_{12} deficiency occurs more frequently from malabsorption syndromes. Pure vegans who do not supplement their diets are at risk of B_{12} deficiency.
- The anemia and GI side effects caused by a deficiency of vitamin B_{12} can be reversed by folic acid. However, the neurologic symptoms persist, and if left untreated, can result in permanent neurologic damage or death.

FOCUS ON **CRITICAL THINKING**

Mr. Bishop is 56 years old, weighs 184 pounds, and is 5′9″. He smokes 2 packs of cigarettes a day and leads a sedentary lifestyle. He was recently divorced and is now living alone, preparing his own meals occasionally, but mostly eating out or getting take-out. The doctor has warned him that his blood pressure is creeping up, with the most recent measurement at 140/95 mm Hg. If Mr. Bishop's blood pressure is not lower at his next office visit, which is scheduled in 3 months, he will have to begin medication. Mr. Bishop has heard that blood pressure medication can have serious side effects, so he says he is determined to get his blood pressure under control. He wonders if fish oil pills will help bring down his blood pressure.

List risk factors that may be contributing to Mr. Bishop's elevated blood pressure.

Before recommending that Mr. Bishop change his eating habits, his usual intake needs to be determined, particularly of which foods or nutrients? List three dietary interventions that may benefit Mr. Bishop. Given his present lifestyle, what does Mr. Bishop need to know to implement the appropriate dietary changes? What would you tell him about using fish oil supplements?

REFERENCES

Adams, S., Maller, O., and Cardello, A. (1995). Consumer acceptance of foods lower in sodium. J Am Diet Assoc, 95, 447–453.

Anderson, J., Smith, B., and Gustafson, N. (1994). Health benefits and practical aspects of high-fiber diets. Am J Clin Nutr, 59(suppl), 1232S–1247S.

CDC/National Center for Health Statistics. (1994). Advance data. Dietary intake of vitamins, minerals, and fiber of persons ages 2 months and over in the United States: Third National Health and Nutrition Examination Survery, Phase 1, 1988–1991.

Chicago Dietetic Association and The South Suburban Dietetic Association (1992). Manual of Clinical Dietetics. 4th ed. Chicago: American Dietetic Association.

Cuddy, R. (1995). Hypertension. Keeping dangerous blood pressure down. Nursing 95, 25(8), 35–41.

Escott-Stump, S. (1992). Nutrition and Diagnosis-Related Care. 3rd ed. Philadelphia: Lea & Febiger.

Fraser, G. (1994). Diet and coronary heart disease: Beyond dietary fats and low-density lipoprotein cholesterol. Am J Clin Nutr, 59(suppl), 1117S–1123S.

Herbert, V. (1992). Everyone should be tested for iron disorders. J Am Diet Assoc, 92, 1502–1509.

Hicks, S. (1994). Standing guard against silent ischemia and infarction. Nursing 94, 24(1), 34–39.

Johannsen, J. (1993). Update: Guidelines for treating hypertension. AJN, 93(3), 42–49.

Leibman, B. (1995a). Heart disease. How to lower your risk. Nutrition Action Health Letter, 22(8), 1, 4–7.

Liebman, B. (1995b). One nation, under pressure. Nutrition Action Health Letter, 22(6), 6–9.

Leibman, B. (1995c). Folic acid: For the young and heart. Nutrition Action Health Letter, 22(7), 1, 4–7.

Leibman, B. and Hurley, J. (1993). The heart of the matter. Nutrition Action Health Letter, 20(8), 5–7.

Lewandowski, D. (1995). Congestive heart failure. AJN, 95(5), 36–37.

Lichtenstein, A. (1995). *Trans* fatty acids and hydrogenated fat—What do we know? Nutrition Today, 30(3), 102–107.

National Cholesterol Education Program (1993a). Second Report of the Expert Panel on Detection, Evaluation, and Treatment of High Blood Cholesterol in Adults (Adult Treatment Panel II). Bethesda: USDHHS, Public Health Service, National Institutes of Health, NIH Publication No. 93-3095.

National Cholesterol Education Program (1993b). Report of the Expert Panel on Population Strategies for Blood Cholesterol Reduction. Executive Summary. USDHHS, Public Health Service, NIH, NHLBI. NIH publication No. 93-3047.

National High Blood Pressure Education Program Working Group (1993). Report on Primary Prevention of Hypertension. Arch Intern Med, 153, 186–208.

Nelson, K. (1995). Therapeutic Nutrition. An alternative approach to coronary heart disease management. Nutrition Today, 30(3), 114–122.

Porth, C (1995). Understanding the cholesterol transport system. Nursing 95, 25(4), 32T–32U.

Posner, B., Cupples, L., Gagnon, D., Wilson, P., Chetwynd, K., and Felix, D. (1993). Healthy People 2000. The rationale and potential efficacy of preventive nutrition in heart disease: The Framingham Offspring-Spouse Study. Arch Intern Med, 153, 1549–1556.

U.S. Department of Agriculture, U.S. Department of Health and Human Services. (1995). Nutrition and Your Healthy. Dietary Guidelines for Americans (4th ed.) Home and Garden Bulletin No. 323.

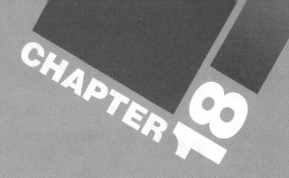

CHAPTER 8

Diabetes Mellitus and Other Endocrine Disorders

Chapter Outline

Key Terms

Cretinism
Diabetes mellitus
Diabetic ketoacidosis (DKA)
Functional hyperinsulinism
Hyperglycemic hyperosmo-
   lar nonketotic syndrome
Hyperthyroidism

Insulin
Insulin-dependent diabetes
   (IDDM or Type I)
Myxedema
Non–insulin-dependent dia-
   betes (NIDDM or Type II)
Organic hyperinsulinism

Primary adrenocortical
   insufficiency
Primary hyperpara-
   thyroidism
Tetraiodothyronine
   (thyroxine)
Triiodothyronine

ENDOCRINE DISORDERS

*T*he endocrine system is composed of ductless glands that secrete hormones into the bloodstream. The endocrine pancreas secretes insulin, the hormone that is involved with the metabolism of not only glucose, but also of protein and fat. Diet management is an integral component of treatment for both insulin-dependent and non–insulin-dependent diabetes. Hormones that are secreted by other endocrine glands, namely the thyroid gland, parathyroid gland, and adrenal cortex, affect nutritional status by regulating nutrient metabolism (Table 18-1). Alterations in hormone secretion can cause nutrient imbalances, weight changes, and unpleasant symptoms that interfere with eating (eg, nausea) or nutrient utilization (eg, diarrhea). Diet management can help alleviate symptoms and may prevent worsening of nutrient imbalances, but it cannot fully compensate for hormone secretion abnormalities. For endocrine assessment guidelines, see the display, General Endocrine Assessment Criteria.

DISORDERS OF THE ENDOCRINE PANCREAS

Diabetes Mellitus

Diabetes mellitus is a chronic heterogeneous disorder that is characterized by elevated blood glucose levels (hyperglycemia) related to a relative or absolute deficiency

Table 18-1
Effect of Various Endocrine Secretions on Nutrient Metabolism

Gland	Secretion	Effect on Nutrient Metabolism
Thyroid 2 lobes located in the anterior portion of the neck	Thyroxine (T_4) and Triiodothyronine (T_3)	Regulates basal metabolic rate (BMR) by regulating the rate of CHO, protein, fat, vitamin, and mineral metabolism; stimulates growth and development
Parathyroid 4 small glands embedded in the posterior section of the thyroid gland	Parathormone (PTH)	Regulates blood calcium and phosphorus levels; increases blood calcium levels by increasing GI absorption, decreasing urinary excretion, and promoting bone resorption; lowers blood phosphorus levels
Adrenals 2 small glands located above and in front of the upper end of each kidney. Consists of the cortex (essential for life) and the medulla (nonessential for life)	Cortex *Glucocorticoids* (cortisone and hydrocortisone) *Mineralocorticoids* (aldosterone)	Influences the metabolism of CHO, protein, and fat Promotes sodium retention and potassium excretion

General Endocrine Assessment Criteria

Weight status, weight changes	Numbness, tingling, paresthesias
Polyphagia	Altered consciousness
Polydipsia	Bone pain
Abdominal pain	Dysuria, polyuria
Anorexia, nausea	Frequent infections
Headache	Fatigue
Seizures	Dry, itchy skin
Syncope	Decreased libido

of insulin. The two major types of diabetes are **insulin-dependent diabetes mellitus (IDDM or type I)** and **non–insulin-dependent diabetes mellitus (NIDDM or type II)**.

Approximately 5% to 6% of the American population has diabetes—only half of whom may be diagnosed (Monk et al, 1995). The prevalence of NIDDM is highest among minorities, such as Hispanic Americans, Native Americans, and African Americans. The exact cause is unknown and the condition may be multifactorial for each type and each client.

NORMAL PHYSIOLOGY

Insulin is the major hormone responsible for maintaining blood glucose levels within the normal range of 70 to 110 mg/dl. It is also required for certain amino acids to enter muscle cells, for protein synthesis, and for fatty acids to enter and be stored in fat cells. As such, it is intricately involved in the metabolism of all body fuels.

Insulin is released by the β cells of the islets of Langerhans in response to elevated blood glucose levels. After eating, blood glucose levels rise. The rise in glucose signals the pancreas to secrete insulin, which binds with special insulin receptors on the surface of fat and muscle cells. This allows circulating glucose to leave the bloodstream and enter the cells. It also enhances the transport of amino acids into the cell and promotes glycogen storage, protein synthesis, and fat formation. As glucose leaves the bloodstream and serum levels drop, insulin secretion falls to keep glucose levels within normal range.

Once inside the cells, glucose can be converted to energy. Glucose that remains after energy needs are met is converted to glycogen (glycogenesis) and stored in the liver and muscles. If glycogen stores are adequate, the remaining glucose is converted to fat (lipogenesis) and stored as adipose.

When serum glucose levels are low, such as during fasting, insulin secretion falls. The fall in insulin causes glycogen stores to release glucose for energy (glycogenolysis) and muscle cells to release amino acids (proteolysis) for their conversion to glucose (gluconeogenesis). This occurs only after glycogen is depleted. If needed, fat stores release fatty acids (lipolysis), which are metabolized to ketone bodies (ketogenesis) and used for energy; the glycerol component of fatty acids can be converted to glucose.

PATHOGENESIS OF INSULIN-DEPENDENT DIABETES

Insulin-dependent diabetes mellitus (IDDM or type I), which is characterized by a lack of insulin secretion, accounts for only about 10% of all diabetes cases. Although it can occur at any age, it is most often detected in childhood; most type I diabetics are within their normal weight range or slightly below. The exact cause of IDDM is unknown; however, it is possible that an autoimmune response, which is triggered by a viral infection, causes the destruction of the β cells in genetically susceptible people, resulting in an inability to produce insulin.

Without insulin, serum glucose levels rise and cells are unable to use glucose for energy. Glucose eventually "spills" over into the urine (glycosuria). To some extent, the body compensates for the lack of usable energy by breaking down protein and fat. Unfortunately, ketone bodies accumulate because the body is not able to completely utilize fat for energy. Ketonuria develops; left untreated, the accumulation of ketones in the blood lowers serum pH, leading to **diabetic ketoacidosis (DKA)**, a potentially fatal form of metabolic acidosis (Reisling, 1995b).

Polyuria and polydipsia, the classic symptoms of diabetes, develop as the body tries to rid itself of excess glucose and ketones. The third hallmark, polyphagia, occurs because the cells are actually starving for energy despite the high glucose levels. Rapid weight loss, muscle wasting, fatigue, weakness, irritability, itchy skin, and poor wound healing may occur.

Although the metabolic derangements may be life-threatening (eg, hyperosmolar coma), the major challenge is to control the progressive vascular damage that occurs over time. Studies indicate that tightly controlled blood glucose levels can significantly reduce the risk of chronic complications that is seen in both type I and type II diabetes (Robertson, 1995). Morphologic changes occur in the small vessels, arteries, pancreas, kidneys, retina, nerves, and other tissues. Atherosclerosis is 50% more common among diabetics than the general population, and the death rate from coronary artery disease is two to three times higher among diabetics than among their age- and sex-matched peers. This increased risk may be partly related to a high incidence of other coronary heart disease risk factors, such as hyperlipidemia, hypertension, and clotting abnormalities. Diabetes is the major cause of renal failure, amputations, and new blindness in the United States. It also leads to neuropathy and neuropathy-induced impotence in men and is the fourth leading cause of death by disease in the United States.

PATHOGENESIS OF NON–INSULIN-DEPENDENT DIABETES

Approximately 90% of the diabetic population has non–insulin-dependent diabetes mellitus (NIDDM or type II). Because it is a slowly progressive disease, the number of diagnosed and undiagnosed cases may be equal. It is most often diagnosed after 40 years of age and occurs more frequently in blacks than whites. The incidence of type II diabetes is strongly correlated to obesity (80% to 90% of type II diabetics are obese) and parental history.

Unlike IDDM, type II diabetes is characterized by normal or above-normal insulin levels; however, there is decreased tissue sensitivity to insulin, primarily in the liver and muscle. The delayed glucose-stimulated insulin response results in ineffective suppression of liver glucose production and decreased glucose uptake by the peripheral tissues. Hyperglycemia results and provides constant stimulation for insulin secretion. Although the amount of insulin secretion may be sufficient, it may take 4 to 5 hours instead of the usual 2 hours for blood glucose levels to return to normal after a meal. Chronic hyperinsulinemia can lead to a decrease in the number of insulin receptors on the cells and a decrease in tissue sensitivity to insulin.

Although it is not a cause of hyperglycemia, obesity complicates the scenario by contributing to insulin resistance. Another risk factor appears to be the distribution of body fat. Obese people with upper body (android) obesity, especially women, are at greater risk for developing diabetes and cardiovascular disease than are obese people with lower body (gynoid) fat distribution. The risk increases in proportion to the degree of obesity.

Many people with type II diabetes are asymptomatic and may not know they have diabetes until a complication develops (see above). However, some people display mild classic symptoms, or experience drowsiness, fatigue, blurred vision, tingling or numbness of the extremities, or frequent infections. Because insulin is available, ketoacidosis does not develop, even though blood glucose levels are high. A complication that may develop rapidly from severe hyperglycemia is **hyperglycemic hyperosmolar nonketotic syndrome (HHNS)**, or **hyperglycemic hyperosmolar nonketotic coma (HHNC)**. The sudden hyperosmolar state that is triggered by extremely high blood glucose levels (ie, >1000 mg/dl) causes severe dehydration and neurologic dysfunction, including coma (Reisling, 1995b).

DIABETES MANAGEMENT

The overall goals of diabetes treatment are to achieve metabolic control as near normal as possible and to prevent or delay the onset of complications. Inherent in those goals are achieving optimal blood lipid levels, attaining or maintaining reasonable weight, avoiding acute complications, and improving overall health through optimal nutrition (ADA, 1994).

Nutrition therapy is the cornerstone of treatment for all diabetics, regardless of the client's weight, blood glucose levels, or use of medication. New diet recommendations issued by the American Diabetes Association in 1994 stress that the diet must be individualized according to assessment data and treatment goals (see display, Nutrition Recommendations for Diabetes). Traditional assumptions that sugar causes diabetics' blood glucose levels to rise too high and too quickly no longer hold true; today, consistency in the total amount of carbohydrate consumed is considered a more important factor influencing blood glucose level than is the type of carbohy-

Nutrition Recommendations for Diabetes

Nutrient	Recommendation
Protein	Should provide 10% to 20% of total calories; there is insufficient evidence to support protein intakes either higher or lower than average protein intake for the general population. Protein should come from both animal and vegetable sources. If nephropathy develops, a protein intake of 0.8 g/kg (normal RDA), or approximately 10% of total calories, is recommended.
Saturated fat	Less than 10% of total calories to reduce the risk of cardiovascular disease.
Polyunsaturated fat	Up to 10% of total calories.
Total fat	The new guidelines recommend a specific amount of saturated fat but not total fat. The distribution of total fat should be based on assessment data and treatment goals. For instance: 30% total calories from fat may be appropriate for clients with normal lipid levels and normal weight. Lower-fat diets may be appropriate for obese clients. Clients with high LDL-cholesterol may benefit from the Step Two Diet (<30% fat, <7% saturated fat, <200 mg cholesterol). If elevated triglycerides are a problem, increasing monounsaturated fats to 20% and providing a more moderate CHO intake may be advised. However, if triglyceride levels exceed 1000 mg/dl, limiting all types of fat is recommended.
Cholesterol	Limit to 300 mg or less to decrease the risk of cardiovascular disease.
Carbohydrate	New recommendations focus on the total amount of CHO rather than the type, which is a significant change from previous recommendations. % contribution is individualized according to the client's eating habits and glucose and lipid goals.
Sucrose	Because scientific evidence shows that the use of sucrose as part of a meal plan does not impair blood glucose control for either type I or type II diabetics, restricting its use is no longer justified, except as part of total CHO. Sucrose and sucrose-containing foods can be substituted for other CHO and foods in the meal plan; they are not to be added as "extras" (ADA, 1994). This shift in thinking may be difficult to accept by long-standing diabetics, and difficult not to abuse (Diabetes Care and Education, 1994).
Fructose	Fructose offers no advantage over sucrose; neither is there a need to avoid naturally occurring fructose (fruits and vegetables) or moderate amounts of fructose-sweetened foods.
Other nutritive sweeteners	There is no evidence that other sweeteners (eg, honey, molasses, corn syrup, dextrose, maltose) have any significant advantage or disadvantage over sucrose.
Nonnutritive sweeteners	Saccharin, aspartame, and acesulfame K are approved for use by the FDA; they are safe for diabetics to consume.
Fiber	Although soluble fiber can delay glucose absorption, the effect of fiber on glycemic control is probably insignificant (ADA, 1994); however, fiber has other benefits, such as increasing the volume of the diet without increasing the calories (a plus for weight management), providing vitamins and minerals, and possibly replacing some fat (Vessby, 1994). The 1994 recommendations for fiber are the same as for the general population; 20–35 g/day, preferably from a wide variety of foods.
Sodium	Because individual sensitivity to sodium differs and is impractical to assess, sodium intake recommendations are the same for diabetics as for the general population: generally no more than 2400 to 3000 mg. For clients with mild to moderate hypertension, sodium intake should not exceed 2400 mg/day.

(continued)

Nutrition Recommendations for Diabetes (Continued)

Nutrient	Recommendation
Alcohol	Under normal circumstances, blood glucose is not affected by moderate use of alcohol when diabetes is well controlled (ADA, 1994).
	Alcohol should be avoided by clients who are pregnant and those with a history of alcohol abuse.
	Alcohol increases the risk of hypoglycemia in clients on insulin or sulfonylureas; those clients should consume alcohol only as part of a meal.
	Alcohol may be contraindicated for other medical conditions (eg, pancreatitis, dyslipidemia, neuropathy).
	Alcohol is best calculated into the meal plan by substituting 1 alcoholic beverage for 2 fat exchanges.
Vitamins and Minerals	Supplements are not necessary if the diet is adequate.

drate (CHO) consumed (see display, Glycemic Index). Rigid guidelines recommending that up to 60% of calories be taken from carbohydrate (mostly complex carbohydrate) and no more than 30% from fat have been replaced by a more flexible approach that is based on the client's usual intake and laboratory data. There is no longer one diabetic diet that is appropriate for all individuals; increased flexibility

Glycemic Index

Diabetic diets have traditionally restricted simple sugars based on the premise that they are absorbed quickly and can cause rapid elevations in blood glucose levels. Most CHO calories are provided by starches, which are digested more slowly than sugars and have less of an impact on blood glucose levels, or so we thought.

Recent studies, however, indicate that a food's glycemic index (the effect of food on blood glucose levels compared to the response of an equivalent amount of glucose) is related to numerous other factors than just whether the food consists of sugar or starch. Fat, fiber (particularly pectin and guar), the action of enzyme inhibitors, protein, protein-starch interactions, and the structure of a food may all influence glycemic index.

Pure sugars, for instance, do raise blood glucose levels; however, high-sugar, high-fat foods like candy bars and ice cream cause less of an increase in blood glucose levels than brown rice or cornflakes. Glycemic indexes vary even among starches; for instance, potatoes have a high glycemic index and legumes have a low glycemic index.

Experts are not concluding that diabetics should eat ice cream instead of brown rice (a high-fat diet may suppress swings in blood glucose levels, but also increases the risk of cardiovascular disease, obesity, and certain types of cancer). Instead, the glycemic index, in addition to a food's nutrient density and composition, may become another factor to consider when choosing carbohydrates. It is feasible that exchange lists of the future may group carbohydrates according to their glycemic index.

necessitates working closely with the client and health care team to customize a nutrition therapy regimen.

Exercise is another important aspect of treatment for both types of diabetes, regardless of weight status, unless it is contraindicated for other medical reasons. Exercise lowers serum glucose levels by increasing the uptake of glucose into muscle cells, and can improve glucose tolerance by increasing the number of insulin receptors (see display, Potential Benefits of Exercise for Diabetics). Insulin sensitivity also improves with exercise, which is an important benefit for both lean and obese type II diabetics.

In addition to diet and exercise, type I diabetics require insulin therapy; type II diabetics who do not achieve glycemic control through diet and exercise may need oral hypoglycemic agents or, if that fails, insulin therapy (see Drug Alert on p. 623).

Medical Nutrition Therapy for Type I Diabetics

A meal plan that is based on the client's typical intake pattern serves as the basis for integrating insulin therapy into eating and exercise patterns (ADA, 1994). Because most type I diabetics are of normal weight, calorie allowances for weight maintenance should be based on the client's age, sex, and activity patterns (see Appendix 10).

The use of insulin necessitates that, to avoid hypoglycemia, meals and snacks be consistent in number, timing, and calorie composition every day. The actual number of feedings and amount of carbohydrate and calories allowed at each meal and snack should be planned to coincide with peak insulin action (Table 18-2). Blood glucose should be monitored throughout the day so that insulin doses can be adjusted for the amount of food consumed (ADA, 1994). Consistent meal timing is less important for clients who receive insulin through a pump or by multiple injections.

Because exercise lowers blood glucose levels, the optimal time for insulin-dependent diabetics to exercise is usually within 2 hours after eating; exercise beyond that time is more likely to cause hypoglycemia. Clients should test their blood glucose before exercising and eat a carbohydrate snack if the level is <100 mg/dl. During exercise, extra food may be needed to avoid hypoglycemia, depending on the duration and intensity of the activity. Although no additional food is indicated for light exercise of short duration, insulin-dependent diabetics may need 10 to 15 g of extra

Potential Benefits of Exercise for Diabetics

Lowered blood glucose levels

Decreased insulin resistance, increased insulin sensitivity

Increased HDL cholesterol, decreased LDL and VLDL cholesterol

Lowered blood pressure

Reduced body fat, when combined with a low-calorie diet

Enhanced weight reduction

Increased work capacity

Improved sense of well-being

Table 18-2
Onset, Peak, and Duration of Insulin Action (Subcutaneous Administration)

Insulin	Onset (hours)	Peak (hours)	Duration (hours)
SHORT-ACTING			
Regular insulin	½–1	2–4	5–7
Semilente	1–3	2–8	12–16
INTERMEDIATE-ACTING			
NPH	3–4	6–12	18–28
Lente	1–3	8–12	18–28
LONG-ACTING			
Ultralente	4–6	8–24	36
MIXTURES			
50%/50% or 70%/30% (regular and NPH)	3–4	6–12	18–28

Source: Reisling, D. (1995). Acute hypoglycemia. Keeping the bottom from falling out. Nursing 95, 25(2), 41–48.

carbohydrate (ie, approximately one serving of fruit or starch) for each hour of moderate exercise such as hunting or golfing, and 20 to 30 g of extra carbohydrate (ie, approximately two servings of fruit or two servings of starch) for each hour of vigorous exercise like digging or playing basketball. Also, because exercise has a prolonged effect on blood glucose, hypoglycemia can occur up to 24 hours after the activity has ceased (Norton, 1995).

Medical Nutrition Therapy for Type II Diabetics

Weight loss has traditionally been the focus of nutrition intervention for type II diabetics. Clinical symptoms may be immediately improved by a low-calorie diet, and even a mild to moderate weight loss (eg, 10 to 20 pounds) can lower blood glucose levels and improve insulin action. Other potential benefits of weight loss include an increase in high-density lipoproteins (the "good" cholesterol) and a decrease in serum triglyceride concentrations. Unfortunately, long-term weight loss is seldom achieved.

The American Diabetes Association's 1994 "Nutrition recommendations and principles for people with diabetes mellitus" represent a change in philosophy regarding the management of clients with type II diabetes. Serum lipid and blood pressure goals have been added to glucose control as the primary goals for overweight type II diabetics. A variety of interventions are advocated to achieve these goals, only one of which is weight loss. Changing the emphasis from weight loss to other parameters can lead to changes that may ultimately result in weight loss (Diabetes Care and Education, 1994). There is no one proven diet that is uniformly recommended (ADA, 1994).

Still, overweight clients should be encouraged to lose weight. Because a gradual weight loss is easier to maintain than a large, rapid weight loss, and because weight fluctuations can be detrimental to long-range goals, a modest calorie-restricted diet that allows for a ½- to 1-pound weight loss/week may be appropriate. For clients who are unwilling or unable to follow a low-calorie diet, a low-fat diet (ie, 20% of total calories) may be an effective alternative that also produces weight loss and improves metabolic control of glucose and lipids.

New to the 1994 recommendations are the options of surgery and pharmacologic therapy for treatment of clients who are resistant to weight loss by traditional dietary, exercise, and behavioral modification methods. Although very-low-calorie diets (VLCD) rarely produce weight loss that is sustained, they do improve blood glucose and lipid levels. In fact, VLCD produce greater improvements in glycemic control than more moderate diets, even if weight losses are the same (Wing, 1995).

Meal spacing should also be a consideration for type II diabetics; eating meals 4 to 5 hours apart allows postprandial glucose levels to return to baseline. Even though meal consistency is especially important for type I diabetics, type II diabetics may avoid glucose fluctuations by eating meals of approximately the same composition at approximately the same time every day.

Like insulin-dependent diabetics, type II diabetics who are treated with oral hypoglycemic agents may experience exercise-induced hypoglycemia. Clients should be encouraged to exercise within 2 hours after eating, and stop activity if signs and symptoms of hypoglycemia develop.

NURSING PROCESS

Assessment

The latest recommendations stress that nutrition therapy should be based on assessment findings. In addition to the general endocrine assessment criteria on page 602, assess for the following factors:

Weight, weight status, and recent weight change; determine desirable or reasonable weight, estimate calorie requirements.

Blood pressure.

Significant laboratory values: serum glucose, serum lipids, glycated hemoglobin.

Identify whether oral hypoglycemics or insulin is used; assess the impact of other medications on nutrition therapy (eg, antihypertensives, lipid-lowering medications, others). See display, Drugs That Commonly Interfere With Blood Glucose Control.

Medical history, particularly history of cardiovascular disease, hypertension, renal disease, neuropathy, or gastrointestinal (GI).

Meal frequency and timing; consider the impact of shiftwork, if appropriate, and weekend deviations. Determine if mealtimes are relatively consistent or variable from day to day.

Usual calorie intake and overall nutritional adequacy.

Drugs That Commonly Interfere With Blood Glucose Control

Potentiates Hypoglycemia	Potentiates Hyperglycemia
• Alcohol	• Corticosteroids, such as prednisone (Deltasone)
• Allopurinol (Lopurin)	• Diuretics, such as furosemide (Lasix) and all thiazide diuretics
• Anticholinergics, such as Dicyclomine (Bentyl)	• Epinephrine (Primatene Mist)
• Beta-adrenergic antagonists, such as atenolol (Tenormin) and metoprolol (Lopressor)	• Estrogens
• Clofibrate (Novofibrate)	• Niacin (Vitamin B_3)
• Haloperidol (Haldol)	• Phenothiazines, such as chlorpromazine (Thorazine)
• H_2-receptor antagonists, such as cimetidine (Tagamet) and ranitidine (Zantac)	• Phenytoin (Dilantin)
• Monoamine oxidase inhibitors, such as phenelzine sulfate (Nardil)	• Rifampin (Rifadin)
• Salicylates, such as aspirin	• Sympathomimetics, such as theophylline (Duraphyl)
• Sulfonamides, such as trimethoprim/sulfamethoxazole (TMP/SMX; Bactrim)	

Type of carbohydrate, protein, and fat usually consumed.

Usual intake of foods high in fiber, especially soluble fiber: oats, oat bran, dried peas and beans, citrus fruits, apples, and certain vegetables.

The client's likes and dislikes, nutritional needs, lifestyle and work schedule, religious or ethnic influences, food budget, and other medical disorders that require diet modification (eg, hypertension, gout, hyperlipidemia).

The client's ability to understand, attitude toward health and nutrition, and readiness to learn.

Previous diet counseling and outcomes.

Level of family and social support.

Activity level; determine how energy expenditure can best be increased, given the client's preferences, lifestyle, medical status, and motivation.

Nursing Diagnosis

Altered Health Maintenance, related to the lack of knowledge of diet management of diabetes mellitus

Planning and Implementation

Before implementing any dietary interventions, quality-of-life issues should be addressed. People who are told to make numerous dietary changes may feel overwhelmed and resentful, especially if their diet is already modified for other chronic diseases like hypertension or heart disease.

Mutually agreed-upon goals between the health care team and client should focus on improved metabolic control and an overall improvement in nutrient intake. However, goals are not static and should change as needed.

The nutrition recommendations for diabetes (see display) are merely guidelines; the actual content of the diet depends on assessment findings and the client's ability and willingness to change eating habits. To maximize compliance, each diet must be individually tailored so that a minimal amount of adjustment is needed.

Diet modifications should be made sequentially rather than simultaneously. Monitoring and evaluation are ongoing; interventions that fail to achieve client goals should be modified. After goals are achieved, periodic monitoring should be continued. Also, the diet should be adjusted as needed to meet the client's changing needs related to lifestyle changes, life cycle changes, and chronic illnesses.

It is important to identify everyday situations that are perceived by the client as obstacles to dietary adherence (see display, Common Obstacles to Adherence to a Diabetic Diet). Ideally, nutritional counseling should include situational problem-solving training to enable the client to overcome obstacles to adherence (Schlundt et al, 1994). For instance, clients who cope with stress by overeating need counseling on stress reduction techniques and alternative coping methods.

Assessment, goals, and interventions for elderly clients may differ from those of younger clients (see display, Elderly Diabetics: Assessment and Teaching Considerations).

Common Obstacles to Adherence to a Diabetic Diet

Negative emotions: Tempted to overeat to cope with stress and negative emotions.

Resisting temptation: Food, food cues, or cravings tempt client to eat inappropriate foods.

Eating out: Eating at restaurants makes dietary adherence difficult.

Feeling deprived: Tempted to give up trying because of feelings of deprivation.

Time pressure: Time pressure makes eating right or treating reactions very difficult.

Tempted to relapse: Consider giving up and no longer trying to eat right.

Planning: Hectic life makes it difficult to plan what and when to eat.

Competing priorities: Responsibilities and obligations get in the way of eating right.

Social events: Parties, holidays, and socializing tempt the client to overeat and make poor food choices.

Family support: Family's behaviors are less than supportive.

Food refusal: When someone offers the client an inappropriate food, the client fears refusing the food would hurt the person's feelings.

Friend's support: Friend's behaviors are less than supportive.

Source: Schlundt, D., et al. (1994). Situational obstacles to dietary adherence for adults with diabetes. J Am Diet Assoc 94(8), 874–879.

Elderly Diabetics: Assessment and Teaching Considerations

Significance of Aging	Assessment and Teaching Considerations
Blood glucose levels rise with age; the reasons are not clear.	Treatment may not be instituted for glucose elevations considered "high" in younger populations, but that may be "normal" for the elderly.
Elderly are more susceptible to severe hypoglycemia.	Target ranges for elderly diabetics may be set higher for good control with decreased risk of hypoglycemia. A fasting level of 120–150 mg/dl may be considered appropriate. The lowest effective dose of oral hypoglycemics may be used to minimize hypoglycemic risk.
Elderly are at greater nutritional risk (eg, poor dentition, physical impairments that make shopping or cooking difficult, poor appetite related to lack of socialization).	Severe calorie-restricted diets have the potential to be more harmful than beneficial. Weight reduction diets may be reserved for clients who are at 150% or more of ideal weight. Often, elderly are simply advised to avoid sugar and eat at regular intervals.
Physical impairments may preclude exercise.	An exercise program may be instituted slowly and gradually progressed as tolerated. Swimming, walking, and riding a stationary bicycle may be safest.
Cognitive impairments (with memory loss, impaired concentration, dementia, depression) may preclude self-management.	Assess for cognitive deficits; determine their severity and impact on client's ability to perform self-care.
Sensory impairments (decreased hearing, poor eyesight, decreased taste and smell) may complicate teaching and self-management	Clients who may clinically benefit from insulin may be treated with oral agents if poor eyesight or decreased manual dexterity preclude self-injection.
	Written teaching materials may not be an option for elderly with visual impairments. Decreased sense of taste and smell can alter appetite and increase the likelihood of irregular eating patterns.

To maximize teaching effectiveness:

Keep teaching sessions short.

Relay only as much information as necessary.

Go slowly and summarize frequently.

Minimize distractions.

Include a spouse or family member.

Speak clearly; face clients who have a hearing impairment.

Use appropriate written materials; don't overload the client with nice-to-know-but-not-essential information.

CLIENT GOALS

The client will:

Consume adequate calories to attain or maintain a reasonable weight.

Maintain blood glucose levels as near normal as possible by balancing food intake with medication (if appropriate) and exercise.

Achieve optimal serum lipid levels.

Achieve blood pressure of <130/85 mm Hg.

Eat meals and snacks on a regular basis; choose appropriate amounts and types of foods according to meal plan.

Avoid acute complications of IDDM, such as hypoglycemia.

Avoid or delay the onset of chronic complications: renal disease, neuropathy, hypertension, cardiovascular disease.

Improve overall health through optimal nutritional intake.

Increase physical activity to promote health.

NURSING INTERVENTIONS

Diet Management

The physician may order a specific calorie level for the client, such as an 1800-calorie ADA (American Diabetes Association) diet (to signify a diabetic diet, which may differ from a plain calorie-controlled diet in the distribution of carbohydrate or provision of one or more snacks). However, sometimes the physician may opt for a No Concentrated Sweets diet, particularly for elderly clients of normal weight.

Calories should be for "reasonable" weight, that is, a weight the client can maintain. Clients within their ideal weight range should maintain their weight; obese clients should be encouraged to lose weight gradually (ie, ½ to 1 pound/week). Clients who are consuming fewer than 1200 calories may require a multivitamin and mineral supplement.

The diet should be individualized as much as possible to correspond with the client's likes, dislikes, and normal eating pattern. Age, physical activity, and medications must also be considered. There is no universal diet for all diabetics; rather, the meal plan must be individualized according to assessment data and the client's willingness to make changes. Guidelines appear in the display, Nutrition Recommendations for Diabetes.

Meals and snacks, if appropriate, should be eaten at approximately the same time every day and contain approximately the same amount and types of food.

Client Teaching

The goal of diet counseling is to facilitate behavior change, not merely to pass along information. Unfortunately, diet counseling is often limited to a preprinted diet sheet that is handed to the client by the physician, nurse, or secretary, with the explanation of "eat what the pattern says." Not only does this approach fail to facilitate behavior change, it doesn't even pass along sufficient information for an extremely well-motivated client to learn.

Goals can best be met by providing information in stages, beginning with basic information and progressing to in-depth details as information is not only understood but also assimilated. Some clients may never progress beyond basic information, which is fine, as long as goals are met. Reinforcement and feedback are also useful.

Basic information includes an overview of nutrition and nutrient requirements and an explanation of both the role of diet in the treatment of diabetes and the importance of meal timing and consistency; survival-skill information, such as label

FOOD *for* THOUGHT

Counting Carbos

Carbohydrate counting is a relatively new meal planning approach that may offer an alternative to the use of traditional exchange lists. Resulting from advances in diabetes management, carbohydrate counting is based on the premise that a carbohydrate is a carbohydrate is a carbohydrate. Emphasis is on consuming a consistent quantity of total carbohydrate, not restricting the type of carbohydrate, as the main priority in establishing glycemic control; published studies indicate no adverse effect when sucrose is substituted for other carbohydrates within the context of a meal plan.

Although carbohydrate counting has the advantage of focusing on a single nutrient (CHO) rather than all the energy-yielding nutrients, protein and fat cannot be disregarded, especially if weight is a concern. Because of its greater flexibility, this method allows the client to feel more in control, and has the potential for improved glucose control. On the minus side, carbohydrate counting requires clients to keep food records initially and periodically; they must also record blood glucose before and after eating. Weighing and measuring foods may be seen as a disadvantage by some clients. In addition, the goals of weight control and healthful eating may be forgotten or foresaken with the emphasis solely on carbohydrate.

The 3 levels of carbohydrate counting as outlined below.

	Goal	Intended Audience
Level I: Getting Started	Carbohydrate consistency, flexible food choices	IDDM, NIDDM, gestational diabetics
Level II: Moving On	Adjustment of medication/food/ activities based on patterns from client's daily records	Any diabetic (diet only, oral agents, IDDM) who has mastered the basics of Level I
Level III: Intensive Diabetes Management Using CHO/Insulin Ratios—Advanced	Adjustment of insulin dose using ratio of CHO/insulin dosage	Clients on intensive insulin therapy; clients who have mastered insulin adjustment and supplementation

reading, how to treat hypoglycemia, and sick day management, must also be conveyed. More in-depth instruction may include how to use exchange lists or carbohydrate counting (see Food for Thought: Counting Carbos). Remember, counseling is not simply a means of imparting information; it should also enable the client to acquire skills needed to change or maintain eating habits (ADA, 1994).

Not all of the following concepts are appropriate for all clients. Instruct the client according to ability and interest

On the appropriate dietary strategies and diet recommendations based on the type of diabetes.

That diet therapy is essential in the treatment of all forms of diabetes and that the diet must be followed permanently, even when no symptoms are apparent.

That medication may be used in addition to diet therapy, not as a substitute.

That the calorie level of the diet is determined by the client's health, energy needs, and activity patterns, and may change as needed.

That eating too much food, stress, acute illness, and certain medications can raise blood sugar levels (hyperglycemia) and can cause excessive urination, increased appetite, increased thirst, confusion, nausea, vomiting, difficulty breathing, and acetone breath.

That not eating enough food while on insulin therapy causes low blood sugar levels (hypoglycemia), which are characterized by nervousness, weakness, sweating, shallow breathing, double vision, and dizziness. To counter hypoglycemic reactions, a readily absorbed form of sugar should be carried at all times (see display, Treatment for Mild Hypoglycemia).

On sick day management:

- Unless otherwise instructed by the physician, clients should maintain their normal medication schedule; monitor blood glucose every 3 to 4 hours. Type I diabetics should monitor their urine for ketones every 3 to 4 hours.
- Clients who are unable to consume a normal diet should rely on liquids to prevent hypoglycemia and to replenish losses that may occur from vomiting or diarrhea.
- Because illness can increase serum glucose levels, precise replacement of all carbohydrate calories may not be required. Generally, 15 g of carbohydrate (ie, 1 starch equivalent or fruit exchange) should be eaten every half-hour and 1½ cups of fluid should be taken every hour. Each of the following have approximately 15 g of carbohydrate and may be acceptable during illness: 6 oz regular ginger ale, ½ cup ice cream, ½ cup apple juice, 1 frozen juice bar, ¼ cup sherbet, ½ cup regular gelatin, ½ cup orange juice, 1 cup creamed soup.

In-depth information

On the use of exchange lists (see displays, Exchanges and Diabetic Diet [American Diabetes Association]; the actual exchange lists appear in Appendix 11).

- Exchange lists simplify meal planning, eliminate the need for daily calculations, ensure a consistent, nutritionally balanced diet, and add variety. However, the exchange lists may not be appropriate or acceptable for all

Treatment for Hypoglycemia

- Test blood sugar.
- Take 10–15 g of readily absorbable CHO (avoid high-fat treatments like candy bars, which work too slowly and may cause very high blood glucose levels hours later). Any of the following will work:
    4 oz regular soft drink
    4 oz orange juice
    8 oz whole or 2% milk

    2 or 3 glucose tablets (5 g each)
    6–8 graham crackers
    5 LifeSavers
- Eat a small, longer-acting snack that provides carbohydrate, protein, and fat, such as crackers and cheese or half of a sandwich.
- Retest blood sugar and repeat the treatment every 15 minutes if symptoms are still present or until blood glucose exceeds 70 mg/dl.

Exchanges

Groups/Lists	Carbohydrate (grams)	Protein (grams)	Fat (grams)	Calories
CARBOHYDRATE GROUP				
Starch	15	3	1 or less	80
Fruit	15	—	—	60
Milk				
Skim	12	8	0–3	90
Low-fat	12	8	5	120
Whole	12	8	8	150
Other carbohydrates	15	varies	varies	varies
Vegetables	5	2	—	25
MEAT AND MEAT SUBSTITUTE GROUP				
Very lean	—	7	0–1	35
Lean	—	7	3	55
Medium-fat	—	7	5	75
High-fat	—	7	8	100
FAT GROUP	—	—	5	45

age, ethnic, and cultural groups; individual adjustments may be vital for compliance.

- The carbohydrate group (which contains the starch, fruit, milk, other carbohydrate, and vegetable exchange lists) is one of three categories on the exchange lists. With the exception of the vegetable list, all other lists within the carbohydrate group contain approximately the same amount of carbohydrate and can generally be substituted for one another.

- The meat and meat substitute group is divided into four groups based on fat content; all four groups provide the same amount of protein and no carbohydrates.

- The fat group supplies only fat; however, it is divided into three sublists: monounsaturated fats, polyunsaturated fats, and saturated fats.

- With the exception of the starch, fruit, milk, and other carbohydrate exchanges, items from one list cannot be exchanged for items in a different exchange list (ie, 1 cup of milk can be exchanged for 1 serving of fruit, but not for 1 serving of meat or fat).

- Portion sizes are important; weigh or measure food until portion sizes can be estimated accurately.

- Based on the client's assessment data, a meal plan is devised that shows how many servings of each exchange the client should have for each meal and snack (see display, Sample Meal Plan). For IDDM, meal size corresponds to peak insulin action. Because of that, it is not a good idea to "save" exchanges from one meal to use at another, especially for clients who are on insulin or oral agents.

Diabetic Diet (American Diabetes Association [ADA] Diet)

OBJECTIVES

Attain and maintain reasonable body weight.

Maintain near normal blood glucose and lipid levels.

Avoid acute complications.

Prevent or delay chronic complications.

Maintain optimal nutritional status.

INDICATIONS

All types of diabetes mellitus.

May also be used for weight reduction in nondiabetics and borderline diabetics.

CHARACTERISTICS OF EXCHANGE LISTS FOR MEAL PLANNING

Foods are grouped into exchange lists according to their composition.

Portion sizes are specified so that each serving within a list contains approximately the same amount of carbohydrates, protein, fat, and calories (see Appendix 11).

The number of servings allowed from each exchange list depends on the calorie content and composition of the diet and should correspond as closely as possible with the client's preferences and food habits.

Meal patterns specify the number of servings from each exchange list allowed for each meal and snack.

POTENTIAL PROBLEM

Noncompliance

RATIONALE/NURSING INTERVENTIONS AND CONSIDERATIONS

1. Emotional trauma related to the diagnosis of diabetes (denial, anger, and depression)
   - Provide support and encouragement. If possible, withhold diet teaching until the client is emotionally ready.
   - Assure the client that his or her usual diet habits and meal patterns, as well as his or her individual tastes, preferences, and food budget, will all be considered during the formulation of an individualized diet plan.
   - Assure the client that it is not necessary to buy special foods and encourage the family to eat the same food/meals as the client.

2. Lack of motivation
   - Encourage the client to attend group learning sessions, which tend to be more effective than individualized instruction.
   - Provide frequent follow-up and feedback over an extended period of time.
   - Enlist family support and involvement and encourage their participation in group sessions.

3. Unwillingness to follow the diet related to a "sweet tooth"
   - Encourage the use of non-nutritive sweeteners (sweeteners that do not contain appreciable amounts of calories), such as saccharin and aspartame.
   - Provide information regarding diabetic cookbooks that include recipes for desserts with the exchange value specified.
   - Advise the client that foods from the Other Carbohydrate list can be substituted for a starch, fruit, or milk, plus fat(s) as specified. Because they are not equivalent nutritionally, they should be used only occasionally, unless calorie needs are high.

4. Intellectually unable to comprehend the reason for the diet and its strategies
   - Encourage family involvement.
   - Tailor the diet instruction to the client's ability; consider using simplified meal patterns, food models, and pictures. Minimize guidelines and restrictions as much as possible.

5. Lack of knowledge related to the misconception that insulin or oral hypoglycemia agents eliminate the need to follow a modified diet
   - Instruct the client that medication and diet work together to control blood sugar levels

(continued)

Diabetic Diet (American Diabetes Association [ADA] Diet) (Continued)

and that medication is not a substitute for diet therapy.

6. Lack of knowledge related to calculating the amount of exchanges from mixed dishes and other foods not listed on the exchange lists
   - Provide the client with appropriate exchange lists, such as those containing ethnic or regional foods, convenience foods, or fast food and restaurant items.
   - Encourage the client to become familiar with the CHO, protein, fat, and calorie content of each of the exchange lists and to use that information to analyze a recipe or food label for its approximate exchange value.

POTENTIAL PROBLEM

Symptoms of hypoglycemia in insulin-dependent diabetics—nervousness, weakness, sweating, shallow breathing, double vision, dizziness, and potential coma. Prolonged hypoglycemia in children can result in permanent neuromotor damage.

RATONALE/NURSING INTERVENTIONS AND CONSIDERATIONS

1. Unbalanced meal selection
   - Stress the importance of using the exchange lists correctly. Although all items within an exchange group can be substituted for each other, items from one group cannot be exchanged for items in another (except for the starch, milk, fruit, and other carbohydrate lists).
   - Advise the client to eat a source of protein and/or fat at each meal and snack to slow the rate of CHO digestion and absorption.
   - Stress the importance of eating the prescribed amount of food at each meal and snack. Food should not be "saved" at one meal so that more can be eaten at the next.
2. Inadequate food intake related to too long an interval between feedings
   - Advise the client not to skip meals and snacks. If a delayed meal is anticipated,

instruct the client to eat part of the meal allowance as a snack at the usual meal time and eat the remaining exchange as soon as possible.
   - Counsel the client to carry a source of rapidly absorbed sugar (hard candy, sugar cubes, and so forth) with him at all times for unexpectedly delayed meals. The client's normal meal should follow as soon as possible.
   - If necessary, modify the meal plan to include more snacks.
3. Inadequate food intake related to decreased appetite
   - Determine the cause of the change in appetite. If the client is not underweight and the change is due to normal causes (decreased activity, decreased metabolic rate related to aging), request a lower calorie allowance and an insulin adjustment from the physician.
   - If the decrease in appetite is related to illness, stress the importance of eating and drinking. Urge the client to attempt to follow the meal plan as closely as possible, using only liquids or soft foods if necessary.
   - Instruct the client to report episodes of vomiting or illnesses lasting more than 2 days to the physician.
4. Decreased insulin requirement related to weight loss
   - Instruct the client to inform the physician of any true weight loss (ie, loss of body fat, not minor, daily, weight fluctuations).
5. An increase in exercise
   - Remind the client to eat extra CHO before moderate and vigorous exercise and to eat a source of sugar if symptoms of hypoglycemia develop while exercising. A change in the meal pattern may be necessary if the increase in exercise is expected to be permanent.

- Certain foods and beverages are considered "free" because they provide less than 5 grams of carbohydrate or less than 20 calories per serving. Some of these items have serving sizes specified; those choices should be limited to three servings per day, preferably spread out over the course of the day. Items without a portion size, like sugar substitutes, may be used as desired.
- A combination foods list gives examples of how mixed dishes can be calculated into a meal plan; components are identified and then classified according to their representative exchange lists. For instance, ¼ of a 10-inch thin crust pizza is listed as 2 starch exchanges (the crust), 2 medium-fat meat exchanges (the cheese), and 1 fat exchange (oil in and on the crust).
- Fast foods are also calculated into a meal plan according to their composition. For instance, one medium submarine sandwich is listed as three starch exchanges (the roll), one vegetable exchange (lettuce, tomato, onion), two medium-fat meat exchanges (two ounces of luncheon meats), and one fat exchange (oil or mayonnaise).
- The use of products that are made with nonnutritive sugar substitutes but that contain other calorie-contributing ingredients must be calculated into the meal plan.
- There is no significant advantage of using sugar alcohols (sorbitol, mannitol, and xylitol) over other nutritive sweeteners; large amounts may have a laxative effect.

If alcohol is consumed, it should be used in moderation. One serving of alcohol (1.5 oz of distilled spirits, 12 oz of beer, or 5 oz of wine) is generally substituted for 2 fat exchanges. Because alcohol can induce hypoglycemia, especially in clients who are taking insulin or sulfonylureas, it should not be consumed in a fasting state. Dry wine and light or "near" beer are preferred because of their reduced calorie and alcohol content. Sugar-free sodas and water are acceptable mixers.

How to order from a menu when dining out:
- Estimate portion sizes of all foods.
- For foods not included on the exchange lists, figure out the number of bread, meat, and fat exchanges by analyzing the ingredients and categorizing them into the appropriate exchange group.
- Choose tomato juice, unsweetened fruit juice, clear broth, bouillon, or consommé as an appetizer instead of sweetened juices, fried vegetables, a seafood cocktail (unless meat exchange is deducted from entrée), or creamed or thick soups.
- Choose fresh vegetable salads and use oil and vinegar or fresh lemon instead of regular salad dressings, or request that the dressing be put on the side. Avoid coleslaw and other salads with the dressing already added.
- Order plain (without gravy or sauce) roasted, baked, or broiled meat, fish, and poultry instead of fried, sautéed, or breaded entrées. Avoid stews and casseroles. Request a doggie bag if the portion exceeds the meal plan allowance.
- Order steamed, boiled, or broiled vegetables.

(Text continues on page 622)

SAMPLE **MEAL PLAN**

Meal Plan for: _____

Dietitian: _____

Date: _____

Phone: _____

	Grams	Percent
Carbohydrate	222	50
Protein	88	20
Fat	59	30
Calories	1771	

Time	Number of Exchanges/Choices	Menu Ideas	Menu Ideas
8:00	4 Carbohydrate group 2 Starch 1 Fruit 1 Milk 0 Meat group 2 Fat group	2 slices wheat toast ½ cup orange juice 1 cup skim milk 2 tsp margarine 2 tsp low-sugar jelly (free)	2 waffles (2 starch plus 2 fat) ½ grapefruit 1 cup skim milk 2 Tbsp sugar-free syrup (free)
12:00	4 Carbohydrate group 3 Starch 1 Fruit _ Milk ✓ Vegetables 3 oz Meat group 2 Fat group	1 cup tomato soup (1 starch) 1 hamburger roll (2 starch) 1 small banana 1 cup tossed salad 3 oz lean hamburger patty (3 med-fat) 2 Tbsp salad dressing (2 fat) 1 Tbsp catsup (free)	2 slices bread 1 cup cantaloupe cubes ½ cup tomato juice 3 oz smoked turkey breast 2 tsp regular mayonnaise ½ cup sugar-free low-fat pudding (1 starch)

Time	Number of Exchanges/Choices	Menu Ideas	Menu Ideas

6:00	Carbohydrate group
	5 ___ Starch
	  4 ___ Starch
	  1 ___ Fruit
	  ___ Milk
	  ✓ Vegetables
	3 oz. Meat group
	2 ___ Fat group
		⅓ cup rice
		½ cup sweet potato
		½ cup peas } 4 starch
		1 plain small dinner roll
		1¼ cup strawberries
		½ cup wax beans
		3 oz skinless chicken breast (lean)
		2 tsp margarine
			1½ cups tuna noodle casserole (3 starch, 3 meat)
			1 sliced kiwi fruit
			½ cup cooked carrots
			1 dinner roll (1 starch)
			2 tsp margarine

HS	1 cup skim milk 1 starch 1 fat	1 cup skim milk 3 cups microwave popcorn (1 starch plus one fat)	1 cup nonfat yogurt sweetened with aspartame 6 butter-type crackers (1 starch, 1 fat)

- Choose plain, baked, mashed, boiled, or steamed potatoes, rice, or noodles.
- Select fresh fruit for dessert.
- Request a sugar substitute for coffee or tea, if desired.
- Diabetic exchange lists are available for fast-food restaurants.
- Most airlines provide diabetic meals if they are requested at the time that flight reservations are made.

On food preparation ideas:
- Food does not have to be prepared separately from the rest of the family's.
- For variety, use margarine or oil from the fat allowance to sauté meat or vegetables.
- Trim all visible fat from meat after cooking and remove the skin from chicken.
- Use diabetic cookbooks for variety; their recipes specify portion sizes and the number of exchanges per portion.

On food purchasing and label reading:
- Buy prepared foods that have nutrition information on the label so that the exchange value can be calculated, or write to the manufacturer to request nutrition information.
- Compare the nutrition information and ingredient labels of different brands of the same product; these can vary greatly.
- Buy fresh, frozen without sugar, or water-packed canned fruit, if possible; if not, rinse sweetened fruit under running water for 1 minute or more to remove sugary syrup.
- Dietetic products are not necessarily calorie-free or specifically intended for diabetics; foods that are labeled "dietetic" may be made without sugar, without salt, with a particular type of fat, or for special food allergies. Read the ingredient label and check with a diet counselor before adding a dietetic food to the diet, or avoid dietetic foods altogether because they are expensive and usually do not taste as good as the foods they are intended to replace.
- Avoid foods that contain coconut oil, palm oil, palm kernel oil, unspecified vegetable oils, and hydrogenated oils because they are high in saturated fats.

Provide the client with the following, if appropriate:
- An individualized meal plan.
- The exchange lists and supplemental exchange lists, if desired (ie, for illnesses, special occasions, ethnic foods, fast-food restaurants, alcoholic beverages).
- Diabetic recipes, titles of diabetic cookbooks.

Monitoring Progress

Monitor for the following signs or symptoms:

Serum glucose, glycosylated hemoglobin, serum lipid levels
Results of self-monitoring of glucose
Weight, weight changes
Compliance with the diet, and the need for follow-up diet counseling

Lifestyle or life cycle changes that necessitate further diet modifications
The onset of complications

Evaluation

Evaluation is ongoing. Provided that the plan of care has not changed, the client will achieve the goals as stated above.

DRUG
ALERT

For type II diabetics, treatment with insulin, and to a lesser degree, oral hypoglycemic agents, can hinder weight loss and actually promote weight gain. Before it is determined that the diet is not effective and that drug therapy is necessary, every attempt should be made to achieve metabolic control through diet alone.

Hyperinsulinism

Hyperinsulinism is characterized by an excessive insulin secretion in response to carbohydrate-rich foods, leading to hypoglycemia (blood glucose levels of 40 mg/dl or less). **Organic hyperinsulinism**, which occurs during fasting, is a rare disorder that is caused by hyperplasia of the islets of Langerhans or by insulin-secreting pancreatic tumors. It is treated by surgical removal of the insulin-secreting tumor, or by pancreatic resection of hyperplastic tissue. The exact cause of **functional hyperinsulinism**, which occurs after eating, is unknown; approximately 15% of cases result in diabetes mellitus. Functional hyperinsulinism may occur after a gastrectomy. Diet management that is designed to avoid stimulating insulin secretion is used to treat functional hyperinsulinism.

NURSING PROCESS

Assessment

In addition to the general endocrine assessment criteria, assess for the following factors:

The relationship between eating and the onset of hypoglycemic symptoms. Observe for weakness, hunger, nervousness, trembling, sweating, and faintness that may occur 2 to 4 hours after eating. Convulsions and loss of consciousness may occur in severe cases.

The impact of carbohydrate ingestion on symptoms—eating carbohydrate should reverse symptoms.

Dietary changes made in response to symptoms (ie, foods avoided, foods preferred).

Nursing Diagnosis

Altered Health Maintenance, related to the lack of knowledge of diet management of functional hyperinsulinism

Planning and Implementation

The diet for functional hyperinsulinism should be nutritionally sound and provide calories for healthy weight; obese clients should be encouraged to lose weight.

To avoid excessive insulin secretion, restrict carbohydrate-rich foods that produce a rapid rise in blood glucose. However, restricting total carbohydrate intake is neither necessary nor practical. Instead, to slow the rise in blood glucose levels, care should be taken to eat protein and/or fat whenever carbohydrates are consumed. A high fiber intake, especially soluble fiber, may be beneficial.

The diet should be liberal in protein, because protein does not stimulate insulin secretion. Fat supplies the remainder of calories.

Small, frequent meals, each containing protein and/or fat, help slow the rate of carbohydrate absorption, decrease the rise in blood glucose levels, and reduce insulin secretion. The diabetic exchange lists may be used for meal planning.

CLIENT GOALS

The client will:

Avoid symptoms of hypoglycemia after eating.

Consume adequate calories and protein to attain or maintain healthy weight.

Describe the principles and rationale of diet management for functional hyperinsulinism, and implement the appropriate dietary changes.

Identify foods and meals that cause hypoglycemic symptoms.

NURSING INTERVENTIONS

Diet Management

Provide calories for healthy weight.

Limit simple sugars and dried fruits. Encourage a high fiber intake, especially foods high in soluble fiber.

Increase protein intake to 1.0 to 1.5 g/kg/day.

Provide three meals and two to three snacks daily, each containing protein and/or fat.

Prohibit alcohol and caffeine.

A sample menu appears in the display, Hyperinsulinism Diet: Sample Menu.

Client Teaching

Instruct the client

On the principles and rationale of diet management for functional hyperinsulinism.

On the use of exchange lists (see section on Client Teaching for Diabetes).

That eliminating sugar also means eliminating foods that are high in sugar, such as syrups, honey, jelly, jam, candy, sweetened snacks (eg, caramel popcorn), and desserts.

That the use of sugar substitutes is allowed.

To carry a source of readily absorbable carbohydrate (such as hard candy or sugar cubes) at all times in case of a hypoglycemic attack.

To avoid alcohol and caffeine, which can aggravate hypoglycemia.

Monitoring Progress

Monitor for the following signs or symptoms:

Weight, weight changes

Compliance with the diet, and evaluate the need for further diet counseling

Effectiveness of the diet, and determine whether additional diet modifications are needed

Signs or symptoms of diabetes mellitus

Evaluation

Evaluation is ongoing. Provided that the plan of care has not changed, the client will achieve the goals as stated above.

SAMPLE **MENU**

Hyperinsulinism Diet

BREAKFAST

½ banana
½ cup oatmeal
1 slice whole-wheat toast with margarine
½ cup 2% milk
Coffee/tea

MIDMORNING SNACK

1 oz cheddar cheese
6 saltine crackers
½ cup 2% milk

LUNCH

Tomato soup
Turkey sandwich
Carrot and celery sticks
1 cup 2% milk
Apple

MIDAFTERNOON SNACK

Peanuts
Sugar-free carbonated beverage

DINNER

Roast beef
Roasted potatoes
Tossed salad
Winter squash
½ cup 2% milk
½ cup rice pudding

BEDTIME SNACK

Popcorn
1 cup 2% milk

THYROID DISORDERS

The thyroid gland secretes two active hormones, **tetraiodothyronine (thyroxine,** or T_4) and triiodothyronine (T_3). Alterations in thyroid hormone secretion cause alterations in the basal metabolic rate, as evidenced by weight changes and changes in bowel elimination.

Hypothyroidism

Hypothyroidism (which may be triggered by idiopathic causes, or occur secondary to surgical removal of the thyroid gland, radioactive iodine therapy, or an autoimmune disorder [Hashimoto's thyroiditis]) is characterized by deficient thyroid hormone secretion that leads to decreased basal metabolic rate, possibly by 15% to 30% or more. **Cretinism** refers to a thyroid deficiency that is present at birth; **myxedema** is the advanced stage of hypothyroidism in adults. Myxedema occurs five times more frequently in women than in men, and it usually occurs between 30 and 60 years of age. Early symptoms include fatigue, menstrual changes (menorrhagia or amenorrhea), hair loss, brittle nails, dry skin, paresthesia of the hands and feet, and thick speech. Later, decreased body temperature and pulse rate; weight gain; physical and mental slowness; an edematous appearance; enlarged tongue, hands, and feet; constipation; and intolerance to cold may develop. Complications of myxedema include rapid onset of atherosclerosis, coronary heart disease, angina pectoris, myocardial infarction, and congestive heart failure. Increased sensitivity to sedatives, opiates, and anesthetic drugs may develop, as well as acute organic psychosis, which is characterized by paranoia and delusions. Hypoventilation, hypothermia, and respiratory acidosis occur with myxedema coma; only 50% of its victims survive.

Hypothyroidism is treated with thyroid hormone replacement and diet management to prevent and/or alleviate symptoms of weight gain and constipation.

Hyperthyroidism

Hyperthyroidism (Graves' disease, thyrotoxicosis, exophthalmic goiter) is characterized by excessive thyroid hormone secretion that leads to increased basal metabolic rate, possibly by 15% to 25% in mild cases, and up to 50% to 75% in severe cases. The exact cause is unknown, but it is believed to be the result of an autoimmune disorder; it may be related to emotional stress or infection. Hyperthyroidism occurs five times more frequently in women than in men, and it most often occurs between 30 and 40 years of age.

Symptoms include nervousness, irritability, apprehension, and decreased attention span; increased pulse rate, palpitations, and increased systolic blood pressure; intolerance to heat and profuse perspiration; flushed, warm, soft, moist skin; bulging eyes (exophthalmos); ravenous appetite accompanied by progressive weight loss;

muscular weakness; amenorrhea; and diarrhea or constipation. Mild cases may be marked by alternating periods of exacerbation and remission, with possible spontaneous recovery within months or years. Emaciation, intense nervousness, delirium, disorientation, and heart disease (tachycardia, atrial fibrillation, congestive heart failure) are possible complications; death occurs in rare instances.

Drug therapy, radiation, or surgical removal of part or all of the thyroid gland may be used to treat hyperthyroidism. The choice of treatment depends on the client's age, the cause and severity of the disease, and the development of complications. Diet management is used to prevent further weight loss and restore normal body weight, to reverse negative nitrogen balance and replenish nutritional losses, and to alleviate diarrhea or constipation.

NURSING PROCESS

Assessment

In addition to the general endocrine assessment criteria, assess for the following factors:

Symptoms of thyroid disorder that directly or indirectly affect nutritional status or intake; assess onset, frequency, severity, interventions attempted and the results.

Dietary changes made in response to thyroid disorder or its symptoms (ie, foods avoided, foods preferred). Determine which foods are best and least tolerated.

Bowel elimination patterns and any recent, significant changes.

Weight status, recent weight changes.

Nursing Diagnosis

Altered Nutrition: More or less than body requirements, related to altered metabolism secondary to hyperthyroidism or hypothyroidism

Planning and Implementation

Provide a well-balanced, nutritionally adequate diet with calories for healthy weight, based on the client's nutritional status, weight status, and symptoms.

Adjust fiber intake to promote normal bowel elimination, as needed.

See Table 18-3 for considerations specific for each thyroid disorder.

CLIENT GOALS

The client will:

Consume adequate calories and protein to attain or maintain healthy body weight and to restore or maintain optimal nutritional status.

Table 18-3
Diet Management Considerations for Hypothyroidism and Hyperthyroidism

Hypothyroidism	Hyperthyroidism
Until normal metabolism is restored, clients with myxedema experience weight gain even if calorie intake is low. However, a low-calorie diet combined with thyroid hormone therapy should enable the client to achieve normal weight.	Calorie requirements may increase to 4500 to 5000 cal or more. A liberal protein intake of 100 g or more combined with a liberal CHO intake is recommended.
A high-fiber diet will not only help alleviate constipation but is useful in weight reduction; high-fiber foods generally are low in calories and provide feeling of fullness	Vitamin and mineral needs increase related to the accelerated rate of metabolism and nutrient utilization. Clients experiencing steady weight loss despite eating large amounts of food are often frustrated and discouraged. Provide emotional support and a pleasant eating environment. Solicit food preferences and encourage the intake of nutritionally dense foods (ie, fortified milk shakes, foods with added milk powder, eggs, cheese, butter, or meat).
Low-fat, modified-fat, or low-sodium diet modifications may be indicated for complications of atherosclerosis and heart disease.	Provide six to eight feedings to maximize intake.
	Eliminate CNS stimulants, such as caffeine and alcohol.
	Clients with hyperthyroidism may experience osteoporosis and an increased risk of bone fractures related to an increase in calcium and phosphorus excretion. Encourage the intake of foods high in calcium (Appendix 12) and provide calcium supplements if needed. Hypothyroidism or hypoparathyroidism resulting from a partial or total thyroidectomy may require diet modification.

Have normal bowel elimination (ie, not have diarrhea or constipation).

Describe the principles and rationale of diet management for hypothyroidism or hyperthyroidism, and implement the appropriate dietary changes.

NURSING INTERVENTIONS

Diet Management

Provide calories for healthy body weight, based on age, sex, and activity.
Modify fiber intake to either promote or reduce bowel stimulation, as indicated.

See Table 18-3 for other diet management considerations.

Client Teaching

Instruct the client

On the principles and rationale of diet management for hypothyroidism or hyperthyroidism.

Monitoring Progress

Monitor for the following signs or symptoms:

Compliance with the diet, and the need for follow-up diet counseling

Effectiveness of the diet (ie, normal weight status, normal bowel elimination), and evaluate the need for further diet modifications

Evaluation

Evaluation is ongoing. Provided that the plan of care has not changed, the client will achieve the goals as stated above.

DRUG
ALERT

Replacement thyroid hormones that are used to treat hypothyroidism can cause elevated blood glucose levels. It may be necessary to restrict the intake of concentrated sweets or to provide a diabetic diet if insulin therapy is used.

Clients who receive iodine in preparation for thyroid surgery may need to restrict their intake of rich sources of iodine—iodized salt, seafood, and bread made with iodate dough conditioners.

PARATHYROID DISORDERS

The parathyroid glands, tiny organs embedded on each side of the thyroid gland, secrete parathyroid hormone (PTH), which regulates calcium and phosphorous metabolism. Parathyroid disorders cause alterations in the calcium content of bones and in serum and urinary calcium levels. Because calcium and phosphorus have an inverse relationship, serum levels of phosphorus are also altered.

Hypoparathyroidism

Hypoparathyroidism occurs most frequently as a result of a thyroidectomy, parathyroidectomy, or radical neck dissection; this is related to suppression of the gland or interference with the blood supply. It may develop immediately after surgery, or within 1 to 2 days, and is usually temporary.

Parathyroid hormone deficiency decreases the mobilization of calcium from the bone; serum phosphorus rises, urinary excretion both of calcium and phosphorus decreases, and hypocalcemia develops. Hypocalcemia increases neuromuscular irritability and can lead to tetany (painful, involuntary muscle spasms); tingling, numbness, and cramping in the extremities; bronchospasms; laryngeal spasms; Trousseau's sign (carpopedal spasm that occurs when circulation is occluded in the arm with a blood pressure cuff); and Chvostek's sign (facial muscle spasms that occur when muscles or branches of facial nerves are tapped). Dysphagia, increased sensitivity to light, cardiac arrhythmias, convulsions, anxiety, irritability, depression, and delirium may develop. Other potential complications include cataracts, psychoses, and permanent brain damage. Heart failure may develop in cases of chronic idiopathic hypoparathyroidism.

In acute hypoparathyroidism (eg, tetany), intravenous calcium gluconate is given to raise serum calcium levels. Sedatives may be needed to control convulsions. For chronic hypoparathyroidism, treatment involves oral calcium and vitamin D supplements, and aluminum hydroxide gel or aluminum carbonate to bind phosphate and increase its excretion.

Hyperparathyroidism

Excessive parathyroid hormone secretion leads to hyperparathyroidism, which may vary from mild to severe. **Primary hyperparathyroidism** is caused by hyperactivity of the parathyroid glands, related to benign or malignant tumor growth, or tissue hyperplasia and hypertrophy; secondary causes include chronic renal disease, rickets, osteomalacia, and acromegaly.

An increase in PTH secretion causes calcium to leave the bones and enter the bloodstream; the rise in serum calcium causes a corresponding drop in serum phosphorus. Hypercalcemia leads to a decrease in neuromuscular irritability, which may be evidenced by apathy, fatigue, depression, paranoia, muscular weakness, nausea, vomiting, constipation, and anorexia. The increase in urinary calcium can lead to numerous renal complications, such as formation of calcium phosphate renal stones, renal obstruction, calcification of renal parenchyma, pyelonephritis, and renal failure. Gastrointestinal complications include pancreatitis and peptic ulcers; these may lead to perforation and hemorrhage. Loss of calcium from the bone can lead to back and joint pain, pain on weight bearing, pathologic fractures, skeletal deformities, and loss of height. Calcium phosphate may precipitate in the lungs, muscles, heart, and eyes.

A hypercalcemic crisis occurs when serum calcium levels exceed 8 to 9 mEq/l. Polyuria, polydipsia, volume depletion, fever, altered consciousness, azotemia, and mental disturbances are frequent symptoms. Cardiac arrest is responsible for the high mortality rate.

Hyperparathyroidism is treated by surgical removal of abnormal tissue, which may result in hypoparathyroidism.

NURSING PROCESS

Assessment

In addition to the general endocrine assessment criteria, assess for the following factors:

Symptoms of parathyroid disorder that directly or indirectly affect nutritional status or intake; assess onset, frequency, severity, interventions attempted and the results.

Dietary changes made in response to parathyroid disorder or its symptoms (ie, foods avoided, foods preferred). Determine which foods are best and least tolerated.

Usual calcium intake: milk and dairy products, green leafy vegetables, and canned fish with bones.

Usual vitamin D intake, and exposure to sunlight.

Nursing Diagnosis

Altered Health Maintenance, related to lack of knowledge of diet management for parathyroid disorders

Planning and Implementation

For both hypoparathyroidism and hyperparathyroidism, diet management may be used to help restore normal calcium balance. However, although the manipulation of dietary calcium may help, in most cases it does not fully compensate for an imbalance of parathyroid hormone. In addition, it is difficult to increase dietary calcium (eg, for hypoparathyroidism) *and* avoid a high phosphorus intake because milk and dairy products are rich sources of both calcium and phosphorus.

In addition to adjusting calcium intake, the diet for hyperparathyroidism may also be modified to alleviate vomiting, constipation, anorexia, and GI upset, as needed (see Chapter 16), or to help prevent renal complications.

CLIENT GOALS

The client will:

Increase or decrease calcium intake to help normalize serum calcium levels in hypoparathyroidism or hyperparathyroidism, respectively.
Modify the diet, as needed, to help prevent or alleviate GI or renal complications.
Identify foods that are high in calcium, phosphorus, and vitamin D.
Consume a nutritionally adequate diet.

NURSING INTERVENTIONS

Diet Management

Increase calcium intake for hypoparathyroidism; use milk and dairy products with caution because they are rich sources of phosphorus. Sources of calcium appear in Appendix 12.
Decrease calcium intake for hyperparathyroidism. After surgery, a high-calcium diet may be indicated.

Other considerations for hypoparathyroidism and hyperparathyroidism are outlined in Table 18-4.

Client Teaching

Instruct the client

On the principles and rationale of diet management for hypoparathyroidism or hyperparathyroidism.
On rich sources of dietary calcium, phosphorus, and vitamin D.
On the role of vitamin D in increasing serum calcium, if appropriate, and to increase daily exposure to the sunlight.
To take supplements only as prescribed by the physician.

Table 18-4
Diet Management Considerations for Hypoparathyroidism and Hyperparathyroidism

Hypoparathyroidism	Hyperparathyroidism
In addition to calcium and vitamin D supplements, a high-calcium, low-phosphorus diet may be prescribed, even though the diet order is not likely to be achieved. Green leafy vegetables are good sources of calcium, but they contain compounds that bind calcium and inhibit its absorption. Milk and dairy products are the best sources of calcium, but they may be allowed only in limited amounts because they are also rich in phosphorus (Appendix 12). Diets lacking in milk and dairy products are not likely to provide the RDA for calcium (800 mg) and certainly cannot meet the needs of clients who may require 1000 to 2000 mg or more of calcium/day.	Increase fluids to 3000 to 4000 ml or more a day to dilute the urine and prevent the precipitation of renal stones. Urge the client to drink large amounts of fluid before bed and periodically through the night to avoid concentrated urine.
Calcium absorption is enhanced by vitamin C and some amino acids because calcium is soluble in an acid medium. More calcium is absorbed when supplements are given in small, divided doses rather than in large individual doses.	Drinking cranberry juice is often recommended to acidify the urine and prevent the precipitation of basic stones, such as calcium. However, it takes at least 1.2 liters of pure cranberry juice (not cranberry juice cocktail, which is a mixture of cranberry juice, water, and sugar) to make a significant change in urinary pH.
	Modify the diet as needed to alleviate anorexia, constipation, GI upset, or ulcers (see Chap. 16).

Monitoring Progress

Monitor for the following signs or symptoms:

Serum calcium and phosphorus; restrict milk and dairy products if phosphorus levels are elevated.

Tolerance of and compliance with the diet, and the need for follow-up diet counseling.

Effectiveness of the diet, and the need for further diet modification.

Evaluation

Evaluation is ongoing. Provided that the plan of care has not changed, the client will achieve the goals as stated above.

ADRENAL CORTEX DISORDERS

The adrenal glands are located above the kidneys. The cortex, or outer portion, secretes corticosteroids, which include glucocorticoids, mineralocorticoids, and small amounts of sex hormones. A deficiency of adrenal cortex hormones primarily affects glucose metabolism and fluid and electrolyte balance.

Primary Adrenocortical Insufficiency (Addison's Disease)

Primary adrenocortical insufficiency is caused by destruction of adrenal cortical tissue, either from idiopathic atrophy or secondary to infections such as tuberculosis. A deficient secretion of glucocorticoid hormones leads to depletion of liver glycogen and hypoglycemia. Mineralocorticoid deficiency (aldosterone) results in increased excretion of sodium, chloride, and water, leading to retention of potassium, acidosis, decreased blood volume, and decreased cardiac output.

With primary adrenocortical insufficiency, adrenal failure occurs over a period of time. Symptoms include muscular weakness, fatigue, weight loss, anorexia, nausea, vomiting, diarrhea, constipation, abdominal pain, and hypotension; symptoms of hypoglycemia, hyponatremia, and hyperkalemia also occur. Diffuse or patchy darkening of the skin is characteristic of Addison's disease; depression, irritability, anxiety, or apprehension may develop. A possible complication of Addison's disease is an addisonian crisis, which is a medical emergency characterized by cyanosis, fever, shock, headache, nausea, abdominal pain, diarrhea, confusion, and restlessness. Circulatory collapse can result from mild overexertion, exposure to cold, acute infection, or decreased salt intake. Death may occur from hypotension and vasomotor collapse.

Addison's disease is treated with hormone replacement: Fludrocortisone is a synthetic corticosteroid that has both glucocorticoid and mineralocorticoid properties. Diet management is used to prevent or treat hypoglycemia and to promote normal fluid and electrolyte balance.

NURSING PROCESS

Assessment

In addition to the general endocrine assessment criteria, assess for the following factors:

Symptoms: onset, frequency, causative factors (if known), severity, interventions attempted and the results.

Dietary changes made in response to symptoms (ie, foods avoided, foods preferred).

Usual sodium intake: convenience foods, processed meats, canned meats, soups, and vegetables; condiments, traditional snack foods, salt-cured foods.

Usual intake of simple sugars.

Usual fluid intake.

Frequency of meals and snacks. Determine if the client frequently skips meals.

Nursing Diagnosis

Fluid Volume Deficit, related to abnormal fluid loss (increased excretion) secondary to primary adrenocortical insufficiency

Planning and Implementation

Depending on the client's fluid and electrolyte status and the type of medication used, the requirements for sodium and potassium may be increased or decreased. Clients who are being treated with cortisone may require a high sodium intake of up to 4 to 6 g/day or more. A high sodium intake is contraindicated for clients who are receiving fludrocortisone because it is a sodium-retaining hormone. Likewise, potassium requirement is determined on an individual basis; although serum potassium levels are elevated in untreated Addison's disease, hormone therapy tends to deplete potassium. A high fluid intake of up to 3 l/day may be indicated to replace losses.

Because hypoglycemia is a recurrent problem, small, frequent meals that are high in protein and moderate in carbohydrate are recommended. The client should consume a large meal at bedtime to avoid early morning hypoglycemia. Concentrated sweets should be avoided.

Supplemental B vitamins and vitamin C may be required for increased metabolism.

CLIENT GOALS

The client will:

Attain or maintain normal fluid and electrolyte balance.
Avoid hypoglycemia by consuming frequent meals, avoiding concentrated sweets, and eating a large meal at bedtime.
Attain or maintain healthy weight.
Describe the principles and rationale of diet management for Addison's disease, and make the appropriate diet changes.
Identify signs and symptoms of hypoglycemia, and carry food at all times.

NURSING INTERVENTIONS

Diet Management

Adjust sodium and potassium intake according to individual requirements.
Provide a high-protein, moderate-carbohydrate diet with calories for healthy weight. Clients who have lost weight should have calories for weight gain. Restrict concentrated sweets.
Increase fluid intake to up to 3 l/day, if indicated.
Provide frequent meals and a large meal at bedtime to prevent hypoglycemia.

Client Teaching

Instruct the client

On the principles and rationale of diet management for Addison's disease, and how to make the appropriate diet changes.

On the signs and symptoms of hypoglycemia. Advise the client to eat frequent meals and to carry food at all times (eg, cheese and crackers).

Monitoring Progress

Monitor for the following signs or symptoms:

Compliance with the diet, and the need for follow-up diet counseling
Effectiveness of the diet, and the need for further diet changes
Weight, weight status
Fluid and electrolyte status; observe for signs of fluid and potassium retention

Evaluation

Evaluation is ongoing. Provided that the plan of care has not changed, the client will achieve the goals as stated above.

DRUG
ALERT *Glucocorticoids*

Glucocorticoids (eg, cortisone, prednisone, dexamethasone) are used to treat Addison's disease and numerous inflammatory, allergic, and immunoreactive disorders. Prolonged or excessive use can cause the following changes in metabolism.

	Dietary Intervention
Increased protein catabolism	Increase protein intake to at least 1 g/kg/day
Negative nitrogen balance, muscle wasting, thinning of the skin, poor wound healing, stunted growth in children	Provide sufficient calories for protein-sparing, especially carbohydrates
Increased gluconeogenesis	Avoid concentrated sweets
Persistent hyperglycemia → diabetes mellitus	Follow diabetic diet if necessary (see Chap. 18)
Increased fat deposition	Not amenable to dietary intervention, unless total calorie intake can be restricted
"Moon face," "buffalo hump," truncal obesity with thin limbs	
Potassium depletion	Increase potassium intake (Appendix 9)
Hypokalemia, arrhythmias, muscular weakness	
Sodium and fluid retention	Restrict sodium intake (see Chap. 17)
Edema, hypertension, complications of hypertension	
Vitamin C depletion from the adrenal glands	Increase vitamin C intake
	Provide vitamin C supplements
Increased HCl secretion	Eat small frequent meals
GI upset, ulcers	Avoid gastric acid stimulants (see Chap. 16)

- Diabetes mellitus is characterized by the absolute or relative deficiency of insulin. Insulin is the hormone that enables glucose to leave the bloodstream and enter cells where it can be metabolized for energy. Insulin also promotes glycogen formation, protein synthesis, and fat formation.

- Type I diabetes, characterized by the lack of insulin secretion, is usually diagnosed during childhood. Its victims are usually at or below normal weight.

- Ninety percent of people with diabetes have type II, which is characterized by normal or above-normal insulin secretion; decreased tissue sensitivity results in hyperglycemia, which provides constant stimulation for insulin secretion. In most cases, obesity contributes to insulin resistance.

- Nutrition therapy is the cornerstone of treatment for all diabetics, regardless of weight status, the use of medication, blood glucose levels, and whether or not symptoms are present. The goals of nutrition therapy are to achieve optimal blood glucose and lipid levels, attain or maintain reasonable weight, and avoid acute and chronic complications.

- Type I diabetics need (1) adequate calories to maintain normal weight; (2) a meal pattern that provides adequate carbohydrate to coincide with peak insulin action; (3) daily consistency in the number, size, and timing of meals and snacks; and (4) extra carbohydrates for moderate and vigorous exercise, especially if exercise occurs more than 2 hours after eating.

- Type II diabetics need to lose weight. Although low-calorie diets have been widely used in the past, their long-term success is low. Other options should be considered, such as a low-fat diet, a very-low-calorie diet, surgery, or pharmacologic therapy. Four to five hours should lapse between meals to allow postprandial glucose levels to return to baseline.

- The American Diabetes Association recommends that diabetics limit their saturated fat intake to less than 10% of total calories, polyunsaturated fat to up to 10% of total calories, and that protein provide 10% to 20% of total calories. The remaining calories are to be divided between carbohydrates and monounsaturated fats, depending on the client's lipid levels, usual dietary pattern, and weight status.

- Diets for diabetics do not come as a "one size fits all." Dietary changes should be made sequentially and restrictions kept to a minimum to maximize the chance of compliance.

- Exchange lists simplify meal planning by allowing clients to make individual selections among food groups and still maintain a relatively consistent intake of carbohydrates, protein, and fat. A meal pattern is used to specify the number of servings from each exchange list allowed for each meal and snack.

- The carbohydrate group contains the following exchange lists: starch, fruit, milk, and other carbohydrate, and vegetable. Except for the vegetable exchange, one exchange from any of the other carbohydrate groups is approximately equivalent in carbohydrate content to any others; these are the only exchange groups that can be substituted one for another.

- Sucrose ("sugar") is no longer considered detrimental to glucose control, as long as it is eaten as part of the meal plan, not as an "extra." However, if weight loss is a goal, high sugar foods should be limited.

- Elderly diabetics may be treated more conservatively than younger diabetics because they are more susceptible to severe hypoglycemia, are at greater nutritional risk, and may have physical or sensory impairments that complicate self-management. Often, a No Concentrated Sweets diet is used in place of a traditional diabetic meal plan.

- To control symptoms of functional hyperinsulinism, it is recommended that 3 meals and 2 to 3 snacks be eaten daily, that protein and/or fat be consumed with every meal and snack, that soluble fiber intake be increased, and that simple sugars, alcohol, and caffeine be avoided.

- Clients with thyroid disorders may need to adjust their calorie intake if weight changes have occurred. Alterations in bowel patterns may be alleviated by adjusting the fiber content of the diet (ie, high fiber for constipation, low fiber for diarrhea).

- Altering dietary calcium intake does not fully compensate for imbalances of parathyroid hormone. Although dairy products are the best source of calcium in the diet, they cannot be used freely by clients with hypoparathyroidism because they are also rich in phosphorus.

- Clients with Addison's disease should eat frequent meals and a large bedtime snack to help avoid hypoglycemia. A high fluid intake is indicated, and sodium and potassium intake may need to be adjusted, depending on the type of medication used.

 FOCUS ON **CRITICAL THINKING**

The doctor you work for has just asked you to teach Mrs. Schultz about a diabetic diet. You know she is 83 years old and the doctor has been watching her blood glucose levels for a couple of years; he's hoping a little diet intervention may effectively control her glucose so that she won't need medication. She is 4'11" tall and weighs 105 pounds. Because the senior services van is on its way to pick her up, you only have about 20 minutes to spend with Mrs. Schultz.

What information should you obtain from Mrs. Schultz's chart? What information do you need to get by interviewing Mrs. Schultz?

What goals would be appropriate for Mrs. Schultz? Does she need to lose weight?

What are the most important points to stress in the limited time you have available?

REFERENCES

American Diabetes Association, American Dietetic Association (1995). Exchange Lists for Meal Planning. Alexandria, VA: American Diabetes Association; Chicago: American Dietetic Association.

American Diabetes Association (1995). 101 Tips for Improving your Blood Sugar. Alexandria, VA: American Diabetes Association.

American Dietetic Association (1994). Nutrition recommendations and principles for people with diabetes mellitus. J Am Diet Assoc, 94(5), 504–506.

Deakins, D. (1994). Teaching elderly patients about diabetes. AJN, 94(4), 39–42.

Diabetes Care and Education, A Practice Group of the American Dietetic Association; Tinker, L., Heins, J., Holler, H. (1994). Commentary and translation: 1994 nutrition recommendations for diabetes. J Am Diet Assoc, 94(5), 507–511.

Miller, J. (1994). Importance of glycemic index in diabetes. Am J Clin Nutr, 59(suppl), 747S–752S.

Monk, A., Barry, B., McClain, K., Weaver, T., Cooper, N., and Franz, M. (1995). Practice guidelines for medical nutrition therapy provided by dietitians for persons with non-insulin-dependent diabetes mellitus. J Am Diet Assoc, 95(9), 999–1006.

Norton, R. (1995). Diabetes 2000. The right mix of diet and exercise. RN, 58(4), 20–24.

Peragallo-Dittko, V. (1995). Diabetes 2000. Acute complications. RN, 58(8), 36–40.

Reisling, D. (1995a). Acute hypoglycemia. Keeping the bottom from falling out. Nursing 95, 25(2), 41–48.

Reisling, D. (1995b). Acute hyperglycemia. Putting a lip on the crisis. Nursing 95, 25(2), 33–40.

Robertson, C. (1995). Diabetes 2000. Chronic complications. RN, 58(9), 34–40.

Schlundt, D., Rea, M., Kline, S., and Pichert, J. (1994). Situational obstacles to dietary adherence for adults with diabetes. J Am Diet Assoc, 94(8), 874–879.

Tinker, L. (1994) Diabetes mellitus—A priority health care issue for women. J Am Diet Assoc, 94(9), 976–983.

Vessby, B. (1994). Dietary carbohydrates in diabetes. Am J Clin Nutr 59(suppl), 742S–746S.

Wing, R. (1995). Use of very-low-calorie diets in the treatment of obese persons with non-insulin-dependent diabetes mellitus. J Am Diet Assoc, 95(5), 569–572.

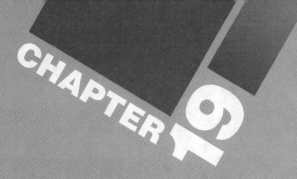

CHAPTER 19

Renal and Urinary Disorders

Chapter Outline

Key Terms

Acid ash diet
Azotemia

Basic ash diet
High biologic value protein

Uremia

The kidneys are two bean-shaped organs that are embedded in fatty tissue and located at the back of the abdominal cavity, one on each side of the spinal column. Each kidney consists of more than a million functional units, called nephrons. Each nephron consists of a glomerulus (tufts of capillaries where blood is filtered) that is attached to a tubule (where reabsorption and secretion occur). About 1.2 liters, or one-fourth of the total cardiac output, is filtered through the kidneys each minute. The kidneys and other organs of the urinary system are depicted in Figure 19-1.

The kidneys perform numerous vital endocrine and exocrine functions. One of their principal functions is to maintain normal blood volume and composition by reabsorbing needed nutrients and excreting wastes through the urine. Urinary excretion is the primary method by which the body rids itself not only of excess water, electrolytes, sulfates, organic acids, toxic substances, and drugs, but also the nitrogenous wastes from exogenous and endogenous protein metabolism, such as ammonia, urea, uric acid, and creatinine. Another kidney function is the regulation of acid–base

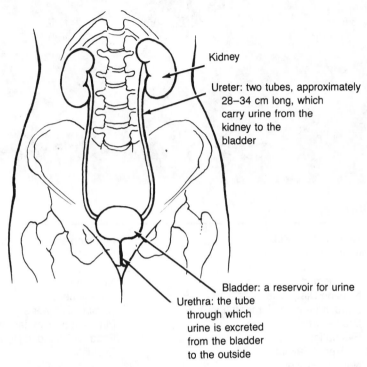

Kidney

Ureter: two tubes, approximately
28–34 cm long, which
carry urine from the
kidney to the
bladder

Bladder: a reservoir for urine

Urethra: the tube
through which
urine is excreted
from the bladder
to the outside

Figure 19-1
Organs of the urinary system.

balance, which is achieved by secreting hydrogen ions to increase pH, or excreting bicarbonate to lower pH. The kidneys also synthesize renin, an enzyme important for blood pressure regulation, and erythropoietin, a hormone that stimulates the bone marrow to produce red blood cells. Vitamin D is converted to its active form (1,25-dihydroxycholecalciferol) in the kidneys; therefore, the kidneys have an important role in maintaining normal metabolism of calcium and phosphorus.

Renal damage and subsequent loss of renal function profoundly affect metabolism, nutritional requirements, and nutritional status. For instance, nitrogenous wastes, fluid, electrolytes, and other compounds in the blood may accumulate to toxic levels as urine output decreases. **Azotemia** refers specifically to high blood concentration of nitrogenous wastes. **Uremia** ("urine in the blood") is a toxic systemic syndrome that is caused by the retention of urea and other nitrogenous waste products that are normally excreted in the urine (see the display, Signs and Symptoms of Uremia). In general, the degree of uremia is related largely to dietary protein intake. Although protein restriction is indicated to reduce uremic symptoms, exactly when protein restriction should be initiated and how severe it should be are controversial. Certainly, protein restriction is contraindicated for clients with protein malnutrition, which often develops with progressive renal failure. Conversely, renal damage can impair the kidney's ability to reabsorb needed nutrients, which are then "wasted" in the urine. Kidney failure impairs gastrointestinal (GI) absorption of certain minerals,

Signs and Symptoms of Uremia

GASTROINTESTINAL

Anorexia
Nausea
Stomatitis
GI ulcerations and bleeding
Metallic taste
Vomiting
Protein–calorie malnutrition
Weight loss
Diarrhea

CARDIOVASCULAR

Congestive heart failure
Hypertension
Retinopathy

NEUROLOGIC

Anxiety
Coma
Convulsions
Decreased mental alertness
Drowsiness
Fatigue
Hallucinations
Headaches
Muscle twitching
Peripheral neuropathy
Personality changes

METABOLIC

Hyperglycemia
Hypermagnesemia
Hypertriglyceridemia
Hyperuricemia
Hypo/hypercalcemia
Hypo/hyperkalemia
Hypo/hypernatremia
Hypo/hyperphosphatemia
Hypothermia
Metabolic acidosis
Volume deficit/overload

RESPIRATORY

Pleuritis
Pulmonary edema

REPRODUCTIVE

Amenorrhea
Impotence
Infertility
Loss of libido

DERMATOLOGIC

Decreased perspiration
Dry itchy skin
Skin discoloration
Pallor

HEMATOLOGIC

Anemia (normocytic and normochromic)
Bleeding tendencies
Decreased resistance to infection
Fatigue

MUSCULOSKELETAL

Calcium deposits in soft tissues
Fractures related to bone demineralization
Muscular irritability and cramping

ENDOCRINE

Hypothyroidism
Impaired growth and development
Renal osteodystrophy
Secondary hyperparathyroidism

like calcium and iron. Impaired synthesis of renin, erythropoietin, and vitamin D can lead to high blood pressure, anemia, and bone demineralization, respectively. Certain peptide hormones, like insulin, parathyroid hormone, and glucagon, are not adequately inactivated, which contributes to altered metabolism. Poor intake related to complex, unpalatable dietary restrictions, anorexia, alterations in taste, nausea, vomiting, stomatitis, depression, or anxiety is common. In addition, nutrients may be lost secondary to drug therapy, dialysis, or renal transplantation. For assessment guidelines, see the display, General Renal and Urinary Assessment Criteria.

The objectives of diet intervention for renal diseases are: 1) to lessen renal workload to forestall or prevent further kidney damage; 2) to restore or maintain optimal nutritional status; and 3) to avoid the symptoms or complications of uremia. The optimal interventions that are needed to meet these objectives vary among individuals and the nature, severity, and stage of the disease. Generally, diet modifications are made in response to symptoms and laboratory values, and therefore require frequent monitoring and adjustment. Nutrients that may be adjusted for clients with renal disease include protein, fluid, sodium, potassium, and phosphorus. Calorie requirements generally increase to spare protein, and supplemental calcium may be needed because of impaired vitamin D metabolism. Multivitamin and mineral supplements may be indicated. In the acute care setting, clients with renal disease may receive a low-sodium diet, a low-protein diet, or a combination diet that restricts protein, sodium, potassium, and phosphorus.

Chronic renal failure (CRF), acute renal failure (ARF), and urolithiasis are discussed in detail. The principles and rationale of diet management for CRF can be applied to other renal diseases that impair renal function. General diet management recommendations for selected kidney disorders are outlined in Table 19-1. However, they are only guidelines—actual nutrient requirements are determined by the client's nutritional status, degree of renal functioning, laboratory values, and clinical presentation. Close monitoring and frequent diet adjustment may be necessary, depending on the client's progress and tolerance.

DISORDERS OF THE KIDNEYS AND URINARY TRACT

Chronic Renal Failure

Chronic renal failure is characterized by the slow, progressive loss of renal function related to irreversible nephron deterioration. The clinical course of renal failure can be divided into three phases. *Diminished renal reserve* is an asymptomatic period in

---

ASSESSMENT CRITERIA

General Renal and Urinary Assessment Criteria

Urine output: volume, abnormal characteristics, pain on voiding

Bone pain; loss of height

Presence of history of urinary tract infection

Treatment measures: hemodialysis, peritoneal dialysis, renal transplant

Signs and symptoms of uremia

Signs and symptoms of fluid overload: hypertension, edema, weight gain, hyponatremia

Anemia

BUN, serum creatinine, serum sodium, serum potassium, Ca^{++}:P ratios, serum triglycerides, cholesterol, hemoglobin, hematocrit

Table 19-1
General Diet Recommendations for Selected Renal Disorders

Disorder	Symptoms/Complications	Diet Management
Acute glomerulonephritis: Inflammation of the glomeruli. Most often caused by an allergic or autoimmune reaction to a streptococcal infection of the throat; may also result from impetigo and scarlet fever.	Nitrogenous waste retention	Decrease protein to 0.2–0.5 g/kg for clients with uremia.
	Oliguria	For oliguria, restrict fluid to 500–700 ml, restrict potassium and phosphorus as needed.
	Edema, hypertension May progress to chronic glomerulonephritis, uremia, and death	For edema or high blood pressure, limit sodium to 500–1000 mg. Increase calories to promote protein sparing.
Nephritis: Kidney inflammation that may be acute or chronic.	Edema, hypertension Uremia; net protein catabolism	Limit sodium to 1–2 g/day. Restrict protein; increase nonprotein calories. Determine fluid allowance: urine output + 500 ml.
Nephrotic syndrome: Increased capillary permeability in the glomeruli leads to leakage of serum proteins into the urine, causing proteinuria, hypoalbuminemia, and massive edema. Hypercholesterolemia may develop for some unknown reason.	Proteinuria	Provide 0.8–1.0 g protein/kg; higher intakes are contraindicated because they increase waste production and glomerular pressure. 60% of protein should be high biologic value. Increase calories to 40–60 cal/kg to spare protein.
	Edema	Limit sodium to 2–4 g or less; fluid restriction is not necessary unless renal failure develops. Provide adequate potassium, as tolerated, and according to diuretic use.
	Hypercholesterolemia, elevated triglycerides	Limit dietary cholesterol and sugar. Emphasize unsaturated fat.
Chronic pyelonephritis: Bacterial invasion of the kidneys leads to fibrosis, scarring, and dilatation of the tubules, and impaired renal function.	Hypertension; possible sodium depletion if sodium is not adequately reabsorbed	Adjust sodium intake according to symptoms.
	Possible hyperkalemia	Limit potassium.
	Possible loss of renal function	Limit protein, accordingly. Encourage appropriate fluid intake.

which homeostasis is maintained despite the loss of 50% of nephrons. *Renal insufficiency* occurs when nephron loss reaches 75%. Serum creatinine may be 8 times greater than normal, the urine becomes more dilute, generalized edema may occur, and mild anemia develops. However, the client is relatively asymptomatic because the remaining nephrons hypertrophy to maintain homeostasis. *End-stage renal disease (ESRD)* occurs when 90% of nephrons are lost; serum creatinine levels steadily increase to about 10 mg/100 ml, overt symptoms develop, and dialysis or a kidney transplant is required.

Chronic renal failure may result from chronic glomerulonephritis, nephrosis, polycystic disease, chronic pyelonephritis, or urinary tract obstruction and infection.

It may also develop secondary to poor circulation related to atherosclerosis or heart failure, or secondary to drugs, nephrotoxic agents, infection, dehydration, diabetic nephropathy, hypertension, lupus erythematosus, or arthritis.

Complications of CRF include anemia, renal osteodystrophy, severe resistant hypertension, edema, congestive heart failure, infection, paresthesia, and alteration in neuromuscular activity. Chronic renal failure results in death unless it is treated with dialysis or renal transplantation; the underlying cause must also be treated.

NURSING PROCESS

Assessment

In addition to the general renal and urinary assessment criteria, assess for the following factors:

Symptoms of uremia (see the display, Signs and Symptoms of Uremia), which develop in response to increasing blood urea nitrogen (BUN) levels and vary with the client's individual tolerance. Generally, all symptoms increase in intensity as uremia progresses.

The impact of symptoms on intake or nutritional status: onset, frequency, severity, interventions attempted and the results.

Dietary changes made in response to CRF or its symptoms (ie, foods avoided, foods preferred). Determine which foods are best and least tolerated.

Usual quantity and quality of protein consumed—whether most of the protein is of high biologic value (generally animal sources) or low biologic value (gelatin and plant sources).

Adequacy of calorie intake; calorie intake becomes increasingly important when protein is restricted to spare body and dietary protein.

The use of salt and intake of high-sodium foods: cold cuts, bacon, frankfurters, smoked meats, sausage, canned meats, chipped or corned beef, buttermilk, cheese, crackers, canned soups and vegetables, convenience products, pickles, condiments. Determine whether a salt substitute is used, and if so, determine its chemical composition.

Weight, weight status. Be aware that fluid retention masks true weight.

Intake and output; observe for signs of fluid and electrolyte imbalance.

Abnormal laboratory values and their significance, especially BUN, creatinine, BUN/creatinine ratio, potassium, phosphorus, hemoglobin, hematocrit.

Nursing Diagnosis

Fluid Volume Excess, related to decreased urine output secondary to CRF

Planning and Implementation

Renal failure produces profound alterations in metabolism, nutrient requirements, and nutritional status. Diet management is the cornerstone of long-term treatment, and daily adjustments in the diet may be necessary to prevent malnutrition and uremic symptoms.

Protein

Debate continues over whether lowering protein intake prevents or delays the onset of renal failure. Data suggest that clients with advanced renal failure may benefit from a low-protein diet; among clients with moderate renal disease, there appears to be no difference in decline of renal function between clients who followed a usual vs. low-protein diet (Gillis et al, 1995). However, because it is noninvasive, decreases physiologic load on the remaining functioning nephrons, and has the potential to be beneficial, protein restriction remains the cornerstone of dietary treatment for renal insufficiency (Beto, 1995).

Table 19-2 outlines dietary parameters in renal failure. Although the most severe level of protein restriction is at, or slightly below, the normal recommended dietary allowance (RDA) for protein (0.8 g/kg), the diet is often viewed as unrealistically restrictive, because most Americans habitually consume more than the RDA for protein.

A narrow margin of error exists with regard to the protein intake of clients with renal failure. Too much protein increases BUN levels and the symptoms of uremia; too little protein results in protein catabolism (which increases serum potassium and BUN levels) and a negative nitrogen balance. However, supplementing very-low-protein diets (30 g or less) with commercial essential amino acid supplements or their keto analogues may promote neutral or positive nitrogen balance, reduce uremic symptoms, and even prevent further kidney damage (see display, Specially Formulated Renal Supplements).

Whenever the quantity of protein is restricted, the quality becomes more important. **High-biologic-value proteins,** which provide adequate amounts of all the essential amino acids, encourage reuse of circulating nonessential amino acids for protein synthesis and minimize urea production (Beto, 1995). At least 60% of total protein intake should be from high biologic sources (Beto, 1995). The protein content of high- and low-biologic-value proteins is listed in the display, Protein Content of High- and Low-Biologic-Value Proteins.

Once dialysis is initiated, protein requirements are increased to above normal levels to ensure adequacy and to compensate for the loss of serum proteins and amino acids in the dialysate. At least half of the protein consumed should be of high biologic value.

Calories

It is extremely important to provide adequate nonprotein calories to prevent hunger, weight loss, and body protein catabolism. However, energy requirements must be individualized. For instance, because calories are absorbed from peritoneal dialysate (average 680 cal/day), calorie adjustment may be necessary. Likewise, sedentary clients and post-transplant clients who are taking immunosuppressive steroids may require fewer calories to avoid excess weight gain.

Pure sugars and pure fats are recommended for calories, even though they are not considered "nutritious" foods (see the display, Sources of Protein-Free Calories and Seasonings). Unfortunately, approximately 50% of CRF clients exhibit glucose intolerance, and many develop hyperlipidemia (elevated triglycerides and very-low-

Table 19-2
Dietary Parameters in Renal Failure

Energy and Nutrients	Renal Insufficiency	Hemodialysis	Peritoneal Dialysis	Transplantation
PROTEIN	0.6–0.8 g/kg per day, >50–60% HBV*, 0.8–1.0 g/kg in nephrotic syndrome	1.2–1.4 g/kg per day, >50–60% HBV	1.2–1.5 g/kg per day, >50–60% HBV	1.3–1.5 g/kg per day after surgery; 1.0 g/kg per day chronic, stable renal function
ENERGY	30–35 cal/kg per day	30–35 kcal/kg per day	25–35 kcal/kg per day, including dialysate energy; 20–25 kcal/kg for weight loss	25–35 kcal/kg per day to maintain desired body weight; limit fat to 30% total energy; <300 mg/day cholesterol
SODIUM	2.0–4.0 g/day; variable with disease etiology and urine output	2.0 g/day	2.0–4.0 g/day	2.0–4.0 g/day after surgery; 3.0–4.0 g/day chronic, stable renal function
POTASSIUM	Not usually restricted until GFR† < 10 ml/minute	2.0–3.0 g/day	3.0–4.0 g/day	Unrestricted; monitor drug effects
PHOSPHORUS	10–12 mg/g dietary protein	12–15 mg/g dietary protein	12–15 mg/g dietary protein	Unrestricted; monitor
CALCIUM	1.0–1.5 g/day	1.0–1.5 g/day	1.0–1.5 g/day	1.0–1.5 g/day
FLUID	Unrestricted until urine output decreases	Urine output plus 1000 ml/day	Monitored; most tolerate 2000 ml/day	Unrestricted unless urine output decreases or fluid overload occurs
VITAMINS AND MINERALS	Daily RDA** of vitamins B, C, and D, iron, zinc; do not supplement vitamin A or magnesium	Daily RDA except: vitamin C = 60–100 mg/day; vitamin B_6 = 5–6 mg/day; folic acid = 0.8–1.0 µg/day; do not supplement vitamin A or magnesium	Daily RDA except vitamin C = 60–100 mg/day; vitamin B_6 = 5–10 mg/day; folic acid = 0.8–1.0 µg/day; do not supplement vitamin A or magnesium	Daily RDA

* HBV = protein of high biologic value.
† GFR = glomerular filtration rate.
** RDA = Recommended Dietary Allowance.

Source: Beto, J. (1995). Which diet for which renal failure: Making sense of the options. © The American Dietetic Association. Reprinted by permission from J Am Diet Assoc, 95(8), 898–903.

density lipoproteins). Emphasis on monounsaturated and polyunsaturated fats, and intake of complex carbohydrates may help to minimize cardiovascular risks.

Sodium and Fluid

Even though clients with renal failure have a decreased ability to reabsorb and regulate sodium, they can usually maintain sodium balance on a moderate sodium intake (2–4 g/day). Sodium allowances for clients who are on peritoneal dialysis are

Specially Formulated Renal Supplements

AMIN-AID (KENDALL McGAW)

Contains free essential amino acids plus histidine in a high-calorie, low-electrolyte supplement. Does not contain vitamins or minerals. Provides 2.0 cal/ml, 4% of calories from protein.

SUPLENA (ROSS LABORATORIES)

Provides complete and balanced nutrition for nondialyzed renal clients. Low in fluid, protein, phosphorus, magnesium, and electrolytes. Provides 2.0 cal/ml, 6% of calories from protein.

TRAVASORB RENAL (CLINTEC)

Contains essential amino acids in a high-calorie, low-protein, electrolyte-free supplement. Does not contain fat-soluble vitamins. Provides 1.4 cal/ml, 7% of calories from protein.

more liberal because fluid removal can be regulated by varying the dextrose concentration of the dialysate (Beto, 1995). See Chapter 17 for foods that are high in sodium and for more information on sodium-restricted diets.

Some clients with advanced renal failure are unable to conserve sodium, and a sodium deficit may occur if sodium intake is restricted. If the client does not have edema, hypertension, or signs of heart failure, increasing sodium intake as tolerated may slightly improve glomerular filtration rate (GFR).

Protein Content of High- and Low-Biologic-Value Proteins

HBV proteins: complete proteins (generally animal sources) that contain sufficient amounts of all the essential amino acids.

Item	Serving Size	Approximate Protein Content (g)
Egg	1	7
Milk and yogurt	½ cup	4
Meat, fish, poultry, cheese	1 oz	7
Tuna, cottage cheese	¼ cup	7

LBV proteins: incomplete proteins (generally plant sources) that lack sufficient amounts of all the essential amino acids

Item	Serving Size	Approximate Protein Content (g)
Bread, regular	1 slice	3
Bread, low protein	1 slice	0.3
Cereals, pasta, rice	½ cup	3
Vegetables	½ cup	<1–4 g
Dried peas and beans	½ cup	6–8 g
Gelatin	½ cup	2
Nuts	1 oz	2–6 g
Peanut butter	2 Tbsp	9
Fruits	½ cup	0.5–1 g

Sources of Protein-Free Calories and Seasonings

PROTEIN-FREE CALORIES

Beverages*
  Alcoholic
  Carbonated
  Cranberry juice cocktail
  Fruit drinks and punches
  Kool-Aid
  Lemonade, limeade
  Tang
Candies
  Buttermints
  Candy corn, fondant
  Chewy fruit snacks
  Cotton candy
  Fruit chews, fruit rollups
  Gum
  Gumdrops
  Jelly beans
  LifeSavers
  Lollipops
  Marshmallows
  Mints
Desserts
  Fruit ice*

Juice bar
Popsicle*
Sorbet
Fats
  Butter and margarine (unsalted)
  Coconut
  Mayonnaise, oils
  Powdered coffee whitener
  Shortening
  Tartar sauce
Sweeteners
  Corn syrup
  Honey
  Jams
  Jellies
  Maple syrup
  Marmalade
  Sugar: confectioners', white, brown

PROTEIN-FREE SEASONINGS

Flavoring extracts
Herbs
Spices
Vinegar

As allowed by fluid restriction.

If blood pressure and serum sodium levels are normal and edema does not occur, fluid intake can exceed 24-hour urine output by 500 ml (the amount of fluid lost through skin, lungs, and perspiration; see the display, Sources of Fluid). Sodium and fluid restrictions are more severe in oliguric or anuric clients who are on dialysis; the goal of approximately 2 pounds per day is the suggested fluid weight gain between hemodialysis treatments (Beto, 1995).

Potassium

Most clients with renal failure can tolerate a normal potassium intake until GFR falls below 10 ml/minute. Some clients develop a gradual tolerance to hyperkalemia and may be asymptomatic. However, an excessive potassium intake, the use of potassium-containing medications, acidosis, inadequate calorie intake, oliguria, and catabolic stress can lead to fatal hyperkalemia. Conversely, clients who are taking potassium-wasting diuretics, or those experiencing severe potassium losses from GI fistulas or gastric suctioning, may need more potassium to avoid hypokalemia.

Phosphorus/Calcium

Vitamin D deficiency is caused by the inability of the kidneys to convert the vitamin to its active form. Consequently, the metabolism of calcium, phosphorus, and magnesium is altered and may result in hyperphosphatemia, bone demineralization,

Sources of Fluid

LIQUIDS

Alcoholic beverages

Carbonated beverages

Cereal beverages

Coffee

Cream

Fruit juices, drinks, and punches

Juice and syrup from canned fruit and vegetables

Liquid medications

Milk

Soup, bouillon, consommé, broth

Tea

Vegetable juices

Water

FOODS THAT LIQUEFY AT ROOM TEMPERATURE

Ice (melts to $9/10$ initial volume)

Ice cream (melts to $1/2$ initial volume)

Ice milk (melts to $1/2$ initial volume)

Gelatin

Popsicles

Sherbet

bone pain, and possible calcification of the soft tissues. Renal osteodystrophy may be prevented by the following measures:

- Limiting phosphorus intake. Low-protein diets are usually low in phosphorus and may control hyperphosphatemia effectively. Allowances are often calculated per gram of protein consumed (eg, 12–15 mg phosphorus/g of protein for clients on dialysis). When serum phosphate level exceeds 5.58 mg/dl, phosphate binders that decrease GI absorption (eg, Amphojel, Basaljel) are required to maintain normal serum levels.
- Providing vitamin D supplements. Clients who are on hemodialysis routinely receive intravenous (IV) supplementation in the form of calcitriol (Beto, 1995).
- Providing calcium supplements. Unfortunately, high-calcium diets are contraindicated because they rely heavily on dairy products, which are high in protein and phosphorus.

Vitamins and Minerals

Water-soluble vitamin deficiencies occur frequently in clients with renal failure and may be caused by inadequate intake related to anorexia or dietary restrictions, altered metabolism related to uremia or medications, or increased losses related to dialysis. With the exception of vitamin C and folic acid, supplements of the water-soluble vitamins at RDA levels are recommended for both nondialyzed and dialyzed clients. Because vitamin C increases the risk of oxalate stones, intake should be less than 100 mg (Beto, 1995). Higher than RDA amounts of folic acid are suggested to promote red blood cell (RBC) production.

Vitamin A supplementation is contraindicated in clients with ESRD because of reported toxicity (Beto, 1995). Requirements for vitamins E and K appear to be the same as for the general population.

Clients who are undergoing dialysis may develop a deficiency of zinc, which could contribute to anorexia and taste alterations. Therapeutic doses of zinc may be added to the dialysate. It is recommended that all other trace elements be routinely removed from the dialysate to prevent toxicities. Dialysate that is contaminated with aluminum has been associated with progressive mental disorders and osteomalacia.

Most clients with ESRD develop serious, disabling anemia that is primarily related to erythropoietin deficiency (Sanders et al, 1994). Other potential contributing factors are as follows:

- Uremic toxins that inhibit RBC production
- Decreased RBC survival rate
- Frequent blood loss related to dialysis treatment and blood sampling. An estimated 2 to 5 liters of blood/year may be lost through hemodialysis treatments (Beto, 1995)
- Catabolism caused by hemodialysis treatments
- Aluminum toxicity, which interferes with RBC generation
- Deficiencies of nutrients that are required for RBC production, such as vitamin B_{12}, folic acid, vitamin B_6, and iron
- Physical factors related to hemodialysis that injure RBC, such as high dialysate temperature

Recombinant human erythropoietin (r-HuEPO) is used to treat anemia; optimal nutritional support is needed to optimize its effectiveness (Sanders et al, 1994). See Drug Alert: Recombinant Human Erythropoietin (r-HuEPO).

Other Considerations

Renal exchange lists (referred to as "choices," rather than "exchanges," to eliminate confusion with diabetic exchanges) are used for ease of meal planning. Allowed foods are grouped into lists based on their protein, sodium, and potassium and phosphorus content; calories are also addressed, and fluids may be considered. Portion sizes are specified so that each serving contains approximately the same amount of protein, sodium, potassium, and phosphorus (Table 19-3). Items within a list may be substituted for each other; substitutions from one list to another are not allowed. An

---

DRUG ALERT *Recombinant Human Erythropoietin (r-HuEPO)*

In clients with ESRD, the kidneys are unable to produce adequate amounts of erythropoietin, the hormone that stimulates the bone marrow to produce RBC. r-HuEPO therapy is used to treat anemia caused by erythropoietin deficiency.

Possible side effects include worsening of hypertension, iron deficiency, increased appetite leading to failure to comply with diet, and possible hyperkalemia; possible seizures, chills, and body aches (Sanders et al, 1994).

Because deficiencies of iron, vitamin B_{12}, and folic acid can cause a poor response to r-HuEPO therapy, it is important to identify and prevent nutritional deficiencies.

Higher hematocrit causes a decrease in phosphorous clearance; an adjustment in dietary phosphorous intake and/or use of phosphate binders may be indicated.

Clients who experience increased appetite, and subsequent worsening of BUN and serum potassium levels, need additional counseling and possible adjustments in their diets.

Table 19-3
Renal Diet "Choice" Lists

Choice	Various Serving Sizes	Nutritional Content				
		g Pro	Calories	mg Na	mg K	mg P
Milk	½ cup milk 1 c low-protein milk ½ cup yogurt, ice cream, or light cream	4	120	80	185	110
Nondairy milk substitutes	½ cup	0.5	140	40	80	30
Meat	1 oz meat, fish, poultry 1 egg ¼ cup cottage cheese	7	65	25	100	65
Starch	1 slice bread ½ bagel or hamburger roll ¾ cup most ready-to-eat cereals ⅓ cup pasta, oatmeal ½ cup rice	2	90	80	35	35
Vegetable	Generally ½ cup, prepared or canned without added salt					
Low potassium		1	25	15	50	20
Medium potassium		1	25	15	150	20
High potassium		1	25	15	270	20
Fruit	Generally ½ cup					
Low potassium		0.5	70	trace	50	15
Moderate potassium		0.5	70	trace	150	15
High potassium		0.5	70	trace	270	15
Fat	1 tsp oil, margarine, butter, mayonnaise 1 tablespoon salad dressing, low-calorie mayonnaise, reduced-calorie margarine, powdered coffee whitener	0	45	55	10	5
High-calorie	Varies 1 cup carbonated beverage, lemonade, fruit-flavored drinks; 1 popsicle, juice bar; 2 fruit roll-ups, 15 gum drops; 2 tablespoons jam, honey, sugar, or syrup; 5 large marshmallows; ½ slice low-protein bread	Trace	100	15	20	5
Salt	Varies ⅛ tsp salt ⅓ cup bouillon 1½ Tbsp catsup 4 tsp mustard 2 medium green olives 2½ tsp steak sauce 2 Tbsp taco sauce	0	0	250	0	0

individualized meal pattern specifies the number of choices that are permitted from each list; allowances are based on laboratory data and clinical symptoms and should correspond as closely as possible with the individual's food preferences and habits (see the display, Sample Renal Failure Menu). The composition, complexity, and number of exchange lists used in the treatment of renal failure vary considerably among institutions.

SAMPLE **MENU**

Sample Renal Failure Menu: 2075 Calories, 42 g Protein, 1785 mg Sodium, 1810 mg Potassium

BREAKFAST	CHOICES
½ cup orange juice	1 high-potassium fruit
¾ cup cornflakes with ½ cup nondairy creamer	1 starch, 1 salt
	1 nondairy milk substitute
1 poached egg	1 meat
1 slice toast	1 starch
2 tsp margarine	2 fats
2 Tbsp jelly	1 high-calorie choice
½ cup coffee*	1 fat
1 Tbsp powdered coffee whitener	

LUNCH	
Sandwich made with	
1 oz turkey	1 meat
2 slices low-protein bread	2 high-calorie choices
2 teaspoons mayonnaise	2 fats
1 cup lettuce	1 low-potassium vegetable
2 Tbsp low-calorie salad dressing	1 fat, 1 salt
1 small apple	1 medium-potassium fruit
2 fruit rollups	1 high-calorie choice

DINNER	
2 oz roast beef	2 meat
2½ tsp steak sauce	1 salt
½ cup unsalted noodles with 2 teaspoons butter and parsley	1 starch, 2 fat
½ cup carrots	1 medium-potassium vegetable
½ cup beets	1 high-potassium vegetable
½ cup blueberries	1 low-potassium fruit
1 cup cola*	1 high-calorie choice
4 sugar wafers	1 starch

SNACKS	
½ cup apple juice*	1 low-potassium fruit
5 large marshmallows	1 high-calorie choice

* As allowed, depending on fluid needs.

Despite the use of "choice" lists, adherence to diet therapies for chronic renal disease is extremely challenging: The diet is complex; modifications are numerous, extensive, and lifelong; and changes are frequent as the disease progresses. Factors associated with adherence appear in the display, Factors Associated with Adherence to Renal Diet. Note that adherence may be improved if counseling focuses on satisfaction with diet (Coyne et al, 1995); clients who are not satisfied with their diets are not likely to maintain long-term adherence to modified protein.

Clients with uremia may experience a deterioration of their appetite as the day progresses. Encourage a good breakfast. Uremia may also cause alterations in taste, so that clients may prefer highly seasoned or strongly flavored foods.

Children with renal failure experience growth failure, which may be permanent if it is not corrected before puberty. An optimal diet prevents depletion of body protein and fat stores in clients of any age.

Enteral nutritional support may be indicated if the client has a functional GI tract but is unable to consume an adequate oral diet; total parental nutrition is used if the GI tract is nonfunctional. The requirements for clients who are receiving parenteral nutrition are controversial, especially regarding amino acids; therefore, total parenteral nutrition solutions should be individualized for each client. High-glucose solutions (hyperosmolar) with lipid emulsions are used to deliver the maximum quantity of calories without increasing the volume.

Clients with renal failure have an increased risk of hypermagnesemia and should avoid magnesium-containing over-the-counter drugs such as antacids, laxatives, and enemas.

After a successful renal transplant, diet modifications to alleviate the side effects of steroids, which are taken to prevent rejection of the new kidney, may be necessary (see Chapter 18, Glucocorticoid Drug Alert). Temporary or permanent rejection of the transplanted kidney may result in uremia, which may require the resumption of chronic renal failure dietary restrictions.

Factors Associated With Adherence to Renal Diet

PSYCHOSOCIAL FACTORS

- Greater knowledge and skills
- More positive attitudes about eating pattern
- More social support
- Eating pattern interfered less often with social activities
- Health interfered less often with ability to adhere
- Higher overall satisfaction with eating pattern
- Self-perception as more successful at adhering

BEHAVIORAL FACTORS

- More frequent self-monitoring of protein intake
- More feedback on self-monitoring records and biochemistry data
- Fewer protein modification guidelines, telephone calls from dietitians, and less frequent review of weighing and measuring techniques
- More low-protein food products received and used
- More food-tasting experiences
- More guidelines for increasing energy

Source: Milas, N., Nowalk, M., Akpele, L., Castaldo, L., Coyne, T., Doroshenko, L., Kigawa, L., Korzec-Ramirez, D., Scherch, L., Snetselaar, L. Factors associated with adherence to the dietary protein intervention in the modification of Diet in Renal Disease Study. © The American Dietetic Association. Reprinted by permission from J Am Diet Assoc, 95(11), 1295–1300, 1995.

CLIENT GOALS

The client will:

Attain and maintain adequate nutritional status.
Avoid symptoms and complications of uremia.
Restore and maintain fluid and electrolyte balance; correct acidosis.
Retard progression of renal failure and postpone the initiation of dialysis.
Minimize tissue catabolism by consuming adequate nonprotein calories.
Describe the rationale and principles in diet management of CRF and implement the appropriate dietary changes.
Practice self-management strategies, especially self-monitoring of protein intake.

NURSING INTERVENTIONS

Diet Management

Modify the diet as outlined in Table 19-2.
Control of protein is the cornerstone of treatment. Approximately two thirds of total protein should be from high-biologic-value sources: milk, eggs, meat.
Provide adequate nonprotein calories. Although exact requirements are not known, a high intake of nonprotein calories is needed when protein intake is restricted to prevent the use of dietary protein for energy, prevent tissue catabolism, and maintain or restore ideal weight. Obese clients may require fewer calories.
Limit sodium intake to 2.0 to 3.0 mg/day if signs of sodium retention occur: sudden weight gain, edema, hypertension, and symptoms of heart failure. Liberalize sodium intake if the client has signs of sodium depletion: unexplained weight loss, low blood pressure, and a further reduction in GFR.
Adjust fluid according to urine output and fluid retention.
Adjust potassium: Actual requirements are based on urine and serum levels of potassium. Foods that are high in potassium include fruit (especially bananas, citrus fruits and juices, melon, raisins), potatoes, tomatoes, dried peas and beans, whole grains, milk, and fresh meat.
Restrict phosphorus intake, if indicated.

Client Teaching

Because diet prescriptions for clients with renal disease are very complex, difficult to fulfill, often unpalatable, and continually changing, thorough diet teaching, ongoing support, and periodic evaluations of the client's (and the family's) knowledge and understanding are vital.
Instruct the client and family

To view the diet as an integral component of treatment and a means of life support. To increase the chance of compliance, self-management is recommended (Gillis et al, 1995). Effective intervention strategies include providing feedback from self-monitoring and/or food records, modeling, particularly by providing low-protein foods, and offering support (Gillis et al, 1995).

That strict adherence to the diet can improve the quality of life and decrease the workload on the kidneys.

That accurate daily weights are necessary to assess fluid balance and diet adequacy. Instruct the client to weigh himself or herself at approximately the same time every day, with the same scale, and while wearing the same amount of clothing. Unexpected weight gain or loss should be reported to the physician.

That a lag time of about 12 hours may exist between when food is eaten and the resultant change in blood chemistries. "Cheating" on the diet is not advised, but if the client chooses to do so, it should occur at least 12 hours before dialysis.

That renal diet cookbooks are available to increase variety in the diet; provide low-protein recipes.

That the vitamin and mineral supplements prescribed by the physician are needed to meet nutritional requirements.

That although eating out is possible, ordering from a restaurant menu requires special attention and planning to comply with the diet restrictions.

On the importance of a consistent, controlled protein intake:

- Too little or too much protein in the diet can cause BUN levels to increase and uremic symptoms to return; therefore, portion sizes should be weighed or measured initially, and thereafter should be periodically spot-checked for accuracy.
- Protein allowance should be spread over the whole day instead of saving it all for one meal.
- Low-protein breads, cereals, cookies, gelatin, and pastas are available to help boost calorie intake without sacrificing protein restriction, although their taste and texture differ from those of the products they are intended to replace, and they are more costly. Because acceptability varies greatly among low-protein products, clients should be encouraged to try a variety. Studies show that providing clients with samples of low-protein and protein-modified foods promotes adherence (Milas et al, 1995).

On the importance of an adequate calorie intake:

- Taking in too few calories can have the same effect as eating too much protein.
- Nonprotein calories, like butter, oils, and allowed sweets, should be used freely.

On the importance of a fluid restriction, if appropriate:

- Sources of fluid include liquids and foods that liquefy at room temperature.
- An easy way to measure fluid intake is to place a pitcher of water that contains a total daily fluid allowance in the refrigerator. As fluids are consumed, the equivalent amount of water should be discarded from the pitcher.
- To relieve thirst try:
  - Hard candies
  - Very cold water instead of tap water
  - Popsicles and ices, as allowed by fluid allowance

- Petroleum jelly applied to the lips, frequent mouth rinsing, and good oral hygiene

On the importance of a sodium-restricted diet, if appropriate (see Chapter 17)

On the importance of a potassium restriction, if appropriate.

- To reduce the potassium content of vegetables and potatoes, cut them in small pieces, soak them overnight, and boil them in fresh water.

Monitoring Progress

Monitor for the following signs or symptoms:

Compliance with the diet, the need for follow-up diet counseling. Studies show that even though substantial and significant reduction in protein intake can be observed in clients who are highly motivated and receive individualized dietary counseling, clients have difficulty in consistently achieving their prescribed levels of protein (The MDRD Study Group, 1994). This may be due to the highly restrictive nature of the diet or because the "choice" listings are imprecise and in some groups, protein content is underestimated (The MDRD Study Group, 1994).

Effectiveness of diet management, and evaluate the need for further diet modifications.

Weight, weight changes.

Intake and output; observe for signs of fluid and electrolyte imbalances and nutritional excesses/deficiencies.

Laboratory values, when available, especially of BUN, creatinine, serum proteins (eg, albumin, transferrin), triglycerides, and electrolytes.

Evaluation

Evaluation is ongoing. Provided that the plan of care has not changed, the client will achieve the goals as stated above.

Acute Renal Failure

Acute renal failure is characterized by a decrease in renal blood flow, or glomerular or tubular damage that leads to sudden loss of renal function, with rising serum levels of urea and other nitrogenous wastes (azotemia) and oliguria or anuria.

Its clinical course begins with an oliguric phase that is characterized by a low urine output of less than 400 to 600 ml/24 hours, which may deteriorate to anuria. Sometimes large amounts of urine are excreted despite the loss of renal function and nitrogenous waste retention (this is called *high-output renal failure*). The oliguric phase may last 10 to 20 days or longer.

The diuretic phase occurs when the kidneys are unable to conserve water. Large volumes of urine are excreted; losses of fluid, sodium, and potassium are extensive. The diuretic phase usually lasts 14 to 21 days. Today, few clients experience the diuretic phase because dialysis is usually performed earlier, thus minimizing extracellular fluid accumulation (Toto, 1992).

The recovery phase is characterized by a gradual improvement in renal function over a 3- to 12-month period; rapid improvement may be noted during the first 1 to 2 weeks, followed by a period of slower improvement (Toto, 1992). Some loss of renal function may be permanent.

Acute renal failure may have *prerenal* causes, such as decreased renal blood flow to the kidney related to shock, trauma, hemorrhage, surgery, burns, hypotension, severe dehydration, or heart failure. Nephron damage related to nephrotoxins, autoimmune disease, infection, or acute glomerulonephritis can cause *intrarenal* failure. *Postrenal* etiologies include obstructed urine outflow from the kidney related to benign prostatic hypertrophy, bladder or prostate cancer, calculi, trauma, or medications.

Complications of ARF include infection, which is the leading cause of death in these clients (Toto, 1992). Hyperkalemia resulting in cardiac arrest, metabolic acidosis, hypercatabolism, circulatory overload (dyspnea, orthopnea, pulmonary congestion, pulmonary edema), hypertension, hypertensive crisis, convulsions, neurologic abnormalities, and permanent loss of some renal function (reduction in glomerular filtration rate, decreased ability to concentrate urine, decreased ability to acidify urine) may also occur. Acute renal failure may progress to CRF; at least 5% of clients with acute tubular necrosis require long-term hemodialysis (Toto, 1992). Acute renal failure is fatal in 50% of cases.

The primary focus of treatment is to correct the underlying disorder. Dialysis is used to keep BUN levels below 100 mg/dl and creatinine levels below 8 mg/dl. Diuretics and other measures to restore fluid and electrolyte balance are used. Symptomatic anemia is treated with transfusions of packed RBC. Diet management may help to lessen the workload of the kidneys and restore optimal nutritional status.

NURSING PROCESS

Assessment

In addition to the general renal and urinary assessment criteria, assess for the following factors:

Symptoms of uremia: onset, causative factors, severity. Assess the impact of those that involve the GI tract (anorexia, nausea, vomiting, diarrhea, erosive gastritis, GI hemorrhage).

Appetite; adequacy of intake.

Intake and output; observe for signs of fluid and electrolyte imbalance.

Weight, and weight changes. Be aware that sudden weight gain or loss indicates sodium retention or depletion, respectively.

Abnormal laboratory values and their significance, especially BUN, creatinine, hemoglobin, hematocrit, albumin, electrolytes; urinalysis for osmolality and protein

Nursing Diagnosis

Fluid Volume Excess, related to decreased urine output secondary to ARF

Planning and Implementation

The optimal diet for clients with acute renal failure is more elusive than the optimal diet for chronic renal failure. Although a high-protein diet is contraindicated because of nitrogenous waste retention, hypercatabolism and infection or sepsis imposed by a major underlying illness increase the need for protein. In addition, catabolism can cause or exacerbate acidosis, and is a significant risk factor for poor outcome (Toto, 1992). Exact nutritional requirements are not known, although it is evident that needs vary among individuals and phases of acute renal failure. Once dialysis is instituted, diet restrictions are liberalized.

Little agreement exists concerning how much protein should be allowed once oral feedings are resumed. When catabolism is not accelerated by an underlying condition, intake may be restricted to 0.55 to 0.60 g/kg of mostly high-biologic-value protein, to lessen the workload of the kidneys. If a more severe protein restriction is ordered, essential amino acid supplements plus histidine (an amino acid shown to be essential for renal clients) are recommended to achieve positive nitrogen balance (see the display, Specially Formulated Renal Supplements). As GFR returns to normal or dialysis is instituted, protein allowance is increased to promote nitrogen balance and tissue healing.

For both the oliguric and diuretic phases of acute renal failure, fluid intake should equal total fluid output (volume of urine plus losses through diarrhea and vomiting plus insensible losses through the skin, lungs, and perspiration, which may be increased due to fever and infection). Generally, fluid allowance during the oliguric phase equals 24-hour urine output plus an additional 400 to 500 ml, depending on the client's hydration status. Up to 3 liters of fluid may be needed daily to replenish losses after diuresis begins.

Life-threatening hyperkalemia that occurs during the oliguric phase of acute renal failure is related to potassium retention and tissue catabolism, which causes potassium to leave the cells and enter the serum. Diets that are low in potassium (2 g or less) and exchange resins may be used during the oliguric phase to reduce serum potassium levels. Intravenous dextrose and insulin may be given as a temporary measure to lower serum potassium (insulin causes dextrose and potassium to leave the serum and enter the cells). Once diuresis begins, large amounts of potassium are excreted and potassium supplements may be necessary to avoid hypokalemia.

Clients who are unable to eat because of critical illness or impaired GI function secondary to ARF may need enteral or parenteral nutrition. Total parenteral nutrition solutions for clients with oliguric acute renal failure may be devoid of potassium, phosphate, and magnesium.

CLIENT GOALS

The client will:

Attain or maintain fluid, electrolyte, and mineral balances.
Avoid progression of renal failure.
Avoid symptoms and complications of uremia.
Lessen renal workload.
Control body catabolism and weight loss.

NURSING INTERVENTIONS

Diet Management

Adjust protein intake according to renal function. Initially, parenteral solutions of amino acids and glucose may be given if the client is unable to eat, although some studies suggest that regular total parenteral nutrition solutions and aggressive dialysis are more effective against uremia and acidosis. Protein allowance may begin at 0.8 g/kg and increase as renal function improves. If the client consumes an oral diet, at least two thirds of the total protein should come from high-biologic-value sources.

Increase calorie intake to approximately 50 cal/kg to promote nitrogen balance and replenish losses. Carbohydrate modules, pure fats, refined sugars, and low-protein starches should be used liberally.

Adjust fluid intake to avoid overhydration and dehydration. Allow urine output +400 to 500 ml/day.

Adjust sodium intake according to urine output, serum sodium level, symptoms of sodium imbalance, and concurrent use of dialysis. Sodium intake may be restricted to 500 to 1000 mg/day during the oliguric phase; sodium requirements increase during the diuretic phase to replace extensive losses.

Adjust potassium intake according to urine output, serum potassium level, and concurrent use of dialysis. Restrict potassium during the anuric phase; liberalize during the diuretic phase.

Provide small, frequent meals and assistance with eating, as needed, for clients receiving an oral diet who are weak or fatigued.

Client Teaching

Instruct the client and family

On the principles and rationale of diet management for ARF, if appropriate.

On the importance of dietary monitoring and restrictions so that the family does not provide the client with inappropriate food and beverages.

Monitoring Progress

Monitor for the following signs or symptoms:

Compliance with the diet, and the need for follow-up diet counseling.

Effectiveness of the diet, and evaluate the need for further diet modifications.

Weight, intake, and output, and observe for changes over 24- to 48-hour periods.

Evaluation

Evaluation is ongoing. Provided that the plan of care has not changed, the client will achieve the goals as stated above.

Urolithiasis

The precipitation of insoluble crystals in the urine leads to the formation of stones (calculi) that vary in size from sandlike "gravel" to large, branching stones.

Although they form most often in the kidney, they can occur anywhere in the urinary system. Generally, stones smaller than 1 cm in diameter are spontaneously voided; larger stones may require removal. Renal stones can lead to infection and obstruction, resulting in renal damage, which may require a nephrectomy.

Renal calculi occur more frequently in men than women, develop most often between the ages of 30 and 50 years, and tend to recur. Approximately 70% to 80% of stones are calcium oxalate crystals; the remaining stones are composed of calcium phosphate salts, uric acid, struvite (magnesium, annomium, phosphate), or cystine (an amino acid). Urolithiasis may be idiopathic, or it may result from certain infections, urinary stasis, metabolic abnormalities, hormone imbalances, or concentrated urine related to inadequate fluid intake. The precipitation of stones also depends on urinary pH. Other causes, specific for the stone's composition, are listed in Table 19-4.

The signs and symptoms of renal stones are dependent on the site of the stones and the presence of obstruction, infection, and edema. Nausea, vomiting, and abdominal pain may occur. Bladder stones may produce symptoms of urinary tract infection, such as chills, fever, or dysuria. Renal pelvic stones may cause renal colic—severe flank pain that radiates down the urinary tract, accompanied by sweating, pallor, nausea, vomiting, and possible abdominal pain and diarrhea. Large amounts of urine that contain blood and pus are voided. An attack may last minutes to several hours. Finally, stones in the ureter may cause ureteral colic—severe, colicky pain that comes in waves and radiates down the thigh and to the genitalia. Although the urge to urinate is frequent, only small amounts of urine, often containing blood, are voided.

The treatment of renal stones involves control of both pain and infection, drug therapy to alter the absorption or excretion of stone components, and diet intervention to dilute the urine and help prevent future stone formation. Extracorporeal

Table 19-4
Possible Causes of Renal Calculi, Based on Composition

Composition	Possible Cause
CALCIUM CALCULI	Hypercalciuria may be related to hyperparathyroidism, immobility, excessive use of alkali antacids, renal disease, or excessive intakes of protein, calcium, or vitamin D. Some clients with calcium stones have idiopathic hypercalciuria related to excess GI calcium absorption or altered renal reabsorption of calcium.
	Calcium oxalate may occur secondary to malabsorption syndrome → GI absorption of dietary oxalate (which normally is excreted in the feces) → hyperoxaluria → risk of calcium oxalate stone formation. Also, regular megadoses of vitamin C (>4 g/day) increase urinary excretion of oxalate and the risk of stone formation.
MAGNESIUM AMMONIUM PHOSPHATE CALCULI (struvite stones)	Sometimes called "infection stones" because they normally accompany urinary tract infections; bacteria that contain urease (an enzyme that converts urea to ammonia) increase the urinary pH, which favors the precipitation of magnesium ammonium phosphate calculi.
CYSTINE CALCULI	Caused by a rare genetic disorder of cystine (an amino acid) metabolism.
URIC ACID CALCULI	Idiopathic causes are characterized by hyperuricosuria and normal serum uric acid levels. May also occur as a side effect of antigout drugs that increase uric acid excretion (ie, probenecid).
	An acidic urine favors the precipitation of uric acid stones.

shock-wave lithotripsy is used to crush stones into particles small enough to be voided. Surgical intervention may be necessary if the stone causes progressive renal damage or obstruction, pain, or infection that does not respond medically.

NURSING PROCESS

Assessment

In addition to the general urinary and renal assessment criteria, assess for the following factors:

Symptoms (eg, nausea, vomiting, severe pain) and their impact on nutritional status and intake; assess onset, frequency, severity, interventions attempted and the results.

Dietary changes made in response to renal stones or symptoms (ie, foods avoided, food preferred). Determine which foods are best and least tolerated.

Usual intake of offending agent (ie, calcium for calcium calculi); relative ash content of the diet.

Adequacy and pattern of fluid intake, especially whether fluid is consumed immediately before bedtime.

Abnormal laboratory values and their significance, especially calcium, uric acid, serum oxalate, BUN, creatinine, phosphate; urinalysis for calcium and stone composition.

Nursing Diagnosis

Altered Health Maintenance, related to the lack of knowledge of dietary management of renal calculi

Planning and Implementation

The most effective diet intervention for the treatment and prevention of renal calculi is to increase fluids to dilute the urine. A high urine output not only helps the client to pass an existing stone, but it also decreases the likelihood that another stone will precipitate out of the urine.

Sometimes acid or basic ash diets are used in conjunction with drugs to alter urine pH (see the display, Acid-Forming, Base-Forming, and Neutral Foods). Acid-forming foods (**acid ash diet**) may help lower urine pH and protect against calcium phosphate and magnesium ammonium phosphate (struvite) stones, which form only in alkaline urine. A diet that is rich in base-forming foods (**basic ash diet**) may help increase urine pH and prevent uric acid and cystine stones. A urine pH of 6.8 is recommended and can be attained in healthy people by purely dietary measures (Remer and Manz, 1995) (see Food for Thought: Urine Distress). Drug therapy, however, has largely replaced diet therapy as an easier and more effective and consistent means of altering urine pH.

Under debate is whether excluding dietary components of the stone is preventive against future stone formation. Often, stones are composed of more than one dietary substance, or they comprise substances that are produced by the body

Acid-Forming, Base-Forming, and Neutral Foods

ACID-FORMING FOODS
Cheese
Meat, fish, poultry, shellfish, eggs
Grains: bread, cereals, crackers, rice, pasta
Cranberries, prunes, plums, and their juices

BASE-FORMING FOODS
All types of milk and noncheese products

Vegetables
All fruits (except cranberries, prunes, and plums)

NEUTRAL FOODS
Butter, margarine, oil, lard
White sugar, honey, syrup
Cornstarch, arrowroot, tapioca
Coffee, tea, Postum

regardless of dietary intake. In those instances, a restrictive diet may be of little value. However, if dietary excesses do contribute to stone formation, a restricted diet may be helpful.

CLIENT GOALS

The client will:

Consume increased fluids to dilute the urine.
Avoid a recurrence.
Describe the principles and rationale of diet management of renal calculi, and make the appropriate dietary changes.
Identify causative factors, if known.

NURSING INTERVENTIONS

Diet Management

For all types of renal stones
- Increase fluid intake to 3 to 4 liters/day.

For calcium oxalate stones (the following modifications are contraindicated for clients with calcium oxalate stones caused by hyperparathyroidism, sarcoidosis, renal tubular acidosis, or primary hyperoxaluria)
- Limit calcium intake to 800 to 1000 mg/day (ie, limit milk to less than 3 cups/day)(see Appendix 12). Avoid vitamin D–fortified foods and vitamin D supplements.
- Avoid excessive protein intake, which increases calcium excretion.
- Increase intake of acid-forming foods.
- Increase fiber intake, which binds with oxalate in the GI tract, thereby decreasing urinary calcium and oxalate.
- Avoid high salt intake, because salt increases urinary calcium excretion.
- Avoid foods high in oxalates (Table 19-5); however, a low-oxalate diet may not be effective if endogenous oxalate production is high.
- Avoid vitamin C supplements, which increase oxalate excretion.

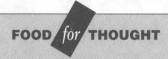

FOOD *for* THOUGHT

Urine Distress

Historically, people with urinary tract infections have been told to drink cranberry juice, based on the rationale that cranberry juice kills bacteria by acidifying the urine. However, because cranberry juice is sold as "cranberry cocktail" that is only about 25% juice, the amount needed to actually change urinary pH is too large to be of practical use.

Although conclusive evidence is lacking, it now appears that, if cranberry juice is effective against urinary tract infections, it is because it contains an ingredient that may prevent bacteria from adhering to the lining of the urinary tract, thus promoting their excretion. Unfortunately, not all bacteria are sensitive to the juice, and protection lasts only as long as the juice is consumed regularly. But, clients who are prone to UTI who like cranberry juice should be encouraged to consume it regularly, just in case. The only other dietary recommendation for urinary tract infections is to increase fluid intake to flush out bacteria.

For magnesium ammonium phosphate stones
- Increase intake of acid-forming foods.

For cystine stones
- Increase intake of base-forming foods.
- Diets low in methionine (an amino acid precursor of cystine) or protein (all protein sources contain cystine) have been used in the past, but they are difficult to follow and unpalatable, and they may not be effective.

Table 19-5
Foods High in Oxalates (>10 mg/½ cup serving)

BEVERAGES		OTHER
Draft beer	Rhubarb	Leeks
Cocoa	Strawberries	Okra
Ovaltine and other	Tangerine	Peppers, green
chocolate beverage		Potatoes, sweet
mixes	**GRAINS**	Rutabagas
Tea	Grits (white corn)	Summer squash
	Soybean crackers	Watercress
FRUITS	Wheat germ	
Blackberries		**OTHER**
Blueberries	**VEGETABLES**	Chocolate
Fruit cocktail	Baked beans canned in tomato sauce	Fruitcake
Green gooseberries	Beans: green, wax, or dried	Marmalade
Grapes, Concord	Beets (tops, roots, greens)	Nuts of any kind
Lemon peel	Celery	Peanut butter
Lime peel	Chive	Tofu
Orange peel	Eggplant	Tomato soup
Raspberries, black	Escarole	Vegetable soup
	Greens of any kind	

Source: Chicago Dietetic Association and the South Suburban Dietetic Association (1992). Manual of Clinical Dietetics 4th ed. Chicago: American Dietetic Association.

For uric acid stones
- Increase intake of base-forming foods.
- Low-purine diets (uric acid precursor) may be used, although they are difficult to follow and are not as effective as drug therapy.
- Limit meat, fish, or poultry intake to 6 to 7 oz /day.
- Restrict or eliminate alcohol.

Client Teaching

Instruct the client

On the principles and rationale of diet management for renal calculi, and how to implement the appropriate diet changes.

On the importance of drinking fluid. Clients should be encouraged to drink 8 oz/hour during waking hours. Encourage fluid intake before bed and during the night to maintain a large, dilute urine output.

Monitoring Progress

Monitor for the following signs or symptoms:

Compliance with the diet, and the need for follow-up diet counseling.
Effectiveness of the diet, and evaluate the need for further diet modifications.

Evaluation

Evaluation is ongoing. Provided that the plan of care has not changed, the client will achieve the goals as stated above.

KEY CONCEPTS

- Loss of renal function profoundly impacts metabolism, nutritional status, and nutritional requirements. The nutrients most affected are protein, calcium, phosphorus, vitamin D, fluid, sodium, and potassium.
- Diet management is an integral component of long-term treatment of chronic renal insufficiency and failure. Diet modifications are often complex, unpalatable, and frequently adjusted according to the client's laboratory values and symptoms.
- Although it has not been proven that protein restriction can slow the decline in renal function, protein restriction remains the cornerstone of dietary treatment for renal insufficiency because it has the potential to lessen renal workload.
- There is a narrow margin of error regarding protein intake: too little protein results in body protein catabolism, which has the same effect as eating too much protein, namely an increase in BUN levels.
- When total protein intake is restricted, protein quality becomes more important. The majority of protein should come from animal sources.
- A high-calorie diet is indicated whenever protein intake is restricted to ensure that the protein consumed will be used for specific protein functions, not for energy requirements.
- Generally, clients with renal insufficiency may tolerate 2 to 4 g of sodium/day. Potassium is usually not rstricted until GFR falls below 10 ml/minute.
- Fluid allowance is based on urine output, plus an additional 400 to 500 ml to account for insensible losses.

- Calcium metabolism is impaired because of faulty vitamin D metabolism secondary to loss of renal function. A high calcium intake is not achievable when protein and phosphorus are restricted.
- When dialysis is instituted, diet restrictions are liberalized; a high protein intake is recommended to compensate for protein lost through the dialysate.
- There is little agreement on the optimal diet for acute renal failure. Although protein needs are usually high because of the effects of any underlying illness, a high-protein diet is contraindicated because of uremia.
- Clients who experience a renal transplant may need to alter their diet to lessen the side effects of steroids. Hyperglycemia, sodium retention, potassium depletion, loss of calcium from the bones, and GI upsets are common side effects.
- A high fluid intake is the most effective diet intervention for the treatment of renal calculi. Ash diets, which are intended to alter urine pH and thus influence stone precipitations, have largely been replaced by more effective and consistent drug therapy.

 FOCUS ON **CRITICAL THINKING**

Michael Murphy is a 42-year-old active male who recently experienced acute renal failure secondary to scleroderma. While he was hospitalized in the intensive care unit, Michael received TPN and dialysis and stayed in a coma for 2 weeks. As his condition improved, he was weaned from TPN and resumed an oral diet; upon discharge, the only dietary advice he received was to avoid salt, limit fluid to 1 quart daily, and limit daily meat intake to 6 ounces. Although he has some urine output, he requires hemodialysis three times each week. Doctors are hopeful that he will eventually regain enough renal function so that he can discontinue dialysis.

Michael has lost 22 pounds since he became ill; his present weight of 168 pounds is the least his 6'2" frame has ever weighed. He complains of fatigue, anorexia, and being "mentally fuzzy." He forces himself to eat, and says the only thing that tastes good to him is ice cream. He has not been gaining any weight between dialysis treatments. As his outpatient dialysis nurse, you find he wants to do whatever he can to feel better and maximize his chance of getting off dialysis treatments.

Is it appropriate that Michael limit his meat intake to 6 ounces daily? How much protein does he require? What other sources of protein might he be eating that would contribute to his daily intake?

Is not gaining weight between dialysis treatments an appropriate goal? What nutrient may he not be getting enough of?

What other nutrients may need to be restricted in Michael's diet?

Explain why he may have symptoms of fatigue, anorexia, and "mental fuzziness."

Michael thought he could eat as much ice cream as he wanted because it's just "a sweet." What would you tell Michael about ice cream to convince him it should not be eaten freely?

Calculate Michael's calorie requirements; list high-calorie foods that he may use to boost his calorie intake. What would you suggest he do to help improve his intake?

REFERENCES

Beto, J. (1995). Which diet for which renal failure: Making sense of the options. J Am Diet Assoc 95(8), 898–903.

Chicago Dietetic Association and the South Suburban Dietetic Association (1992). Manual of Clinical Dietetics. 4th ed. Chicago: American Dietetic Association.

Coyne, T., Olson, M., Bradham, K. et al. (1995). Dietary satisfaction correlated with adherence in the Modification of Diet in Renal Disease Study. J Am Diet Assoc, 95(11), 1301–1306.

Escott-Stump, S. (1992). Nutrition and Diagnosis-Related Care. 3rd ed. Philadelphia: Lea & Febiger.

Gillis, B., et al. (1995). Nutrition intervention program of the Modification of Diet in Renal Disease Study: A self-management approach. J Am Diet Assoc, 91(11), 1288–1294.

Milas, N., et al. (1995). Factors associated with adherence to the dietary protein intervention in the Modification of Diet in Renal Disease Study. J Am Diet Assoc, 95(11), 1295–1300.

MDRD Study Group (1994). Reduction of dietary protein and phosphorus in the Modification of Diet in Renal Disease Feasibility Study. J Am Diet Assoc, 94(9), 986–990.

Remer, T. and Manz, F. (1995). Potential renal acid load of foods and its influence on urine pH. J Am Diet Assoc, 95(7), 791–797.

Renal Dietitians Dietetic Practice Group, National Kidney Foundation Council on Renal Nutrition (1993). National Renal Diet: Professional Guide. Chicago: American Dietetic Association.

Sanders, H., Rabb, H., Bittle, P. and Ramirez, G. (1994). Nutritional implications of recombinant human erythropoietin therapy in renal disease. J Am Diet Assoc, 94(9), 1023–1029.

Schardt, D. (1994). Take two walnuts. Nutrition Action Health Letter, 21(2), 8–9.

Stark, J. (1994). Interpreting BUN/creatinine levels. Nursing 94, 24(9), 58–61.

Toto, K. (1992). Acute renal failure: A question of location. AJN, 92(11), 44–53.

CHAPTER 20

Musculoskeletal Disorders

Chapter Outline

Key Terms

Peak bone mass
Purines

SYSTEM COMPONENTS AND FUNCTIONS

*B*ones support and shape the body, protect vital organs and other soft tissues, store minerals, play a role in red blood cell production, and act as levers to make movement possible. Collagen (connective tissue protein) serves as the bone matrix, which is strengthened and hardened by deposits of mineral salts. Calcium phosphate and calcium carbonate, which together are called hydroxyapatite, are the most abundant mineral salts.

Bone formation and maintenance depend on an adequate supply of nutrients and are regulated by hormones (see the display, Role of Nutrients and Hormones in Bone Formation and Maintenance) Bone remodeling occurs continuously as new bone is formed and existing bone is resorbed. Before age 30 to 35 years, when peak bone mass is attained, bone formation exceeds bone resorption. Thereafter, bone resorption exceeds bone formation and all people lose bone with age.

The contact point between two or more bones is called a joint (or articulation). Joints usually are formed of fibrous connective tissue and cartilage and are classified as immovable, slightly movable, or freely movable.

ROLE OF DIET THERAPY

Joint disorders often affect nutritional status by interfering with intake, and some disorders may be relieved by diet therapy (weight reduction for osteoarthritis). Diet intervention that is initiated early in life may help protect against osteoporosis, a prevalent bone disorder among postmenopausal women; once osteoporosis develops, diet therapy is used routinely in its treatment. Other conditions, such as bone fracture and prolonged immobility, require diet modification because of increased nutritional requirements and altered body metabolism.

Guidelines for musculoskeletal assessment are listed in the display, General Musculoskeletal Assessment Criteria.

Role of Nutrients and Hormones in Bone Formation and Maintenance

NUTRIENTS

Calcium and phosphorus are components of hydroxyapatite, the organic salt that provides strength and rigidity to bones and teeth.

Fluoride, magnesium, sodium, and chloride are components of bone in small amounts.

Vitamin A is necessary for bone growth and development because of its role in bone cell differentiation and protein synthesis.

Vitamin C and protein are necessary for the production and integrity of collagen, the protein matrix of bones.

HORMONES

Parathyroid hormone (PTH) prevents serum calcium levels from falling by:
- Stimulating the release of calcium from the bone (resorption)
- Increasing intestinal absorption of calcium
- Enhancing calcium retention by the kidneys
- Reducing serum phosphorus levels

Excessive PTH secretion → bone demineralization

Calcitonin lowers serum calcium levels by:
- Stimulating bone deposition of calcium
- Inhibiting bone resorption of calcium
- Reducing tubular reabsorption of calcium and phosphorus

Vitamin D functions as a hormone to increase the amount of calcium and phosphorus available to mineralize the surface of the bone by:
- Stimulating intestinal calcium absorption
- Increasing resorption of calcium and phosphate from bone

Sex hormones aid in the growth of new bone.

ASSESSMENT CRITERIA

General Musculoskeletal Assessment Criteria

Weight status, weight loss	Weakness in the extremities
Loss of height	Contractures
Pain or edema in muscles, joints, bone	Anorexia
Decreased range of motion; decreased mobility; unsteady gait	Easy fatigue
	Insomnia

JOINT DISORDERS

Rheumatoid Arthritis

Rheumatoid arthritis is a chronic, debilitating, systemic inflammatory disease that is characterized by progressive joint deformity and destruction, and systemic manifestations such as anemia, Sjögren's syndrome, and bone disease. The cause of rheumatoid arthritis is not known, but it is believed to be an autoimmune disorder. Inflammation of the synovial tissues is the cardinal manifestation; gradual pathologic changes eventually lead to joint immobility and destruction. The onset is insidious and occurs at any age, but the condition most often affects adults between the ages of 20 to 40 years. As many as 5 to 8 million Americans have rheumatoid arthritis, 75% of whom are women (Schardt, 1994). It is estimated that the incidence rate in women over 60 years of age may be as high as 15%.

Complications of rheumatoid arthritis include severe weight loss, fever, anemia, muscle atrophy, osteoporosis, dry eyes, dry mouth, and liver or spleen enlargement. In addition, degenerative changes that lead to ischemia and thrombosis may occur in the lungs, heart, muscles, blood vessels, pleura, and tendons, and vasculitis may develop in the eyes, nervous system, and skin. Rheumatoid arthritis is characterized by periods of exacerbation and remission.

Drug therapy to control the inflammatory process is the cornerstone of treatment. There are several primary drug classifications used to treat rheumatoid arthritis; actual drug choice depends on the client's tolerance, response, and compliance (see Drug Alert). Rest and exercise and application of heat and cold may help relieve pain. Diet intervention may be needed to improve overall nutritional status or to counter the side effects of drug therapy.

NURSING PROCESS

Assessment

In addition to the general musculoskeletal assessment criteria, assess for the following factors:

Affected joints that may appear painful, stiff, swollen, red, warm, and tender; observe for impaired range of motion and strength, and assess impact on the client's ability to procure, prepare, and eat meals.

Symptoms of fatigue, weakness, anorexia, and low-grade fever; assess onset, frequency, severity, interventions attempted and the results.

Dietary changes made in response to arthritis or its symptoms (ie, foods avoided, foods preferred). Determine which foods are best and least tolerated.

The use of unorthodox or unproven dietary remedies to treat arthritis, and the potential impact on nutritional status.

Medications used, and their side effects.

Weight, weight changes.

Abnormal laboratory values and their significance, especially hemoglobin, hematocrit.

Nursing Diagnosis

Altered Nutrition: Less than body requirements, related to inability to prepare meals adequately secondary to pain and limited motion in the fingers and hands

Planning and Implementation

It is estimated that arthritis sufferers spend $8 to $10 billion each year in search of relief. The chronic, debilitating nature of rheumatoid arthritis makes its victims vulnerable to claims of nutritional cures and fad diets. Low-carbohydrate diets, high-protein diets, vegetarian diets, no-dairy-products diets, supplemental B vitamins, vitamin C, vitamin A, and sulfur all have been used unsuccessfully in the treatment of arthritis. Cod liver oil, alfalfa, apple cider vinegar, pokeberries, and blackstrap molasses all have been touted as "cures" for arthritis. As yet, there is no conclusive evidence that diet therapy can prevent or cure rheumatoid arthritis. However, some studies suggest that about 5% of cases of rheumatoid arthritis may be caused by a food allergy (Buchanan et al, 1991), with milk and milk products, corn, cereals, citrus fruits, and tomatoes proposed as possible offenders. Eliminating the suspected food and then reintroducing it and observing symptoms can subjectively measure sensitivity.

Other studies suggest that fish oil supplements may help relieve joint tenderness and fatigue, possibly because omega-3 fatty acids decrease prostaglandin synthesis and thus inhibit the inflammatory response. Although the use of fish oil supplements is not recommended, eating more fatty fish may be prudent.

Although no specific diet is recommended for rheumatoid arthritis, diet intervention is useful for restoring optimal nutritional status and helping to alleviate arthritis symptoms and medication side effects. For instance, clients with rheumatoid arthritis often are poorly nourished. The process of inflammation can increase nutritional requirements by increasing metabolic rate, and also may cause malabsorption of nutrients by altering the gastrointestinal mucosa. Chronic inflammation can cause carbohydrate intolerance in some clients. Intake may be impaired because of gastrointestinal upset and peptic ulcers, which may develop as a result of arthritis or secondary to drug therapy. Pain and medications contribute to anorexia. Dry mouth, a complication of rheumatoid arthritis, may cause difficulty in swallowing and increase the risk of dental decay. Bone and joint deformities and loss of function often hinder physical preparation of meals.

Clients with Sjögren's syndrome may have chewing and swallowing difficulties and are at increased risk for dental decay. Moist, texture-modified foods and cold liquids may facilitate swallowing; concentrated sweets should be avoided. Unsweetened lemon may be used to help stimulate salivation, and good oral hygiene is encouraged.

Although a multivitamin and mineral supplement may be indicated to help restore optimal nutritional status, clients should be advised not to self-prescribe megadoses of vitamins to "cure" arthritis.

Hypochromic anemia may be an inherent characteristic of arthritis and may not respond to iron supplementation.

Be aware of the potential side effects of drug therapy and the appropriate dietary interventions to relieve those side effects.

CLIENT GOALS

The client will:

Experience fewer symptoms of arthritis and its complications, and fewer side effects of arthritis medication, as appropriate.

Consume adequate calories and protein to attain or maintain "healthy" weight and to restore or maintain optimal nutritional status.

Describe the principles and rationale of diet management to relieve the symptoms of arthritis and the side effects of medications.

NURSING INTERVENTIONS

Diet Management

Provide adequate calories and protein to attain or maintain "healthy" weight. Calorie requirements increase in response to inflammation when the disease is active and decline when the disease is in remission; adjust calories accordingly.

Increase protein during active disease to 1.5 to 2.0 g/kg to reverse negative nitrogen balance and restore nutritional status.

Modify the diet as needed to alleviate anorexia, peptic ulcer, and difficulty in swallowing (see Chapter 16) (eg, eliminate food intolerances if gastric irritation exists, provide soft or thick puréed foods as needed, if the client has dysphagia).

Client Teaching

Instruct the client

On the principles and rationale of diet management to relieve symptoms of arthritis and the side effects of medications, as indicated, and how to implement the appropriate dietary changes.

That there is no dietary cure for arthritis. Advise the client to avoid unproven diets and supplements, which may not only be costly but also may be potentially dangerous.

That because the oils in fish may help decrease joint inflammation, it may be prudent to eat more fatty fish like mackerel, herring, and salmon.

On joint-saving ideas for food preparation (see the display, Joint-Saving Ideas for Food Preparation).

Joint-Saving Ideas for Food Preparation

KITCHEN ORGANIZATION IDEAS

Keep utensils that are used most often within easy reach and place duplicates at strategic locations around the kitchen.

Wear an apron with several pockets to keep small utensils handy.

Hang pots and pans on a wall rack to avoid bending and stretching.

Use lazy Susans and pull-out shelves.

Use drawer dividers to create vertical filing so that items can be located easily without moving others.

Training or financial assistance for kitchen remodeling and equipment may be available from the local Division of Vocational Rehabilitation.

MEAL PREPARATION IDEAS

Take advantage of "good" days by making double or triple portions and freezing the extras.

Use one-dish meals and convenience foods whenever possible.

Invest in labor-saving appliances such as a food processor, blender, mixer, electric knife, and electric can opener.

Prepare meals while sitting on a moveable swivel stool and use a wheeled cart to move heavy items.

Use lightweight cooking utensils and bowls, such as aluminum and plastic.

Use nonstick cookware and soak dishes and pans immediately after use to reduce clean-up.

Whenever possible, use paper plates, napkins, and tablecloths.

Don't overdo it, and ask for help from family and friends.

Assistance may be available from community resources, such as Meals on Wheels and volunteer shoppers.

JOINT PROTECTION IDEAS

Tie a looped rope around cabinet, drawer, refrigerator, and oven handles and open by slipping the forearm through the loop and pulling.

Use a rubber gripper to open lids by twisting with the palm or heel of the hand placed flat on the top of the lid.

Build up utensil handles with foam rubber to make them easier to hold.

Open pull-top cans with a knife or screwdriver inserted through the metal ring.

Lay boxes flat on their side and open by cutting with a knife.

Anchor bowls with a rubber mat in the corner of the sink to make stirring easier.

Beat eggs with a whisk instead of a fork or spoon, because whisks offer less resistance.

Tongs release food more easily than a fork.

Use cookware with two handles.

Boil foods in a wire mesh basket inserted in a pot; when the food is done, simply remove the basket rather than lifting the whole pot.

Use an oven shovel or wooden rack jack to reduce bending while retrieving hot items from the oven.

Use a toaster oven or stove-top oven if using the oven is difficult.

For clean-up, use sponge mitts instead of a hand-held sponge.

Select joint protection gadgets, such as open-handled knives and jar openers, suited to meet your needs.

Numerous eating aids, such as utensils with built-up plastic handles, scooper bowls with nonskid bases, plate guards, swivel spoons, and large-handled mugs are available to simplify eating.

Arthritis Health Professions Section of the Arthritis Foundation: Self-Help Manual for Patients with Arthritis. Atlanta: Arthritis Foundation, 1980.

Monitoring Progress

Monitor for the following signs or symptoms:

Tolerance to oral feedings (eg, ability to swallow for clients with Sjögren's syndrome)

Compliance with the diet, and the need for follow-up diet counseling

Effectiveness of diet (ie, attains "healthy" weight, avoids side effects of medications), and the need for further diet modification

Evaluation

Evaluation is ongoing. Provided that the plan of care has not changed, the client will achieve the goals as stated above.

Rheumatoid Arthritis

Aspirin is the treatment of choice for rheumatoid arthritis. Nonsteroidal antiinflammatory drugs, steroidal antiinflammatories, and gold compounds have a higher incidence of adverse side effects and are used only after aspirin therapy fails (see the display, Rheumatoid Arthritis: Drug Alert on page 674).

Degenerative Joint Disease (Osteoarthritis)

Osteoarthritis is a chronic, progressive, noninflammatory joint disorder that is characterized by destruction of joint cartilage, spur and bone cyst formation, pain, and impaired joint movement. It most often affects weight-bearing joints (knees, hips, ankles, and spine) and fingers.

Osteoarthritis, which affects more than 16 million people, is the most common form of arthritis. As much as 80% of the population over 55 years of age may be affected, and it is equally prevalent in men and women. Approximately twice as many obese people as people of normal weight have osteoarthritis; however, it is not known whether obesity is an etiologic factor or whether it occurs secondary to reduced activity related to osteoarthritis.

Osteoarthritis is believed to result from prolonged mechanical stress, although it probably does not have a single cause. Predisposing factors include aging, congenital abnormalities, trauma, obesity, and systemic disease.

Drug therapy to control pain and discomfort and physical therapy are used to treat osteoarthritis. Surgical intervention may be used if medical treatment fails to control pain, or if joint destruction is severe. Although anecdotal "evidence" of nutritional remedies is abundant, no scientific evidence links diet to relief of osteoarthritis (see Food for Thought: Knocking Nightshades). Adjunctively, diet intervention is used to promote weight loss in obese clients, thereby reducing strain on weight-bearing joints.

Rheumatoid Arthritis: Drug Alert

Drug	Possible Side Effects	Diet Interventions
SALICYLATES		
Aspirin	High doses or chronic use can cause gastric pain and bleeding, peptic ulcer, heartburn, nausea, vomiting, increased excretion of vitamin C, potassium depletion, iron deficiency anemia, delayed blood clotting	GI problems may be avoided by taking aspirin with food, milk, or a full glass of water, or by using enteric coated types. Buffered compounds containing sodium may be contraindicated for clients on sodium restricted diets. Encourage the intake of foods high in vitamin C and folic acid and provide supplements if needed.
NONSTEROIDAL ANTI-INFLAMMATORIES		
Indomethacin Phenylbutazone Ibuprofen Fenoprofen Sulindac Naproxen Tolmetin	Dyspepsia, dizziness, nausea, GI bleeding, epigastric pain, heartburn, diarrhea, stomatitis, duodenal ulcer, constipation, anemia	Administer with food, milk, or a full glass of water. Avoiding or eliminating the following foods may help reduce GI distress: citrus fruits and juices, tomatoes, alcohol, and caffeine.
Methotrexate	Folic acid antagonist. May cause stomatitis, nausea, vomiting, and megaloblastic anemia.	1 mg supplemental folic acid/day can reduce GI side effects of low-dose therapy.
Gold salts Myochrysine	Nephrotoxic. May cause nephrosis and protein deficiency.	Increase protein and calories if nephrosis or protein deficiency occurs.
STEROID ANTI-INFLAMMATORIES: MAY BE TAKEN ORALLY OR AS LOCAL INJECTIONS		
Prednisone	Sodium retention; edema Increased potassium excretion Protein catabolism, delayed wound healing, muscle wasting; negative nitrogen balance Impaired glucose tolerance GI upset, duodenal ulcer Increased need for vitamin B_6, vitamin C, folic acid, and vitamin D Decreased calcium and phosphorus absorption, decreased bone formation, osteoporosis	Possible modifications: Decrease sodium Increase potassium Increase protein Diabetic diet Small, frequent meals Provide multivitamin and mineral supplements.
Penicillamine Cuprimine	May cause zinc deficiency with altered taste, anorexia, and weight loss. Vitamin B_6 antagonist.	Increase foods rich in zinc (meat, seafood, egg yolks, legumes, whole grains); supplemental zinc may be indicated. A daily supplement of 25 mg of vitamin B_6 is advised.

Source: Roe, D. (1994). Handbook on Drugs & Nutrient Interactions. 5th ed. Chicago: American Dietetic Association.

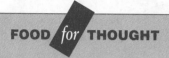

FOOD *for* THOUGHT

Knocking Nightshades

Back in the early 1960s, a horticulture professor at Rutgers University named Norman Childers noticed that his joints and muscles became sore within an hour or two after eating vegetables of the nightshade family, like potatoes, tomatoes, eggplant, and bell peppers. He spread the word in newspapers across the country, urging arthritis sufferers to stop eating nightshade vegetables. Over the next 10 years, he heard from thousands who had tried his idea; most claimed at least some improvement in symptoms.

Childers concluded that about 10% of arthritis sufferers are sensitive to something in nightshade vegetables. Unfortunately, his "study" was not scientific, and there have been no controlled studies since then linking anything in the diet to osteoarthritis.

As for eliminating nightshades to lessen the pain of osteoarthritis, as long as the diet is nutritionally adequate, it could do no harm, and may help, even if it is only a placebo effect.

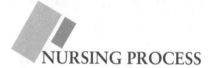

NURSING PROCESS

Assessment

In addition to the general musculoskeletal assessment criteria, assess for the following factors:

Limitation of motion, contractures, and muscle spasms, and determine the impact on procuring, preparing, and eating meals.

Dietary changes made in response to arthritis or its symptoms (ie, foods avoided, foods preferred). Determine which foods are best and least tolerated.

The use of unorthodox or unproven dietary remedies to treat arthritis, and the potential impact on nutritional status.

Medications and their side effects.

Weight, weight status.

Nursing Diagnosis

Altered Health Maintenance, related to lack of knowledge of diet intervention for osteoarthritis

Planning and Implementation

Clients with osteoarthritis are often obese, which contributes to strain on the weight-bearing joints. For some unexplained reason, weight reduction has been shown to eliminate symptoms of osteoarthritis throughout the body, not just in the weight-bearing joints. However, weight loss may be hindered because of impaired physical mobility and exercise-related pain. Provide emotional support and periodic diet follow-up.

Arthritis that affects finger joints may impair ability to prepare meals.

With the exception of oral steroidal antiinflammatories, osteoarthritis may be treated with the same drugs as rheumatoid arthritis (see rheumatoid arthritis Drug Alert). Local injections of corticosteroids may be given.

CLIENT GOALS

The client will:

Lose weight, if overweight, to lessen the strain on weight-bearing joints.
Consume a well-balanced, nutritionally adequate diet.
Describe the principles and rationale of diet intervention for osteoarthritis, and implement the appropriate dietary changes.
Modify the diet, as needed, to minimize the side effects of drug therapy.

NURSING INTERVENTIONS

Diet Management

Decrease calories to attain and maintain "healthy" weight (see Appendix 10).
Modify the diet, as needed, to minimize the side effects of drug therapy.

Client Teaching

Instruct the client

On the principles and rationale of diet management for osteoarthritis, and how to implement the appropriate dietary changes.
To avoid unorthodox dietary "cures" for arthritis, which are unfounded and may be potentially dangerous.
On joint-saving ideas for food preparation (see the display, Joint-Saving Ideas for Food Preparation).

Monitoring Progress

Monitor for the following signs or symptoms:

Compliance with the diet, and the need for follow-up diet counseling
Effectiveness of the diet (ie, achieves weight loss, avoids side effects of medication), and the need for additional diet modification

Evaluation

Evaluation is ongoing. Provided that the plan of care has not changed, the client will achieve the goals as stated above.

Gout

Gout, which affects almost 2 million Americans, is characterized by the overproduction or underexcretion of uric acid (or a combination of both), leading to hyperuricemia, precipitation of uric acid crystals in joints and connective tissue, and inflammation. Tophi, which are relatively painless deposits of urate crystals on the ears, fingers, hands, forearms, or feet, may form, depending on the duration of the disease, the degree of hyperuricemia, and renal functional status.

The sudden onset of severe pain in one or more peripheral joints, most often the joints of the large toe, foot, ankle, knee, wrist, and elbow, signals an acute attack. Usually the affected joints return to normal within 1 week. Recurrent attacks occur at irregular intervals and may be precipitated by fasting, weight loss, low carbohydrate intake, alcohol, stress, or the use of aspirin and thiazide diuretics. Attacks become more frequent and last longer as the disease worsens.

Chronic gout leads to bone and joint erosion, which can result in gross deformities, loss of joint function, chronic pain, and progressive renal dysfunction. Left untreated, gout can lead to chronic renal disease secondary to urate kidney stones.

Primary gout is caused by either a genetic defect of purine metabolism or a renal defect that decreases uric acid excretion; it most often affects men in their 50s and is associated with obesity. Gout may also occur secondary to other disorders, such as polycythemia or leukemia, or it may be precipitated by prolonged use of thiazide diuretics and aspirin, trauma, or treatment of myeloproliferative diseases.

Gout is treated with drug therapy that includes colchicine, analgesics, and antiinflammatory drugs. Rest and elevation of the affected joint may help relieve pain during an acute attack. A high fluid intake is indicated to help flush the kidneys, and high-purine foods may be eliminated from the diet.

NURSING PROCESS

Assessment

In addition to the general musculoskeletal assessment criteria, assess for the following factors:

Symptoms (possible headache, fever, malaise, and anorexia); onset, frequency, severity, interventions attempted and the results.

Dietary changes made in response to gout (ie, foods avoided, foods preferred). Determine if unorthodox dietary practices are followed. Determine if a relationship exists between an acute attack and diet—whether attack was precipitated by fasting, weight loss, a low-carbohydrate diet, or alcohol.

Nursing Diagnosis

Altered Health Maintenance, related to a lack of knowledge of the dietary management of gout

Planning and Implementation

Uric acid is the end-product of **purine** metabolism; purines are found in nucleoproteins, which are most abundant in high-protein foods but are present to some degree in all foods. The body also synthesizes purines from dietary carbohydrate, protein, and fat, and from endogenous purine breakdown.

Severe purine-restricted diets have been replaced largely by drug therapy. From a practical standpoint, a low-purine diet is difficult to achieve; some foods are rich in purines and all foods contain nucleoproteins, from which purines are derived. Also, restricting purine intake does not affect endogenous uric acid synthesis and has little impact on serum uric acid levels. Instead of following a rigid low-purine diet, clients may benefit from avoiding those foods that are extremely high in purines.

The most effective diet intervention in the treatment of gout is to increase fluid intake (to at least 2–3 liters/day) to promote uric acid excretion and dilute the urine, thereby avoiding kidney stone formation.

Weight loss also is effective at reducing serum uric acid levels but must be undertaken gradually to avoid precipitating an acute attack of gouty arthritis. Fasting, low-carbohydrate diets, and rapid weight loss should be avoided; all favor the formation of ketones, which inhibit uric acid excretion.

An acidic urine favors the precipitation of uric acid stones and should be avoided. However, it is not likely that the client's usual consumption of acid-ash foods (cranberries, cranberry juice, prunes, prune juice, cheese, meat, fish, and poultry) is sufficient for this intervention to produce a significant decrease in urine pH.

A high-fat diet favors the renal retention of uric acid and should therefore be avoided. In addition, many clients with primary gout have hypertriglyceridemia and may benefit from a low-fat diet (Chicago Dietetic Association, 1992).

Generally, high-carbohydrate diets tend to increase uric acid excretion; however, a high fructose intake (fruit sugar) may increase uric acid production and should be avoided.

In the past, clients with gout were instructed to avoid coffee, tea, and cocoa based on the rationale that they contain compounds that are readily converted to uric acid. However, there is no scientific evidence to support the elimination of coffee, tea, and cocoa from a purine-restricted diet.

Because alcohol increases purine production, alcohol intake should be moderated—it should be consumed with meals or diluted (Chicago Dietetic Association, 1992).

If chronic renal disease develops, additional diet modifications are necessary (see Chapter 19).

CLIENT GOALS

The client will:

Consume appropriate calories and protein to attain or maintain a "healthy" weight; if weight reduction is indicated, client will lose weight gradually (ie, ½ to 1 pounds/week) to avoid precipitating an attack.

Increase fluid intake to at least 2 to 3 liters/day to promote the excretion of uric acid.

Modify the diet, as needed, to minimize the side effects of drug therapy.

Describe the principles and rationale of diet management for gout, and implement the appropriate dietary changes.

Identify factors that contribute to an acute attack, when known.

Avoid chronic renal failure as a complication of gout.

NURSING INTERVENTIONS

Diet Management

Increase fluid intake to at least 2 to 3 quarts/day.

Decrease calories for gradual weight loss of ½ to 1 pounds/week, if overweight.

Eliminate high-purine foods (more than 150 mg of purine/100 g of food): anchovies, dried peas and beans, lentils, beef kidney, liver, brains, herring, mackerel, meat extracts (meat drippings, gravy, broth, consommeé), sardines, scallops, sweetbreads.

Moderate protein intake should not exceed .75 to 1.0 g/kg of ideal body weight/day. Limit meat intake to 3 to 4 oz/meal. Cheese, eggs, milk, and vegetables are low in nucleoproteins and should fulfill most of the moderate protein allowance. Fish, meat, meat-based soups, poultry, and shellfish are higher in purines and may be restricted during acute attacks.

Eliminate/restrict alcohol.

Client Teaching

Instruct the client

On the principles and rationale of diet management for gout.

To increase fluid intake to at least 2 to 3 liters/day. Encourage fluid intake before bed and during the night to avoid concentrated urine, which is more conducive to stone formation.

To avoid alcohol, or to use moderate amounts infrequently that are diluted with other liquids or foods, because excessive alcohol consumption reduces uric acid excretion.

To avoid fasting, which may precipitate an attack.

Monitoring Progress

Monitor for the following signs or symptoms:

Compliance with the diet, and the need for follow-up diet counseling
Effectiveness of diet, and evaluate the need for further dietary changes
Weight, weight status

Evaluation

Evaluation is ongoing. Provided that the plan of care has not changed, the client will achieve the goals as stated above.

DRUG ALERT

Anti-Gout Drugs

Drugs that are used in the treatment of gout are aimed at reducing serum uric acid levels (uricosuric agents) and providing symptomatic relief for acute attacks of gouty arthritis.

Be aware of the potential side effects associated with the use of antiinflammatory agents (indomethacin, phenylbutazone) in the treatment of acute attacks of gouty arthritis (see Rheumatoid Arthritis Drug Alert on page 674).

Drug	Possible Side Effects	Diet Interventions
Colchicine decreases uric acid deposition	Nausea, vomiting, diarrhea Abdominal pain Malabsorption of sodium, potassium, fat, carotene, and vitamin B_{12} Decreased lactase activity Loss of appetite	Take with water immediately before, with, or after meals to avoid GI upset. Encourage high fluid intake (greater than 2000 ml/day) to reduce risk of urate kidney stone formation.
Allopurinol controls hyperuricemia from - overproduction of uric acid	Skin rash Vomiting, diarrhea, abdominal pain Enhances iron absorption and hepatic iron stores	Encourage high fluid intake (greater than 2000 ml/day) to reduce the risk of urate kidney stone formation.
Probenecid: Promotes urinary excretion of uric acid	GI irritation and nausea (initially worsens symptoms of acute gouty arthritis)	Encourage high fluid intake (greater than 2000 ml/day) to reduce the risk of urate kidney stone formation.
Sulfinpyrazone: Promotes urinary excretion of uric acid	Nausea, epigastric pain, burning, dyspepsia	Take with water immediately before, during, or after meals to avoid GI upset.

BONE DISORDERS

Osteoporosis

Osteoporosis is a disease that is characterized by a decrease in total bone mass and deterioration of bone tissue, which leads to increased bone fragility and risk of fracture (McBean et al, 1994). Osteoporosis most often affects the spine, hips, and forearms.

Osteoporosis is the most frequent skeletal disorder in the world, and is estimated to affect 25 million Americans, mostly women. It is considered to be a pediatric disease with a geriatric outcome (McBean et al, 1994). Approximately half of all 45-year-old women have some degree of osteoporosis, and by 80 years of age, bone mass may be decreased by 30% to 60%. A woman's chance of developing osteoporosis is said to be equal to her combined risks of developing breast, ovarian, and uterine cancer, yet it is preventable (McBean et al, 1994).

Throughout life, bone tissue is constantly being destroyed and rebuilt, a process known as remodeling. In the first few decades of life, net gain exceeds net loss as bone mass is accrued. Between 30 and 35 years of age, **peak bone mass**, which is the most bone mass a person will ever have, is attained. Thereafter, all people lose more bone than is gained; the rate of bone loss appears to be accelerated by a calcium deficiency and to be retarded by a high calcium intake. During the first 5 years or so after onset of menopause, women experience rapid bone loss that is related to estrogen deficiency. After that, bone loss continues at a slower rate. Unfortunately, neither calcium nor exercise can stop bone loss that results from estrogen withdrawal.

Progressive bone loss that occurs over a long time may not be detected until a fracture occurs; vertebral, hip, and wrist fractures are the hallmarks of osteoporosis. Each year, about 1.5 million fractures are related to osteoporosis; of patients with hip fractures, 20% die within a year, and half of the survivors never walk independently again (McBean et al, 1994). Other long-term effects of decreased stature and deformity include decreased thoracic and abdominal volume, chronic back pain, early dietary satiety, and decreased tolerance to exercise related to decreased lung capacity. Quality of life is significantly impaired, both physically and emotionally. It is estimated that osteoporosis has an annual national cost of $10 billion.

Although primary osteoporosis is complex and multifactorial, low peak bone mass and estrogen deficiency appear to be the most important risk factors in its development. Premature menopause is a strong predictor of osteoporosis. Other risk factors appear in the display, Osteoporosis: Risk Factors. Secondary osteoporosis may result from endocrine, gastrointestinal, and renal diseases, neoplasms of the bone marrow, excessive use of corticosteroids, prolonged immobility, radiation therapy, and long-term use of heparin.

The treatment of osteoporosis is neither totally effective nor completely safe. Although long-standing calcium deficiency plays a role in the development of osteoporosis, a high calcium intake cannot replace bone once it is lost. Estrogen replacement is the most effective method of treating osteoporosis; however, it is associated with an increased risk of endometrial cancer. Pain resulting from fractures may be treated with bed rest and analgesics.

Because prevention is more effective than treatment, efforts should focus on maximizing peak bone mass: The greater the peak bone mass, the greater the bone mass in old age. Weight-bearing exercise is important for building and strengthening bones, as is dietary calcium. Studies show a positive link between drinking milk in childhood and peak bone mass (McBean et al, 1994). It appears that peak periods for calcium retention for girls are in the pre- and early pubertal periods (Abrams and Stuff, 1994). Although the biggest impact on preventing osteoporosis may be made between 4 and 20 years of age (Liebman, 1994a), an adequate calcium intake throughout life is important for bone health.

Osteoporosis: Risk Factors

	Rationale
Female sex	Women have 30% less bone mass than men, which may also be influenced by hereditary factors, inactivity, and low calcium intakes. Osteoporosis is four times more common among women than men, and women tend to develop it earlier and more severely.
Natural or surgically induced menopause	After the onset of menopause, bone loss is rapidly accelerated for 3 to 5 years and continues for 20 years. Estrogen deficiency appears to increase calcium requirement by decreasing its absorption and retention. Studies have shown that fair-skinned women have less estrogen than dark-skinned women, which increases their risk of osteoporosis.
Long-standing calcium deficiency	Studies suggest osteoporotics have lower calcium intakes than nonosteoporotics and that an inadequate calcium intake contributes to bone loss.
	Also, inadequate calcium intake prior to age 30 to 35 may prevent attainment of peak bone mass.
Inactivity/Immobility	The rate of bone resorption exceeds bone formation when normal weight-bearing and muscle tension is impaired.
Positive family history	Although conclusive evidence is lacking, studies on twins suggest osteoporosis may be related to genetic factors.
Smoking and alcohol abuse	Associated with decreased estrogen levels; excessive alcohol promotes calcium excretion.
Long-term use of steroids or anticonvulsants	Altered calcium metabolism related to decreased absorption (steroids) or vitamin D deficiency (anticonvulsant Dilantin, phenobarbital).

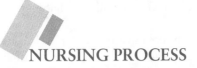

NURSING PROCESS

Assessment

In addition to the general musculoskeletal assessment criteria, assess for the following factors:

Symptoms that may affect intake (eg, anorexia related to pain, mild ileus related to T10 and L2 fractures); onset, frequency, causative factors, severity, interventions attempted and the results.

Dietary changes made in response to osteoporosis (ie, foods avoided, foods preferred).

Usual calcium intake. Determine if the client is taking supplemental calcium; if so, find out what type, how much, how often, and whether the client experiences any unpleasant side effects.

Adequacy of vitamin D intake and exposure to sunlight.

Frequency and intensity of weight-bearing exercise.

Use of tobacco and alcohol.

Intake of wheat bran: large amounts impair calcium absorption.

Use of medications that decrease calcium availability, such as aluminum antacids and glucocorticoids.

Nursing Diagnosis

Altered Health Maintenance, related to lack of knowledge of the dietary management of osteoporosis

Planning and Implementation

The optimal amount of calcium that is needed to slow or prevent the progression of osteoporosis is not known, although many experts agree that intakes of calcium and vitamin D above the current recommended dietary allowance (RDA) may be necessary (McBean et al, 1994). See Table 20-1 for the National Institutes of Health calcium recommendations.

Increasing dietary calcium is safe and effective and is preferred over use of pharmacologic supplements because dietary calcium is better absorbed and contains the correct proportion of calcium to protein, phosphorus, and vitamin D. Milk and dairy products are the richest sources of calcium; four cups of milk or its equivalent supplies about 1200 mg of calcium. However, clients with lactose intolerance who must restrict their intake of calcium to low-lactose sources (hard cheese, yogurt, buttermilk, lactose-reduced milk, and possibly small, frequent servings of milk [see Chapter 16]) may not be able to consume adequate calcium through diet alone. And

Table 20-1
Optimal Calcium Intake

The National Institutes of Health Consensus Development Panel on Optimal Calcium Intake has issued the following recommendations for calcium intake in milligrams (mg) per day:

Age/Gender	NIH Recommendations	Current RDA
Birth–1 yr	400–600 mg	400–600 mg
1–5 yrs	800 mg	800 mg
6–10 yrs	800–1200 mg	1200 mg
11–24 yrs	1200–1500 mg	1200 mg
Females, 25–49 yrs	1000 mg	800 mg
Females, pregnant/nursing	1200–1500 mg	1200 mg
Females, postmenopausal, 50–64 yrs:		
On estrogen replacement therapy	1000 mg	800 mg
Not on estrogen replacement therapy	1500 mg	800 mg
Males, 25–64 yrs	1000 mg	800 mg
Males/females, 65 yrs+	1500 mg	800 mg

Source: IFIC Foundation, Auld, E. ed. Calcium: Make no bones about it. Food Insight Sept/Oct 1994 pg 4.

unfortunately, many women voluntarily restrict their intake of dairy products because they believe they are high in cholesterol and calories and cause gastrointestinal (GI) discomfort (Chapman et al, 1995).

Food consumption surveys indicate that a large percentage of Americans fail to consume the RDA for calcium. In one study of 351 women, 43.2% had calcium intakes below 60% of the RDA (Chapman et al, 1995). Data from the latest National Health and Nutrition Examination Survey (NHANES III) indicate that more than half of all American children fail to consume recommended calcium intakes (Auld [ed], 1994). At all ages, men consume more calcium than women. Also, calcium intake decreases with age, as does calcium absorption, for both normal and osteoporotic people.

Vitamin D promotes calcium absorption; in the absence of vitamin D, less than 10% of dietary calcium may be absorbed (NIH, 1994). A deficiency of vitamin D is most likely to occur in the elderly because of inadequate intakes, inadequate exposure to sunlight, and decreased nutrient absorption and synthesis. Besides supplements, sources of vitamin D include sunlight, fortified liquid dairy products, fortified cereals, cod liver oil, and fatty fish. Vitamin D and calcium do not need to be taken together to be effective. Some studies suggest that the current RDA for vitamin D of 5.0 micrograms/day for postmenopausal women is too low, and that although as much as 20 micrograms/day may not be needed, it is safe and effective (Dawson-Hughes et al, 1995). Although vitamin D supplements may be appropriate in high-risk clients, caution is advised because excessive doses can lead to hypercalciuria and hypercalcemia.

Calcium availability is decreased by several dietary factors. High intakes of caffeine, alcohol, sodium, and protein increase urinary calcium excretion. Large amounts of wheat bran impair calcium absorption (NIH, 1994).

Smoking affects bone health by impairing calcium absorption, reducing estrogen production, speeding estrogen metabolism, and promoting early menopause (ADA, 1995).

Calcium supplements are indicated for clients who cannot or will not consume adequate calcium. Supplements differ significantly in their calcium content (Table 20-2) and rate of absorption. Calcium carbonate generally is recommended because it is the least expensive and contains the largest percentage of calcium by weight. However, one study found that calcium citrate maleate, which is currently available only in fortified orange juice, prevented loss of spine bone, whereas calcium carbonate, the most common calcium supplement, did not.

Calcium intakes up to 1.5 g/day appear to be safe for most people. In fact, calcium intakes up to 2.0 g/day are safe for most people who do not have other medical conditions that cause hypercalcemia (hyperparathyroidism, sarcoidosis), and for those who are not prone to renal stones. As a precaution against possible calcium oxalate stones, a high fluid intake (ie, 10 to 20 oz of fluid with each calcium dose) is recommended during the first 3 months of supplementation to dilute urinary calcium. Supplements may be contraindicated for clients who are predisposed to urinary calculi.

Table 20-2
Calcium Supplements

	% of Calcium	Comments
Calcium carbonate (eg, Tums)	40	Most concentrated and least expensive calcium source (ie, fewest number of tablets required). High incidence of constipation and "gas"; if gastric acid secretion is impaired (ie, elderly), calcium carbonate should be taken with food.
Tricalcium phosphate (eg, Posture)	39	Occasional GI upset.
Calcium chloride	36	Administer with food to reduce GI irritation.
Bone meal	33	Not recommended because of possible lead and mercury contamination.
Dibasic calcium phosphate (dihydrate dicalcium phosphate)	23	Administer with food to reduce GI irritation.
Dolomite	22	Not recommended because of possible lead and mercury contamination.
Calcium citrate	21	Better absorbed than calcium carbonate in people who lack stomach acid and who are fasting. Not better absorbed than calcium carbonate in most people. Lower incidence of constipation and gas than calcium carbonate.
Calcium lactate	13	Lactose may enhance absorption. Administer with food to reduce GI irritation.
Calcium gluconate	9	GI irritation is minimal, but may cause constipation.
Calcium glubionate (eg, Neo-Calglucon)	6.5	Rare incidence of GI disturbances. Administer before meals to enhance absorption.

Malseed RT: Pharmacology, Drug Therapy, and Nursing Considerations, 3rd ed. Philadelphia: JB Lippincott, 1990.

Another concern is that calcium supplements (except those containing citrate and ascorbic acid) can decrease iron absorption by as much as 50% (NIH, 1994). To minimize their impact on iron absorption, calcium supplements should not be taken with meals.

The prolonged or frequent use of aluminum-containing antacids should be discouraged because they may contribute to bone loss by increasing bone resorption, depleting phosphorus and calcium, and impairing fluoride absorption.

Because bone remodeling is a relatively slow process, it may take months to years before any improvement is noted.

CLIENT GOALS

The client will:

Consume at least 1200 to 1500 mg of calcium daily, preferably from dairy products and other food sources.

Describe the rationale and principles of diet management for osteoporosis, and implement the appropriate dietary changes.

Identify risk factors, if known (eg, smoking, sedentary lifestyle, low calcium intake).

NURSING INTERVENTIONS

Diet Management

Promote a well-balanced diet that contains at least 1000 mg calcium (see Appendix 12 for sources of calcium).

Avoid excessive sodium and protein intake, which promote calcium excretion.

Avoid excessive caffeine and alcohol intake because they promote calcium excretion and can contribute to negative calcium balance.

Client Teaching

Instruct the client

On the principles and rationale of diet management for osteoporosis, and how to implement the appropriate dietary changes.

That calcium supplements may be necessary if fewer than three servings of dairy products are consumed daily. Advise the client to drink at least 10 to 20 oz of water with each supplement, unless the client also is taking thiazide, and to take the supplements between meals. Explain that calcium supplements may not be effective for protecting against calcium loss in all types of bone, and that they are not a panacea against osteoporosis.

To modify the diet, as needed, to minimize the side effects of calcium supplements, if appropriate.

To practice other preventive measures, as appropriate: Increase weight-bearing exercise, quit smoking, avoid excessive alcohol intake.

Monitoring Progress

Monitor for the following signs or symptoms:

Tolerance to increased intake of dairy products, if appropriate (ie, absence of gas, distention, cramping, and diarrhea after consuming milk and milk products)

Compliance with the diet, and the need for follow-up diet counseling

Effectiveness of the diet in minimizing side effects of calcium supplements, if appropriate, and evaluate the need for further diet modification

Evaluation

Evaluation is ongoing. Provided that the plan of care has not changed, the client will achieve the goals as stated above.

Estrogen Therapy

Although estrogen therapy has been shown to reduce bone loss, especially during the 5 to 10 years after menopause, its use is still controversial because estrogen therapy increases the risk of endometrial cancer. Frequent side effects include nausea, fluid retention, and breast fullness or tenderness.

Prolonged Immobilization

Prolonged immobilization that results from bone fracture and other types of trauma can lead to numerous nutritional problems. The objectives of diet therapy are to promote healing and to avoid complications related to altered body metabolism (see the display, Prolonged Immobilization).

NURSING CONSIDERATIONS

During the acute phase that follows trauma, clients often are anorexic and may benefit from small, frequent meals.

Thirst may not be a valid indicator of fluid need in clients who are immobilized; monitor intake and output. If bladder training is indicated, give fluids at regular, specified intervals.

Provide adequate vitamin C and zinc to promote healing (if appropriate) and prevent skin breakdown.

Observe for signs and symptoms of hypercalcemia, which may develop insidiously or rapidly: anorexia, nausea, vomiting, abdominal cramps, constipation, headache, malaise, lethargy, and possible polydipsia and polyuria. Untreated hypercalcemia can result in renal insufficiency, hypertension, seizures, and hearing loss.

Prolonged Immobilization

Diet Recommendations	Rationale
Increase protein intake to 1.2 g/kg body weight	Both prolonged bed rest and stress increase nitrogen excretion and result in a negative nitrogen balance.
	A high protein intake is needed to prevent skin breakdown, decubitus ulcers, infection, and to restore nitrogen balance.
Adjust calorie intake periodically according to need	In the acute phase following trauma, calorie requirements are high due to the effect of stress hormones and the need for protein-sparing calories.
	Calorie requirements level off in the chronic phase and should be adjusted to prevent excessive weight gain.
	Clients with paraplegia, hemiplegia, and paralysis have decreased energy requirements.
Maintain normal calcium intake, despite increased bone resorption, hypercalcemia, and hypercalciuria	Decreased activity → increased calcium resorption and bone loss (osteopenia) → elevated levels of serum and urinary calcium.
	Calcium kidney stones and calcification of the kidney and other soft tissues may also occur.
	Altered calcium metabolism is not nutritionally related and cannot be prevented or treated by diet intervention.
Calcium requirements may increase after mobility is resumed	Normal calcium metabolism is restored only after remobilization, and bone losses are replenished only if sufficient calcium is available.
Increase fluid intake	High fluid intake is necessary to dilute urine and prevent the formation of calcium kidney stones.
Increase fiber	To help prevent constipation.

KEY CONCEPTS

- Although there is no known dietary cause or cure for rheumatoid arthritis, food allergy may contribute to a small percentage of cases.
- Clients with rheumatoid arthritis are often malnourished; a diet adequate in calories and protein and modified to minimize GI side effects of the disease may be indicated.
- Clients with osteoarthritis are often obese; weight loss can relieve symptoms of osteoarthritis throughout the body, not just in weight-bearing joints.
- Drugs used to treat arthritis can have side effects with nutritional implications.
- Clients with gout should consume a high fluid intake to promote uric acid excretion and keep the urine dilute. A gout attack may be precipitated by fasting, rapid weight loss, and a low carbohydrate diet.
- Prevention of osteoporosis is far more effective than treatment. The biggest impact on osteoporosis prevention may be made between 4 and 20 years of age; however, adequate calcium intake throughout life is important for bone health.
- Although it is not known precisely how much calcium is needed to prevent osteoporosis, many experts believe the current RDA is inadequate for all people 11 years of age and older.
- The calcium in milk and milk products is better absorbed than the calcium in pharmacologic supplements because it contains the ideal proportion of calcium to proetin, phosphorus, and vitamin D. The equivalent of 4 cups of milk provides 1200 mg of calcium.
- Most adult American women do not consume the RDA for calcium.
- High intakes of caffeine, alcohol, and protein increase urinary excretion of calcium. Calcium absorption is impaired by large amounts of wheat bran.
- Calcium carbonate (ie, Tums) is the most concentrated and least expensive calcium supplement. Calcium supplements interfere with iron absorption and may increase the risk of renal calculi in susceptible people.
- Depending on its duration and the development of side effects, clients experiencing prolonged immobilization may require adjustment in their intake of calories, protein, calcium, fluid, and fiber.

 FOCUS ON **CRITICAL THINKING**

Mrs. Oakland is 48 years old, 5′3″ tall, and weighs 118 pounds. Her last menstrual period was 3 years ago. Because she was bothered by hot flashes and has a positive family history for osteoporosis, Mrs. Oakland is taking estrogen, which she claims made her gain 10 pounds. Her doctor has urged her to drink more milk, but she says she can't afford the calories, and that too much milk gives her "gas." She's been taking Dolomite on the advice of the health food store salesperson.

(continued)

FOCUS ON **CRITICAL THINKING** (Continued)

What risk factors does Mrs. Oakland have for osteoporosis?

How much calcium should Mrs. Oakland be consuming? What points would you be sure to include in counseling Mrs. Oakland about consuming adequate calcium? What sources would you recommend, and how many servings of each per day? How could she maximize her tolerance to milk?

What would you tell Mrs. Oakland about Dolomite? If she is unwilling to consume the high-calcium foods you recommended, what calcium supplement would you recommend? What instructions would you give her about when and how much to take?

REFERENCES

Abrams, S. and Stuff, J. (1994). Calcium metabolism in girls: Current dietary intakes lead to low rates of calcium absorption and retention during puberty. Am J Clin Nutr, 60, 739–743.

American Dietetic Association (1995). Position of the American Dietetic Association and the Canadian Dietetic Association: Women's health and nutrition. J Am Diet Assoc, 95(3), 362–366.

Auld, E., ed. (1994). Calcium: Make no bones about it. Food Insight, Sept/Oct, 1, 4.

Buchanan, H., Preston, S., Brooks, P. et al. (1991). Is diet important in rheumatoid arthritis? Br J Rheumatol, 30(2), 125–134.

Chapman, K., Chan, M., and Clark, C. (1995). Factors influencing dairy calcium intake in women. J Am Coll Nutr, 14, 336–340.

Chicago Dietetic Association and The South Suburban Dietetic Association (1992). Manual of Clinical Dietetics. 4th ed. Chicago: American Dietetics Association.

Dawson-Hughes, B., Harris, S., Krall, E., Dallal, G., Falconer, G., and Green, C. (1995). Rates of bone loss in postmenopausal women randomly assigned to one of two dosages of vitamin D. Am J Clin Nutr 61, 1140–1145.

Escott-Stump, S. (1992). Nutrition and Diagnosis-Related Care. 3rd ed. Philadelphia: Lea & Febiger.

Heaney, R. (1993). Protein intake and the calcium economy. J Am Diet Assoc, 93(11), 1259–1260.

Liebman, B. (1994a). Calcium: After the craze. Nutrition Action Health Letter, 21(5), 1, 5–7.

Liebman, B. (1994b). Just the calcium facts. Nutrition Action Health Letter, 21(5), 8–9.

McBean, L., Forgac, T., and Finn, S. (1994). Osteoporosis: Visions for care and prevention— A conference report. J Am Diet Assoc, 94(6), 668–671.

National Institutes of Health, Office of the Director (1994). NIH Consensus Statement. Optimal Calcium Intake. Vol 12, No. 4. Bethesda: USDHHS, Public Health Service.

Schardt, D. (1994). Take two walnuts. Nutrition Action Health Letter, 21(2), 8–9.

Scherer, J. and Timby, B. (1995). Introductory Medical-Surgical Nursing. 6th ed. Philadelphia: JB Lippincott.

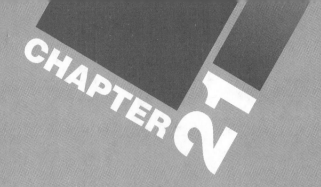

CHAPTER 21

Cancer and Immunodeficiency

Chapter Outline

Key Terms

Acute HIV infection
Anticipatory nausea and
   vomiting
Cachexia

Opportunistic infections
Persistent generalized
   lymphadenopathy (PGL)

Wasting syndrome

*T*he relationship between diet, nutritional status, and cancer is complex and multifaceted. Nutrition education in the well population should focus on cancer prevention. For clients who are being aggressively treated for cancer, diet intervention plays a vital role in maintaining nutritional status and optimizing the chance for successful cancer treatment; it also may decrease morbidity and mortality. Palliative nutritional support for the terminally ill may improve the quality of life and enhance the client's sense of well-being.

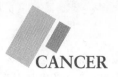

CANCER

Cancer, neoplasm, and malignant tumor are used interchangeably to describe a group of diseases characterized by the uncontrolled growth and spread of abnormal cells. Although the general course of the disease and its metabolic effects are predictable, cancer is not a single disease with one cause but represents a group of distinct diseases with different causes, manifestations, treatments, and prognoses. Because the chance of curing cancer lessens with each advancing stage ("staging" may classify cancer from stage 1 through stage 4, with ascending degrees of size, involvement, and metastasis), health teaching should emphasize prevention and early detection. General cancer assessment criteria, including cancer's seven warning signals, are also useful for screening and early detection (see display, General Cancer Assessment Criteria).

Cancer develops when an *initiating* event (eg, repeated or prolonged exposure to carcinogens or radiation) changes the deoxyribonucleic acid (DNA) structure, or reproductive code, of normal cells. Exactly why this change in normal cell structure occurs is not known. After a latent period of usually 5 to 30 years, a *promoting* event (eg, a favorable hormonal environment) transforms initiated cells into cancer cells, which autonomously proliferate, then infiltrate and destroy surrounding tissues. Eventually, cancer cells detach from the tumor mass and migrate, or are transported, to a distant site, where they lodge and grow (metastasize) in the new location to form a secondary tumor mass. Left unchecked, cancer ends in death.

Incidence and Etiology

Two out of every five Americans will develop cancer in their lifetime (Liebman, 1995). Cancer does not discriminate against age, sex, race, or any body organ.

ASSESSMENT CRITERIA

General Cancer Assessment Criteria

Weight, weight changes

Anorexia, nausea, vomiting

Seven warning signals:

- **C** hange in bowel or bladder habits
- **A** sore that does not heal
- **U** nusual bleeding or discharge
- **T** hickening or lump on the breast or elsewhere
- **I** ndigestion or difficulty swallowing
- **O** bvious change in the size or color of a wart or mole
- **N** agging cough or hoarseness

Today, 40% of Americans who get cancer will be alive 5 years after diagnosis; how-ever, in 1995, an estimated 547,00 people died from cancer. Cancer accounts for 20% of all deaths in the United States (American Cancer Society, 1995).

There is no single etiology of cancer in humans. External causes include chemi-cals, radiation, and viruses; hormones, immune conditions, and inherited mutations account for internal causes. Fortunately, many cancers are curable if detected early, and the risk of getting cancer can be greatly reduced by lifestyle changes. As many as 80% of all cases of cancer may be related to environmental causes, such as smoking, exposure to the sun, and diet, and thus may be preventable (Table 21-1). Numerous animal, clinical, and epidemiologic studies suggest that diet may cause or prevent the development of certain types of cancer; it is estimated that 30% to 35% of all can-cers may be diet-related and therefore potentially preventable by changes in eating habits (American Institute for Cancer Research, 1992).

DIETARY FACTORS

Food may contain carcinogens or procarcinogens that can be converted under the proper conditions to cancer-causing agents. Nitrates, nitrites, some naturally occur-ring compounds, and intentional and accidental additives all may be carcinogenic.

Table 21-1
Major and Lesser Cancer Risks

Major Factors	Risk	Risk Reduction
Tobacco	Causes approximately 30% of all cancer deaths, and 85% of all lung cancer deaths (leading cause of cancer death among men and women). Smokeless tobacco increases the risk of mouth and throat cancer.	Don't use tobacco in any form.
Sun	Accounts for 30% of all cancers and approximately 1%–2% of cancer deaths.	Limit exposure to the sun, especially between 10 AM and 3 PM. Wear protective clothing. Use a sunscreen with SPF of 15 or more.
Lesser Risks		
Occupational exposure to carcinogens	Accounts for 4% of all cancer deaths. Known car-cinogens include asbestos (risk potentiated by smoking), nickel, vinyl chloride, and chromate.	Find out if these hazards exist in your workplace. Wear recommended safety gear and follow precautions.
Radon	May contribute to 2%–3% of all cancer deaths (risk may be potentiated by smoking).	Test for radon in your home. If high, take neces-sary steps to reduce or correct problem.
Emissions and air pollution	Account for about 3% of all cancer deaths.	Use your car less. Keep your car well tuned.
Chemicals like dioxin	May be responsible for 1% or fewer cancer deaths.	Eat more fruits, vegetables, and fiber, which may be protective.
Medical x-rays	Account for 0.5% of all cancer deaths.	Avoid unnecessary x-rays. Wear a protective shield to cover other parts of the body, if possible.

Source: Everything Doesn't Cause Cancer. Washington, DC: American Institute for Cancer Research, 1992.

Aflatoxin B, a substance produced by mold that grows on improperly stored grains and nuts, has been implicated as the cause of liver cell cancer.

Other diet-related cancers may be due to nutritional excesses or deficiencies that alter the body's ability to defend against cancer (altered immunocompetence), or that may alter enzymes, gastrointestinal (GI) flora, and hormone levels to create an environment favorable to cancer promotion. Epidemiologic and animal studies indicate a strong correlation between high-fat diets and a high incidence of colon, breast, prostate, and ovarian cancers. High intakes of calories, cholesterol, and animal protein may also be involved in promoting some cancers.

Vitamin A, especially beta-carotene (the vegetable form of Vitamin A), helps to maintain the body's immune system and its ability to defend against cancer, and also may be protective against epithelial cancers. Vitamin C may decrease the risk of gastric and esophageal cancers. Fiber, folic acid, compounds found in cruciferous vegetables (eg, broccoli, cabbage, brussels sprouts), selenium, and other trace minerals are being investigated for their anticancer effects.

Current evidence suggests that the risk of cancer can be reduced by changing eating habits. A varied diet and moderation in all things seem prudent. Although they are not guaranteed to prevent cancer in all people, the American Cancer Society's Dietary Guidelines for reducing the risk of cancer appear in Table 21-2.

OTHER ETIOLOGIC FACTORS

In addition to environmental causes, genetic factors may be involved in cancer incidence; a familial tendency exists for breast, stomach, colon, ovarian, and lung cancers. For instance, new research has identified a gene that is responsible for familial breast cancer and genes that increase the susceptibility to colon cancer (American Cancer Society, 1995). Familially linked cancers appear to have a younger age of onset and an increased incidence of bilateral development.

Viral factors, such as Epstein-Barr virus, also have been linked to the development of certain cancers, such as Burkitt's lymphoma. Although evidence is lacking, viruses are suspected of being able to invade cells and alter their genetic code for reproduction.

Effect of Cancer and Cancer Treatments on Nutritional Status

Unless aggressive nutritional support is initiated early, cancer and its treatments can have profound and devastating effects on nutritional status, often resulting in cachexia and death.

LOCAL EFFECTS

Some cancers cause localized nutritional problems, depending on their site. For instance, cancers of the GI tract can cause partial or total obstruction at one or more sites; this obstruction may impair intake, digestion, and absorption (see display, Some Potential Local Effects of GI Cancers).

Table 21-2
Dietary Guidelines for Reducing the Risk of Cancer

Recommendation	Rationale
Avoid obesity.	Obesity is correlated to cancers of the breast and endometrium, possibly due to an alteration in hormone levels.
Cut fat intake to 30% of total calories or less.	High-fat diets generally are high-calorie diets, which increase the risk of obesity.
	A high-fat diet may promote colon cancer. Although the exact mechanism is unknown, fat may promote cancer by stimulating the secretion of bile acids into the intestines; bile acids and their byproducts are structurally similar to certain carcinogens.
	A high-fat diet may also promote breast, prostate, pancreatic, and ovarian cancer.
Eat more high-fiber foods.	Fiber may help protect against colon cancer, possibly by diluting the intestinal contents and decreasing transit time.
Include foods rich in vitamins A and C in your daily diet.	Vitamin A, or possibly beta-carotene, may reduce the risk of cancers of the lung, esophagus, larynx, and bladder, possibly through its function as an antioxidant.
	Vitamin C prevents nitrites from combining with amines to form nitrosamines, which are carcinogens that increase the risk of stomach, and esophageal cancers.
Include cruciferous (cabbage family) vegetables in your diet.	Cruciferous vegetables produce powerful enzymes in the liver, which may break down cancer-promoting chemicals. They may reduce the risk of cancers of the stomach, colon, rectum, and lung.
Cut down on salt-cured, smoked, and nitrite-cured foods.	Salt-cured, smoked, and nitrite-cured foods are considered cancer promoters, and they also tend to be high in fat.
Keep alcohol consumption moderate, if you do drink.	Heavy drinking increases the risk of breast and liver cancer; smoking and drinking greatly increases the risk of cancers of the mouth, larynx, throat, and esophagus.

SYSTEMIC EFFECTS: CANCER CACHEXIA

Cancer exerts systemic effects on metabolism, and these effects lead to nutritional problems of a pervasive nature. Although metastatic cancers may produce more pronounced changes, even cancers that are limited to one site can produce generalized effects. The result of these alterations—increased energy expenditure, increased protein catabolism and whole-body protein turnover (the reuse of amino acids that are generated by protein metabolism), increased lipolysis, and preferential use of fat as an energy source—is impaired nutritional status that contributes to cancer **cachexia.**

Cancer cachexia is a wasting syndrome that is characterized by early satiety, anorexia, severe weight loss, anemia, muscle weakness, loss of immunocompetence, and emaciation. It leads to a decreased sense of well-being and diminished quality of life, impaired wound healing, and increased risks of infection, morbidity, and mortality. Alterations in metabolism, fluid and electrolyte balance, enzyme and endocrine functions, and immune system integrity distinguish cancer cachexia from malnutrition related to other causes.

Some Potential Local Effects of GI Cancers

GI tract obstruction can produce

Weight loss related to poor intake

Fluid and electrolyte imbalance related to vomiting or diarrhea

Dysphagia, pain, and anemia can also occur

Malabsorption, resulting from

Blind loop syndrome secondary to partial obstruction of the upper small bowel leading to bacterial overgrowth, steatorrhea, and vitamin B_{12} deficiency

Fistulous bypass of the small bowel. The degree of malabsorption depends on the site and completeness of the fistula

Liver metastasis, resulting in an increase in serotonin, histamines, and other substances that promote periodic watery diarrhea

Protein-losing enteropathy secondary to obstruction and dilation of the lymphatics within the intestinal villi

Maldigestion secondary to decrease in pancreatic enzymes due to pancreatic cancer

Cachexia affects approximately two thirds of all cancer clients and is responsible for more deaths than cancer itself. Anorexia, altered metabolism, and increased nutrient losses can contribute to the development of cachexia; each of these factors can result from cancer or cancer treatments and may be multifactorial in origin (Fig. 21-1). Cachexia appears to be caused by changes that are induced by the tumor itself; removing the tumor can reverse the cachexia.

Neither the incidence nor the severity of cachexia can be related directly to calorie intake (cachexia can develop even if calorie intake is high), tumor weight, or tumor cell type. Cachexia has developed in clients whose tumors weighed less than 500 g. Cancers of the GI tract, pancreas, lung, and prostate, and some lymph node cancers are more likely to cause cachexia than breast cancer or sarcomas.

CANCER TREATMENTS

Cancer may be treated with chemotherapy, radiation, surgery, immunotherapy, or a combination of therapies. Some hematologic cancers are treated with bone marrow transplants. Each of these treatment modalities can cause significant nutritional problems related to systemic or localized side effects that interfere with intake, increase nutrient losses, or alter metabolism. Actual response to each of these therapies depends on the individual and the type, and extent of treatment.

Nutritional support that is used as an adjuvant to effective cancer therapy helps sustain the client through adverse side effects and reduces morbidity and mortality. Studies show that improved nutritional status can reverse weight loss, restore or maintain immunocompetence, help restore normal metabolism, enhance tolerance for antineoplastic therapy, maintain body composition during nutritional repletion, and reduce postoperative morbidity. However, for nutritional support to improve the results of cancer therapy, the therapy itself must have a reasonable chance of success. Evidence suggests that aggressive nutritional support may be of little value, or even detrimental, when it is used in conjunction with ineffective cancer treatment.

Oncology

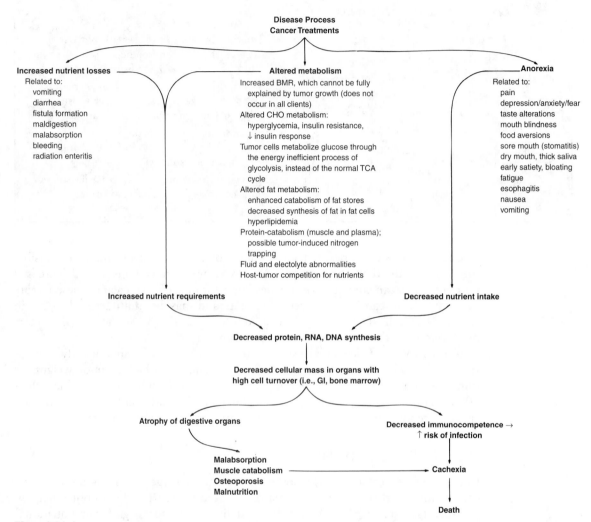

Figure 21-1
The causes of cachexia.

Chemotherapy

Chemotherapy damages the reproductive ability of both malignant and normal cells, especially rapidly dividing cells, such as well-nourished cancer cells and normal cells of the GI tract, respiratory system, bone marrow, skin, and gonadal tissue. Cyclical administration of multiple drugs is given in maximum tolerated doses.

The side effects of chemotherapy vary with the type of drug or combination of drugs used, dose, rate of excretion, duration of treatment, and individual tolerance. Generally, chemotherapy side effects are more widespread than those associated with other forms of treatment. The most frequent side effects are anorexia, nausea and vomiting, taste changes, sore mouth or throat, diarrhea, and constipation. Some combinations of chemotherapeutic drugs may produce severe and long-lasting GI complications. Table 21-3 lists side effects of various chemotherapeutic drugs.

Nausea and vomiting are considered by clients to be the the most distressing side effects of chemotherapy, and may affect 70% to 80% of those who do not receive antiemetics (Jenns, 1994). Acute nausea and vomiting can develop within 2 hours of drug administration and last up to 24 hours. Some drugs can produce delayed nausea and vomiting beyond the day of chemotherapy, which may last for 3 to 5 days

Table 21-3
Side Effects of Various Chemotherapeutic Drugs

	Anorexia	Nausea and Vomiting	Mucositis/Stomatitis	Diarrhea	Abdominal Pain	Nephrotoxic	Intestinal Ulceration	Constipation	Other
Asparaginase	√√	√√				√√			
Azacitidine	√√	√√		√√					
Bleomycin	√	√	√√						
Carmustine	√	√√				√			May cause glycosuria
Chlorambucil	√	√							
Cisplatin	√	√√				√√			May cause Mg⁺⁺ depletion
Cyclophosphamide	√	√√							
Cytarabine	√	√√	√						
Dacarbazine	√	√√		√					
Dactinomycin	√	√√	√	√					
Doxorubicin	√	√	√						
Etoposide									Oral dose may cause nausea and vomiting
Fluorouracil	√	√	√√	√√					
Hexamethylmelamine	√	√√							
Hydroxyurea	√	√	√						
Idarubicin	√	√	√						
Mercaptopurine	√	√√	√	√					
Methotrexate	√	√	√√	√√	√	√√	√		
Pentostatin	√	√√		√		√√			
Procarbazine	√	√√							
Streptozocin	√	√√					√		
Teniposide		√	√	√					
Taxol	√	√	√	√					
Vinblastine		√	√	√				√	
Vincristine					√			√√	

√ = low potential; √√ = moderate to high potential.

or even up to 3 weeks. Rarely, nausea and vomiting persist from one cycle of chemotherapy to the next (Jenns, 1994). Clients who experience poor control of emesis may suffer from **anticipatory nausea and vomiting**, defined as nausea and vomiting that occur prior to or during chemotherapy, at a time when symptoms would normally not be expected (Jenns, 1994). Dehydration, decreased renal elimination of drugs, malnutrition, esophageal tears, and aspiration pneumonia are potential consequences of vomiting. Nausea may persist even when vomiting is controlled, and can have a more devastating impact on quality of life than vomiting. Should the client refuse or postpone subsequent chemotherapy treatments because of nausea and vomiting, long-term survival may be affected.

Radiation

Radiation causes cell death as particles of radioactive energy break chemical bonds, disrupting reproductive ability. Although radiation injures all rapidly dividing cells, it is most lethal for the poorly differentiated and rapidly proliferating cells of cancer tissue. Recovery from sublethal doses of radiation occurs in the interval between the first dose and subsequent doses. Fortunately, normal tissue appears to recover more quickly from radiation damage than cancerous tissue.

Side effects are specific for the area irradiated, usually develop within 1 to 2 days after treatment is given, and may last for 2 weeks. The type and intensity of radiation side effects depend on the type of radiation used, the site, the volume of tissue irradiated, the dose of radiation, the duration of therapy, and individual tolerance. The rapidly growing cells of the GI mucosa, skin, and bone marrow are particularly vulnerable. General weakness, fatigue, and anorexia are frequent side effects, regardless of the site, amount, and duration of therapy. Radiation to the abdomen may produce acute side effects of nausea, vomiting, and diarrhea that resolve shortly after radiation is discontinued. However, delayed side effects can develop years after radiation is completed. Surgical and nutritional intervention may be required to alleviate progressive diarrhea, malabsorption, and malnutrition. Potential complications of radiation appear in Table 21-4.

Surgery

Surgery may be better tolerated (shorter postoperative hospital stay and fewer complications) by people who have good nutritional status before treatment. Postsurgical nutrition requirements increase for protein, calories, vitamin C, B vitamins, and iron to replenish losses and promote healing (see Chapter 15). Actual side effects incurred depend on the location and extent of surgery (Table 21-5).

Immunotherapy

Immunotherapy seeks to enhance the body's immune system to help control cancer. Products currently being studied for their effectiveness are interferon, interleukin-2, and tumor necrosis factor. Potential adverse effects include nausea and vomiting, diarrhea, anorexia, and fluid retention.

Table 21-4
Potential Complications of Radiation

Area	Potential Complications
Head and neck	Altered or loss of taste ("mouth blindness")
	Decreased salivary secretions → dry mouth
	Thick salivary secretions
	Difficulty swallowing and chewing
	Loss of teeth
Lower neck and midchest	Acute: esophagitis with dysphagia
	Delayed: fibrosis → esophageal stricture → difficulty swallowing
Abdomen and pelvis	Extensive radiation to the upper or mid-abdomen → nausea and vomiting
	Acute or chronic bowel damage → cramps, steatorrhea, malabsorption, disaccharidase deficiency, protein-losing enteropathy; bowel constriction, obstruction, or fistula formation
	Chronic blood loss from intestine and bladder
	Pelvic radiation → increased urinary frequency, urgency, and dysuria

Bone Marrow Transplants

Bone marrow transplants are used primarily to treat hematologic cancers and are used experimentally to treat solid tumors such as breast cancer. Bone marrow transplants are preceded by high-dose chemotherapy and total body irradiation; these are used to suppress immune function and destroy cancer cells. Nausea, vomiting, and diarrhea are frequent side effects, which may last 24 to 48 hours. Other complications include delayed mucositis, stomatitis, esophagitis, taste alterations, and intestinal damage that prevents oral intake; total parenteral nutrition (TPN) may be needed for 1 to 2 months after bone marrow transplants.

NURSING PROCESS

Assessment

In addition to general cancer assessment criteria (see display, General Cancer Assessment Criteria), assess for the following factors:

Physical:

Side effects that interfere with intake or metabolism, such as nausea, vomiting, anorexia, diarrhea, alterations in taste, dry or sore mouth, pain, fatigue, and so forth; onset, frequency, duration, severity, interventions attempted and results.

The client's emotional state and presence of outside support systems.

Weight changes. Severe weight loss, defined as a loss of 10% or more of body weight within 6 months, or an unintentional weight loss of 2 lbs per week, is associated with an increase in morbidity and mortality. Total parenteral nutrition may be used when weight loss exceeds 20% of body weight and progno-

Table 21-5
Potential Complications of Surgery

Type	Potential Complications
Head and neck resection	Difficulty chewing and swallowing Tube feeding dependency
Esophagectomy or esophageal resection	Early satiety Regurgitation Vagotomy → decreased stomach motility, decreased HCl production, diarrhea, steatorrhea
Gastrectomy	"Dumping syndrome": crampy diarrhea that develops quickly after eating accompanied by flushing, dizziness, weakness, pain, distention, and vomiting Hypoglycemia Malabsorption Achlorhydria Vitamin B_{12} malabsorption related to a lack of intrinsic factor
Removal of part of the small intestine	Early satiety
Jejunum	Malnutrition related to generalized malabsorption
Ileum	Vitamin B_{12} malabsorption Decreased absorption of bile salts → fat malabsorption and steatorrhea Fluid and electrolyte imbalance Diarrhea Hyperoxaluria → increased risk of renal oxalate stone formation and increased excretion of calcium Calcium and magnesium deficiency Malabsorption of fat-soluble vitamins
Massive bowel resection	Steatorrhea Malnutrition related to severe generalized malabsorption Metabolic acidosis Dehydration
Ileostomy or colostomy	Fluid and electrolyte imbalance Blind loop syndrome
Pancreatectomy	Generalized malabsorption Diabetes mellitus

sis is good. Loss of 30% of body weight usually is fatal. Note that fluid retention and dehydration can mask true weight status.

Signs of malnutrition, such as skin changes, edema, easy fatigability, and tissue wasting.

Intake and output, and observe for signs of fluid and electrolyte balance.

Presence of preexisting conditions that require diet intervention, such as endocrine, cardiac, renal, or liver disorders.

Biochemical:

Protein status, such as serum albumin, serum transferrin, thyroxine-bound prealbumin, and retinol-binding protein; nitrogen balance; creatinine–height index, if available.

Other abnormal laboratory values. Keep in mind that cancer and cancer therapies can cause low values for hemoglobin, hematocrit, and total lymphocyte count; therefore they are not valid indicators of poor nutritional status in cancer clients.

Dietary:

Adequacy of usual intake.

Dietary changes made in response to symptoms or side effects of cancer or cancer treatment (ie, foods avoided, foods preferred). Determine which foods are best and least tolerated.

The use of unorthodox products, diets, or supplements with unproven nutritional benefits.

Nursing Diagnosis

Altered Nutrition: Less than body requirements, related to anorexia, dysphagia, and nausea secondary to cancer/cancer therapy

Planning and Implementation

Malnutrition and cachexia are not inevitable results of cancer and cancer therapy; they may be prevented by early and aggressive nutritional support (complete or supplemental enteral or parenteral nutrition). The increased risks of morbidity and mortality associated with cachexia make preventive nutrition intervention imperative; early and ongoing nutritional assessment, planning, implementation, and evaluation are vital.

Used as an adjunct to cancer treatment, aggressive nutritional support can improve cachexia and reduce morbidity and mortality by stimulating weight gain, reversing negative nitrogen balance, improving immunocompetence, and increasing the sense of well-being. However, it is likely that some characteristics of cachexia are not caused simply by an inadequate intake; therefore, it is possible that some cachectic clients may not respond to aggressive nutritional support.

In clients whose prognosis is terminal, the value of nutritional support is a controversial ethical issue. No benefit is derived from "force-feeding" a client whose cancer is not being treated, because both body weight gain and tumor growth are stimulated. Instead, enteral nutrition should be maintained as an integral component of palliative care with the goals of providing comfort and improving the quality of life. See display, Eight Golden Rules for Nutrition Care of the Terminally Ill.

An overall goal of diet intervention for all cancer clients is to keep the client out of the hospital whenever possible. Specifically, nutrition support should seek to attain and maintain desirable weight; identify, prevent, or correct nutritional deficiencies; and enhance the quality of life. Because cachexia is easier to prevent than to treat, nutritional support should be initiated before the downhill spiral of malnutrition develops.

For clients with cancer, nutritional needs increase as appetite decreases. However, because a "typical" cancer client does not exist, the diet must be individualized and continually evaluated and revised according to the client's needs and ability to eat. Diet management objectives and interventions are based on the client's treatment

Eight Golden Rules for Nutrition Care of the Terminally Ill

Success of the medical treatment for controlling pain, constipation, and troublesome secondary effects of the narcotic analgesics such as nausea, vomiting, and heartburn.

Respect for the patient's wishes concerning the level of nutrition support desired at the various stages of illness, and their goals for treatment.

Success of the systematic and intensive mouth care for controlling dryness of the mouth and thirst.

Respect for personal tastes and eating habits of the patient.

Respect for conviviality—the importance of the meal environment and the meal distribution.

Appropriate texture of the food offered.

Attractive presentation of the meals.

Cooperation of an informed medical and nursing staff.

Feuz, A. and Rapin, C. (1994). An observational study of the role of pain control and food adaptation of elderly patients with terminal cancer. © The American Dietetic Association. Reprinted by permission from J Am Diet Assoc, 94(7), 770.

goals; diet for clients who are receiving aggressive treatment to arrest or cure the disease differs from diet for clients who are receiving palliative care for comfort and improved quality of life.

If the client has, or is at risk for, nausea and vomiting related to chemotherapy, administer antiemetics as necessary at least an hour before chemotherapy begins. To help avoid nausea, advise the client to take antiemetics as prescribed for 72 hours, even when symptoms are absent. Highly seasoned foods, fatty foods, and caffeine should be avoided 24 hours before and 72 hours after chemotherapy.

Nutritional support is one area of treatment in which the client can be an active participant. The client and health care team may "contract" for an acceptable amount of weight loss. As long as the client does not lose more weight than was agreed on, the client is in charge of his own nutritional care.

It is more effective and practical to teach the client how to increase the nutrient density of his diet (increase the protein and calorie content of his diet without increasing the volume of food eaten) and alleviate eating problems than it is to provide a therapeutic diet that specifies exact amounts and rigid guidelines.

Loss of dignity and control, change in sexuality and body image, and loss of appetite can create a frustrating, seemingly hopeless situation for the client, and food may be used to express anger and frustration. Allow the client and family to verbalize feelings, and emphasize a positive, supportive, team-effort approach. The client's rights and preferences should be respected at all times.

Although the client may need the encouragement and support of family and friends, putting them in a position of "force-feeding" the client may add tension to an already stressful situation.

Decreased intake and increased requirements may necessitate the use of multivitamin and mineral supplements.

CLIENT GOALS

Clients who are receiving aggressive nutritional support will

Modify the diet as needed to lessen the side effects of cancer and cancer therapies.
Consume adequate calories and protein to prevent or correct significant weight loss and prevent or correct nutritional deficiencies.
Describe the principles and rationale of diet management during aggressive cancer treatment and nutritional support.

Clients who are receiving palliative nutritional support will

Maintain activity level, if possible.
Modify the diet as needed to lessen cancer side effects.

NURSING INTERVENTIONS

Diet Management

Aggressive nutritional support

Increase protein intake to 1.5 to 2.0 g/kg to prevent body protein catabolism.
Increase calorie intake to meet increased metabolic demands and to replace nutritional losses related to cancer or its treatment. At least 25 to 35 cal/kg are needed to maintain weight and 40 to 50 cal/kg are required to replenish body stores (see display, Ways to Increase Nutrient Density With Protein and Calories).
Modify the diet as needed to alleviate problems that interfere with appetite and intake (Table 21-6; see Chapter 16 for diet recommendations, nursing considerations, and client teaching for general GI problems such as nausea, vomiting, diarrhea, constipation, esophagitis and heartburn, malabsorption, and lactose intolerance).
Clients who are receiving chemotherapy, especially those with low platelet counts, may be advised to avoid fresh vegetables, nuts, and other difficult-to-digest foods that can injure the GI tract.
Encourage small, frequent meals and snacks to help maximize intake.
If oral intake is inadequate or contraindicated, use enteral tube feedings or TPN as a supplemental or complete feeding (see Chapter 14).

Palliative nutritional support

Encourage eating as a source of pleasure. The client's requests and preferences are more important than the nutritional quality of the diet.
Modify the diet as needed to alleviate problems that interfere with appetite and intake (see Table 21-6; see Chapter 16 for diet recommendations and nursing considerations for general GI problems). Modify the texture, as needed, to facilitate swallowing in clients with weakness, dry mouth, or stomatitis.
Use tube feedings only if the client is unable to eat; TPN rarely is indicated.

(Text continues on page 707)

Ways to Increase Nutrient Density With Protein and Calories

Skim milk powder
    Add to milk and milk-based drinks for a fortified beverage.
    Use on hot or cold cereals.
    Add to scrambled eggs, soups, gravies, casseroles, desserts, and baked products.

Milk
    Substitute milk, evaporated milk, or heavy cream for water in recipes.
    Dip meat, poultry, and fish in eggs or milk and coat with bread or cereal crumbs before baking, broiling, or pan frying.
    Choose desserts made with eggs or milk: sponge cake, angel food cake, custard, puddings.

Cheese
    Add grated or cubed cheese, or diced or ground meats, fish, or poultry to soups, omelets, casseroles, vegetable dishes, and sauces.
    Melt on sandwiches, bread, muffins, rice, meats, vegetables, and eggs.

Cream cheese
    Mix with butter and spread on hot bread, rolls, biscuits, and muffins.
    Add to vegetables.

Peanut butter
    Use as a spread on slices of apple, banana, pears, crackers, and waffles.
    Stuff celery with it.
    Combine with cream cheese and use as a sandwich filling.
    Add to milk drinks and milk shakes.
    Blend into soft ice cream or yogurt.

Eggs
    Add chopped, hard-cooked eggs to salads and dressings, vegetables, casseroles, and creamed meats.
    Beat eggs into mashed potatoes, vegetable purees, and sauces.
    Add extra egg yolks to quiches, scrambles, custards, puddings, pancakes, French toast batter, and milkshakes.

    Dip meat, fish, and poultry into eggs and coat with bread or cereal crumbs before baking, broiling, or pan frying.

Butter
    Whenever possible, add butter to hot foods: bread, rolls, pancakes, waffles, soups, vegetables, potatoes, cooked cereal, rice, pasta.

Mayonnaise
    Use in place of salad dressing in salads, eggs, casseroles, sandwiches.

Honey
    Use on toast and cereal.
    Add to coffee and tea.

Sour cream or yogurt
    Sweeten with sugar or honey and use as a sauce for desserts and fruit.
    Use as a sauce on vegetables.
    Use in gravies and dips.

Nuts, seeds, and wheat germ
    Sprinkle on fruit, cereal, ice cream, yogurt, vegetables, salads, and toast.
    Use in place of bread crumbs.
    Add to casseroles, breads, muffins, pancakes, cookies, and waffles.

Whipped cream
    Use as a topping on hot chocolate, pies, fruit, pudding, gelatin, ice cream, and other desserts.
    Add to coffee and tea.

Marshmallows
    Use in hot chocolate, on fruit, and in desserts.

Food preparation
    Bread meat and vegetables before cooking.
    Sauté and fry foods when possible to add more calories.
    Add sauces or gravies.

Snack frequently on nuts, dried fruit, candy, buttered popcorn, cheese and crackers, granola, ice cream.

(United States Department of Health and Human Services: Eating Hints, Tips and Recipes for Better Nutrition During Cancer Treatment. NIH Publication No. 91-2079. Washington, DC: Government Printing Office, revised April 1990)

Table 21-6

Nursing Interventions and Considerations for Problems That Interfere with Appetite and Intake

Potential Problem	Nursing Interventions and Considerations
Anorexia (total lack of appetite)	Anorexia may be continuous or sporadic.
	Encourage the client to overeat during "good" days and to eat whenever hungry.
	Provide small frequent meals seasoned according to individual taste. Snacks of nutrient-dense liquids (instant breakfast, milk shakes, commercial supplements) can provide significant amounts of protein and calories, are easily consumed, and tend to leave the stomach quickly.
	The appearance and aroma of food are more important when appetite is lacking. Attractive food, a bright, cheerful environment, soft music, and company can help make eating a pleasant experience.
	Clients with anorexia should not be expected to order food for the following day. If possible, allow spontaneous meal selections and honor day-to-day requests.
	Provide emotional support and encouragement to the client and family.
	Encourage the family to bring food from home.
	Appetite is often best in the morning and deteriorates gradually throughout the day. Encourage a high-protein, high-calorie, nutrient-dense breakfast.
	Use appropriate medications to control pain, nausea, and depression. If tolerated, a small amount of alcohol before mealtime may stimulate appetite.
Nausea	Provide small, frequent meals; provide liquids between meals to avoid bloating at mealtime.
	Foods served cold or at room temperature may be better tolerated; hot foods may contribute to nausea.
	Try high-carbohydrate, low-fat foods, like toast, crackers, yogurt, sherbet, cooked cereal, soft or canned fruits, watermelon, banana, fruit juices, and angel food cake.
	Advise the client to avoid foods that are fatty, greasy, fried, or strongly seasoned.
	Encourage the client to keep track of foods that cause nausea so that they can be avoided.
	Advise the client to avoid eating 1–2 hours before chemotherapy or radiotherapy to decrease the likelihood of nausea.
	Request an antiemetic be ordered to control nausea.
Pain	Administer analgesics or appropriate pain medication prior to mealtime.
	Relaxation techniques, distraction, and biofeedback may help control pain.
Depression/anxiety/fear	Provide emotional support and give the client a reason to eat: tolerance to treatments and the effectiveness of therapy may be increased if nutritional status is maintained.
	Use appropriate medications to control depression and anxiety.
Taste alterations	Taste changes may be due to cancer or cancer treatments. Radiation-induced taste alterations usually develop by the 3rd week of therapy and return to normal within 1 year.
	Clients who experience taste changes are more likely to lose weight. Conversely, clients who lose weight may be more likely to develop taste alterations.
	Elemental zinc has been shown to correct taste abnormalities. If prescribed, zinc should be taken with food or milk to decrease the risk of GI irritation.
	Clients may experience a decreased threshold for urea (bitter), increased threshold for sucrose (sweet), or both.
	Chemotherapy may cause a metallic taste. Clients who complain of a bitter taste while receiving chemotherapy should be advised to suck on hard candy during therapy. Use plastic utensils and dishes. Tart foods like citrus juices, cranberry juice, pickles, or relish may help overcome metallic taste.
	Encourage good oral hygiene before eating to eliminate unpleasant tastes.
	Encourage the client to experiment with a variety of seasonings, especially if oral mucosa is not impaired.

(continued)

Table 21-6 (Continued)

Nursing Interventions and Considerations for Problems That Interfere with Appetite and Intake

Potential Problem	Nursing Interventions and Considerations
Taste alterations (continued)	Advise the client to avoid anything that tastes unpleasant.
	Reassure the client that taste changes are not uncommon and encourage him or her to verbalize feelings.
Decreased threshold for urea → bitter taste	Red meats, particularly beef and pork, are frequently said to have a "bad," "rotten," or fecal taste. Aversions may also include poultry, fish, coffee, and chocolate.
	Meats may be better tolerated if served cold or at room temperature, or if highly flavored with strong seasonings, sweet marinades, or sauces.
	Assure the client that red meat is not essential in the diet. Encourage the intake of other high-protein foods, such as eggs, cheese, mild fish, nuts, and dried peas and beans. If those sources are not tolerated, milk shakes, eggnogs, puddings, ice cream, and commercial supplements can provide sufficient protein and calories.
Increased threshold for sucrose	Season foods according to individual taste.
Lack of taste (mouth blindness)	Appearance and aroma become more important when taste is absent: Serve attractively presented, steaming food in a bright, cheerful environment.
Food aversions	Food aversions may be intermittent or may worsen as the day progresses.
	To avoid learned aversions, instruct the client to avoid his or her favorite foods or fast completely before receiving radiation or chemotherapy. If nausea and vomiting tend to occur around the same time each day, withholding food beforehand may help avoid learned aversions.
Sore mouth (stomatitis)	Good oral hygiene (thorough cleaning with a soft bristle tooth brush or cotton swabs plus frequent mouth rinses with normal saline and water or baking soda and water) may help prevent or minimize stomatitis. Commercial mouthwashes containing alcohol may burn the oral mucosa.
	Stomatitis may produce taste alterations, mouth blindness, or the association between eating and pain. Topical anesthetics may help relieve discomfort.
	Cut food into small portions.
	Clients with stomatitis are more susceptible to *Candida albicans* infections, which may cause ulcerated white or yellow patches on the oral mucosa and further diminish taste sensation.
	Instruct the client to avoid spices, acidic foods, coarse foods, alcohol, and smoking, which can aggravate an already irritated oral mucosa.
	Encourage the client to eat a soft or liquid bland diet, drink plenty of fluids, and avoid hot food and beverages. Cold items may help numb the oral mucosa. Try bananas, applesauce, canned fruit, watermelon, cottage cheese, yogurt, mashed potatoes, macaroni and cheese, custards, pudding, scrambled eggs, cooked cereals, and liquids.
	Straws may ease swallowing.
	Caution the client against wearing ill-fitting dentures.
Dry mouth/thick saliva	Clients with decreased saliva production are susceptible to dental caries. Encourage good oral hygiene, frequent mouth rinsing, and the avoidance of concentrated sweets.
	Artificial saliva and the use of straws may facilitate swallowing. Petroleum jelly applied to the lips may help prevent drying.
	Provide mouth care immediately before mealtime for added moisture.
	Advise the client to avoid dry coarse foods, and to use gravies, sauces, and sugar-free jellies liberally. Some clients may require a liquid diet.
	Offer high-calorie liquids in between meals.
	Encourage the client to use ice chips and sugar-free hard candies and gum between meals to relieve dryness.

(continued)

Table 21-6 (Continued)
Nursing Interventions and Considerations for Problems That Interfere with Appetite and Intake

Potential Problem	Nursing Interventions and Considerations

Early satiety/bloating	Instruct the client to avoid
	    High-fat foods (gravies, rich sauces, greasy foods, excessive butter)
	    Gas-forming foods such as onions, garlic, and vegetables in the cabbage family
	    Liquids with meals
	    Empty-calorie foods and beverages
	Encourage the client to chew foods thoroughly and to eat small frequent meals.
	Recommend moderate exercise before and after eating.

Fatigue	Encourage the client to rest before meals. Position the client so that all food and utensils are within easy reach. Provide easy-to-eat foods that can be prepared with a minimal amount of effort. Commercial prepared oral supplements, like Ensure and Sustacal, may boost protein and calorie intake with a minimum of effort. Enlist the help of family and friends to help with meal preparation at home. Encourage the use of convenience foods and labor-saving appliances (blender, crock-pot, toaster oven, microwave oven, dishwasher). Assistance may be available from Meals On Wheels or other community services. Encourage a good breakfast, since fatigue may worsen as the day progresses.
Hiccups	If hiccups cannot be managed medically, provide small, frequent meals when the client is hiccup-free.

Client Teaching

Instruct the client and family

That an adequate nutritional status reduces the side effects of treatment, may make cancer cells more receptive to treatment, improves quality of life, and may increase survival rate. Poor nutritional status may potentiate chemotherapeutic drug toxicity.

That the client is in charge of his or her nutritional care.

To view food as a medicine, rather than a social pleasure, that must be "taken" even when the desire to eat is lacking.

To eat frequently and as much as possible, unless the client is nauseated.

On how to add protein and calories to his or her diet to increase the nutrient density (see display, Ways to Increase Nutrient Density With Protein and Calories).

On how to alleviate eating problems that may develop from the disease process or cancer treatments (see Table 21-6).

That it is necessary to drink ample fluids 1 to 2 days before and after chemotherapy to enhance excretion of the drugs and to decrease the risk of renal toxicity.

That no diets or nutritional supplements can cure cancer and that starving the tumor will also starve the body.

Monitoring Progress

Monitor for the following signs or symptoms:

Tolerance to oral feedings (ie, absence of mouth pain; ability to swallow; absence of nausea, vomiting, and indigestion).

Compliance with the diet and the need for follow-up diet counseling.

Effectiveness of the diet, and evaluate the need for further diet modification.

Weight and weight changes, as appropriate. Unless weight status is needed to adjust drug doses, continued weight loss in a terminal client need not be monitored.

The development of complications related to disease progression or side effects of cancer therapy.

Protein status, when available.

Evaluation

Evaluation is ongoing. Provided that the plan of care has not changed, the client will achieve the goals as stated above.

NUTRITION AND IMMUNODEFICIENCY

Nutritional status and immunity are interrelated. People with impaired nutritional status have suboptimal immunity, which may lead to infection, and further deterioration in both nutritional status and immunity (Timbo and Tollefson, 1994). Although the relationship between malnutrition and the progression of human immunodeficiency virus (HIV) disease is not clearly understood, malnutrition appears to hasten the progression of HIV to acquired immunodeficiency syndrome (AIDS). (See Food for Thought: Nutritional Immunology: Looking for the Magic Bullet.)

ACQUIRED IMMUNODEFICIENCY SYNDROME (AIDS)

AIDS is an end-stage immune disorder that is caused by an infection with the retrovirus known as HIV. HIV is transmitted through the direct exchange of infected body fluids from one person to another, such as through sexual intercourse and use of contaminated needles or blood products, and from mother to infant during pregnancy, delivery, or lactation.

Once in the body, the virus attaches itself to cells that have a specific protein on their cell membranes, called CD4 surface markers. T4 lymphocytes have CD4 surface markers and are targeted by the virus. The virus' genetic material becomes permanently incorporated into the T4 lymphocytes, rendering them incapable of normal immune function, but able to replicate HIV. Eventually, T4 lymphocytes are

FOOD *for* THOUGHT

Nutritional Immunology: Looking for the Magic Bullet

Clearly, nutrition plays a role in immune function. Studies have shown that simple protein–calorie malnutrition negatively affects immune function by impairing the effectiveness of phagocytes, reducing the number and function of T lymphocytes, and decreasing the production of antibodies.

Nutritional immunology has been an area of accelerated research within the last decade, especially since the discovery of HIV. Human and animal studies have shown that abnormalities in the immune system can be improved by adjusting specific types of micro- and macro-nutrients in the diet (Timbo and Tollefson, 1994). Although advances are being made, there is still much to be learned. Future research will likely focus on specialized formulas and specific immunotherapy for defined groups of clients. Futuristic "magic bullets" may include:

Specific amino acids. In animal and human studies, the amino acid arginine has been shown to stimulate cell-mediated immune response, and in animals, protect against bacterial challenges. Arginine appears to have a direct stimulatory effect on the number of T lymphocytes and natural killer cells (Timbo and Tollefson, 1994). Clinical studies have shown improved immune function in cancer clients who are fed arginine, leading some researchers to recommend that arginine comprise 25% of the total protein content of enteral and parenteral formulas, instead of the current level of 5%.

Glutamine has been shown to be beneficial for gut function and intestinal mucosal integrity. It is also an important substrate for rapidly proliferating cells, including lymphocytes. Enteral gluta-mine has been shown to preserve and improve muscle cellularity in the small bowel, which may prevent the translocation of gut bacteria into the lymph nodes, other organs, and the bloodstream.

Nucleotides. Dietary sources of preformed purines and pyrimidines seem to be important for optimal cellular immune response, probably because they are necessary for the development and activation of T cells. Because lymphoid cells have a limited capacity to synthesize nucleotides, dietary sources of purines and pyrimides are essential (Rudolph et al, 1994). Defined formulas for enteral and parenteral formulas should contain preformed nucleotides.

Lipids. Large megadoses of saturated fatty acids have been found to inhibit in vivo antibody responses to certain antigens (Timbo and Tollefson, 1994). Omega-3 fatty acids have been shown to improve immune function, probably through an alteration of prostaglandin synthesis or by changes in the phospholipid content of cell membranes.

Micronutrients. Some studies have shown that supplements of beta-carotene increase natural killer cells and have a positive effect on certain immune cells (Jacobson, 1993). Large doses of vitamin E may also boost immunity. Conversely, decreased immunity and increased infection are associated with iron deficiency anemia. Zinc deficiency also appears to impair immune response that is reversed when adequate zinc is provided. However, large amounts of zinc, as well as megadoses of iron, vitamin A, and selenium, impair immune system function and can increase the risk of infection. Exact amounts and proportions have yet to be determined.

destroyed and depleted, leading to immunodeficiency and **opportunistic infections** (infections caused by microorganisms found in the environment that normally do not cause infection) and malignancies. Another cardinal feature and defining criterion of AIDS is the **wasting syndrome**, which is characterized by the loss of 10% or more of usual body weight.

The clinical course of HIV disease may begin with an acute illness, followed by an asymptomatic period, which progresses to advanced immunodeficiency with opportunistic disease. Clinically, HIV progresses as CD4 cell count decreases (Table 21-7). The rate at which HIV progresses to AIDS varies with age and how HIV was acquired (Chaussin in Mandell et al, 1995). Some studies estimate that HIV infection takes 6.5 to 13 years to progress to AIDS, with an average of 8 to 9 years. Not all clients follow this pattern; some may appear asymptomatic for years; others progress very rapidly.

Acute HIV infection is characterized by a mononucleosislike illness with variable and nonspecific symptoms. Fever, lymphadenopathy, night sweats, muscle pain, rash, malaise, lethargy, sore throat, anorexia, nausea, vomiting, diarrhea, and headache may occur (Chamberlain in Mandell et al, 1995). Fifty to seventy percent or more of people who are infected with HIV experience an acute illness, which typically occurs 2 to 4 weeks after exposure and lasts 1 to 2 weeks. A relatively asymptomatic period follows, during which nonspecific symptoms may persist: fatigue, seborrhea, eczema, intermittent fever, diarrhea, muscle pain, night sweats, weight loss, oral candidiasis, herpes zoster, and other non–life-threatening opportunistic infections. After becoming antibody-positive, many infected individuals develop **persistent generalized lymphadenopathy (PGL)**, characterized by enlarged lymph glands at two or more extrainguinal sites. Symptoms of PGL vary in intensity among individuals, but become more numerous and severe with time.

HIV has progressed to AIDS when the CD4 cell count is 200 cells/mm³ or less, and opportunistic infections occur. Symptoms of AIDS include fever, unproductive cough, malaise, shortness of breath, significant weight loss, anorexia, and diarrhea. Kaposi's sarcoma (cancer of the connective tissues that support blood vessels) and T-cell lymphoma of the skin are common malignancies. *Pneumocystis carinii* pneumonia, HIV wasting syndrome, and candidiasis of the esophagus are the most common frequent indicators of AIDS (Mandell et al, 1995). Gynecologic problems are common, and cognitive, motor, and visual impairments may occur. Various opportunistic infections and their symptoms appear in the display, Some Common Opportunistic Infections and Their Symptoms. AIDS ultimately ends in death.

Table 21-7
Clinical Stages of HIV Infection

CD4 Cell Count	Stage	Comment
>500	Early	Risk of disease low. Response to routine immunizations and PPD skin testing reliable.
200–500	Middle	Risk of minor signs and symptoms high; risk of opportunistic disease moderate. May benefit from antiretroviral therapy.
50–200	Late	Risk of opportunistic disease high. Benefit from *Pneumocystis* prophylaxis and antiretroviral therapy.
<50	Advanced	Risk of opportunistic disease and death high. Benefit from *Pneumocystis, Mycobacterium avium* complex, and fungal prophylaxis. May benefit from antiretroviral therapy.

Some Common Opportunistic Infections and Their Symptoms

BACTERIAL INFECTIONS

Mycobacterium avium-intracellulare (MAI)
Disseminated infection; fever, severe weight loss, abdominal pain, diarrhea, malabsorption

Mycobacterium tuberculosis
Pneumonia, cerebral tuberculosis

Enteric infections:
Salmonella
Diarrhea and nonspecific symptoms such as fever, anorexia, fatigue, weight loss, malaise
Shigella
Severe diarrhea with fever
Campylobacter
Diarrhea that is frequently bloody, abdominal cramping, fever

FUNGAL INFECTIONS

Candida albicans
Oral (thrush)
Anorexia, thick coating on the mouth and tongue, mouth pain, taste alterations
Esophageal
Burning pain, difficulty swallowing
Proctal
Rectal pain, weeping lesions

Cryptococcus neoformans
Major cause of meningitis in HIV disease; low-grade fever, severe headache, stiff neck, double vision, nausea and vomiting

May also cause local organ dysfunction and disseminated disease

Histoplasma capsulatum
Fever, weight loss, meningitis

PROTOZAN INFECTIONS

Cryptosporidium enteritis
Bowel is the major target; severe, protracted, watery diarrhea; weight loss, electrolyte imbalances, abdominal cramps, nausea and vomiting, fever. Lactose intolerance and malabsorption may occur

Pneumocystis carinii pneumonia (PCP)
Fever, cough, chest pain, dyspnea, fatigue, weight loss, weakness

Taxoplasma gondii
Persistent headache, fever, seizures, altered consciousness, encephalitis, retinitis, enteritis

VIRAL INFECTIONS

Cytomegalovirus (CMV)
Blindness or retinitis
GI involvement may produce stomatitis, esophagitis, gastritis, colitis
CNS involvement may cause encephalitis
Pulmonary involvement may cause pneumonitis

Herpes simplex
Painful oral, genital, or perianal lesions

Herpes zoster (shingles)
Skin lesions

The Centers for Disease Control and Prevention estimates that approximately one million Americans, or one in every 250 people, are infected with HIV (ADA, 1994). In 1990, HIV infection was the tenth leading cause of death for Americans of all ages; by the year 2000, AIDS is expected to rank third. Although homosexual and bisexual men constitute a major portion of HIV infections, trends indicate that the rate of HIV infection is growing in women, adolescents, children, intravenous drug users, the incarcerated, and the poor and homeless (ADA, 1994).

As yet, there is no cure for AIDS. Treatment focuses on forestalling the onset of AIDS symptoms, preserving independence, and maintaining quality of life. Drugs are used to inhibit HIV replication and prevent and treat infection (see Drug Alert).

DRUG
ALERT

HIV Drugs

Multiple drug regimens are often used not only to inhibit HIV replication, but also to prevent or treat opportunistic infections. Some commonly used medications, their uses, and possible adverse effects include:

Drug	Use	Possible Effects
Zidovudine (Retrovir, commonly known as ZDV or AZT)	Inhibits HIV replication	Nausea and vomiting; taste changes; decrease in serum B_{12}, zinc, and copper Absorption is decreased and delayed with high-fat meals
Zalcitabine (Hivid, also known as ddC)	Inhibits HIV replication	Nausea and vomiting, diarrhea, pancreatitis, esophageal ulcers
Didanosine (Videx, commonly known as ddI)	Inhibits HIV replication	Pancreatitis, hypokalemia, hypocalcemia, hypomagnesemia, mouth sores Needs basic stomach for absorption; buffer is added, which may cause diarrhea
Sulfamethoxazole-trimethoprim (TMP/SMX) (Bactrim)	*Pneumocystis carnii* pneumonia (PCP), *Taxoplasma gondii*	Nausea and vomiting, anorexia, pruritus, rash, epigastric pain, glossitis, stomatitis, hyponatremia
Dapsone	With sulfamethoxazole for PCP	Nausea, rash, altered taste, dizziness
Isoniazid (INH)	*M. tuberculosis*	B_6 and niacin deficiency, impaired calcium absorption, epigastric pain
Rifampin (Rifadin)	*M. tuberculosis*	Nausea and vomiting, anorexia, diarrhea, heartburn, impaired calcium absorption
Rifabutin (Mycobutin)	*Mycobacterium avium* complex	Nausea, flatulence, rash
Fluconazole (Diflucan)	*Candida* *Cryptococcus neoformans*	Nausea and vomiting, diarrhea
Ketoconazole (Nizoral)	*Candida*	Nausea, anorexia, requires gastric acidity for absorption
Acyclovir (Zovirax)	*Herpes simplex* *Herpes zoster*	Nausea and vomiting (rarely), diarrhea
Famciclovir (Famvir)	Acute *Herpes zoster*	Headache, nausea, diarrhea, fatigue

Source: Anastasi, J. and Rivera, J. (1994). Understanding prophylactic therapy for HIV infections. AJN 94(2), 36–41, and Centers for Disease Control and Prevention: "USPHS/ IDSA Guidelines for the Prevention of Opportunistic Infections in persons infected with Human Immunodeficiency Virus: A summary . . . Morbidity and Mortality Weekly Report, 44(RR-8):24–25, July 1995.

Chemotherapeutic drugs may be used to combat any malignancies that develop (see Table 21-3). Improved treatment methods have greatly prolonged survival, which has led to the view that HIV is a chronic process (Gorbach et al, 1993).

Effect of HIV and AIDS on Nutritional Status

HIV has a devastating impact on nutritional status. Opportunistic infections, malignancies, and therapies can produce a progressive and profound loss of 30% to 50% of preillness weight (Gorbach et al, 1993). Even in clients who do not appear malnourished, lean body mass is often decreased (Risser et al, 1995). Appetite and intake are often significantly impaired. It is estimated that malnutrition occurs in 80% or more of people with HIV or AIDS; malnourished clients may progress to AIDS more quickly than their well-nourished counterparts because malnutrition may potentiate immunosuppression related to AIDS (Cameron, 1994). Clearly, malnutrition itself, without HIV infection, impairs immune system function and the ability to fight infection; conversely, infection increases the risk for malnutrition.

Like cancer cachexia, the cause of malnutrition in AIDS is multifactorial; inadequate intake, malabsorption, and altered metabolism may be contributing factors (Table 21-8). In the early stages of HIV, subclinical signs of malnutrition may exist,

Table 21-8
Possible Causes of Malnutrition in HIV/AIDS

Inadequate intake related to:
 Infections
 Fever
 Fatigue
 Mouth ulcers
 Depression, fear, anxiety
 Nausea and vomiting
 Drug therapy
 Difficulty swallowing
 Dry mouth
 AIDS dementia complex
 Impaired taste
 Esophageal ulcerations or obstructions
 Shortness of breath; difficulty breathing
Malabsorption related to:
 AIDS enteropathy (diarrhea caused by no diagnosable pathogen)
 Intestinal infections that alter GI integrity
 Drug therapy; long-term use of antibiotics
 Low serum albumin
 GI malignancies
Altered metabolism related to:
 Fever
 Drug therapy
 Infections
 Cancer

but are frequently overlooked. Deficiencies in vitamins A, B_6, B_{12}, E, and B_2, copper, selenium, and zinc have been reported in asymptomatic clients, as well as a decline in body cell mass (Anastasi and Sun Lee, 1994). As the process advances, the cumulative effect of more numerous and severe infections, combined with unmet nutritional needs, promotes the downward spiral of wasting, with a disproportionate loss of lean body mass to fat. The amount of wasting, rather than the specific cause of weight loss, has been shown to be the primary determinant of death in AIDS (Luder et al, 1995). However, weight loss and malnutrition are not inevitable consequences of HIV; some studies suggest that early nutrition intervention in clients with HIV infection can favorably influence both nutritional and clinical outcomes, even though it cannot stop the progression of AIDS (Chlebowski et al, 1995). At the very least, nutrition intervention can help improve quality of life (eg, minimizing diarrhea, maintaining weight).

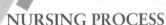

NURSING PROCESS

Assessment

In addition to the general HIV assessment criteria (see display, General HIV/AIDS Assessment Criteria), assess for the following factors:

Physical

Usual weight, recent weight change. Weight loss 10% or more of usual weight is indicative of wasting.
The client's ability to perform self-care activities, including cooking and eating.
Observe for signs of fluid and electrolyte imbalance.

Biochemical

Depleted visceral protein status, as indicated by low albumin, prealbumin, and retinol-binding protein.
Serum cholesterol level. Hypocholesterolemia is associated with adverse clinical outcomes (Chlebowski, 1995).

ASSESSMENT CRITERIA

General HIV/AIDS Assessment Criteria

Use of drugs and medications

Alterations in skin and mucous membranes, including decreased turgor and ulcerations

Vital signs, especially temperature

Neurologic impairments, including the tendency to choke, forgetfulness

Fluid and electrolyte balance

Presence of edema

Respiratory status

Emotional status

Lymph node enlargement

Muscle wasting

Infectious process, sepsis

Other abnormal laboratory values and their significance.

Dietary

Adequacy of intake.

Symptoms that interfere with eating, such as nausea, vomiting, diarrhea, dysphagia, altered taste, difficulty chewing, shortness of breath; assess onset, frequency, severity, interventions attempted and the results.

Dietary changes made in response to symptoms (ie, foods avoided, food preferred). Determine which foods are best and least tolerated.

The use of unorthodox or unproven dietary remedies to combat HIV/AIDS, and the potential impact on nutritional status (see display, Nutritional Therapies for HIV.

The use of vitamin and mineral supplements; determine dosage.

Usual intake of alcohol; alcohol can displace the intake of nutrient-rich food and alter nutrient metabolism and excretion to further compromise nutritional status.

Nursing Diagnosis

Altered nutrition: Less than body requirement, related to anorexia

---

Nutritional Therapies for HIV

The following are a sampling of nutritional therapies that may be used by people with HIV/AIDS; none can stop the progression of HIV, and some may be potentially harmful. Be aware of the potential complications, and "work around" the therapy whenever possible to ensure an adequate intake.

Dr. Berger's Immune Power Diet. An elimination-type diet is implemented over a 21-day period, followed by the reintroduction phase and 4-day cycle maintenance diet. Because cow's milk, wheat, corn, yeast, soy, sugar, and eggs are targeted, this diet can cause undernutrition, especially of calories and protein.

Yeast-free diet. With the rationale that limiting yeast will help prevent candidiasis and other infections, foods that contain yeast and high concentrations of simple sugars are eliminated. This diet can compromise calorie intake and therefore promote weight loss.

Macrobiotic diet. Based on yin and yang ideology and the belief that AIDS is caused by an imbalance in the body, the macrobiotic diet purports to maintain balance and thus cure AIDS. This highly restrictive diet is comprised of brown rice and other whole grains, vegetables, seaweed, legumes, miso, soup, and a little fish. This diet is likely to be deficient in calories, complete protein, iron, calcium, vitamin D, vitamin B_{12}, folic acid, riboflavin, and vitamin C.

Km (Matol Corporation). A high-potassium supplement that contains herbal extracts and claims to detoxify and speed the rate of chemical reactions in the blood. Nausea, diarrhea, lightheadedness, and headache are adverse effects.

Cleansing rituals. Fasting and starvation may be used to "starve" the infection; unfortunately, the body is also starved. Enemas may be used with the idea that they cleanse the bowel and body by removing toxins and bacteria; they can compound problems with malabsorption and alter fluid and electrolyte balance.

Planning and Implementation

It is possible that maintaining good nutritional status can slow the progression of AIDS and improve the effectiveness of drug therapy. The ultimate goal of diet intervention is to help preserve the client's independence (eg, allowing him to stay at home) and quality of life.

Nutrition assessment should occur as soon as HIV is diagnosed, and be repeated periodically. Nutrition intervention that is aimed at preserving weight status should begin before the client exhibits any symptoms of HIV, and even if intake appears adequate. Once the client is ill enough to need hospital care, the effectiveness of diet intervention may be limited.

Although exact nutrient requirements for HIV and AIDS have not yet been established, it appears that calorie needs are higher than normal, even in the absence of malabsorption, possibly related to altered metabolism. Protein requirements are also increased, especially in clients with serum protein depletion and loss of lean body tissue. Vitamin and mineral requirements are not known; however, clients should consume at least 100% of the Recommended Dietary Allowance (RDA) for these nutrients.

Clients with HIV or AIDS may experience problems with appetite and intake similar to those of cancer clients (see Table 21-6). Every attempt should be made to maximize oral intake and tolerance; clients should be encouraged to consume small, frequent, nutritionally dense meals and supplements throughout the day.

Clients who are unable to consume an adequate oral intake may require tube feeding for supplemental or complete nutrition. Because many formulas have the potential to cause diarrhea, the client's tolerance should be closely monitored. Clients with intractable vomiting, severe secretory diarrhea, bowel obstruction, or those at risk for aspiration may be candidates for TPN. However, the use of TPN is controversial because it may not be able to stop progressive wasting in clients who have systemic infections. Some studies have found that TPN increases body fat without increasing body cell mass (Cameron, 1994).

Clients with malabsorption may need to limit fat intake and use supplemental medium-chain triglyceride (MCT) oil for additional calories (MCT oil comprises medium-chain triglycerides, does not require pancreatic lipase or bile for digestion and absorption, and thus can be absorbed easily by people with impaired digestion or absorption). An added complication may be lactose or gluten intolerance; modify the diet, as needed (see Chapter 16).

Decreased intake and increased requirements may necessitate the use of a multivitamin and mineral supplement, in doses of one to two times the RDA.

Clients should be taught safe food handling practices to help avoid food-borne illnesses (see display, Safe Food Handling, Chapter 8).

CLIENT GOALS

The client will

Consume adequate calories and protein to prevent or correct weight loss, protein depletion, and malnutrition.

Modify the diet as needed to lessen side effects or complications (eg, anorexia, nausea and vomiting, diarrhea, malabsorption, dysphagia, chewing difficulties).

NURSING INTERVENTIONS

Diet Management

Increase calorie intake to 35 to 45 cal/kg (see display, Ways to Increase Nutrient Density with Protein and Calories).

Increase protein intake to 1.0 to 2.0 g/kg to replenish losses and help maintain lean body mass.

Increase fluid intake in response to diarrhea, fever, and vomiting; exact requirements vary with the number and severity of complications.

Modify the diet as needed to alleviate problems that interfere with appetite and intake (see Table 21-6).

If malabsorption exists, limit fat and consider the use of MCT oil.

Encourage small, frequent feedings to help maximize intake. Liquid commercial supplements tend to leave the stomach quickly, are easy to consume, and provide significant quantities of calories and protein (see display, Liquid Supplements; for more details, see Appendix 7). If the client can tolerate milk, homemade milkshakes and instant breakfasts made with whole milk are nutritionally comparable and less expensive.

Client Teaching

Instruct the client

On the importance of consuming a balanced, nutrient-dense intake to help preserve independence, maintain quality of life, and possibly slow the progression

---

Liquid Supplements

The following is an incomplete list of commercial supplements that may be used to boost calorie and protein intake. Experiment with different brands to find the one best accepted.

Lactose-Free
  Ensure (Ross)
  Ensure HN (Ross)
  Ensure Plus (Ross)
  Nutren (Clintec)
  Promote (Ross)
  Resource (Sandoz)
  Sustacal (Mead Johnson)
  Sustacal HC (Mead Johnson)

Containing Lactose (may aggravate diarrhea)
  Carnation Instant Breakfast (Clintec)
  Delmark Instant Breakfast (Delmark)
  Forta Shake (Ross)
  Meritene powder (Sandoz)
  Sustacal powder (Mead Johnson)

of AIDS. Clients should be encouraged to eat at regular intervals, even when appetite is lacking.

To make extra food on "good" days and freeze for later use.

On how to avoid food-borne illnesses through the use of safe food handling.

How to modify the diet as needed to alleviate side effects and complications of HIV and AIDS.

That nutritional "cures" for HIV and AIDS do not exist. Caution the client against the use of unorthodox nutritional therapies (see display, Nutritional Therapies for HIV).

That other forms of nutritional support are available when the client is unable to consume enough food orally. The client should be counseled on the potential risks and benefits of both tube feedings and parenteral nutrition.

Monitoring Progress

Monitor for the following signs or symptoms

Adequacy of oral intake, as evidenced by weight, weight changes.

Tolerance to oral intake.

Effectiveness of diet modifications to alleviate side effects and complications, and the need for follow-up diet counseling.

The client's self-care abilities and the need for home care or support services.

Evaluation

Evaluation is ongoing. Provided that the plan of care has not changed, the client will achieve the goals as stated above.

KEY CONCEPTS

- Nutrition intervention in clients aggresively treated for cancer can increase the chance for successful cancer treatment and can reduce morbidity and mortality.
- Diet may play a role in a 30% to 35% of all cancers, either directly (providing carcinogens or procarcinogens) or indirectly (promoting cancer through its effect on immunocompetence, enzymes, or hormones).
- Without early and aggressive nutrition intervention, cancer and its treatments can have profound and devastating effects on nutritional status, often resulting in cachexia and death.
- Localized effects of GI cancers can impair intake, digestion, and absorption. Systemic effects are much more far reaching, and may occur even when cancer is limited to one site. Systemic effects include increased energy expenditure, increased protein catabolism, and increased fat metabolism.
- Cancer cachexia is a wasting syndrome that causes more deaths than cancer itself. Neither the incidence nor severity of cachexia can be related directly to calorie intake or tumor weight. Cachexia is easier to prevent than treat.
- Cancer treatments can produce local and systemic effects that profoundly impact nutritional status and requirements. Most people undergoing chemotherapy consider nausea and vomiting to be the most distressing side effects.

- The goal of diet intervention for cancer clients is to keep them out of the hospital whenever possible. Attaining and maintaining desirable weight and correcting nutrient deficiencies can improve quality of life.
- Generally, a high-protein, high-calorie diet modified to minimize GI side effects is indicated for clients treated for cancer. Small frequent meals are recommended.
- Increasing the calorie and protein density of the diet is generally more acceptable than increasing the volume of food served.
- No benefit is derived from force-feeding a client whose cancer is not being aggresively treated.
- There is no cure for AIDS. Treatment, including nutrition intervention, focuses on delaying the onset of AIDS symptoms, preserving independence, and maintaining the quality of life.
- As many as 80% of clients with HIV or AIDS have malnutrition; malnutrition may speed the progression from HIV to AIDS.
- Nutrient requirements for people with HIV and AIDS have not been determined, but it appears calorie and protein needs are increased.
- Clients with HIV or AIDS may have anorexia similar to that experienced by cancer clients. Malabsorption may complicate nutritional support.
- Cancer and HIV and AIDS clients are susceptible to nutrition "cures" and may use unorthodox diets or supplements that may be detrimental to their health.

FOCUS ON **CRITICAL THINKING**

Irene is a 58-year-old woman who was recently diagnosed with colon cancer with metastasis to the liver. After surgical removal of part of her colon, she began chemotherapy, which was to be given for 30 minutes each day for 7 days, followed by 21 days off. This cycle was to be repeated for 3 months.

Irene lost 12 pounds while hospitalized for her surgery. When she began chemotherapy, she weighed 128 pounds; she is 5'5" tall. Within days of beginning chemotherapy, Irene developed stomatitis and stopped eating. She has always been fearful of nausea, and believes fasting is the most effective approach to avoiding nausea. She is complaining of tremendous mouth pain, and told her daughter she will not continue with chemotherapy if these problems persist. Because her mother is so fatigued, Irene's daughter brought her a large pot of homemade vegetable soup that she could simply heat up when she is too tired to cook.

How many calories and grams of protein should Irene be consuming to meet her estimated requirements while undergoing chemotherapy? What types of food should you encourage Irene to eat in order to meet her nutritional requirements, keeping in mind that she has mouth pain and nausea? Plan a day's menu that Irene could follow.

In counseling Irene about the importance of eating, what important points should you stress?

Was homemade soup a good choice for premade meals? Why or why not? Name foods that you would encourage her daughter to make for Irene.

REFERENCES

American Cancer Society (1995). Cancer Facts and Figures—1995. Atlanta, GA: American Cancer Society.

American Dietetic Association (1994). Position of the American Dietetic Association and the Canadian Dietetic Association: Nutrition intervention in the care of persons with human immunodeficiency virus infection. J Am Diet Assoc 94(10), 1042–1045.

American Institute for Cancer Research (1992): Everything Doesn't Cause Cancer. Washington, DC: American Institute for Cancer Research.

Anastasi, J. and Rivera, J. (1994). Understanding prophylactic therapy for HIV infections. AJN 94(2), 36–41.

Anastasi, J. and Sun Lee, V. (1994). HIV wasting. How to stop the cycle. AJN 94(6), 18–25.

Bass, F. and Cox, R. (1995). The need for dietary counseling of cancer patients as indicated by nutrient and supplement intake. J Am Diet Assoc, 95, 1319–1321.

Cameron, A., ed. (1994). Nutrition in HIV/AIDS. Dietetic Currents 21(3), 11–16.

Chlebowski, R., Grosvenor, M., Lillington, L., et al. (1995). Dietary intake and counseling, weight maintenance, and the course of HIV infection. J Am Diet Assoc, 95(4), 428–432, 435.

DeVita, V., Hellman, S., and Rosenberg, S., eds. (1992). AIDS. Etiology, Diagnosis, Treatment, and Prevention. 3rd ed. Philadelphia: JB Lippincott.

Feuz, A. and Rapin, C. (1994). An observational study of the role of pain control and food adaptation of elderly patients with terminal cancer. J Am Diet Assoc, 94, 767–770.

Gorbach, S., Knox, T., and Roubenoff, R. (1993). Interactions between nutrition and infection with human immunodeficiency virus. Nutrition Reviews, 51(8), 226–234.

Haller, D. (1994). Weight gain in patients with AIDS-related cachexia: Is bigger better? Ann Intern Med 121(6), 462–463.

Held, J. (1994). Managing fatigue: How to help your patients cope with persistent fatigue during their cancer treatments. Nursing 94, 26.

Jacobson, M., ed. (1993). Pumping immunity. Nutrition Action Health Letter 20(3), 5–7.

Jenns, K. (1994). Importance of nausea. Cancer Nursing 17, 488–493.

Liebman, B. (1995). Dodging cancer with diet. Nutrition Action Health Letter 22(1), 4–7.

Luder, E., Godfrey, E, Godbold, J., and Simpson, D. (1995). Assessment of nutritional, clinical, and immunologic status of HIV-infected, inner-city patients with multiple risk factors. J Am Diet Assoc, 95(6), 655–660.

Mandell, G., Dolin, R., and Bennett, J., eds. (1995). Principles and Practice of Infectious Diseases. 4th ed. New York: Churchill Livingstone, Inc.

McKinley, M., Goodman-Block, J., Lesser, M., and Salbe, A. (1994). Improved body weight status as a result of nutrition intervention in adult, HIV-positive outpatients. J Am Diet Assoc 94(10), 1014–1017.

Risser, J., Rabeneck, L. and Foote, L., (1995). Prevalence of wasting in men infected with human immunodeficiency virus seeking routine medical care in an outpatient clinic. J Am Diet Assoc 95(9), 1025–1026.

Rudolph, R, Chandra, S., et al. (1994). Symposium: Dietary nucleotides: A recently demonstrated requirement for cellular development and immune function. Journal of Nutrition 124(8S), 1431S–1442S.

Shils, M., Olson, J., and Shike, M (1994). Modern Nutrition in Health and Disease. 8th ed. Philadelphia: Lea & Febiger.

Timbo, B. and Tollefson, L. (1994). Nutrition: A cofactor in HIV disease. J Am Diet Assoc 94(10), 1018–1022.

Weber, M. (1995). Chemotherapy-induced nausea and vomiting. AJN, 95(4), 34–35.

Appendices

Appendix 1
Nutritive Value of the Edible Part of Food*
(footnotes on pp. 768–769; nutrients in indicated quantity)

Item	Foods, Approximate Measures, Units, and Weight (Weight of Edible Portion Only)	Weight (g)	Water (%)	Food Energy (kcal)	Protein (g)	Fat (g)	Fatty Acids Saturated (g)	Monounsaturated (g)	Polyunsaturated (g)	Cholesterol (mg)	Carbohydrate (g)	Calcium (mg)	Phosphorus (mg)	Iron (mg)	Potassium (mg)	Sodium (mg)	Vitamin A Value (IU)	(RE)	Thiamine (mg)	Riboflavin (mg)	Niacin (mg)	Ascorbic Acid (mg)
BEVERAGES																						
Alcoholic																						
Beer																						
Regular	12 fl oz	360	92	150	1	0	0.0	0.0	0.0	0	13	14	50	0.1	115	18	0	0	0.02	0.09	1.8	0
Light	12 fl oz	355	95	95	1	0	0.0	0.0	0.0	0	5	14	43	0.1	64	11	0	0	0.03	0.11	1.4	0
Gin, rum, vodka, whiskey																						
80-proof	1½ fl oz	42	67	95	0	0	0.0	0.0	0.0	0	Tr	Tr	Tr	Tr	1	Tr	0	0	Tr	Tr	Tr	0
86-proof	1½ fl oz	42	64	105	0	0	0.0	0.0	0.0	0	Tr	Tr	Tr	Tr	1	Tr	0	0	Tr	Tr	Tr	0
90-proof	1½ fl oz	42	62	110	0	0	0.0	0.0	0.0	0	Tr	Tr	Tr	Tr	1	Tr	0	0	Tr	Tr	Tr	0
Wines																						
Dessert	3½ fl oz	103	77	140	Tr	0	0.0	0.0	0.0	0	8	8	9	0.2	95	9	(¹)	(¹)	0.01	0.02	0.2	0
Table																						
Red	3½ fl oz	102	88	75	Tr	0	0.0	0.0	0.0	0	3	8	18	0.4	113	5	(¹)	(¹)	0.00	0.03	0.1	0
White	3½ fl oz	102	87	80	Tr	0	0.0	0.0	0.0	0	3	9	14	0.3	83	5	(¹)	(¹)	0.00	0.01	0.1	0
Carbonated[2]																						
Club soda	12 fl oz	355	100	0	0	0	0.0	0.0	0.0	0	0	18	0	Tr	0	78	0	0	0.00	0.00	0.0	0
Cola type																						
Regular	12 fl oz	369	89	160	0	0	0.0	0.0	0.0	0	41	11	52	0.2	7	18	0	0	0.00	0.00	0.0	0
Diet, artificially sweetened	12 fl oz	355	100	Tr	0	0	0.0	0.0	0.0	0	Tr	14	39	0.2	7	³32	0	0	0.00	0.00	0.0	0
Ginger ale	12 fl oz	366	91	125	0	0	0.0	0.0	0.0	0	32	11	0	0.1	4	29	0	0	0.00	0.00	0.0	0
Grape	12 fl oz	372	88	180	0	0	0.0	0.0	0.0	0	46	15	0	0.4	4	48	0	0	0.00	0.00	0.0	0
Lemon-lime	12 fl oz	372	89	155	0	0	0.0	0.0	0.0	0	39	7	0	0.4	4	33	0	0	0.00	0.00	0.0	0
Orange	12 fl oz	372	88	180	0	0	0.0	0.0	0.0	0	46	15	4	0.3	7	52	0	0	0.00	0.00	0.0	0
Pepper type	12 fl oz	369	89	160	0	0	0.0	0.0	0.0	0	41	11	41	0.1	4	37	0	0	0.00	0.00	0.0	0
Root beer	12 fl oz	370	89	165	0	0	0.0	0.0	0.0	0	42	15	0	0.2	4	48	0	0	0.00	0.00	0.0	0
Cocoa and chocolate-flavored beverages																						
See Dairy Products.																						

(continued)

(Continuation of a nutrient-value table. The numeric column headers are not printed on this page; the value columns appear in the following order: weight (g), water (%), food energy, protein (g), fat (g), saturated fat (g), monounsaturated fat (g), polyunsaturated fat (g), cholesterol (mg), carbohydrate (g), calcium (mg), phosphorus (mg), iron (mg), potassium (mg), sodium (mg), vitamin A (IU), vitamin A (RE), thiamin (mg), riboflavin (mg), niacin (mg), ascorbic acid (mg).)

Coffee

Food	Measure	(g)	water	energy	prot	fat	sat	mono	poly	chol	carb	Ca	P	Fe	K	Na	A(IU)	A(RE)	thia	ribo	niac	asc
Brewed	6 fl oz	180	100	Tr	Tr	0	Tr	Tr	Tr	0	Tr	4	2	Tr	124	2	0	0	0.00	0.02	0.4	0
Instant, prepared (2 tsp powder plus 6 fl oz water)	6 fl oz	182	99	Tr	Tr	0	Tr	Tr	Tr	0	1	2	6	0.1	71	Tr	0	0	0.00	0.03	0.6	0

Fruit drinks, noncarbonated

Canned

Food	Measure	(g)	water	energy	prot	fat	sat	mono	poly	chol	carb	Ca	P	Fe	K	Na	A(IU)	A(RE)	thia	ribo	niac	asc
Fruit punch drink	6 fl oz	190	88	85	Tr	0	0.0	0.0	0.0	0	22	15	2	0.4	48	15	20	2	0.03	0.04	Tr	⁴61
Grape drink	6 fl oz	187	86	100	Tr	0	0.0	0.0	0.0	0	26	2	2	0.3	9	11	Tr	Tr	0.01	0.01	Tr	⁴64
Pineapple-grapefruit juice drink	6 fl oz	187	87	90	Tr	Tr	Tr	Tr	Tr	0	23	13	7	0.9	97	24	60	6	0.06	0.04	0.5	⁴110

Frozen

Food	Measure	(g)	water	energy	prot	fat	sat	mono	poly	chol	carb	Ca	P	Fe	K	Na	A(IU)	A(RE)	thia	ribo	niac	asc
Lemonade concentrate — Undiluted	6 fl oz	219	49	245	Tr	Tr	Tr	Tr	Tr	0	112	9	13	0.4	153	4	40	4	0.04	0.07	0.7	66
Diluted with 4⅓ parts water by volume	6 fl oz	185	89	80	Tr	Tr	Tr	Tr	Tr	0	21	2	2	0.1	30	1	10	1	0.01	0.02	0.2	13
Limeade concentrate — Undiluted	6 fl oz	218	50	410	Tr	Tr	Tr	Tr	Tr	0	108	11	13	0.2	129	Tr	Tr	Tr	0.02	0.02	0.2	26
Diluted with 4⅓ parts water by volume	6 fl oz	185	89	75	Tr	Tr	Tr	Tr	Tr	0	20	2	2	Tr	24	Tr	Tr	Tr	Tr	Tr	Tr	4

Fruit juices

See type under Fruits and Fruit juices.

Milk beverages

See Dairy Products.

Tea

Food	Measure	(g)	water	energy	prot	fat	sat	mono	poly	chol	carb	Ca	P	Fe	K	Na	A(IU)	A(RE)	thia	ribo	niac	asc
Brewed	8 fl oz	240	100	Tr	Tr	0	Tr	Tr	Tr	0	Tr	0	2	Tr	36	1	0	0	0.00	0.03	Tr	0
Instant, powder, prepared — Unsweetened (1 tsp powder plus 8 fl oz water)	8 fl oz	241	100	Tr	Tr	0	Tr	Tr	Tr	0	1	1	4	Tr	61	1	0	0	0.00	0.02	Tr	0
Sweetened (3 tsp powder plus 8 fl oz water)	8 fl oz	262	91	85	Tr	0	Tr	Tr	Tr	0	22	1	3	Tr	49	Tr	0	0	0.00	0.04	0.1	0

DAIRY PRODUCTS

Butter

See Fats and Oils.

Cheese

Natural

Food	Measure	(g)	water	energy	prot	fat	sat	mono	poly	chol	carb	Ca	P	Fe	K	Na	A(IU)	A(RE)	thia	ribo	niac	asc
Blue	1 oz	28	42	100	6	8	5.3	2.2	0.2	21	1	150	110	0.1	73	396	200	65	0.01	0.11	0.3	0
Camembert (3 wedges per 4-oz container)	1 wedge	38	52	115	8	9	5.8	2.7	0.3	27	Tr	147	132	0.1	71	320	350	96	0.01	0.19	0.2	0
Cheddar — Cut pieces	1 oz	28	37	115	7	9	6.0	2.7	0.3	30	Tr	204	145	0.2	28	176	300	86	0.01	0.11	Tr	0
Cut pieces	1 in³	17	37	70	4	6	3.6	1.6	0.2	18	Tr	123	87	0.1	17	105	180	52	Tr	0.06	Tr	0
Shredded	1 cup	113	37	455	28	37	23.8	10.6	1.1	119	1	815	579	0.8	111	701	1,200	342	0.03	0.42	0.1	0

Appendix 1 (Continued)
Nutritive Value of the Edible Part of Food*

Item	Foods, Approximate Measures, Units, and Weight (Weight of Edible Portion Only)	Weight (g)	Water (%)	Food Energy (kcal)	Protein (g)	Fat (g)	Fatty Acids Saturated (g)	Monounsaturated (g)	Polyunsaturated (g)	Cholesterol (mg)	Carbohydrate (g)	Calcium (mg)	Phosphorus (mg)	Iron (mg)	Potassium (mg)	Sodium (mg)	Vitamin A Value (IU)	Vitamin A Value (RE)	Thiamine (mg)	Riboflavine (mg)	Niacin (mg)	Ascorbic Acid (mg)
Cottage (curd not pressed down)																						
Creamed (cottage cheese, 4% fat)																						
Large curd	1 cup	225	79	235	28	10	6.4	2.9	0.3	34	6	135	297	0.3	190	911	370	108	0.05	0.37	0.3	Tr
Small curd	1 cup	210	79	215	26	9	6.0	2.7	0.3	31	6	126	277	0.3	177	850	340	101	0.04	0.34	0.2	Tr
With fruit	1 cup	226	72	280	22	8	4.9	2.2	0.2	25	30	108	236	0.2	151	915	280	81	0.04	0.29	0.2	Tr
Lowfat (2%)	1 cup	226	79	205	31	4	2.8	1.2	0.1	19	8	155	340	0.4	217	918	160	45	0.05	0.42	0.3	Tr
Uncreamed (cottage cheese dry curd, less than 1/2% fat)	1 cup	145	80	125	25	1	0.4	0.2	Tr	10	3	46	151	0.3	47	19	40	12	0.04	0.21	0.2	0
Cream	1 oz	28	54	100	2	10	6.2	2.8	0.4	31	1	23	30	0.3	34	84	400	124	Tr	0.06	Tr	0
Feta	1 oz	28	55	75	4	6	4.2	1.3	0.2	25	1	140	96	0.2	18	316	130	36	0.04	0.24	0.3	0
Mozzarella, made with																						
Whole milk	1 oz	28	54	80	6	6	3.7	1.9	0.2	22	1	147	105	0.1	19	106	220	68	Tr	0.07	Tr	0
Part skim milk (low moisture)	1 oz	28	49	80	8	5	3.1	1.4	0.1	15	1	207	149	0.1	27	150	180	54	0.01	0.10	Tr	0
Muenster	1 oz	28	42	105	7	9	5.4	2.5	0.2	27	Tr	203	133	0.1	38	178	320	90	Tr	0.09	Tr	0
Parmesan, grated																						
Cup, not pressed down	1 cup	100	18	455	42	30	19.1	8.7	0.7	79	4	1,376	807	1.0	107	1,861	700	173	0.05	0.39	0.3	0
Tablespoon	1 tbsp	5	18	25	2	2	1.0	0.4	Tr	4	Tr	69	40	Tr	5	93	40	9	Tr	0.02	Tr	0
Ounce	1 oz	28	18	130	12	9	5.4	2.5	0.2	22	1	390	229	0.3	30	528	200	49	0.01	0.11	0.1	0
Provolone	1 oz	28	41	100	7	8	4.8	2.1	0.2	20	1	214	141	0.1	39	248	230	75	0.01	0.09	Tr	0
Ricotta, made with																						
Whole milk	1 cup	246	72	430	28	32	20.4	8.9	0.9	124	7	509	389	0.9	257	207	1,210	330	0.03	0.48	0.3	0
Part skim milk	1 cup	246	74	340	28	19	12.1	5.7	0.6	76	13	669	449	1.1	307	307	1,060	278	0.05	0.46	0.2	0
Swiss	1 oz	28	37	105	8	8	5.0	2.1	0.3	26	1	272	171	Tr	31	74	240	72	0.01	0.10	Tr	0
Pasteurized process cheese																						
American	1 oz	28	39	105	6	9	5.6	2.5	0.3	27	Tr	174	211	0.1	46	406	340	82	0.01	0.10	Tr	0
Swiss	1 oz	28	42	95	7	7	4.5	2.0	0.2	24	1	219	216	0.2	61	388	230	65	Tr	0.08	Tr	0
Pasteurized process cheese food, American	1 oz	28	43	95	6	7	4.4	2.0	0.2	18	2	163	130	0.2	79	337	260	62	0.01	0.13	Tr	0
Pasteurized process cheese spread, American	1 oz	28	48	80	5	6	3.8	1.8	0.2	16	2	159	202	0.1	69	381	220	54	0.01	0.12	Tr	0

Cream, sweet

Food	Measure	Grams	Water (%)	Food energy (Cal)	Protein (g)	Fat (g)	Saturated fat (g)	Monounsaturated (g)	Polyunsaturated (g)	Cholesterol (mg)	Carbohydrate (g)	Calcium (mg)	Phosphorus (mg)	Iron (mg)	Potassium (mg)	Sodium (mg)	Vitamin A (IU)	Vitamin A (RE)	Thiamin (mg)	Riboflavin (mg)	Niacin (mg)	Ascorbic acid (mg)
Half-and-half (cream and milk)	1 cup	242	81	315	7	28	17.3	8.0	1.0	89	10	254	230	0.2	314	98	1,050	259	0.08	0.36	0.2	2
	1 tbsp	15	81	20	Tr	2	1.1	0.5	0.1	6	1	16	14	Tr	19	6	70	16	0.01	0.02	Tr	Tr
Light, coffee, or table	1 cup	240	74	470	6	46	28.8	13.4	1.7	159	9	231	192	0.1	292	95	1,730	437	0.08	0.36	0.1	2
	1 tbsp	15	74	30	Tr	3	1.8	0.8	0.1	10	1	14	12	Tr	18	6	110	27	Tr	0.02	Tr	Tr
Whipping, unwhipped (volume about double when whipped)																						
Light	1 cup	239	64	700	5	74	46.2	21.7	2.1	265	7	166	146	0.1	231	82	2,690	705	0.06	0.30	0.1	1
	1 tbsp	15	64	45	Tr	5	2.9	1.4	0.1	17	Tr	10	9	Tr	15	5	170	44	Tr	0.02	Tr	Tr
Heavy	1 cup	238	58	820	5	88	54.8	25.4	3.3	326	7	154	149	0.1	179	89	3,500	1,002	0.05	0.26	0.1	1
	1 tbsp	15	58	50	Tr	6	3.5	1.6	0.2	21	Tr	10	9	Tr	11	6	220	63	Tr	0.02	Tr	Tr
Whipped topping, (pressurized)	1 cup	60	61	155	2	13	8.3	3.9	0.5	46	7	61	54	Tr	88	78	550	124	0.02	0.04	Tr	0
	1 tbsp	3	61	10	Tr	1	0.4	0.2	Tr	2	Tr	3	3	Tr	4	4	30	6	Tr	Tr	Tr	0
Cream, sour	1 cup	230	71	495	7	48	30.0	13.9	1.8	102	10	268	195	0.1	331	123	1,820	448	0.08	0.34	0.2	2
	1 tbsp	12	71	25	Tr	3	1.6	0.7	0.1	5	1	14	10	Tr	17	6	90	23	Tr	0.02	Tr	Tr
Cream products, imitation (made with vegetable fat)																						
Sweet																						
Creamers																						
Liquid (frozen)	1 tbsp	15	77	20	Tr	1	1.4	Tr	Tr	0	2	1	10	Tr	29	12	[5]510	[5]1	0.00	0.00	0.0	0
Powdered	1 tsp	2	2	10	Tr	1	0.7	Tr	Tr	0	1	Tr	8	Tr	16	4	Tr	Tr	0.00	0.00	0.0	0
Whipped topping																						
Frozen	1 cup	75	50	240	1	19	16.3	1.2	0.4	0	17	5	6	0.1	14	19	[5]650	[5]65	0.00	0.00	0.0	0
	1 tbsp	4	50	15	Tr	1	0.9	0.1	Tr	0	1	Tr	Tr	Tr	1	1	[5]30	[5]3	0.00	0.00	0.0	0
Powdered, made with whole milk	1 cup	80	67	150	3	10	8.5	0.7	0.2	8	13	72	69	Tr	121	53	[5]290	[5]39	0.02	0.09	Tr	1
	1 tbsp	4	67	10	Tr	Tr	0.4	Tr	Tr	Tr	1	4	3	Tr	6	3	[5]10	[5]2	Tr	Tr	Tr	Tr
Pressurized	1 cup	70	60	185	1	16	13.2	1.3	0.2	0	11	4	13	Tr	13	43	[5]330	[5]33	0.00	0.00	0.0	0
	1 tbsp	4	60	10	Tr	1	0.8	0.1	Tr	0	1	Tr	1	Tr	1	2	[5]20	[5]2	0.00	0.00	0.0	0
Sour dressing (filled cream type product, nonbutterfat)	1 cup	235	75	415	8	39	31.2	4.6	1.1	13	11	266	205	0.1	380	113	20	5	0.09	0.38	0.2	2
	1 tbsp	12	75	20	Tr	2	1.6	0.2	0.1	1	1	14	10	Tr	19	6	Tr	Tr	Tr	0.02	Tr	Tr
Ice cream See Milk desserts, frozen.																						
Ice milk See Milk desserts, frozen.																						
Milk																						
Fluid																						
Whole (3.3% fat)	1 cup	244	88	150	8	8	5.1	2.4	0.3	33	11	291	228	0.1	370	120	310	76	0.09	0.40	0.2	2
Lowfat (2%)																						
No milk solids added	1 cup	244	89	120	8	5	2.9	1.4	0.2	18	12	297	232	0.1	377	122	500	139	0.10	0.40	0.2	2
Milk solids added, label claims less than 10 g of protein per cup	1 cup	245	89	125	9	5	2.9	1.4	0.2	18	12	313	245	0.1	397	128	500	140	0.10	0.42	0.2	2

(continued)

Appendix 1 (Continued)
Nutritive Value of the Edible Part of Food*

Item	Foods, Approximate Measures, Units, and Weight (Weight of Edible Portion Only)	Weight (g)	Water (%)	Food Energy (kcal)	Protein (g)	Fat (g)	Saturated (g)	Monounsaturated (g)	Polyunsaturated (g)	Cholesterol (mg)	Carbohydrate (g)	Calcium (mg)	Phosphorus (mg)	Iron (mg)	Potassium (mg)	Sodium (mg)	Vitamin A Value (IU)	Vitamin A Value (RE)	Thiamine (mg)	Riboflavine (mg)	Niacin (mg)	Ascorbic Acid (mg)
Lowfat (1%)																						
No milk solids added	1 cup	244	90	100	8	3	1.6	0.7	0.1	10	12	300	235	0.1	381	123	500	144	0.10	0.41	0.2	2
Milk solids added, label claim less than 10 g of protein per cup	1 cup	245	90	105	9	2	1.5	0.7	0.1	10	12	313	245	0.1	397	128	500	145	0.10	0.42	0.2	2
Nonfat (skim)																						
No milk solids added	1 cup	245	91	85	8	Tr	0.3	0.1	Tr	4	12	302	247	0.1	406	126	500	149	0.09	0.34	0.2	2
Milk solids added, label claim less than 10 g of protein per cup	1 cup	245	90	90	9	1	0.4	0.2	Tr	5	12	316	255	0.1	418	130	500	149	0.10	0.43	0.2	2
Buttermilk	1 cup	245	90	100	8	2	1.3	0.6	0.1	9	12	285	219	0.1	371	257	80	20	0.08	0.38	0.1	2
Canned																						
Condensed, sweetened	1 cup	306	27	980	24	27	16.8	7.4	1.0	104	166	868	775	0.6	1,136	389	1,000	248	0.28	1.27	0.6	8
Evaporated																						
Whole milk	1 cup	252	74	340	17	19	11.6	5.9	0.6	74	25	657	510	0.5	764	267	610	136	0.12	0.80	0.5	5
Skim milk	1 cup	255	79	200	19	1	0.3	0.2	Tr	9	29	738	497	0.7	845	293	1,000	298	0.11	0.79	0.4	3
Dried																						
Buttermilk	1 cup	120	3	465	41	7	4.3	2.0	0.3	83	59	1,421	1,119	0.4	1,910	621	260	65	0.47	1.89	1.1	7
Nonfat, instantized																						
Envelope, 3.2 oz, net wt.[6]	1 envelope	91	4	325	32	1	0.4	0.2	Tr	17	47	1,120	896	0.3	1,552	499	[7]2,160	[7]646	0.38	1.59	0.8	5
Cup	1 cup	68	4	245	24	Tr	0.3	0.1	Tr	12	35	837	670	0.2	1,160	373	[7]1,610	[7]483	0.28	1.19	0.6	4
Milk beverages																						
Chocolate milk (commercial)																						
Regular	1 cup	250	82	210	8	8	5.3	2.5	0.3	31	26	280	251	0.6	417	149	300	73	0.09	0.41	0.3	2
Lowfat (2%)	1 cup	250	84	180	8	5	3.1	1.5	0.2	17	26	284	254	0.6	422	151	500	143	0.09	0.41	0.3	2
Lowfat (1%)	1 cup	250	85	160	8	3	1.5	0.8	0.1	7	26	287	256	0.6	425	152	500	148	0.10	0.42	0.3	2
Cocoa and chocolate-flavored beverages																						
Powder containing nonfat dry milk	1 oz	28	1	100	3	1	0.6	0.3	Tr	1	22	90	88	0.3	223	139	Tr	Tr	0.03	0.17	0.2	Tr
Prepared (6 oz water plus 1 oz powder)	1 serving	206	86	100	3	1	0.6	0.3	Tr	1	22	90	88	0.3	223	139	Tr	Tr	0.03	0.17	0.2	Tr

Food	Amount																					
Powder without nonfat dry milk	¾ oz	21	1	75	1	1	0.3	0.2	Tr	0	19	7	26	0.7	136	56	Tr	Tr	Tr	0.03	0.1	Tr
Prepared (8 oz whole milk plus ¾ oz powder)	1 serving	265	81	225	9	9	5.4	2.5	0.3	33	30	298	254	0.9	508	176	310	76	0.10	0.43	0.3	3
Eggnog (commercial)	1 cup	254	74	340	10	19	11.3	5.7	0.9	149	34	330	278	0.5	420	138	890	203	0.09	0.48	0.3	4
Malted milk																						
Chocolate																						
Powder	¾ oz	21	2	85	1	1	0.5	0.3	0.1	1	18	13	37	0.4	130	49	20	5	0.04	0.04	0.4	0
Prepared (8 oz whole milk plus ¾ oz powder)	1 serving	265	81	235	9	9	5.5	2.7	0.4	34	29	304	265	0.5	500	168	330	80	0.14	0.43	0.7	2
Natural																						
Powder	¾ oz	21	3	85	3	2	0.9	0.5	0.3	4	15	56	79	0.2	159	96	70	17	0.11	0.14	1.1	0
Prepared (8 oz whole milk plus ¾ oz powder)	1 serving	265	81	235	11	10	6.0	2.9	0.6	37	27	347	307	0.3	529	215	380	93	0.20	0.54	1.3	2
Shakes, thick																						
Chocolate	10 oz	283	72	335	9	8	4.8	2.2	0.2	30	60	374	357	0.9	634	314	240	59	0.13	0.63	0.4	0
Vanilla	10 oz	283	74	315	11	9	5.3	2.5	0.3	33	50	413	326	0.3	517	270	320	79	0.08	0.55	0.4	0
Milk desserts, frozen																						
Ice cream, vanilla																						
Regular (about 11% fat)																						
Hardened	½ gal	1,064	61	2,155	38	115	71.3	33.1	4.3	476	254	1,406	1,075	1.0	2,052	929	4,340	1,064	0.42	2.63	1.1	6
	1 cup	133	61	270	5	14	8.9	4.1	0.5	59	32	176	134	0.1	257	116	540	133	0.05	0.33	0.1	1
	3 fl oz	50	61	100	2	5	3.4	1.6	0.2	22	12	66	51	Tr	96	44	200	50	0.02	0.12	0.1	Tr
Soft serve (frozen custard)	1 cup	173	60	375	7	23	13.5	6.7	1.0	153	38	236	199	0.4	338	153	790	199	0.08	0.45	0.2	1
Rich (about 16% fat),																						
hardened	½ gal	1,188	59	2,805	33	190	118.3	54.9	7.1	703	256	1,213	927	0.8	1,771	868	7,200	1,758	0.36	2.27	0.9	5
	1 cup	148	59	350	4	24	14.7	6.8	0.9	88	32	151	115	0.1	221	108	900	219	0.04	0.28	0.1	1
Ice milk, vanilla																						
Hardened (about 4% fat)	½ gal	1,048	69	1,470	41	45	28.1	13.0	1.7	146	232	1,409	1,035	1.5	2,117	836	1,710	419	0.61	2.78	0.9	6
	1 cup	131	69	185	5	6	3.5	1.6	0.2	18	29	176	129	0.2	265	105	210	52	0.08	0.35	0.1	1
Soft serve (about 3% fat)	1 cup	175	70	225	8	5	2.9	1.3	0.2	13	38	274	202	0.3	412	163	175	44	0.12	0.54	0.2	1
Sherbet (about 2% fat)	½ gal	1,542	66	2,160	17	31	19.0	8.8	1.1	113	469	827	594	2.5	1,585	706	1,480	308	0.26	0.71	1.0	31
	1 cup	193	66	270	2	4	2.4	1.1	0.1	14	59	103	74	0.3	198	88	190	39	0.03	0.09	0.1	4
Yogurt																						
With added milk solids																						
Made with lowfat milk																						
Fruit-flavored[8]	8 oz	227	74	230	10	2	1.6	0.7	0.1	10	43	345	271	0.2	442	133	100	25	0.08	0.40	0.2	1
Plain	8 oz	227	85	145	12	4	2.3	1.0	0.1	14	16	415	326	0.2	531	159	150	36	0.10	0.49	0.3	2
Made with nonfat milk	8 oz	227	85	125	13	Tr	0.3	0.1	Tr	4	17	452	355	0.2	579	174	20	5	0.11	0.53	0.3	2
Made with whole milk	8 oz	227	88	140	8	7	4.8	2.0	0.2	29	11	274	215	0.1	351	105	280	68	0.07	0.32	0.2	1
Without added milk solids																						
EGGS																						
Eggs, large (24 oz per dozen)																						
Raw																						
Whole, without shell	1	50	75	75	6	5	1.6	1.9	0.7	213	1	25	89	0.7	60	63	320	95	0.03	0.25	Tr	0
White	1	33	88	15	4	Tr	0.0	0.0	0.0	0	Tr	2	4	Tr	48	55	0	0	Tr	0.15	Tr	0
Yolk	1	17	49	60	3	5	1.6	1.9	0.7	213	Tr	23	81	0.6	16	7	320	97	0.04	0.07	Tr	0

Appendix 1 (Continued)
Nutritive Value of the Edible Part of Food*

Item	Foods, Approximate Measures, Units, and Weight (Weight of Edible Portion Only)	Weight (g)	Water (%)	Food Energy (kcal)	Protein (g)	Fat (g)	Fatty Acids Saturated (g)	Monounsaturated (g)	Polyunsaturated (g)	Cholesterol (mg)	Carbohydrate (g)	Calcium (mg)	Phosphorus (mg)	Iron (mg)	Potassium (mg)	Sodium (mg)	Vitamin A Value (IU)	Vitamin A Value (RE)	Thiamine (mg)	Riboflavin (mg)	Niacin (mg)	Ascorbic Acid (mg)
Cooked																						
Fried in margarine	1	46	69	90	6	7	1.9	2.7	1.3	211	1	25	89	0.7	61	162	390	114	0.03	0.24	Tr	0
Hard-cooked, shell removed	1	50	75	75	6	5	1.6	2.0	0.7	213	1	25	86	0.6	63	62	280	84	0.03	0.26	Tr	0
Poached	1	50	75	75	6	5	1.5	1.9	0.7	212	1	25	89	0.7	60	140	320	95	0.02	0.22	Tr	0
Scrambled (milk added) in margarine	1	61	73	100	7	7	2.2	2.9	1.3	215	1	44	104	0.7	84	171	420	119	0.03	0.27	Tr	Tr
FATS AND OILS																						
Butter (4 sticks per lb)																						
Stick	1/2 cup	113	16	810	1	92	57.1	26.4	3.4	247	Tr	27	26	0.2	29	[9]933	[10]3,460	[10]852	0.01	0.04	Tr	0
	1 tbsp	14	16	100	Tr	11	7.1	3.3	0.4	31	Tr	3	3	Tr	4	[9]116	[10]430	[10]106	Tr	Tr	Tr	0
Tablespoon (1/2 stick) Pat (1 in square, 1/3 in high; 90 per lb)	1	5	16	35	Tr	4	2.5	1.2	0.2	11	Tr	1	1	Tr	1	[9]41	[10]150	[10]38	Tr	Tr	Tr	0
Fats, cooking (vegetable shortenings)	1 cup	205	0	1,810	0	205	51.3	91.2	53.5	0	0	0	0	0.0	0	0	0	0	0.00	0.00	0.0	0
	1 tbsp	13	0	115	0	13	3.3	5.8	3.4	0	0	0	0	0.0	0	0	0	0	0.00	0.00	0.0	0
Lard	1 cup	205	0	1,850	0	205	80.4	92.5	23.0	195	0	0	0	0.0	0	0	0	0	0.00	0.00	0.0	0
	1 tbsp	13	0	115	0	13	5.1	5.9	1.5	12	0	0	0	0.0	0	0	0	0	0.00	0.00	0.0	0
Margarine																						
Imitation (about 40% fat), soft	8 oz	227	58	785	1	88	17.5	35.6	31.3	0	1	40	31	0.0	57	[12]2,178	[12]7,510	[12]2,254	0.01	0.05	Tr	Tr
	1 tbsp	14	58	50	Tr	5	1.1	2.2	1.9	0	Tr	2	2	0.0	4	[11]134	[12]460	[12]139	Tr	Tr	Tr	Tr
Regular (about 80% fat)																						
Hard (4 sticks per lb)																						
Stick	1/2 cup	113	16	810	1	91	17.9	40.5	28.7	0	1	34	26	0.1	48	[11]1,066	[12]3,740	[12]1,122	0.01	0.04	Tr	Tr
Tablespoon (1/2 stick)	1 tbsp	14	16	100	Tr	11	2.2	5.0	3.6	0	Tr	4	3	Tr	6	[11]132	[12]460	[12]139	Tr	0.01	Tr	Tr
Pat (1 in square, 1/3 in high; 90 per lb)	1	5	16	35	Tr	4	0.8	1.8	1.3	0	Tr	1	1	Tr	2	[1]47	[12]170	[12]50	Tr	Tr	Tr	Tr
Soft	8 oz	227	16	1,625	2	183	31.3	64.7	78.5	0	1	60	46	0.0	86	[12]2,449	[12]7,510	[12]2,254	0.02	0.07	Tr	Tr
	1 tbsp	14	16	100	Tr	11	1.9	4.0	4.8	0	Tr	4	3	0.0	5	[11]151	[12]460	[12]139	Tr	Tr	Tr	Tr

(continued)

Food	Measure	Grams	Water (%)	Calories	Protein (g)	Fat (g)	Saturated (g)	Mono-unsat. (g)	Poly-unsat. (g)	Cholesterol (mg)	Carbo-hydrate (g)	Calcium (mg)	Phosphorus (mg)	Iron (mg)	Potassium (mg)	Sodium (mg)	Vit. A (IU)	Vit. A (RE)	Thiamin (mg)	Riboflavin (mg)	Niacin (mg)	Ascorbic acid (mg)
Spread (about 60% fat)																						
Hard (4 sticks per lb)																						
Stick	1/2 cup	113	37	610	1	69	15.9	29.4	20.5	0	0	24	18	0.0	34	[11]1,123	[11]3,740	[12]1,122	0.01	0.03	Tr	Tr
Tablespoon (1/8 stick)	1 tbsp	14	37	75	Tr	9	2.0	3.6	2.5	0	0	3	2	0.0	4	[11]139	[11]460	[12]139	Tr	Tr	Tr	Tr
Pat (1 in square, 1/3 in high; 90 per lb)	1	5	37	25	Tr	3	0.7	1.3	0.9	0	0	1	1	0.0	1	[11]50	[11]170	[12]50	Tr	Tr	Tr	Tr
Soft	8 oz	227	37	1,225	1	138	29.1	71.5	31.3	0	0	47	37	0.0	68	[11]2,256	[11]7,510	[12]2,254	0.02	0.06	Tr	Tr
	1 tbsp	14	37	75	Tr	9	1.8	4.4	1.9	0	0	3	2	0.0	4	[11]139	[11]460	[12]139	Tr	Tr	Tr	Tr
Oils, salad or cooking																						
Corn	1 cup	218	0	1,925	0	218	27.7	52.8	128.0	0	0	0	0	0.0	0	0	0	0	0.00	0.00	0.0	0
	1 tbsp	14	0	125	0	14	1.8	3.4	8.2	0	0	0	0	0.0	0	0	0	0	0.00	0.00	0.0	0
Olive	1 cup	216	0	1,910	0	216	29.2	159.2	18.1	0	0	0	0	0.0	0	0	0	0	0.00	0.00	0.0	0
	1 tbsp	14	0	125	0	14	1.9	10.3	1.2	0	0	0	0	0.0	0	0	0	0	0.00	0.00	0.0	0
Peanut	1 cup	216	0	1,910	0	216	36.5	99.8	69.1	0	0	0	0	0.0	0	0	0	0	0.00	0.00	0.0	0
	1 tbsp	14	0	125	0	14	2.4	6.5	4.5	0	0	0	0	0.0	0	0	0	0	0.00	0.00	0.0	0
Safflower	1 cup	218	0	1,925	0	218	19.8	26.4	162.4	0	0	0	0	0.0	0	0	0	0	0.00	0.00	0.0	0
	1 tbsp	14	0	125	0	14	1.3	1.7	10.4	0	0	0	0	0.0	0	0	0	0	0.00	0.00	0.0	0.0
Soybean oil, hydrogenated (partially hardened)	1 cup	218	0	1,925	0	218	32.5	93.7	82.0	0	0	0	0	0.0	0	0	0	0	0.00	0.00	0.0	0
	1 tbsp	14	0	125	0	14	2.1	6.0	5.3	0	0	0	0	0.0	0	0	0	0	0.00	0.00	0.0	0
Soybean-cottonseed oil blend, hydrogenated	1 cup	218	0	1,925	0	218	39.2	64.3	104.9	0	0	0	0	0.0	0	0	0	0	0.00	0.00	0.0	0
	1 tbsp	14	0	125	0	14	2.5	4.1	6.7	0	0	0	0	0.0	0	0	0	0	0.00	0.00	0.0	0
Sunflower	1 cup	218	0	1,925	0	218	22.5	42.5	143.2	0	0	0	0	0.0	0	0	0	0	0.00	0.00	0.0	0
	1 tbsp	14	0	125	0	14	1.4	2.7	9.2	0	0	0	0	0.0	0	0	0	0	0.00	0.00	0.0	0
Salad dressings																						
Commercial																						
Blue cheese	1 tbsp	15	32	75	1	8	1.5	1.8	4.2	3	1	12	11	Tr	6	164	30	10	Tr	0.02	Tr	Tr
French — Regular	1 tbsp	16	35	85	Tr	9	1.4	4.0	3.5	0	1	2	1	Tr	9	188	Tr	Tr	Tr	Tr	Tr	Tr
French — Low calorie	1 tbsp	16	75	25	Tr	2	0.2	0.3	1.0	0	2	2	5	Tr	13	306	Tr	Tr	Tr	Tr	Tr	Tr
Italian — Regular	1 tbsp	15	34	80	Tr	9	1.3	3.7	3.2	0	1	1	1	Tr	5	162	30	3	Tr	Tr	Tr	Tr
Italian — Low calorie	1 tbsp	15	86	5	Tr	Tr	Tr	Tr	Tr	0	2	1	1	Tr	4	136	Tr	Tr	Tr	Tr	Tr	Tr
Mayonnaise — Regular	1 tbsp	14	15	100	Tr	11	1.7	3.2	5.8	8	Tr	3	4	0.1	5	80	40	12	0.00	0.00	Tr	0
Mayonnaise — Imitation	1 tbsp	15	63	35	Tr	3	0.5	0.7	1.6	4	2	2	Tr	0.0	2	75	0	0	0.00	0.00	Tr	0
Mayonnaise type	1 tbsp	15	40	60	Tr	5	0.7	1.4	2.7	4	4	2	4	Tr	4	107	30	13	0.00	Tr	Tr	0
Tartar sauce	1 tbsp	14	34	75	Tr	8	1.2	2.6	3.9	4	1	3	4	0.1	11	182	30	9	Tr	Tr	Tr	Tr
Thousand Island — Regular	1 tbsp	16	46	60	Tr	6	1.0	1.3	3.2	4	2	2	3	0.1	18	112	50	15	Tr	Tr	Tr	0
Thousand Island — Low calorie	1 tbsp	15	69	25	Tr	2	0.2	0.4	0.9	2	2	2	3	0.1	17	150	50	14	Tr	Tr	0.0	0
Prepared from home recipe																						
Cooked type[13]	1 tbsp	16	69	25	1	2	0.5	0.6	0.3	9	2	13	14	0.1	19	117	70	20	0.01	0.02	Tr	Tr
Vinegar and oil	1 tbsp	16	47	70	0	8	1.5	2.4	3.9	0	Tr	0	0	0.0	1	Tr	0	0	0.00	0.00	0.0	0

FISH AND SHELLFISH

Food	Measure	Grams	Water (%)	Calories	Protein (g)	Fat (g)	Saturated (g)	Mono-unsat. (g)	Poly-unsat. (g)	Cholesterol (mg)	Carbo-hydrate (g)	Calcium (mg)	Phosphorus (mg)	Iron (mg)	Potassium (mg)	Sodium (mg)	Vit. A (IU)	Vit. A (RE)	Thiamin (mg)	Riboflavin (mg)	Niacin (mg)	Ascorbic acid (mg)
Clams																						
Raw, meat only	3 oz	85	82	65	11	1	0.3	0.3	0.3	43	2	59	138	2.6	154	102	90	26	0.09	0.15	1.1	9
Canned, drained solids	3 oz	85	77	85	13	2	0.5	0.5	0.4	54	2	47	116	3.5	119	102	90	26	0.01	0.09	0.9	3

Appendix 1 (Continued)
Nutritive Value of the Edible Part of Food*

Item	Foods, Approximate Measures, Units, and Weight (Weight of Edible Portion Only)	Weight (g)	Water (%)	Food Energy (kcal)	Protein (g)	Fat (g)	Saturated (g)	Monounsaturated (g)	Polyunsaturated (g)	Cholesterol (mg)	Carbohydrate (g)	Calcium (mg)	Phosphorus (mg)	Iron (mg)	Potassium (mg)	Sodium (mg)	Vitamin A Value (IU)	Vitamin A Value (RE)	Thiamine (mg)	Riboflavine (mg)	Niacin (mg)	Ascorbic Acid (mg)
Crabmeat																						
Canned	1 cup	135	77	135	23	3	0.5	0.8	1.4	135	1	61	246	1.1	149	1,350	50	14	0.11	0.11	2.6	0
Fish sticks																						
Frozen, reheated, (stick 4 by 1 by ½ in)	1	28	52	70	6	3	0.8	1.4	0.8	26	4	11	58	0.3	94	53	20	5	0.03	0.05	0.6	0
Flounder or sole																						
Baked, with lemon juice																						
With butter	3 oz	85	73	120	16	6	3.2	1.5	0.5	68	Tr	13	187	0.3	272	145	210	54	0.05	0.08	1.6	1
With margarine	3 oz	85	73	120	16	6	1.2	2.3	1.9	55	Tr	14	187	0.3	273	151	230	69	0.05	0.08	1.6	1
Without added fat	3 oz	85	78	80	17	1	0.3	0.2	0.4	59	Tr	13	197	0.3	286	101	30	10	0.05	0.08	1.7	1
Haddock																						
Breaded, fried[14]	3 oz	85	61	175	17	9	2.4	3.9	2.4	75	7	34	183	1.0	270	123	70	20	0.06	0.10	2.9	0
Halibut																						
Broiled, with butter and lemon juice	3 oz	85	67	140	20	6	3.3	1.6	0.7	62	Tr	14	206	0.7	441	103	610	174	0.06	0.07	7.7	1
Herring																						
Pickled	3 oz	85	59	190	17	13	4.3	4.6	3.1	85	0	29	128	0.9	85	850	110	33	0.04	0.18	2.8	0
Ocean perch																						
Breaded, fried[14]	1 fillet	85	59	185	16	11	2.6	4.6	2.8	66	7	31	191	1.2	241	138	70	20	0.10	0.11	2.0	0
Oysters																						
Raw, meat only (13–19 medium Selects)	1 cup	240	85	160	20	4	1.4	0.5	1.4	120	8	226	343	15.6	290	175	740	223	0.34	0.43	6.0	24
Breaded, fried[14]	1	45	65	90	5	5	1.4	2.1	1.4	35	5	49	73	3.0	64	70	150	44	0.07	0.10	1.3	4
Salmon																						
Canned (pink), solids and liquid	3 oz	85	71	120	17	5	0.9	1.5	2.1	34	0	[15]167	243	0.7	307	443	60	18	0.03	0.15	6.8	0
Baked (red)	3 oz	85	67	140	21	5	1.2	2.4	1.4	60	0	26	269	0.5	305	55	290	87	0.18	0.14	5.5	0
Smoked	3 oz	85	59	150	18	8	2.6	3.9	0.7	51	0	12	208	0.8	327	1,700	260	77	0.17	0.17	6.8	0
Sardines																						
Atlantic, canned in oil, drained solids	3 oz	85	62	175	20	9	2.1	3.7	2.9	85	0	[15]371	424	2.6	349	425	190	56	0.03	0.17	4.6	0

Scallops																						
Breaded, frozen, reheated	6	90	59	195	15	10	2.5	2.5	2.5	70	10	39	203	2.0	369	298	70	21	0.11	0.11	1.6	0
Shrimp																						
Canned, drained solids	3 oz	85	70	100	21	1	0.2	0.2	0.4	128	1	98	224	1.4	104	1,955	50	15	0.01	0.03	1.5	0
French fried (7 medium)[16]	3 oz	85	55	200	16	10	2.5	4.1	2.6	168	11	61	154	2.0	189	384	90	26	0.06	0.09	2.8	0
Trout																						
Broiled, with butter and lemon juice	3 oz	85	63	175	21	9	4.1	2.9	1.6	71	Tr	26	259	1.0	297	122	230	60	0.07	0.07	2.3	1
Tuna																						
Canned, drained solids																						
Oil pack, chunk light	3 oz	85	61	165	24	7	1.4	1.9	3.1	55	0	7	199	1.6	298	303	70	20	0.04	0.09	10.0	0
Water pack, solid white	3 oz	85	63	135	30	1	0.3	0.2	0.3	48	0	17	202	0.6	255	468	110	32	0.03	0.10	13.4	0
Tuna salad[17]	1 cup	205	63	375	33	19	3.3	4.9	9.2	80	19	31	281	2.5	531	877	230	53	0.06	0.14	13.3	6

FRUITS AND FRUIT JUICES

Apples																						
Raw																						
Unpeeled, without cores 2¾-in diam. (about 3 per lb with cores)	1	138	84	80	Tr	Tr	Tr	Tr	0.1	0	21	10	10	0.2	159	Tr	70	7	0.02	0.02	0.1	8
3¼-in diam. (about 2 per lb with cores)	1	212	84	125	Tr	1	0.1	Tr	0.2	0	32	15	15	0.4	244	Tr	110	11	0.04	0.03	0.2	12
Peeled, sliced	1 cup	110	84	65	Tr	Tr	Tr	Tr	0.1	0	16	4	8	0.1	124	Tr	50	5	0.02	0.01	0.1	4
Dried, sulfured	10 rings	64	32	155	1	Tr	Tr	Tr	0.1	0	42	9	24	0.9	288	[18]56	0	0	0.00	0.10	0.6	2
Apple juice																						
Bottled or canned[19]	1 cup	248	88	115	Tr	Tr	Tr	Tr	0.1	0	29	17	17	0.9	295	7	Tr	Tr	0.05	0.04	0.2	[20]2
Applesauce																						
Canned																						
Sweetened	1 cup	255	80	195	Tr	Tr	0.1	Tr	0.1	0	51	10	18	0.9	156	8	30	3	0.03	0.07	0.5	[20]4
Unsweetened	1 cup	244	88	105	Tr	Tr	Tr	Tr	Tr	0	28	7	17	0.3	183	5	70	7	0.03	0.06	0.5	[20]3
Apricots																						
Raw, without pits (about 12 per lb with pits)	3	106	86	50	1	Tr	Tr	Tr	0.1	0	12	15	20	0.6	314	1	2,770	277	0.03	0.04	0.6	11
Canned (fruit and liquid)																						
Heavy syrup pack	1 cup	258	78	215	1	Tr	Tr	Tr	Tr	0	55	23	31	0.8	361	10	3,170	317	0.05	0.06	1.0	8
	3 halves	85	78	70	Tr	Tr	Tr	Tr	Tr	0	18	8	10	0.3	119	3	1,050	105	0.02	0.02	0.3	3
Juice pack	1 cup	248	87	120	2	Tr	Tr	Tr	Tr	0	31	30	50	0.7	409	10	4,190	419	0.04	0.05	0.9	12
	3 halves	84	87	40	1	Tr	Tr	Tr	Tr	0	10	10	17	0.3	139	3	1,420	142	0.02	0.02	0.3	4
Dried																						
Uncooked (28 large or 37 medium halves per cup)	1 cup	130	31	310	5	1	Tr	0.3	0.1	0	80	59	152	6.1	1,791	13	9,410	941	0.01	0.20	3.9	3
Cooked, unsweetened, fruit and liquid	1 cup	250	76	210	3	Tr	Tr	0.2	0.1	0	55	40	103	4.2	1,222	8	5,910	591	0.02	0.08	2.4	4
Apricot nectar																						
Canned	1 cup	251	85	140	1	Tr	Tr	0.1	Tr	0	36	18	23	1.0	286	8	3,300	330	0.02	0.04	0.7	[20]2
Avocados																						
Raw, whole, without skin and seed																						

(continued)

Appendix 1 (Continued)
Nutritive Value of the Edible Part of Food*

Item	Foods, Approximate Measures, Units, and Weight (Weight of Edible Portion Only)	Weight (g)	Water (%)	Food Energy (kcal)	Protein (g)	Fat (g)	Fatty Acids Saturated (g)	Monounsaturated (g)	Polyunsaturated (g)	Cholesterol (mg)	Carbohydrate (g)	Calcium (mg)	Phosphorus (mg)	Iron (mg)	Potassium (mg)	Sodium (mg)	Vitamin A Value (IU)	Vitamin A Value (RE)	Thiamine (mg)	Riboflavine (mg)	Niacin (mg)	Ascorbic Acid (mg)
California (about 2 per lb with skin and seed)	1	173	73	305	4	30	4.5	19.4	3.5	0	12	19	73	2.0	1,097	21	1,060	106	0.19	0.21	3.3	14
Florida (about 1 per lb with skin and seed)	1	304	80	340	5	27	5.3	14.8	4.5	0	27	33	119	1.6	1,484	15	1,860	186	0.33	0.37	5.8	24
Bananas																						
Raw, without peel																						
Whole (about 2½ per lb with peel)	1	114	74	105	1	1	0.2	Tr	0.1	0	27	7	23	0.4	451	1	90	9	0.05	0.11	0.6	10
Sliced	1 cup	150	74	140	2	1	0.3	0.1	0.1	0	35	9	30	0.5	594	2	120	12	0.07	0.15	0.8	14
Blackberries																						
Raw	1 cup	144	86	75	1	1	0.2	0.1	0.1	0	18	46	30	0.8	282	Tr	240	24	0.04	0.06	0.6	30
Blueberries																						
Raw	1 cup	145	85	80	1	1	Tr	0.1	0.3	0	20	9	15	0.2	129	9	150	15	0.07	0.07	0.5	19
Frozen, sweetened	10 oz	284	77	230	1	Tr	Tr	0.1	0.2	0	62	17	20	1.1	170	3	120	12	0.06	0.15	0.7	3
	1 cup	230	77	185	1	Tr	Tr	Tr	0.1	0	50	14	16	0.9	138	2	100	10	0.05	0.12	0.6	2
Cantaloupe																						
See Melons																						
Cherries																						
Sour, red, pitted, canned, water pack	1 cup	244	90	90	2	Tr	0.1	0.1	0.1	0	22	27	24	3.3	239	17	1,840	184	0.04	0.10	0.4	5
Sweet, raw, without pits and stems	10	68	81	50	1	1	0.1	0.2	0.2	0	11	10	13	0.3	152	Tr	150	15	0.03	0.04	0.3	5
Cranberry juice cocktail																						
Bottled, sweetened	1 cup	253	85	145	Tr	Tr	Tr	Tr	0.1	0	38	8	3	0.4	61	10	10	1	0.01	0.04	0.1	[21]108
Cranberry sauce																						
Sweetened, canned, strained	1 cup	277	61	420	1	Tr	Tr	0.1	0.2	0	108	11	17	0.6	72	80	60	6	0.04	0.06	0.3	6
Dates																						
Whole, without pits	10	83	23	230	2	Tr	Tr	Tr	Tr	0	61	27	33	1.0	541	2	40	4	0.07	0.08	1.8	0
Chopped	1 cup	178	23	490	4	1	0.1	0.2	Tr	0	131	57	71	2.0	1,161	5	90	9	0.16	0.18	3.9	0
Figs																						
Dried	10	187	28	475	6	2	0.4	0.5	1.0	0	122	269	127	4.2	1,331	21	250	25	0.13	0.16	1.3	1

(continued)

Food	Measure	Grams	Water (%)	Food energy (cal)	Protein (g)	Fat (g)	Saturated (g)	Monounsat. (g)	Polyunsat. (g)	Cholesterol (mg)	Carbohydrate (g)	Calcium (mg)	Phosphorus (mg)	Iron (mg)	Potassium (mg)	Sodium (mg)	Vitamin A (IU)	Thiamin (mg)	Riboflavin (mg)	Niacin (mg)	Ascorbic acid (mg)
Fruit cocktail																					
Canned, fruit and liquid																					
Heavy syrup pack	1 cup	255	80	185	1	Tr	Tr	Tr	0.1	0	48	15	28	0.7	224	15	520	0.05	0.05	1.0	5
Juice pack	1 cup	248	87	115	1	Tr	Tr	Tr	Tr	0	29	20	35	0.5	236	10	760	0.03	0.04	1.0	7
Grapefruit																					
Raw, without peel, membrane and seeds (3¾-in diam., 1 lb 1 oz, whole, with refuse)	½	120	91	40	1	Tr	Tr	Tr	Tr	0	10	14	10	0.1	167	Tr	[22]10	0.04	0.02	0.3	41
Canned, sections with syrup	1 cup	254	84	150	1	Tr	Tr	Tr	0.1	0	39	36	25	1.0	328	5	Tr	0.10	0.05	0.6	54
Grapefruit juice																					
Raw	1 cup	247	90	95	1	Tr	Tr	Tr	0.1	0	23	22	37	0.5	400	2	20	0.10	0.05	0.5	94
Canned																					
Unsweetened	1 cup	247	90	95	1	Tr	Tr	Tr	0.1	0	22	17	27	0.5	378	2	20	0.10	0.05	0.6	72
Sweetened	1 cup	250	87	115	1	Tr	Tr	Tr	0.1	0	28	20	28	0.9	405	5	20	0.10	0.06	0.8	67
Frozen concentrate, unsweetened																					
Undiluted	6 fl oz	207	62	300	4	1	0.1	Tr	0.2	0	72	56	101	1.0	1,002	6	60	0.30	0.16	1.6	248
Diluted with 3 parts water by volume	1 cup	247	89	100	1	Tr	Tr	Tr	0.1	0	24	20	35	0.3	336	2	20	0.10	0.05	0.5	83
Grapes																					
European type (adherent skin), raw																					
Thompson seedless	10	50	81	35	Tr	Tr	0.1	Tr	0.1	0	9	6	7	0.1	93	1	40	0.05	0.03	0.2	5
Tokay and Emperor, seeded types	10	57	81	40	Tr	Tr	0.1	Tr	0.1	0	10	6	7	0.1	105	1	40	0.05	0.03	0.2	6
Grape juice																					
Canned or bottled	1 cup	253	84	155	1	Tr	0.1	Tr	0.1	0	38	23	28	0.6	334	8	20	0.07	0.09	0.7	[20]Tr
Frozen concentrate, sweetened:																					
Undiluted	6 fl oz	216	54	385	1	1	0.2	Tr	0.2	0	96	28	32	0.8	160	15	60	0.11	0.20	0.9	[21]179
Diluted with 3 parts water by volume	1 cup	250	87	125	Tr	Tr	0.1	Tr	0.1	0	32	10	10	0.3	53	5	20	0.04	0.07	0.3	[21]60
Kiwifruit																					
Raw, without skin (about 5 per lb with skin)	1	76	83	45	1	Tr	Tr	0.1	0.1	0	11	20	30	0.3	252	4	130	0.02	0.04	0.4	74
Lemons																					
Raw, without peel and seeds (about 4 per lb with peel and seeds)	1	58	89	15	1	Tr	Tr	Tr	Tr	0	5	15	9	0.3	80	1	20	0.02	0.01	0.1	31
Lemon juice																					
Raw	1 cup	244	91	60	1	Tr	Tr	Tr	Tr	0	21	17	15	0.1	303	2	50	0.07	0.02	0.2	112
Canned or bottled, unsweetened	1 cup	244	92	50	1	1	0.1	Tr	0.2	0	16	27	22	0.3	249	[25]51	40	0.10	0.02	0.5	61
	1 tbsp	15	92	5	Tr	Tr	Tr	Tr	Tr	0	1	2	1	Tr	15	[25]3	Tr	0.01	Tr	Tr	4
Frozen, single-strength, unsweetened	6 fl oz	244	92	55	1	1	0.1	Tr	0.2	0	16	20	20	0.3	217	2	30	0.14	0.03	0.3	77

Appendix 1 (Continued)
Nutritive Value of the Edible Part of Food*

Item / Foods, Approximate Measures, Units, and Weight (Weight of Edible Portion Only)		Weight (g)	Water (%)	Food Energy (kcal)	Protein (g)	Fat (g)	Saturated (g)	Monounsaturated (g)	Polyunsaturated (g)	Cholesterol (mg)	Carbohydrate (g)	Calcium (mg)	Phosphorus (mg)	Iron (mg)	Potassium (mg)	Sodium (mg)	Vitamin A Value (IU)	Vitamin A Value (RE)	Thiamine (mg)	Riboflavine (mg)	Niacin (mg)	Ascorbic Acid (mg)
Lime juice																						
Raw	1 cup	246	90	65	1	Tr	Tr	Tr	0.1	0	22	22	17	0.1	268	2	20	2	0.05	0.02	0.2	72
Canned, unsweetened	1 cup	246	93	50	1	1	0.1	0.1	0.2	0	16	30	25	0.6	185	²39	40	4	0.08	0.01	0.4	16
Mangos																						
Raw, without skin and seed (about 1½ per lb with skin and seed)	1	207	82	135	1	1	0.1	0.2	0.1	0	35	21	23	0.3	323	4	8,060	806	0.12	0.12	1.2	57
Melons																						
Raw, without rind and cavity contents																						
Cantaloupe, orange-fleshed (5-in diam, 2⅓ lb, whole, with rind and cavity contents)	½	267	90	95	2	1	0.1	0.1	0.3	0	22	29	45	0.6	825	24	8,610	861	0.10	0.06	1.5	113
Honeydew (6½-in diam., 5¼ lb, whole, with rind and cavity contents)	1/10	129	90	45	1	Tr	Tr	Tr	0.1	0	12	8	13	0.1	350	13	50	5	0.10	0.02	0.8	32
Nectarines																						
Raw, without pits (about 3 per lb with pits)	1	136	86	65	1	1	0.1	0.2	0.3	0	16	7	22	0.2	288	Tr	1,000	100	0.02	0.06	1.3	7
Oranges																						
Raw																						
Whole, without peel and seeds (2⅝-in diam., about 2½ per lb, with peel and seeds)	1	131	87	60	1	Tr	Tr	Tr	Tr	0	15	52	18	0.1	237	Tr	270	27	0.11	0.05	0.4	70
Sections without membranes	1 cup	180	87	85	2	Tr	Tr	Tr	Tr	0	21	72	25	0.2	326	Tr	370	37	0.16	0.07	0.5	96
Orange juice																						
Raw, all varieties	1 cup	248	88	110	2	Tr	0.1	0.1	0.1	0	26	27	42	0.5	496	2	500	50	0.22	0.07	1.0	124
Canned, unsweetened	1 cup	249	89	105	1	Tr	Tr	Tr	0.1	0	25	20	35	1.1	436	5	440	44	0.15	0.07	0.8	86
Chilled	1 cup	249	88	110	2	1	0.1	0.1	0.2	0	25	25	27	0.4	473	2	190	19	0.28	0.05	0.7	82

Food item	Measure																					
Frozen concentrate																						
Undiluted	6 fl oz	213	58	340	5	Tr	0.1	0.1	0.1	0	81	68	121	0.7	1,436	6	59	590	0.60	0.14	1.5	294
Diluted with 3 parts water by volume	1 cup	249	88	110	2	Tr	Tr	Tr	Tr	0	27	22	40	0.2	473	2	19	190	0.20	0.04	0.5	97
Orange and grapefruit juice																						
Canned	1 cup	247	89	105	1	Tr	Tr	Tr	Tr	0	25	20	35	1.1	390	7	29	290	0.14	0.07	0.8	72
Papayas																						
Raw, ½-in cubes	1 cup	140	86	65	1	Tr	Tr	0.1	Tr	0	17	35	12	0.3	247	9	40	400	0.04	0.04	0.5	92
Peaches																						
Raw																						
Whole, 2½-in diam., peeled, pitted (about 4 per lb with peels and pits)	1	87	88	35	1	Tr	Tr	Tr	Tr	0	10	4	10	0.1	171	Tr	47	470	0.01	0.04	0.9	6
Sliced	1 cup	170	88	75	1	Tr	0.1	0.1	0.1	0	19	9	20	0.2	335	Tr	91	910	0.03	0.07	1.7	11
Canned, fruit and liquid																						
Heavy syrup pack	1 cup	256	79	190	1	Tr	0.1	0.1	0.1	0	51	8	28	0.7	236	15	85	850	0.03	0.06	1.6	7
	1 half	81	79	60	Tr	Tr	Tr	Tr	Tr	0	16	2	9	0.2	75	5	27	270	0.01	0.02	0.5	2
Juice pack	1 cup	248	87	110	2	Tr	Tr	Tr	Tr	0	29	15	42	0.7	317	10	94	940	0.02	0.04	1.4	9
	1 half	77	87	35	Tr	Tr	Tr	Tr	Tr	0	9	5	13	0.2	99	3	29	290	0.01	0.01	0.4	3
Peaches																						
Dried																						
Uncooked	1 cup	160	32	380	6	1	0.1	0.4	0.6	0	98	45	190	6.5	1,594	11	346	3,460	Tr	0.34	7.0	8
Cooked, unsweetened, fruit and liquid	1 cup	258	78	200	3	1	0.1	0.2	0.3	0	51	23	98	3.4	826	5	51	510	0.01	0.05	3.9	10
Frozen, sliced, sweetened	10 oz	284	75	265	2	Tr	Tr	0.1	0.2	0	68	9	31	1.1	369	17	81	810	0.04	0.10	1.9	268[21]
	1 cup	250	75	235	2	Tr	0.1	0.1	0.2	0	60	8	28	0.9	325	15	71	710	0.03	0.09	1.6	236[21]
Pears																						
Raw, with skin, cored																						
Bartlett, 2½-in diam (about 2½ per lb with cores and stems)	1	166	84	100	1	1	Tr	0.1	0.1	0	25	18	18	0.4	208	Tr	3	30	0.03	0.07	0.2	7
Bosc, 2½-in diam. (about 3 per lb with cores and stems)	1	141	84	85	1	1	Tr	0.1	0.1	0	21	16	16	0.4	176	Tr	3	30	0.03	0.06	0.1	6
D'Anjou, 3-in diam. (about 2 per lb with cores and stems)	1	200	84	120	1	1	0.2	0.2	0.2	0	30	22	22	0.5	250	Tr	4	40	0.04	0.08	0.2	8
Canned, fruit and liquid																						
Heavy syrup pack	1 cup	255	80	190	1	Tr	Tr	0.1	0.1	0	49	13	18	0.6	166	13	1	10	0.03	0.06	0.6	3
	1 half	79	80	60	Tr	Tr	Tr	Tr	Tr	0	15	4	6	0.2	51	4	Tr	Tr	0.01	0.02	0.2	1
Juice pack	1 cup	248	86	125	1	Tr	Tr	Tr	Tr	0	32	22	30	0.7	238	10	1	10	0.03	0.03	0.5	4
	1 half	77	86	40	Tr	Tr	Tr	Tr	Tr	0	10	7	9	0.2	74	3	Tr	Tr	0.01	0.01	0.2	1
Pineapple																						
Raw, diced	1 cup	155	87	75	1	1	Tr	0.2	0.2	0	19	11	11	0.6	175	2	4	40	0.14	0.06	0.7	24
Canned, fruit and liquid																						
Heavy syrup pack:																						
Crushed, chunks, tidbits	1 cup	255	79	200	1	Tr	Tr	Tr	Tr	0	52	36	18	1.0	265	3	4	40	0.23	0.06	0.7	19
Slices	1	58	79	45	Tr	Tr	Tr	Tr	Tr	0	12	8	4	0.2	60	1	1	10	0.05	0.01	0.2	4

(continued)

Appendix 1 (Continued)
Nutritive Value of the Edible Part of Food*

Item / Foods, Approximate Measures, Units, and Weight (Weight of Edible Portion Only)	Weight (g)	Water (%)	Food Energy (kcal)	Protein (g)	Fat (g)	Fatty Acids Saturated (g)	Monounsaturated (g)	Polyunsaturated (g)	Cholesterol (mg)	Carbohydrate (g)	Calcium (mg)	Phosphorus (mg)	Iron (mg)	Potassium (mg)	Sodium (mg)	Vitamin A Value (IU)	(RE)	Thiamine (mg)	Riboflavin (mg)	Niacin (mg)	Ascorbic Acid (mg)
Juice pack																					
Chunks or tidbits, 1 cup	250	84	150	1	Tr	Tr	Tr	0.1	0	39	35	15	0.7	305	3	100	10	0.24	0.05	0.7	24
Slices, 1	58	84	35	Tr	Tr	Tr	Tr	Tr	0	9	8	3	0.2	71	1	20	2	0.06	0.01	0.2	6
Pineapple juice *Unsweetened, canned*																					
1 cup	250	86	140	1	Tr	Tr	Tr	Tr	0	34	43	20	0.7	335	3	10	1	0.14	0.06	0.6	27
Plantains *Without peel*																					
Raw, 1	179	65	220	2	1	0.3	0.1	0.1	0	57	5	61	1.1	893	7	2,020	202	0.09	0.10	1.2	33
Cooked, boiled, sliced, 1 cup	154	67	180	1	Tr	0.1	Tr	0.1	0	48	3	43	0.9	716	8	1,400	140	0.07	0.08	1.2	17
Plums *Without pits*																					
Raw																					
2⅛-in diam. (about 6½ per lb with pits), 1	66	85	35	1	Tr	Tr	0.3	0.1	0	9	3	7	0.1	114	Tr	210	21	0.03	0.06	0.3	6
1½-in diam. (about 15 per lb with pits), 1	28	85	15	Tr	Tr	Tr	0.1	Tr	0	4	1	3	Tr	48	Tr	90	9	0.01	0.03	0.1	3
Canned, purple, fruit and liquid Heavy syrup pack																					
1 cup	258	76	230	1	Tr	Tr	0.2	0.1	0	60	23	34	2.2	235	49	670	67	0.04	0.10	0.8	1
3	133	76	120	Tr	Tr	Tr	0.1	Tr	0	31	12	17	1.1	121	25	340	34	0.02	0.05	0.4	1
Juice pack																					
1 cup	252	84	145	1	Tr	Tr	Tr	Tr	0	38	25	38	0.9	388	3	2,540	254	0.06	0.15	1.2	7
3	95	84	55	Tr	Tr	Tr	Tr	Tr	0	14	10	14	0.3	146	1	960	96	0.02	0.06	0.4	3
Prunes *Dried*																					
Uncooked, 4 extra large or 5 large	49	32	115	1	Tr	Tr	0.2	0.1	0	31	25	39	1.2	365	2	970	97	0.04	0.08	1.0	2
Cooked, unsweetened, fruit and liquid, 1 cup	212	70	225	2	Tr	Tr	0.3	0.1	0	60	49	74	2.4	708	4	650	65	0.05	0.21	1.5	6
Prune juice *Canned or bottled*																					
1 cup	256	81	180	2	Tr	Tr	0.1	Tr	0	45	31	64	3.0	707	10	10	1	0.04	0.18	2.0	10
Raisins *Seedless*																					
Cup, not pressed down, 1 cup	145	15	435	5	1	0.2	Tr	0.2	0	115	71	141	3.0	1,089	17	10	1	0.23	0.13	1.2	5
Packet, ½ oz (1½ tbsp), 1	14	15	40	Tr	Tr	Tr	Tr	Tr	0	11	7	14	0.3	105	2	Tr	Tr	0.02	0.01	0.1	Tr

	Measure	Weight (g)	Water (%)	Food energy (cal)	Protein (g)	Fat (g)	Saturated (g)	Monounsaturated (g)	Polyunsaturated (g)	Cholesterol (mg)	Carbohydrate (g)	Calcium (mg)	Phosphorus (mg)	Iron (mg)	Potassium (mg)	Sodium (mg)	Vitamin A (IU)	Vitamin A (RE)	Thiamin (mg)	Riboflavin (mg)	Niacin (mg)	Ascorbic acid (mg)
Raspberries																						
Raw	1 cup	123	87	60	1	1	Tr	0.1	0.4	0	14	27	15	0.7	187	Tr	160	16	0.04	0.11	1.1	31
Frozen, sweetened	10 oz	284	73	295	2	Tr	Tr	Tr	0.3	0	74	43	48	1.8	324	3	170	17	0.05	0.13	0.7	47
	1 cup	250	73	255	2	Tr	Tr	Tr	0.2	0	65	38	43	1.6	285	3	150	15	0.05	0.11	0.6	41
Rhubarb																						
Cooked, added sugar	1 cup	240	68	280	1	Tr	Tr	Tr	0.1	0	75	348	19	0.5	230	2	170	17	0.04	0.06	0.5	8
Strawberries																						
Raw, capped, whole	1 cup	149	92	45	1	1	Tr	0.1	0.3	0	10	21	28	0.6	247	1	40	4	0.03	0.10	0.3	84
Frozen, sweetened, sliced	10 oz	284	73	275	2	Tr	Tr	Tr	0.2	0	74	31	37	1.7	278	9	70	7	0.05	0.14	1.1	118
	1 cup	255	73	245	1	Tr	Tr	Tr	0.2	0	66	28	33	1.5	250	8	60	6	0.04	0.13	1.0	106
Tangerines																						
Raw, without peel and seeds (2⅜-in diam., about 4 per lb, with peel and seeds)	1	84	88	35	1	Tr	Tr	Tr	Tr	0	9	12	8	0.1	132	1	770	77	0.09	0.02	0.1	26
Canned, light syrup, fruit and liquid	1 cup	252	83	155	1	Tr	Tr	Tr	0.1	0	41	18	25	0.9	197	15	2,120	212	0.13	0.11	1.1	50
Tangerine juice																						
Canned, sweetened	1 cup	249	87	125	1	Tr	Tr	Tr	0.1	0	30	45	35	0.5	443	2	1,050	105	0.15	0.05	0.2	55
Watermelon																						
Raw, without rind and seeds: Piece (4 by 8 in wedge with rind and seeds; 1/16 or 32⅔-lb melon, 10 by 16 in)	1	482	92	155	3	2	0.3	0.2	1.0	0	35	39	43	0.8	559	10	1,760	176	0.39	0.10	1.0	46
Diced	1 cup	160	92	50	1	1	0.1	0.1	0.3	0	11	13	14	0.3	186	3	590	59	0.13	0.03	0.3	15

GRAIN PRODUCTS

	Measure	Weight (g)	Water (%)	Food energy (cal)	Protein (g)	Fat (g)	Saturated (g)	Monounsaturated (g)	Polyunsaturated (g)	Cholesterol (mg)	Carbohydrate (g)	Calcium (mg)	Phosphorus (mg)	Iron (mg)	Potassium (mg)	Sodium (mg)	Vitamin A (IU)	Vitamin A (RE)	Thiamin (mg)	Riboflavin (mg)	Niacin (mg)	Ascorbic acid (mg)
Bagels																						
Plain or water, enriched, 3½-in diam.[24]	1	68	29	200	7	2	0.3	0.5	0.7	0	38	29	46	1.8	50	245	0	0	0.26	0.20	2.4	0
Barley																						
Pearled, light, uncooked	1 cup	200	11	700	16	2	0.3	0.2	0.9	0	158	32	378	4.2	320	6	0	0	0.24	0.10	6.2	0
Biscuits																						
Baking powder, 2-in diam. *(enriched flour, vegetable shortening):*																						
From home recipe	1	28	28	100	2	5	1.2	2.0	1.3	Tr	13	47	36	0.7	32	195	10	3	0.08	0.08	0.8	Tr
From mix	1	28	29	95	2	3	0.8	1.4	0.9	Tr	14	58	128	0.7	56	262	20	4	0.12	0.11	0.8	Tr
From refrigerated dough	1	20	30	65	1	2	0.6	0.9	0.6	1	10	4	79	0.5	18	249	0	0	0.08	0.05	0.7	0
Breadcrumbs																						
Enriched:																						
Dry, grated	1 cup	100	7	390	13	5	1.5	1.6	1.0	5	73	122	141	4.1	152	736	0	0	0.35	0.35	4.8	0
Soft, See White bread.																						
Breads																						
Boston brown bread, canned, slice, 3¼ in by ½ in[25]	1	45	45	95	2	1	0.3	0.1	0.1	3	21	41	72	0.9	131	113	0[26]	0	0.06	0.04	0.7	0

(continued)

737

Appendix 1 (Continued)
Nutritive Value of the Edible Part of Food*

Item (Foods, Approximate Measures, Units, and Weight — Weight of Edible Portion Only)	Weight (g)	Water (%)	Food Energy (kcal)	Protein (g)	Fat (g)	Saturated (g)	Monounsaturated (g)	Polyunsaturated (g)	Cholesterol (mg)	Carbohydrate (g)	Calcium (mg)	Phosphorus (mg)	Iron (mg)	Potassium (mg)	Sodium (mg)	Vitamin A (IU)	Vitamin A (RE)	Thiamine (mg)	Riboflavine (mg)	Niacin (mg)	Ascorbic Acid (mg)
Cracked-wheat bread (²/₃ enriched wheat flour, ¹/₃ cracked wheat flour)[25]																					
Loaf, 1 lb	454	35	1,190	42	16	3.1	4.3	5.7	0	227	295	581	12.1	608	1,966	Tr	Tr	1.73	1.73	15.3	Tr
Slice (18 per loaf)	25	35	65	2	1	0.2	0.2	0.3	0	12	16	32	0.7	34	106	Tr	Tr	0.10	0.09	0.8	Tr
Toasted	21	26	65	2	1	0.2	0.2	0.3	0	12	16	32	0.7	34	106	Tr	Tr	0.07	0.09	0.8	Tr
French or Vienna bread, enriched[25]																					
Loaf, 1 lb	454	34	1,270	43	18	3.8	5.7	5.9	0	230	499	386	14.0	409	2,633	Tr	Tr	2.09	1.59	18.2	Tr
Slice French, 5 by 2½ by 1 in	35	34	100	3	1	0.3	0.4	0.5	0	18	39	30	1.1	32	203	Tr	Tr	0.16	0.12	1.4	Tr
Vienna, 4¾ by 4 by ½ in	25	34	70	2	1	0.2	0.3	0.3	0	13	28	21	0.8	23	145	Tr	Tr	0.12	0.09	1.0	Tr
Italian bread, enriched																					
Loaf, 1 lb	454	32	1,255	41	4	0.6	0.3	1.6	0	256	77	350	12.7	336	2,656	0	0	1.80	1.10	15.0	0
Slice, 4½ by 3¼ by ¾ in	30	32	85	3	Tr	Tr	Tr	0.1	0	17	5	23	0.8	22	176	0	0	0.12	0.07	1.0	0
Mixed grain bread, enriched[25]																					
Loaf, 1 lb	454	37	1,165	45	17	3.2	4.1	6.5	0	212	472	962	14.8	990	1,870	Tr	Tr	1.77	1.73	18.9	Tr
Slice (18 per loaf)	25	37	65	2	1	0.2	0.2	0.4	0	12	27	55	0.8	56	106	Tr	Tr	0.10	0.10	1.1	Tr
Toasted	23	27	65	2	1	0.2	0.2	0.4	0	12	27	55	0.8	56	106	Tr	Tr	0.08	0.10	1.1	Tr
Oatmeal bread, enriched[25]																					
Loaf, 1 lb	454	37	1,145	38	20	3.7	7.1	8.2	0	212	267	563	12.0	707	2,231	0	0	2.09	1.20	15.4	0
Slice (18 per loaf)	25	37	65	2	1	0.2	0.4	0.5	0	12	15	31	0.7	39	124	0	0	0.12	0.07	0.9	0
Toasted	23	30	65	2	1	0.2	0.4	0.5	0	12	15	31	0.7	39	124	0	0	0.09	0.07	0.9	0
Pita bread, enriched, white, 6½-in diam.	60	31	165	6	1	0.1	0.1	0.4	0	33	49	60	1.4	71	339	0	0	0.27	0.12	2.2	0
Pumpernickel (²/₃ rye flour, ¹/₃ enriched wheat flour)[25]																					
Loaf, 1 lb	454	37	1,160	42	16	2.6	3.6	6.4	0	218	322	990	12.4	1,966	2,461	0	0	1.54	2.36	15.0	0
Slice, 5 by 4 by ⅜ in	32	37	80	3	1	0.2	0.3	0.5	0	16	23	71	0.9	141	177	0	0	0.11	0.17	1.1	0
Toasted	29	28	80	3	1	0.2	0.3	0.5	0	16	23	71	0.9	141	177	0	0	0.09	0.17	1.1	0

(continued)

Food	Measure	Grams	Water (%)	Food energy (cal)	Protein (g)	Fat (g)	Saturated (g)	Monounsat. (g)	Polyunsat. (g)	Cholesterol (mg)	Carbohydrate (g)	Calcium (mg)	Phosphorus (mg)	Iron (mg)	Potassium (mg)	Sodium (mg)	Vitamin A (IU)	Thiamin (mg)	Riboflavin (mg)	Niacin (mg)	Ascorbic acid (mg)
Raisin bread, enriched[25]																					
Loaf, 1 lb	1	454	33	1,260	37	18	4.1	6.5	6.7	0	239	463	395	14.1	1,058	1,657	Tr	1.50	2.81	18.6	Tr
Slice (18 per loaf)	1	25	33	65	2	1	0.2	0.3	0.4	0	13	25	22	0.8	59	92	Tr	0.08	0.15	1.0	Tr
Toasted	1	21	24	65	2	1	0.2	0.3	0.4	0	13	25	22	0.8	59	92	Tr	0.06	0.15	1.0	Tr
Rye bread, light (²⁄₃ enriched wheat flour, ¹⁄₃ rye flour)[25]																					
Loaf, 1 lb	1	454	37	1,190	38	17	3.3	5.2	5.5	0	218	363	658	12.3	926	3,164	0	1.86	1.45	15.0	0
Slice, 4¾ by 3¾ by 7/16 in	1	25	37	65	2	1	0.2	0.3	0.3	0	12	20	36	0.7	51	175	0	0.10	0.08	0.8	0
Toasted	1	22	28	65	2	1	0.2	0.3	0.3	0	12	20	36	0.7	51	175	0	0.08	0.08	0.8	0
Wheat bread, enriched[25]																					
Loaf, 1 lb	1	454	37	1,160	43	19	3.9	7.3	4.5	0	213	572	835	15.8	627	2,447	Tr	2.09	1.45	20.5	Tr
Slice (18 per loaf)	1	25	37	65	2	1	0.2	0.4	0.3	0	12	32	47	0.9	35	138	Tr	0.12	0.08	1.2	Tr
Toasted	1	23	28	65	3	1	0.2	0.4	0.3	0	12	32	47	0.9	35	138	Tr	0.10	0.08	1.2	Tr
White bread, enriched[25]																					
Loaf, 1 lb	1	454	37	1,210	38	18	5.6	6.5	4.2	0	222	572	490	12.9	508	2,334	Tr	2.13	1.41	17.0	Tr
Slice (18 per loaf)	1	25	37	65	2	1	0.3	0.4	0.2	0	12	32	27	0.7	28	129	Tr	0.12	0.08	0.9	Tr
Toasted	1	22	28	65	2	1	0.3	0.4	0.2	0	12	32	27	0.7	28	129	Tr	0.09	0.08	0.9	Tr
Slice (22 per loaf)	1	20	37	55	2	1	0.2	0.3	0.2	0	10	25	21	0.6	22	101	Tr	0.09	0.06	0.7	Tr
Toasted	1	17	28	55	2	1	0.2	0.3	0.2	0	10	25	21	0.6	22	101	Tr	0.07	0.06	0.7	Tr
Cubes	1 cup	30	37	80	2	1	0.4	0.4	0.3	0	15	38	32	0.9	34	154	Tr	0.14	0.09	1.1	Tr
Crumbs, soft	1 cup	45	37	120	4	2	0.6	0.6	0.4	0	22	57	49	1.3	50	231	Tr	0.21	0.14	1.7	Tr
Whole-wheat bread[25]																					
Loaf, 1 lb	1	454	38	1,110	44	20	5.8	6.8	5.2	0	206	327	1,180	15.5	799	2,887	Tr	1.59	0.95	17.4	Tr
Slice (16 per loaf)	1	28	38	70	3	1	0.4	0.4	0.3	0	13	20	74	1.0	74	180	Tr	0.10	0.06	1.1	Tr
Toasted	1	25	29	70	3	1	0.4	0.4	0.3	0	13	20	74	1.0	74	180	Tr	0.08	0.06	1.1	Tr
Bread stuffing (from enriched bread), prepared from mix																					
Dry type	1 cup	140	33	500	9	31	6.1	13.3	9.6	0	50	92	136	2.2	126	1,254	910	0.17	0.20	2.5	0
Moist type	1 cup	203	61	420	9	26	5.3	11.3	8.0	67	40	81	134	2.0	118	1,023	850	0.10	0.18	1.6	0
Breakfast cereals																					
Hot type, cooked																					
Corn (hominy) grits																					
Regular and quick, enriched	1 cup	242	85	143	3	Tr	Tr	0.1	0.2	0	31	0	29	[27]1.5	53	[29]0	[29]0	[27]0.24	[27]0.15	[27]2.0	0
Instant, plain	1 pkt	137	85	80	2	Tr	Tr	Tr	0.1	0	18	7	16	[27]1.0	29	343	0	[27]0.18	[27]0.08	[27]1.3	0
Cream of Wheat																					
Regular, quick, instant	1 cup	244	86	140	4	Tr	0.1	Tr	0.2	0	29	[30]54	[31,35]43	[30]10.9	46	0	0	[27]0.24	[30]0.07	[30]1.5	0
Mix'n Eat, plain	1 pkt	142	82	100	3	Tr	Tr	Tr	0.1	0	21	[30]20	[30]20	[30]8.1	38	[30]1,250	[30]1,335	[30]0.43	[30]0.28	[30]5.0	0
Malt-O-Meal	1 cup	240	88	120	4	Tr	Tr	Tr	0.1	0	26	5	24	[30]9.6	31	0	[30]2	[30]0.48	[30]0.24	[30]5.8	0
Oatmeal or rolled oats																					
Regular, quick, instant, nonfortified	1 cup	234	85	145	6	2	0.4	0.8	1.0	0	25	19	178	16	131	1	40	0.26	0.05	0.3	0
Instant, fortified																					
Plain	1 pkt	177	86	105	4	2	0.3	0.6	0.7	0	18	[27]163	133	[27]6.3	99	[27]1,510	[27]453	[27]0.53	[27]0.28	[27]5.5	0
Flavored	1 pkt	164	76	160	5	2	0.3	0.7	0.8	0	31	[27]168	148	[27]6.7	137	[27]1,530	[27]460	[27]0.53	[27]0.38	[27]5.9	Tr

Nutritive Value of the Edible Part of Food*

Fatty Acids

Item	Measure	Weight (g)	Water (%)	Food Energy (kcal)	Protein (g)	Fat (g)	Saturated (g)	Monounsaturated (g)	Polyunsaturated (g)	Cholesterol (mg)	Carbohydrate (g)	Calcium (mg)	Phosphorus (mg)	Iron (mg)	Potassium (mg)	Sodium (mg)	Vitamin A Value (IU)	Vitamin A Value (RE)	Thiamine (mg)	Riboflavine (mg)	Niacin (mg)	Ascorbic Acid (mg)
Ready to eat																						
All-Bran (about 1/3 cup)	1 oz	28	3	70	4	1	0.1	0.1	0.3	0	21	23	264	[30]4.5	350	320	[30]1,250	[30]375	[30]0.37	[30]0.43	[30]5.0	[30]15
Cap'n Crunch (about 3/4 cup)	1 oz	28	3	120	1	3	1.7	0.3	0.4	0	23	5	36	[27]7.5	37	213	40	4	[27]0.50	[27]0.55	[27]6.6	0
Cheerios (about 1 1/4 cup)	1 oz	28	5	110	4	2	0.3	0.6	0.7	0	20	48	134	[30]4.5	101	307	[30]1,250	[30]375	[30]0.37	[30]0.43	[30]5.0	[30]15
Corn Flakes (about 1 1/4 cup)																						
Kellogg's	1 oz	28	3	110	2	Tr	Tr	Tr	Tr	0	24	1	18	[30]1.8	26	351	[30]1,250	[30]375	[30]0.37	[30]0.43	[30]5.0	15
Toasties	1 oz	28	3	110	2	Tr	Tr	Tr	Tr	0	24	1	12	[27]0.7	33	297	[30]1,250	[30]375	[30]0.37	[30]0.43	[30]5.0	0
40% Bran Flakes																						
Kellogg's (about 3/4 cup)	1 oz	28	3	90	4	1	0.1	0.1	0.3	0	22	14	139	[30]8.1	180	264	[30]1,250	[30]375	[30]0.37	[30]0.43	[30]5.0	0
Post (about 2/3 cup)	1 oz	28	3	90	3	Tr	0.1	0.1	0.2	0	22	12	179	[30]4.5	151	260	[30]1,250	[30]375	[30]0.37	[30]0.43	[30]5.0	0
Fruit Loops (about 1 cup)	1 oz	28	3	110	2	1	0.2	0.1	0.1	0	25	3	24	[30]4.5	26	145	[30]1,250	[30]375	[30]0.37	[30]0.43	[30]5.0	[30]15
Golden Grahams (about 3/4 cup)	1 oz	28	2	110	2	1	0.7	0.1	0.2	Tr	24	17	41	[30]4.5	63	346	[30]1,250	[30]375	[30]0.37	[30]0.43	[30]5.0	[30]15
Grape-Nuts (about 1/4 cup)	1 oz	28	3	100	3	Tr	Tr	Tr	0.1	0	23	11	71	1.2	95	197	[30]1,250	[30]375	[30]0.37	[30]0.43	[30]5.0	0
Honey Nut Cheerios (about 3/4 cup)	1 oz	28	3	105	3	1	0.1	0.3	0.3	0	23	20	105	[30]4.5	99	257	[30]1,250	[30]375	[30]0.37	[30]0.43	[30]5.0	[30]15
Lucky Charms (about 1 cup)	1 oz	28	3	110	3	1	0.2	0.4	0.4	0	23	32	79	[0]4.5	59	201	[30]1,250	[30]375	[30]0.37	[30]0.43	[30]5.0	[30]15
Nature Valley Granola (about 1/3 cup)	1 oz	28	4	125	3	5	3.3	0.7	0.7	0	19	18	89	0.9	98	58	20	2	0.10	0.05	0.2	0
100% Natural Cereal (about 1/4 cup)	1 oz	28	2	135	3	6	4.1	1.2	0.5	Tr	18	49	104	0.8	140	12	20	2	0.09	0.15	0.6	0
Product 19 (about 3/4 cup)	1 oz	28	3	110	3	Tr	Tr	Tr	0.1	0	24	3	40	[30]18.0	44	325	[30]5,000	[30]1,501	[30]1.50	[30]1.70	[30]20.0	[30]60
Raisin Bran																						
Kellogg's (about 3/4 cup)	1 oz	28	8	90	3	1	0.1	0.1	0.3	0	21	10	105	[30]3.5	147	207	[30]960	[30]288	[30]0.28	[30]0.34	[30]3.9	0
Post (about 1/2 cup)	1 oz	28	9	85	3	1	0.1	0.1	0.3	0	21	13	119	[30]4.5	175	185	[30]1,250	[30]375	[30]0.37	[30]0.43	[30]5.0	0
Rice Krispies (about 1 cup)	1 oz	28	2	110	2	Tr	Tr	Tr	0.1	0	25	4	34	[30]1.8	29	340	[30]1,250	[30]375	[30]0.37	[30]0.43	[30]5.0	[30]15
Shredded Wheat (about 2/3 cup)	1 oz	28	5	100	3	1	0.1	0.1	0.3	0	23	11	100	1.2	102	3	0	0	0.07	0.08	1.5	0
Special K (about 1 1/3 cup)	1 oz	28	2	110	6	Tr	Tr	Tr	Tr	Tr	21	8	55	[30]4.5	49	265	[30]1,250	[30]375	[30]0.37	[30]0.43	[30]5.0	[30]15
Sugar Frosted Flakes, Kellogg's (about 3/4 cup)	1 oz	28	3	110	1	Tr	Tr	Tr	Tr	0	26	1	21	[30]1.8	18	230	[30]1,250	[30]375	[30]0.37	[30]0.43	[30]5.0	[30]15
Sugar Smacks (about 3/4 cup)	1 oz	28	3	105	2	1	0.1	0.1	0.2	0	25	3	31	[30]1.8	42	75	[30]1,250	[30]375	[30]0.37	[30]0.43	[30]5.0	[30]15
Super Sugar Crisp (about 7/8 cup)	1 oz	28	2	105	2	Tr	Tr	Tr	0.1	0	26	6	52	[30]1.8	105	25	[30]1,250	[30]375	[30]0.37	[30]0.43	[30]5.0	0

Food	Measure	Weight (g)	Water (%)	Energy (cal)	Protein (g)	Fat (g)	Satur. (g)	Mono. (g)	Poly. (g)	Cholest. (mg)	Carb. (g)	Calcium (mg)	Phos. (mg)	Iron (mg)	Potas. (mg)	Sodium (mg)	Vit A (IU)	Vit A (RE)	Thiamin (mg)	Ribo. (mg)	Niacin (mg)	Asc. acid (mg)
Total (about 1 cup)	1 oz	28	4	100	3	1	0.1	0.1	0.3	0	22	48	118	[30]18.0	106	352	[30]5,000	[30]1,501	[30]1.50	[30]1.70	[30]20.0	[30]60
Trix (about 1 cup)	1 oz	28	3	110	2	2	0.2	0.1	0.1	0	25	6	19	[30]4.5	27	181	[30]1,250	[30]375	[30].37	[30].43	[30]5.0	[30]15
Wheaties (about 1 cup)	1 oz	28	5	100	3	1	0.1	Tr	0.2	0	23	43	98	[30]4.5	106	354	[30]1,250	[30]375	[30].37	[30].43	[30]5.0	[30]15
Buckwheat flour Light, sifted	1 cup	98	12	340	6	1	0.2	0.4	0.4	0	78	11	86	1.0	314	2	0	0	0.08	0.04	0.4	0
Bulgur Uncooked	1 cup	170	10	600	19	3	1.2	0.3	1.2	0	129	49	575	9.5	389	7	0	0	0.48	0.24	7.7	0
Cakes prepared from cake mixes with enriched flour[33] *Angel food* Whole cake, 9¾-in diam. tube cake	1	635	38	1,510	27	2	0.4	0.2	1.0	0	342	527	1,086	2.7	845	3,226	0	0	0.32	1.27	1.6	0
Piece, 1/12 of cake	1	53	38	125	5	Tr	Tr	Tr	0.1	0	29	44	91	0.2	71	269	0	0	0.03	0.11	0.1	0
Coffeecake, crumb Whole cake, 7¾ by 5⅝ by 1¼ in	1	430	30	1,385	27	41	11.8	16.7	9.6	279	225	262	748	7.3	469	1,853	690	194	0.82	0.90	7.7	1
Piece, 1/6 of cake	1	72	30	230	5	7	2.0	2.8	1.6	47	38	44	125	1.2	78	310	120	32	0.14	0.15	1.3	Tr
Devil's food with chocolate frosting Whole, 2-layer cake, 8- or 9-in diam.	1	1,107	24	3,755	49	136	55.6	51.4	19.7	598	645	653	1,162	22.1	1,439	2,900	1,660	498	1.11	1.66	10.0	1
Piece, 1/16 of cake	1	69	24	235	3	8	3.5	3.2	1.2	37	40	41	72	1.4	90	181	100	31	0.07	0.10	0.6	Tr
Cupcake, 2½-in diam.	1	35	24	120	2	4	1.8	1.6	0.6	19	20	21	37	0.7	46	92	50	16	0.04	0.05	0.3	Tr
Gingerbread Whole cake, 8 in square	1	570	37	1,575	18	39	9.6	16.4	10.5	6	291	513	570	10.8	1,562	1,733	0	0	0.86	1.03	7.4	1
Piece, 1/9 of cake	1	63	37	175	2	4	1.1	1.8	1.2	1	32	57	63	1.2	173	192	0	0	0.09	0.11	0.8	Tr
Cakes prepared from cake mixes with enriched flour[35] *Yellow with chocolate frosting* Whole, 2-layer cake, 8- or 9-in diam.	1	1,108	26	3,735	45	125	47.8	48.8	21.8	576	638	1,008	2,017	15.5	1,208	2,515	1,550	465	1.22	1.66	11.1	1
Piece, 1/16 of cake	1	69	26	235	3	8	3.0	3.0	1.4	36	40	63	126	1.0	75	157	100	29	0.08	0.10	0.7	Tr
Cakes prepared from home recipes using enriched flour *Carrot, with cream cheese frosting[36]* Whole cake, 10-in diam. tube cake	1	1,536	23	6,175	63	328	66.0	135.2	107.5	1183	775	707	998	21.0	1,720	4,470	2,240	246	1.83	1.97	14.7	23
Piece, 1/16 of cake	1	96	23	385	4	21	4.1	8.4	6.7	74	48	44	62	1.3	108	279	140	15	0.11	0.12	0.9	1
Fruitcake, dark[36] Whole cake, 7½-in diam., 2¼-in high tube cake	1	1,361	18	5,185	74	228	47.6	113.0	51.7	640	783	1,293	1,592	37.6	6,138	2,123	1,720	422	2.41	2.55	17.0	504
Piece, 1/32 of cake, ⅔-in arc	1	43	18	165	2	7	1.5	3.6	1.6	20	25	41	50	1.2	194	67	50	13	0.08	0.08	0.5	16

(continued)

Appendix 1 (Continued)
Nutritive Value of the Edible Part of Food*

Item (Foods, Approximate Measures, Units, and Weight — Weight of Edible Portion Only)		Weight (g)	Water (%)	Food Energy (kcal)	Protein (g)	Fat (g)	Saturated (g)	Monounsaturated (g)	Polyunsaturated (g)	Cholesterol (mg)	Carbohydrate (g)	Calcium (mg)	Phosphorus (mg)	Iron (mg)	Potassium (mg)	Sodium (mg)	Vitamin A Value (IU)	Vitamin A Value (RE)	Thiamine (mg)	Riboflavine (mg)	Niacin (mg)	Ascorbic Acid (mg)
Plain sheet cake[37]																						
Without frosting																						
Whole cake, 9-in square	1	777	25	2,830	35	108	29.5	45.1	25.6	552	434	497	793	11.7	614	2,331	1,320	373	1.24	1.40	10.1	2
Piece, 1/9 of cake	1	86	25	315	4	12	3.3	5.0	2.8	61	48	55	88	1.3	68	258	150	41	0.14	0.15	1.1	Tr
With uncooked white frosting																						
Whole cake, 9-in square	1	1,096	21	4,020	37	129	41.6	50.4	26.3	636	694	548	822	11.0	669	2,488	2,190	647	1.21	1.42	9.9	2
Piece, 1/9 of cake	1	121	21	445	4	14	4.6	5.6	2.9	70	77	61	91	1.2	74	275	240	71	0.13	0.16	1.1	Tr
Pound[38]																						
Loaf, 8½ by 3½ by 3¼ in	1	514	22	2,025	33	94	21.1	40.9	26.7	555	265	339	473	9.3	483	1,645	3,470	1,033	0.93	1.08	7.8	1
Slice, 1/17 of loaf	1	30	22	120	2	5	1.2	2.4	1.6	32	15	20	28	0.5	28	96	200	60	0.05	0.06	0.5	Tr
Cakes, commercial, made with enriched flavor																						
Pound																						
Loaf, 8½ by 3½ by 3 in	1	500	24	1,935	26	94	52.0	30.0	4.0	1100	257	146	517	8.0	443	1,857	2,820	715	0.96	1.12	8.1	0
Slice, 1/17 of loaf	1	29	24	110	2	5	3.0	1.7	0.2	64	15	8	30	0.5	26	108	160	41	0.06	0.06	0.5	0
Snack cakes																						
Devil's food with creme filling (2 small cakes per pkg)	1	28	20	105	1	4	1.7	1.5	0.6	15	17	21	26	1.0	34	105	20	4	0.06	0.09	0.7	0
Sponge with creme filling (2 small cakes per pkg)	1	42	19	155	1	5	2.3	2.1	0.5	7	27	14	44	0.6	37	155	30	9	0.07	0.06	0.6	0
White with white frosting																						
Whole cake, 2-layer cake, 8- or 9-in diam.	1	1,140	24	4,170	43	148	33.1	61.6	42.2	46	670	536	1,585	15.5	832	2,827	640	194	3.19	2.05	27.6	0
Piece, 1/16 of cake	1	71	24	260	3	9	2.1	3.8	2.6	3	42	33	99	1.0	52	176	40	12	0.20	0.13	1.7	0
Yellow with chocolate frosting																						
Whole cake, 2-layer cake, 8- or 9-in diam.	1	1,108	23	3,895	40	175	92.0	58.7	10.0	609	620	366	1,884	19.9	1,972	3,080	1,850	488	0.78	2.22	10.0	0
Piece, 1/16 of cake	1	69	23	245	2	11	5.7	3.7	0.6	38	39	23	117	1.2	123	192	120	30	0.05	0.14	0.6	0
Cheesecake																						
Whole cake, 9-in diam.	1	1,110	46	3,350	60	213	119.9	65.5	14.4	2053	317	622	977	5.3	1,088	2,464	2,820	833	0.33	1.44	5.1	56
Piece, 1/12 of cake	1	92	46	280	5	18	9.9	5.4	1.2	170	26	52	81	0.4	90	204	230	69	0.03	0.12	0.4	5

(continued)

Cookies made with enriched flour

Brownies with nuts

Food	Measure	Grams	Water (%)	Food energy (cal)	Protein (g)	Fat (g)	Saturated (g)	Monounsat. (g)	Polyunsat. (g)	Cholesterol (mg)	Carbohydrate (g)	Calcium (mg)	Phosphorus (mg)	Iron (mg)	Potassium (mg)	Sodium (mg)	Vit. A (IU)	Vit. A (RE)	Thiamin (mg)	Riboflavin (mg)	Niacin (mg)	Ascorbic (mg)
Commercial with frosting, 1½ by 1¾ by ⅞ in	1	25	13	100	1	4	1.6	2.0	0.6	14	16	13	26	0.6	50	59	70	18	0.08	0.07	0.3	Tr
From home recipe, 1¾ by 1¾ by ⅞ in[36]	1	20	10	95	1	6	1.4	2.8	1.2	18	11	9	26	0.4	35	51	20	6	0.05	0.05	0.3	Tr
Chocolate chip Commercial, 2¼-in diam., ⅜ in thick	4	42	4	180	2	9	2.9	3.1	2.6	5	28	13	41	0.8	68	140	50	15	0.10	0.23	1.0	Tr
Chocolate chip From home recipe, 2⅓-in diam.[25]	4	40	3	185	2	11	3.9	4.3	2.0	18	26	13	34	1.0	82	82	20	5	0.06	0.06	0.6	0
From refrigerated dough, 2¼-diam., ⅜ in thick	4	48	5	225	2	11	4.0	4.4	2.0	22	32	13	34	1.0	62	173	30	8	0.06	0.10	0.9	0
Fig bars, square, 1⅝ by 1⅝ by ⅜ in or rectangular, 1½ by 1¾ by ½ in	4	56	12	210	2	4	1.0	1.5	1.0	27	42	40	34	1.4	162	180	60	6	0.08	0.06	0.7	Tr
Oatmeal with raisins, 2⅝-in diam., ¼ in thick	4	52	4	245	3	10	2.5	4.5	2.8	2	36	18	58	1.4	90	148	40	12	0.09	0.06	1.0	0
Peanut butter cookie, from home recipe, 2⅝-in diam.[25]	4	48	3	245	3	14	4.0	5.8	2.8	22	28	21	60	1.1	110	142	20	5	0.07	0.07	1.9	0
Sandwich type (chocolate or vanilla), 1¾-in diam., ⅜ in thick	4	40	2	195	2	8	2.0	3.6	2.2	0	29	28	28	1.4	66	189	0	0	0.09	0.07	0.8	0
Shortbread Commercial	4	32	6	155	2	8	2.9	3.0	1.1	27	20	13	39	0.8	38	123	30	8	0.10	0.09	0.9	0
From home recipe[38]	2	28	3	145	2	8	1.3	2.7	3.4	0	17	6	31	0.6	18	125	300	89	0.08	0.06	0.7	Tr
Sugar cookie, from refrigerated dough, 2½-in diam., ¼ in thick	4	48	4	235	2	12	2.3	5.0	3.6	29	31	35	52	0.9	33	261	40	11	0.09	0.06	1.1	0
Vanilla wafers, 1¾-in diam., ¼ in thick	10	40	4	185	2	7	1.8	3.0	1.8	25	29	16	36	0.8	50	150	50	14	0.07	0.10	1.0	0
Corn chips	1 oz	28	1	155	1	9	1.4	2.4	3.7	0	16	36	52	0.5	52	233	110	11	0.04	0.05	0.4	1
Cornmeal *Whole-ground, unbolted, dry form*	1 cup	122	12	435	11	5	0.5	1.1	2.5	0	90	24	312	2.2	346	1	620	62	0.46	0.13	2.4	0
Bolted (nearly whole-grain), dry form	1 cup	122	12	440	11	5	0.5	0.9	2.2	0	91	21	272	2.2	303	1	590	59	0.37	0.10	2.3	0
Degermed, enriched Dry form	1 cup	138	12	500	11	2	0.2	0.4	0.9	0	108	8	137	5.9	166	1	610	61	0.61	0.36	4.8	0
Cooked	1 cup	240	88	120	3	Tr	Tr	0.1	0.2	0	26	2	34	1.4	38	0	140	14	0.14	0.10	1.2	0
Crackers[39] *Cheese* Plain, 1 in square	10	10	4	50	1	3	0.9	1.2	0.3	6	6	11	17	0.3	17	112	20	5	0.05	0.04	0.4	0
Sandwich type (peanut butter)	1	8	3	40	2	1	0.4	0.8	0.3	1	5	7	25	0.3	17	90	Tr	Tr	0.04	0.03	0.6	0
Graham, plain, 2½ in square	2	14	5	60	1	1	0.4	0.6	0.4	0	11	6	20	0.4	36	86	0	0	0.02	0.03	0.6	0

Item	Foods, Approximate Measures, Units, and Weight (Weight of Edible Portion Only)	Weight (g)	Water (%)	Food Energy (kcal)	Protein (g)	Fat (g)	Fatty Acids Saturated (g)	Monounsaturated (g)	Polyunsaturated (g)	Cholesterol (mg)	Carbohydrate (g)	Calcium (mg)	Phosphorus (mg)	Iron (mg)	Potassium (mg)	Sodium (mg)	Vitamin A Value (IU)	(RE)	Thiamine (mg)	Riboflavine (mg)	Niacin (mg)	Ascorbic Acid (mg)
Melba toast, plain	1	5	4	20	1	Tr	0.1	0.1	0.1	0	4	6	10	0.1	11	44	0	0	0.01	0.01	0.1	0
Rye wafers, whole-grain, 1⅞ by 3½ in	2	14	5	55	1	1	0.3	0.4	0.3	0	10	7	44	0.5	65	115	0	0	0.06	0.03	0.5	0
Saltines[a]	4	12	4	50	1	1	0.5	0.4	0.2	4	9	3	12	0.5	17	165	0	0	0.06	0.05	0.6	0
Snack-type, standard	1	3	3	15	Tr	1	0.2	0.4	0.1	0	2	3	6	0.1	4	30	Tr	Tr	0.01	0.01	0.1	0
Wheat, thin	4	8	3	35	1	1	0.5	0.5	0.4	0	5	3	15	0.3	17	69	Tr	Tr	0.04	0.03	0.4	0
Whole-wheat wafers	2	8	4	35	1	2	0.5	0.6	0.4	0	5	3	22	0.2	31	59	0	0	0.02	0.03	0.4	0
Croissants																						
Made with enriched flour, 4½ by 4 by 1¾ in	1	57	22	235	5	12	3.5	6.7	1.4	13	27	20	64	2.1	68	452	50	13	0.17	0.13	1.3	0
Danish pastry																						
Made with enriched flour																						
Plain without fruit or nuts																						
Packaged ring, 12 oz	1	340	27	1,305	21	71	21.8	28.6	15.6	292	152	360	347	6.5	316	1,302	360	99	0.95	1.02	8.5	Tr
Round piece, about 4¼-in diam., 1 in high	1	57	27	220	4	12	3.6	4.8	2.6	49	26	60	58	1.1	53	218	60	17	0.16	0.17	1.4	Tr
Ounce	1 oz	28	27	110	2	6	1.8	2.4	1.3	24	13	30	29	0.5	26	109	30	8	0.08	0.09	0.7	Tr
Fruit, round piece	1	65	30	235	4	13	3.9	5.2	2.9	56	28	17	80	1.3	57	233	40	11	0.16	0.14	1.4	Tr
Doughnuts																						
Made with enriched flour																						
Cake type, plain, 3⅓-in diam., 1 in high	1	50	21	210	3	12	2.8	5.0	3.0	20	24	22	111	1.0	58	192	20	5	0.12	0.12	1.1	Tr
Yeast-leavened, glazed, 3¾-in diam., 1¼ in high	1	60	27	235	4	13	5.2	5.5	0.9	21	26	17	55	1.4	64	222	Tr	Tr	0.28	0.12	1.8	0
English muffins																						
Plain, enriched	1	57	42	140	5	1	0.3	0.2	0.3	0	27	96	67	1.7	331	378	0	0	0.26	0.19	2.2	0
Toasted	1	50	29	140	5	1	0.3	0.2	0.3	0	27	96	67	1.7	331	378	0	0	0.23	0.19	2.2	0
French toast																						
From home recipe	1	65	53	155	6	7	1.6	2.0	1.6	112	17	72	85	1.3	86	257	110	32	0.12	0.16	1.0	Tr

Macaroni
Enriched, cooked (cut lengths, elbows, shells)

Food	Measure																			
Firm stage (hot)	1 cup	130	64	190	7	1	0.1	0.1	0.3	0	39	14	85	2.1	103	1	0	0.23	0.13	1.8	0
Tender stage																					
Cold	1 cup	105	72	115	4	Tr	0.1	0.1	0.1	0	24	8	53	1.3	64	1	0	0.15	0.08	1.2	0
Hot	1 cup	140	72	155	5	1	0.1	0.1	0.2	0	32	11	70	1.7	85	1	0	0.20	0.11	1.5	0

Muffins made with enriched flour
2½-in diam., 1½ in high

Food	Measure																			
From home recipe																					
Blueberry[25]	1	45	37	135	3	5	1.5	2.1	1.2	19	20	54	46	0.9	47	198	9	0.10	0.11	0.9	1
Bran[34]	1	45	35	125	3	6	1.4	1.6	2.3	24	19	60	125	1.4	99	189	30	0.11	0.13	1.3	3
Corn (enriched, degermed cornmeal and flour)[25]	1	45	33	145	3	5	1.5	2.2	1.4	23	21	66	59	0.9	57	169	80	0.11	0.11	0.9	Tr
From commercial mix (egg and water added)																					
Blueberry	1	45	33	140	3	5	1.4	2.0	1.2	45	22	15	90	0.9	54	225	11	0.10	0.17	1.1	Tr
Bran	1	45	28	140	4	4	1.3	1.6	1.0	28	24	27	182	1.7	50	385	14	0.08	0.12	1.9	0
Corn	1	45	30	145	3	6	1.7	2.3	1.4	42	22	30	128	1.3	31	291	16	0.09	0.09	0.8	Tr

Noodles

Food	Measure																			
(Egg noodles), enriched, cooked	1 cup	160	70	200	7	2	0.5	0.6	0.6	50	37	16	94	2.6	70	3	110	0.22	0.13	1.9	0
Chow mein, canned	1 cup	45	11	220	6	11	2.1	7.3	0.4	5	26	14	41	0.4	33	450	0	0.05	0.03	0.6	0

Pancakes, 4-in diam.

Food	Measure																			
Buckwheat, from mix (with buckwheat and enriched flours), egg and milk added	1	27	58	55	2	2	0.9	0.9	0.5	20	6	59	91	0.4	66	125	60	0.04	0.05	0.2	Tr
Plain																					
From home recipe using enriched flour	1	27	50	60	2	2	0.5	0.8	0.5	16	9	27	38	0.5	33	115	10	0.06	0.07	0.5	Tr
From mix (with enriched flour), egg, milk, and oil added	1	27	54	60	2	2	0.5	0.9	0.5	16	8	36	71	0.7	43	160	7	0.09	0.12	0.8	Tr

Piecrust
Made with enriched flour and vegetable shortening, baked

Food	Measure																			
From home recipe, 9-in diam.	1 piecrust for 2-crust pie	180	15	900	11	60	14.8	25.9	15.7	0	79	25	90	4.5	90	1,100	0	0.54	0.40	5.0	0
From mix, 9-in diam.	1 piecrust for 2-crust pie	320	19	1,485	20	93	22.7	41.0	25.0	0	141	131	272	9.3	179	2,602	0	1.06	0.80	9.9	0

Pies, piecrust made with enriched flour, vegetable shortening, 9-in diam.

Apple

Food	Measure																			
Whole	1	945	48	2,420	21	105	27.4	44.4	26.5	0	360	76	206	9.5	756	2,844	280	1.04	0.76	9.5	9
Piece, ⅙ of pie	1	158	48	405	3	18	4.6	7.4	4.4	0	60	13	35	1.6	126	476	50	0.17	0.13	1.6	2

(continued)

Nutritive Value of the Edible Part of Food*

Item / Foods, Approximate Measures, Units, and Weight (Weight of Edible Portion Only)	Weight (g)	Water (%)	Food Energy (kcal)	Protein (g)	Fat (g)	Fatty Acids Saturated (g)	Monounsaturated (g)	Polyunsaturated (g)	Cholesterol (mg)	Carbohydrate (g)	Calcium (mg)	Phosphorus (mg)	Iron (mg)	Potassium (mg)	Sodium (mg)	Vitamin A Value (IU)	(RE)	Thiamine (mg)	Riboflavine (mg)	Niacin (mg)	Ascorbic Acid (mg)
Blueberry																					
Whole, 1	945	51	2,285	23	102	25.5	44.4	27.4	0	330	104	217	12.3	945	2,533	850	85	1.04	0.85	10.4	38
Piece, 1/6 of pie, 1	158	51	380	4	17	4.3	7.4	4.6	0	55	17	36	2.1	158	423	140	14	0.17	0.14	1.7	6
Cherry																					
Whole, 1	945	47	2,465	25	107	28.4	46.3	27.4	0	363	132	236	9.5	992	2,873	4,160	416	1.13	0.85	9.5	0
Piece, 1/6 of pie, 1	158	47	410	4	18	4.7	7.7	4.6	0	61	22	40	1.6	166	480	700	70	0.19	0.14	1.6	0
Creme																					
Whole, 1	910	43	2,710	20	139	90.1	23.7	6.4	46	351	273	919	6.8	796	2,207	1,250	391	0.36	0.89	6.4	0
Piece, 1/6 of pie, 1	152	43	455	3	23	15.0	4.0	1.1	8	59	46	154	1.1	133	369	210	65	0.06	0.15	1.1	0
Custard																					
Whole, 1	910	58	1,985	56	101	33.7	40.0	19.1	1010	213	874	1,028	9.1	1,247	2,612	2,090	573	0.82	1.91	5.5	0
Piece, 1/6 of pie, 1	152	58	330	9	17	5.6	6.7	3.2	169	36	146	172	1.5	208	436	350	96	0.14	0.32	0.9	0
Lemon meringue																					
Whole, 1	840	47	2,140	31	86	26.0	34.4	17.6	857	317	118	412	8.4	420	2,369	1,430	395	0.59	0.84	5.0	25
Piece, 1/6 of pie, 1	140	47	355	5	14	4.3	5.7	2.9	143	53	20	69	1.4	70	395	240	66	0.10	0.14	0.8	4
Peach																					
Whole, 1	945	48	2,410	24	101	24.6	43.5	26.5	0	361	95	274	11.3	1,408	2,533	6,900	690	1.04	0.95	14.2	28
Piece, 1/6 of pie, 1	158	48	405	4	17	4.1	7.3	4.4	0	60	16	46	1.9	235	423	1,150	115	0.17	0.16	2.4	5
Pies Piecrust made with enriched flour, vegetable shortening, 9-in diam.																					
Pecan																					
Whole, 1	825	20	3,450	42	189	28.1	101.5	47.0	569	423	388	850	27.2	1,015	1,823	1,320	322	1.82	0.99	6.6	0
Piece, 1/6 of pie, 1	138	20	575	7	32	4.7	17.0	7.9	95	71	65	142	4.6	170	305	220	54	0.30	0.17	1.1	0
Pumpkin																					
Whole, 1	910	59	1,920	36	102	38.2	40.0	18.2	655	223	464	628	8.2	1,456	1,947	22,480	2,493	0.82	1.27	7.3	0
Piece, 1/6 of pie, 1	152	59	320	6	17	6.4	6.7	3.0	109	37	78	105	1.4	243	325	3,750	416	0.14	0.21	1.2	0
Fried																					
Apple, 1	85	43	255	2	14	5.8	6.6	0.6	14	31	12	34	0.9	42	326	30	3	0.09	0.06	1.0	1
Cherry, 1	85	42	250	2	14	5.8	6.7	0.6	13	32	11	41	0.7	61	371	190	19	0.06	0.06	0.6	1

Food	Measure	Grams	Water (%)	Food energy (cal)	Protein (g)	Fat (g)	Saturated (g)	Monounsat. (g)	Polyunsat. (g)	Cholesterol (mg)	Carbohydrate (g)	Calcium (mg)	Phosphorus (mg)	Iron (mg)	Potassium (mg)	Sodium (mg)	Vitamin A (IU)	Thiamin (mg)	Riboflavin (mg)	Niacin (mg)	Ascorbic acid (mg)
Popcorn																					
Popped																					
Air-popped, unsalted	1 cup	8	4	30	1	Tr	Tr	0.1	0.2	0	6	1	22	0.2	20	Tr	10	0.03	0.01	0.2	0
Popped in vegetable oil, salted	1 cup	11	3	55	1	3	0.5	1.4	1.2	0	6	3	31	0.3	19	86	20	0.01	0.02	0.1	0
Sugar syrup coated	1 cup	35	4	135	2	1	0.1	0.3	0.6	0	30	2	47	0.5	90	Tr	30	0.13	0.02	0.4	0
Pretzels																					
Made with enriched flour																					
Stick, 2¼ in long	10	3	3	10	Tr	Tr	Tr	Tr	Tr	0	2	1	3	0.1	3	48	0	0.01	0.01	0.1	0
Twisted, dutch, 2¾ by 2⅝ in	1	16	3	65	2	1	0.2	0.4	0.2	0	13	4	15	0.3	16	258	0	0.05	0.04	0.7	0
Twisted, thin, 3¼ by 2¼ by ¼ in	10	60	3	240	6	2	0.4	0.8	0.6	0	48	16	55	1.2	61	966	0	0.19	0.15	2.6	0
Rice																					
Brown, cooked, served hot	1 cup	195	70	230	5	1	0.3	0.3	0.4	0	50	23	142	1.0	137	0	0	0.18	0.04	2.7	0
White, enriched																					
Commercial varieties, all types																					
Raw	1 cup	185	12	670	12	1	0.2	0.3	0.3	0	149	44	174	5.4	170	9	0	0.81	0.06	6.5	0
Cooked, served hot	1 cup	205	73	225	4	Tr	0.1	0.1	0.1	0	50	21	57	1.8	57	0	0	0.23	0.02	2.1	0
Instant, ready-to-serve, hot	1 cup	165	73	180	4	0	0.1	0.1	0.1	0	40	5	31	1.3	0	0	0	0.21	0.02	1.7	0
Parboiled																					
Raw	1 cup	185	10	685	14	1	0.1	0.1	0.1	0	150	111	370	5.4	278	17	0	0.81	0.07	6.5	0
Cooked, served hot	1 cup	175	73	185	4	Tr	Tr	Tr	Tr	0	41	33	100	1.4	75	0	0	0.19	0.02	2.1	0
Rolls, enriched																					
Commercial																					
Dinner, 2½-in diam., 2 in high	1	28	32	85	2	2	0.5	0.8	0.6	Tr	14	33	44	0.8	36	155	Tr	0.14	0.09	1.1	Tr
Frankfurter and hamburger (8 per 11½-oz pkg.)	1	40	34	115	3	2	0.5	0.8	0.6	Tr	20	54	44	1.2	56	241	Tr	0.20	0.13	1.6	Tr
Hard, 3¾-in diam., 2 in high	1	50	25	155	5	2	0.4	0.5	0.6	Tr	30	24	46	1.4	49	313	0	0.20	0.12	1.7	0
Hoagie or submarine, 11½ by 3 by 2½ in	1	135	31	400	11	8	1.8	3.0	2.2	Tr	72	100	115	3.8	128	683	0	0.54	0.33	4.5	0
From home recipe																					
Dinner, 2½-in diam., 2 in high	1	35	26	120	3	3	0.8	1.2	0.9	12	20	16	36	1.1	41	98	30	0.12	0.12	1.2	0
Spaghetti																					
Enriched, cooked																					
Firm stage, "al dente," served hot	1 cup	130	64	190	7	1	0.1	0.1	0.3	0	39	14	85	2.0	103	1	0	0.23	0.13	1.8	0
Tender stage, served hot	1 cup	140	73	155	5	1	0.1	0.1	0.2	0	32	11	70	1.7	85	1	0	0.20	0.11	1.5	0
Toaster pastries	1	54	13	210	2	6	1.7	3.6	0.4	0	38	104	104	2.2	91	248	520	0.17	0.18	2.3	4
Tortillas																					
Corn	1	30	45	65	2	1	0.1	0.3	0.6	0	13	42	55	0.6	43	1	80	0.05	0.03	0.4	0
Waffles																					
Made with enriched flour, 7-in diam.																					
From home recipe	1	75	37	245	7	13	4.0	4.9	2.6	102	26	154	135	1.5	129	445	140	0.18	0.24	1.5	Tr
From mix, egg and milk added	1	75	42	205	7	8	2.7	2.9	1.5	59	27	179	257	1.2	146	515	170	0.14	0.23	0.9	Tr

(continued)

Appendix 1 (Continued)
Nutritive Value of the Edible Part of Food*

Item	Foods, Approximate Measures, Units, and Weight (Weight of Edible Portion Only)	Weight (g)	Water (%)	Food Energy (kcal)	Protein (g)	Fat (g)	Saturated (g)	Monounsaturated (g)	Polyunsaturated (g)	Cholesterol (mg)	Carbohydrate (g)	Calcium (mg)	Phosphorus (mg)	Iron (mg)	Potassium (mg)	Sodium (mg)	Vitamin A Value (IU)	Vitamin A Value (RE)	Thiamine (mg)	Riboflavin (mg)	Niacin (mg)	Ascorbic Acid (mg)
Wheat flours																						
All-purpose or family flour, enriched																						
Sifted, spooned	1 cup	115	12	420	12	1	0.2	0.1	0.5	0	88	18	100	5.1	109	2	0	0	0.73	0.46	6.1	0
Unsifted, spooned	1 cup	125	12	455	13	1	0.2	0.1	0.5	0	95	20	109	5.5	119	3	0	0	0.80	0.50	6.6	0
Cake or pastry flour, enriched, sifted, spooned	1 cup	96	12	350	7	1	0.1	0.1	0.3	0	76	16	70	4.2	91	2	0	0	0.58	0.38	5.1	0
Self-rising, enriched, unsifted, spooned	1 cup	125	12	440	12	1	0.2	0.1	0.5	0	93	331	583	5.5	113	1,349	0	0	0.80	0.50	6.6	0
Whole-wheat, from hard wheats, stirred	1 cup	120	12	400	16	2	0.3	0.3	1.1	0	85	49	446	5.2	444	4	0	0	0.66	0.14	5.2	0
LEGUMES, NUTS, AND SEEDS																						
Almonds, shelled																						
Slivered, packed	1 cup	135	4	795	27	70	6.7	45.8	14.8	0	28	359	702	4.9	988	15	0	0	0.28	1.05	4.5	1
Whole	1 oz	28	4	165	6	15	1.4	9.6	3.1	0	6	75	147	1.0	208	3	0	0	0.06	0.22	1.0	Tr
Beans																						
Dry																						
Cooked, drained																						
Black	1 cup	171	66	225	15	1	0.1	0.1	0.5	0	41	47	239	2.9	608	1	Tr	Tr	0.43	0.05	0.9	0
Great Northern	1 cup	180	69	210	14	1	0.1	0.1	0.6	0	38	90	266	4.9	749	13	0	0	0.25	0.13	1.3	0
Lima	1 cup	190	64	260	16	1	0.2	0.1	0.5	0	49	55	293	5.9	1,163	4	0	0	0.25	0.11	1.3	0
Pea (navy)	1 cup	190	69	225	15	1	0.1	0.1	0.7	0	40	95	281	5.1	790	13	0	0	0.27	0.13	1.3	0
Pinto	1 cup	180	65	265	15	1	0.1	0.1	0.5	0	49	86	296	5.4	882	3	Tr	Tr	0.33	0.16	0.7	0
Canned, solids and liquid																						
White with																						
Frankfurters (sliced)	1 cup	255	71	365	19	18	7.4	8.8	0.7	30	32	94	303	4.8	668	1,374	330	33	0.18	0.15	3.3	Tr
Pork and tomato sauce	1 cup	255	71	310	16	7	2.4	2.7	0.7	10	48	138	235	4.6	536	1,181	330	33	0.20	0.08	1.5	5
Pork and sweet sauce	1 cup	255	66	385	16	12	4.3	4.9	1.2	10	54	161	291	5.9	536	969	330	33	0.15	0.10	1.3	5
Red kidney	1 cup	255	76	230	15	1	0.1	0.1	0.6	0	42	74	278	4.6	673	968	10	1	0.13	0.10	1.5	0

Food	Measure																					
Black-eye peas																						
Dry, cooked (with residual cooking liquid)	1 cup	250	80	190	13	1	0.2	Tr	0.3	0	35	43	238	3.3	573	20	30	3	0.40	0.10	1.0	0
Brazil nuts																						
Shelled	1 oz	28	3	185	4	19	4.6	6.5	6.8	0	4	50	170	1.0	170	1	Tr	Tr	0.28	0.03	0.5	Tr
Carob flour	1 cup	140	3	255	6	Tr	Tr	0.1	0.1	0	126	390	102	5.7	1,275	24	Tr	Tr	0.07	0.07	2.2	Tr
Cashew nuts																						
Salted																						
Dry roasted	1 cup	137	2	785	21	63	12.5	37.4	10.7	0	45	62	671	8.2	774	[41]877	0	0	0.27	0.27	1.9	0
	1 oz	28	2	165	4	13	2.6	7.7	2.2	0	9	13	139	1.7	160	[41]181	0	0	0.06	0.06	0.4	0
Roasted in oil	1 cup	130	4	750	21	63	12.4	36.9	10.6	0	37	53	554	5.3	689	[42]814	0	0	0.55	0.23	2.3	0
	1 oz	28	4	165	5	14	2.7	8.1	2.3	0	8	12	121	1.2	150	[42]177	0	0	0.12	0.05	0.5	0
Chestnuts																						
European (Italian), roasted, shelled	1 cup	143	40	350	5	3	0.6	1.1	1.2	0	76	41	153	1.3	847	3	30	3	0.35	0.25	1.9	37
Chickpeas																						
Cooked, drained	1 cup	163	60	270	15	4	0.4	0.9	1.9	0	45	80	273	4.9	475	11	Tr	Tr	0.18	0.09	0.9	0
Coconut																						
Raw																						
Piece, about 2 by 2 by ½ in	1	45	47	160	1	15	13.4	0.6	0.2	0	7	6	51	1.1	160	9	0	0	0.03	0.01	0.2	1
Shredded or grated	1 cup	80	47	285	3	27	23.8	1.1	0.3	0	12	11	90	1.9	285	16	0	0	0.05	0.02	0.4	3
Dried, sweetened, shredded	1 cup	93	13	470	3	33	29.3	1.4	0.4	0	44	14	99	1.8	313	244	0	0	0.03	0.02	0.4	1
Filberts																						
(Hazelnuts), chopped	1 cup	115	5	725	15	72	5.3	56.5	6.9	0	18	216	359	3.8	512	3	80	8	0.58	0.13	1.3	1
	1 oz	28	5	180	4	18	1.3	13.9	1.7	0	4	53	88	0.9	126	1	20	2	0.14	0.03	0.3	Tr
Lentils																						
Dry, cooked	1 cup	200	72	215	16	1	0.1	0.2	0.5	0	38	50	238	4.2	498	26	40	4	0.14	0.12	1.2	0
Macadamia nuts																						
Roasted in oil, salted	1 cup	134	2	960	10	103	15.4	80.9	1.8	0	17	60	268	2.4	441	[43]348	10	1	0.29	0.15	2.7	0
	1 oz	28	2	205	2	22	3.2	17.1	0.4	0	4	13	57	0.5	93	[43]74	Tr	Tr	0.06	0.03	0.6	0
Mixed nuts																						
With peanuts, salted																						
Dry roasted	1 oz	28	2	170	5	15	2.0	8.9	3.1	0	7	20	123	1.0	169	[44]190	Tr	Tr	0.06	0.06	1.3	0
Roasted in oil	1 oz	28	2	175	5	16	2.5	9.0	3.8	0	6	31	131	0.9	165	[44]185	10	1	0.14	0.06	1.4	Tr
Peanuts																						
Roasted in oil, salted	1 cup	145	2	840	39	71	9.9	35.5	22.6	0	27	125	734	2.8	1,019	[45]626	0	0	0.42	0.15	21.5	0
	1 oz	28	2	165	8	14	1.9	6.9	4.4	0	5	24	143	0.5	199	[45]122	0	0	0.08	0.03	4.2	0
Peanut butter	1 tbsp	16	1	95	5	8	1.4	4.0	2.5	0	3	5	60	0.3	110	75	0	0	0.02	0.02	2.2	0
Peas																						
Split, dry, cooked	1 cup	200	70	230	16	1	0.1	0.1	0.3	0	42	22	178	3.4	592	26	80	8	0.30	0.18	1.8	0
Pecans																						
Halves	1 cup	108	5	720	8	73	5.9	45.5	18.1	0	20	39	314	2.3	423	1	140	14	0.92	0.14	1.0	2
	1 oz	28	5	190	2	19	1.5	12.0	4.7	0	5	10	83	0.6	111	Tr	40	4	0.24	0.04	0.3	1
Pine nuts																						
(Pinyons), shelled	1 oz	28	6	160	3	17	2.7	6.5	7.3	0	5	2	10	0.9	178	20	10	1	0.35	0.06	1.2	1

(continued)

749

Appendix 1 (Continued)
Nutritive Value of the Edible Part of Food*

Item	Foods, Approximate Measures, Units, and Weight (Weight of Edible Portion Only)	Weight (g)	Water (%)	Food Energy (kcal)	Protein (g)	Fat (g)	Fatty Acids Saturated (g)	Monounsaturated (g)	Polyunsaturated (g)	Cholesterol (mg)	Carbohydrate (g)	Calcium (mg)	Phosphorus (mg)	Iron (mg)	Potassium (mg)	Sodium (mg)	Vitamin A Value (IU)	Vitamin A Value (RE)	Thiamine (mg)	Riboflavin (mg)	Niacin (mg)	Ascorbic Acid (mg)
Pistachio nuts																						
Dried, shelled	1 oz	28	4	165	6	14	1.7	9.3	2.1	0	7	38	143	1.9	310	2	70	7	0.23	0.05	0.3	Tr
Pumpkin and squash kernels																						
Dry, hulled	1 oz	28	7	155	7	13	2.5	4.0	5.9	0	5	12	333	4.2	229	5	110	11	0.06	0.09	0.5	Tr
Refried beans																						
Canned	1 cup	290	72	295	18	3	0.4	0.6	1.4	0	51	141	245	5.1	1,141	1,228	0	0	0.14	0.16	1.4	17
Sesame seeds																						
Dry, hulled	1 tbsp	8	5	45	2	4	0.6	1.7	1.9	0	1	11	62	0.6	33	3	10	1	0.06	0.01	0.4	0
Soybeans																						
Dry, cooked, drained	1 cup	180	71	235	20	10	1.3	1.9	5.3	0	19	131	322	4.9	972	4	50	5	0.38	0.16	1.1	0
Soy products																						
Miso	1 cup	276	53	470	29	13	1.8	2.6	7.3	0	65	188	853	4.7	922	8,142	110	11	0.17	0.28	0.8	0
Tofu, piece 2½ by 2¾ by 1 in	1	120	85	85	9	5	0.7	1.0	2.9	0	3	108	151	2.3	50	8	0	0	0.07	0.04	0.1	0
Sunflower seeds																						
Dry, hulled	1 oz	28	5	160	6	14	1.5	2.7	9.3	0	5	33	200	1.9	195	1	10	1	0.65	0.07	1.3	Tr
Tahini	1 tbsp	15	3	90	3	8	1.1	3.0	3.5	0	3	21	119	0.7	69	5	10	1	0.24	0.02	0.8	1
Walnuts																						
Black, chopped	1 cup	125	4	760	30	71	4.5	15.9	46.9	0	15	73	580	3.8	655	1	370	37	0.27	0.14	0.9	Tr
	1 oz	28	4	170	7	16	1.0	3.6	10.6	0	3	16	132	0.9	149	Tr	80	8	0.06	0.03	0.2	Tr
English or Persian, pieces or chips	1 cup	120	4	770	17	74	6.7	17.0	47.0	0	22	113	380	2.9	602	12	150	15	0.46	0.18	1.3	4
	1 oz	28	4	180	4	18	1.6	4.0	11.1	0	5	27	90	0.7	142	3	40	4	0.11	0.04	0.3	1

MEAT AND MEAT PRODUCTS

Beef, cooked
Cuts braised, simmered, or pot roasted
Relatively fat such as chuck blade

Item	Foods, Approximate Measures, Units, and Weight	Weight (g)	Water (%)	Food Energy (kcal)	Protein (g)	Fat (g)	Saturated (g)	Monounsaturated (g)	Polyunsaturated (g)	Cholesterol (mg)	Carbohydrate (g)	Calcium (mg)	Phosphorus (mg)	Iron (mg)	Potassium (mg)	Sodium (mg)	Vit A (IU)	Vit A (RE)	Thiamine (mg)	Riboflavin (mg)	Niacin (mg)	Ascorbic Acid (mg)
Lean and fat, piece, 2½ by 2½ by ¾ in	3 oz	85	43	325	22	26	10.8	11.7	0.9	87	0	11	163	2.5	163	53	Tr	Tr	0.06	0.19	2.0	0
Lean only	2.2 oz	62	53	170	19	9	3.9	4.2	0.3	66	0	8	146	2.3	163	44	Tr	Tr	0.05	0.17	1.7	0

Food	Measure	Grams	Water (%)	Food energy (cal)	Protein (g)	Fat (g)	Saturated (g)	Monounsaturated (g)	Polyunsaturated (g)	Cholesterol (mg)	Carbohydrate (g)	Calcium (mg)	Phosphorus (mg)	Iron (mg)	Potassium (mg)	Sodium (mg)	Vitamin A (IU)	Vitamin A (RE)	Thiamin (mg)	Riboflavin (mg)	Niacin (mg)	Ascorbic acid (mg)
Relatively lean, such as bottom round																						
Lean and fat, piece, 4⅛ by 2¼ by ½ in	3 oz	85	54	220	25	13	4.8	5.7	0.5	81	0	5	217	2.8	248	43	Tr	Tr	0.06	0.21	3.3	0
Lean only	2.8 oz	78	57	175	25	8	2.7	3.4	0.3	75	0	4	212	2.7	240	40	Tr	Tr	0.06	0.20	3.0	0
Ground beef, broiled, patty, 3 by ⅝ in																						
Lean	3 oz	85	56	230	21	16	6.2	6.9	0.6	74	0	9	134	1.8	256	65	Tr	Tr	0.04	0.18	4.4	0
Regular	3 oz	85	54	245	20	18	6.9	7.7	0.7	76	0	9	144	2.1	248	70	Tr	Tr	0.03	0.16	4.9	0
Heart, lean, braised	3 oz	85	65	150	24	5	1.2	0.8	1.6	164	0	5	213	6.4	198	54	Tr	Tr	0.12	1.31	3.4	5
Liver, fried, slice, 6½ by 2⅜ by ⅜ in[17]	3 oz	85	56	185	23	7	2.5	3.6	1.3	410	7	9	392	5.3	309	90	[48]30,690	[48]9,120	0.18	3.52	12.3	23
Roast, oven cooked, no liquid added																						
Relatively fat, such as rib																						
Lean and fat, 2 pieces, 4⅛ by 2¼ by ¼ in	3 oz	85	46	315	19	26	10.8	11.4	0.9	72	0	8	145	2.0	246	54	Tr	Tr	0.06	0.16	3.1	0
Lean only	2.2 oz	61	57	150	17	9	3.6	3.7	0.3	49	0	5	127	1.7	218	45	Tr	Tr	0.05	0.13	2.7	0
Relatively lean, such as eye of round																						
Lean and fat, 2 pieces, 2½ by 2½ by ⅜ in	3 oz	85	57	205	23	12	4.9	5.4	0.5	62	0	5	177	1.6	308	50	Tr	Tr	0.07	0.14	3.0	0
Lean only	2.6 oz	75	63	135	22	5	1.9	2.1	0.2	52	0	3	170	1.5	297	46	Tr	Tr	0.07	0.13	2.8	0
Steak																						
Sirloin, broiled																						
Lean and fat, piece, 2½ by 2½ by ¾ in	3 oz	85	53	240	23	15	6.4	6.9	0.6	77	0	9	186	2.6	306	53	Tr	Tr	0.10	0.23	3.3	0
Lean only	2.5 oz	72	59	150	22	6	2.6	2.8	0.3	64	0	8	176	2.4	290	48	Tr	Tr	0.09	0.22	3.1	0
Beef, canned corned	3 oz	85	59	185	22	10	4.2	4.9	0.4	80	0	17	90	3.7	51	802	Tr	Tr	0.02	0.20	2.9	0
Beef, dried chipped	2.5 oz	72	48	145	24	4	1.8	2.0	0.2	46	0	14	287	2.3	142	3,053	Tr	Tr	0.05	0.23	2.7	0
Lamb, Cooked																						
Chops, (3 per lb with bone):																						
Arm, braised																						
Lean and fat	2.2 oz	63	44	220	20	15	6.9	6.0	0.9	77	0	16	132	1.5	195	46	Tr	Tr	0.04	0.16	4.4	0
Lean only	1.7 oz	48	49	135	17	7	2.9	2.6	0.4	59	0	12	111	1.3	162	36	Tr	Tr	0.03	0.13	3.0	0
Loin, broiled																						
Lean and fat	2.8 oz	80	54	235	22	16	7.3	6.4	1.0	78	0	16	162	1.4	272	62	Tr	Tr	0.09	0.21	5.5	0
Lean only	2.3 oz	64	61	140	19	6	2.6	2.4	0.4	60	0	12	145	1.3	241	54	Tr	Tr	0.08	0.18	4.4	0
Leg, roasted																						
Lean and fat, 2 pieces, 4⅛ by 2¼ by ¼ in	3 oz	85	59	205	22	13	5.6	4.9	0.8	78	0	8	162	1.7	273	57	Tr	Tr	0.09	0.24	5.5	0
Lean only	2.6 oz	73	64	140	20	6	2.4	2.2	0.4	65	0	6	150	1.5	247	50	Tr	Tr	0.08	0.20	4.6	0
Rib, roasted																						
Lean and fat, 3 pieces, 2½ by 2½ by ¼ in	3 oz	85	47	315	18	26	12.1	10.6	1.5	77	0	19	139	1.4	224	60	Tr	Tr	0.08	0.18	5.5	0
Lean only	2 oz	57	60	130	15	7	3.2	3.0	0.5	50	0	12	111	1.0	179	46	Tr	Tr	0.05	0.13	3.5	0

(continued)

Appendix 1 (Continued)
Nutritive Value of the Edible Part of Food*

Item	Foods, Approximate Measures, Units, and Weight (Weight of Edible Portion Only)	Weight (g)	Water (%)	Food Energy (kcal)	Protein (g)	Fat (g)	Saturated (g)	Monounsaturated (g)	Polyunsaturated (g)	Cholesterol (mg)	Carbohydrate (g)	Calcium (mg)	Phosphorus (mg)	Iron (mg)	Potassium (mg)	Sodium (mg)	Vitamin A Value (IU)	Vitamin A Value (RE)	Thiamine (mg)	Riboflavine (mg)	Niacin (mg)	Ascorbic Acid (mg)
Pork, cured, cooked																						
Bacon																						
Regular slice	3	19	13	110	6	9	3.3	4.5	1.1	16	Tr	2	64	0.3	92	303	0	0	0.13	0.05	1.4	6
Canadian-style slice	2	46	62	85	11	4	1.3	1.9	0.4	27	1	5	136	0.4	179	711	0	0	0.38	0.09	3.2	10
Ham, light cure, roasted																						
Lean and fat, 2 pieces, 4⅛ by 2¼ by ¼ in	3 oz	85	58	205	18	14	5.1	6.7	1.5	53	0	6	182	0.7	243	1,009	0	0	0.51	0.19	3.8	0
Lean only	2.4 oz	68	66	105	17	4	1.3	1.7	0.4	37	0	5	154	0.6	215	902	0	0	0.46	0.17	3.4	0
Ham, canned, roasted, 2 pieces, 4⅛ by 2¼ by ¼ in	3 oz	85	67	140	18	7	2.4	3.5	0.8	35	Tr	6	188	0.9	298	908	0	0	0.82	0.21	4.3	[49]19
Luncheon meat																						
Canned, spiced or unspiced, slice, 3 by 2 by ½ in	2	42	52	140	5	13	4.5	6.0	1.5	26	1	3	34	0.3	90	541	0	0	0.15	0.08	1.3	Tr
Chopped ham (8 slices per 6 oz pkg)	2	42	64	95	7	7	2.4	3.4	0.9	21	0	3	65	0.3	134	576	0	0	0.27	0.09	1.6	[49]8
Cooked ham (8 slices per 8-oz pkg)																						
Regular	2	57	65	105	10	6	1.9	2.8	0.7	32	2	4	141	0.6	189	751	0	0	0.49	0.14	3.0	[49]16
Extra lean	2	57	71	75	11	3	0.9	1.3	0.3	27	1	4	124	0.4	200	815	0	0	0.53	0.13	2.8	[49]15
Pork, fresh, cooked																						
Chop, loin (cut 3 per lb with bone)																						
Broiled																						
Lean and fat	3.1 oz	87	50	275	24	19	7.0	8.8	2.2	84	0	3	184	0.7	312	61	10	3	0.87	0.24	4.3	Tr
Lean only	2.5 oz	72	57	165	23	8	2.6	3.4	0.9	71	0	4	176	0.7	302	56	10	1	0.83	0.22	4.0	Tr
Pan fried																						
Lean and fat	3.1 oz	89	45	335	21	27	9.8	12.5	3.1	92	0	4	190	0.7	323	64	10	3	0.91	0.24	4.6	Tr
Lean only	2.4 oz	67	54	180	19	11	3.7	4.8	1.3	72	0	3	178	0.7	305	57	10	1	0.84	0.22	4.0	Tr
Ham (leg), roasted																						
Lean and fat, piece, 2½ by 2½ by ¾ in	3 oz	85	53	250	21	18	6.4	8.1	2.0	79	0	5	210	0.9	280	50	10	2	0.54	0.27	3.9	Tr
Lean only	2.5 oz	72	60	160	20	8	2.7	3.6	1.0	68	0	5	202	0.8	269	46	10	1	0.50	0.25	3.6	Tr

Food	Measure	Grams	Water (%)	Calories	Protein (g)	Fat (g)	Sat. (g)	Mono. (g)	Poly. (g)	Cholesterol (mg)	Carbohydrate (g)	Calcium (mg)	Phosphorus (mg)	Iron (mg)	Potassium (mg)	Sodium (mg)	Vit A (IU)	Vit A (RE)	Thiamin (mg)	Riboflavin (mg)	Niacin (mg)	Ascorbic acid (mg)
Rib, roasted																						
Lean and fat, piece, 2½ by ¾ in	3 oz	85	51	270	21	20	7.2	9.2	2.3	69	0	9	190	0.8	313	37	10	3	0.50	0.24	4.2	Tr
Lean only	2.5 oz	71	57	175	20	10	3.4	4.4	1.2	56	0	8	182	0.7	300	33	10	2	0.45	0.22	3.8	Tr
Shoulder cut, braised																						
Lean and fat, 3 pieces, 2½ by 2½ by ¼ in	3 oz	85	47	295	23	22	7.9	10.0	2.4	93	0	6	162	1.4	286	75	10	3	0.46	0.26	4.4	Tr
Lean only	2.4 oz	67	54	165	22	8	2.8	3.7	1.0	76	0	5	151	1.3	271	68	10	1	0.40	0.24	4.0	Tr
Sausages																						
(See also Luncheon meats.)																						
Bologna, slice (8 per 8-oz pkg)	2	57	54	180	7	16	6.1	7.6	1.4	31	2	7	52	0.9	103	581	0	0	0.10	0.08	1.5	[49]12
Braunschweiger, slice (6 per 6-oz pkg)	2	57	48	205	8	18	6.2	8.5	2.1	89	2	5	96	5.3	113	652	8,010	2,405	0.14	0.87	4.8	[49]6
Brown and serve (10–11 per 8-oz pkg), browned	1	13	45	50	2	5	1.7	2.2	0.5	9	Tr	1	14	0.1	25	105	0	0	0.05	0.02	0.4	0
Frankfurter (10 per 1-lb pkg), cooked (reheated)	1	45	54	145	5	13	4.8	6.2	1.2	23	1	5	39	0.5	75	504	0	0	0.09	0.05	1.2	[49]12
Pork link (16 per 1-lb pkg), cooked[50]	1	13	45	50	3	4	1.4	1.8	0.5	11	Tr	4	24	0.2	47	168	0	0	0.10	0.03	0.6	Tr
Salami																						
Cooked type, slice (8 per 8-oz pkg)	2	57	60	145	8	11	4.6	5.2	1.2	37	1	7	66	1.5	113	607	0	0	0.14	0.21	2.0	[49]7
Dry type, slice (12 per 4-oz pkg)	2	20	35	85	5	7	2.4	3.4	0.6	16	1	2	28	0.3	76	372	0	0	0.12	0.06	1.0	[49]5
Sandwich spread (pork, beef)	1 tbsp	15	60	35	1	3	0.9	1.1	0.4	6	2	2	9	0.1	17	152	10	1	0.03	0.02	0.3	0
Vienna sausage (7 per 4-oz can)	1	16	60	45	2	4	1.5	2.0	0.3	8	Tr	Tr	8	0.1	16	152	0	0	0.01	0.02	0.3	0
Veal																						
Medium fat, cooked, bone removed Cutlet, 4⅛ by 2¼ by ½ in, braised or broiled	3 oz	85	60	185	23	9	4.1	4.1	0.6	109	0	9	196	0.8	258	56	Tr	Tr	0.06	0.21	4.6	0
Rib, 2 pieces, 4⅛ by 2¼ by ¼ in, roasted	3 oz	85	55	230	23	14	6.0	6.0	1.0	109	0	10	211	0.7	259	57	Tr	Tr	0.11	0.26	6.6	0

MIXED DISHES AND FAST FOODS

Food	Measure	Grams	Water (%)	Calories	Protein (g)	Fat (g)	Sat. (g)	Mono. (g)	Poly. (g)	Cholesterol (mg)	Carbohydrate (g)	Calcium (mg)	Phosphorus (mg)	Iron (mg)	Potassium (mg)	Sodium (mg)	Vit A (IU)	Vit A (RE)	Thiamin (mg)	Riboflavin (mg)	Niacin (mg)	Ascorbic acid (mg)
Mixed dishes																						
Beef and vegetable stew, from home recipe	1 cup	245	82	220	16	11	4.4	4.5	0.5	71	15	29	184	2.9	613	292	5,690	568	0.15	0.17	4.7	17
Beef potpie, from home recipe, baked, piece, ⅓ of 9-in diam. pie[51]	1	210	55	515	21	30	7.9	12.9	7.4	42	39	29	149	3.8	334	596	4,220	517	0.29	0.29	4.8	6
Chicken a la king, cooked, from home recipe	1 cup	245	68	470	27	34	12.9	13.4	6.2	221	12	127	358	2.5	404	760	1,130	272	0.10	0.42	5.4	12
Chicken and noodles, cooked, from home recipe	1 cup	240	71	365	22	18	5.1	7.1	3.9	103	26	26	247	2.2	149	600	430	130	0.05	0.17	4.3	Tr
Chicken chow mein																						
Canned	1 cup	250	89	95	7	Tr	0.1	0.1	0.8	8	18	45	85	1.3	418	725	150	28	0.05	0.10	1.0	13
From home recipe	1 cup	250	78	255	31	10	4.1	4.9	3.5	75	10	58	293	2.5	473	718	280	50	0.08	0.23	4.3	10

(continued)

Appendix 1 (Continued)
Nutritive Value of the Edible Part of Food*

Item	Foods, Approximate Measures, Units, and Weight (Weight of Edible Portion Only)	Weight (g)	Water (%)	Food Energy (kcal)	Protein (g)	Fat (g)	Fatty Acids Saturated (g)	Monounsaturated (g)	Polyunsaturated (g)	Cholesterol (mg)	Carbohydrate (g)	Calcium (mg)	Phosphorus (mg)	Iron (mg)	Potassium (mg)	Sodium (mg)	Vitamin A Value (IU)	Vitamin A Value (RE)	Thiamine (mg)	Riboflavine (mg)	Niacin (mg)	Ascorbic Acid (mg)
Chicken potpie, from home recipe, baked, piece, 1/3 of 9-in diam. pie[51]	1	232	57	545	23	31	10.3	15.5	6.6	56	42	70	232	3.0	343	594	7,220	735	0.32	0.32	4.9	5
Chili con carne with beans, canned	1 cup	255	72	340	19	16	5.8	7.2	1.0	28	31	82	321	4.3	594	1,354	150	15	0.08	0.18	3.3	8
Chop suey with beef and pork, from home recipe	1 cup	250	75	300	26	17	4.3	7.4	4.2	68	13	60	248	4.8	425	1,053	600	60	0.28	0.38	5.0	33
Macaroni (enriched) and cheese																						
Canned[62]	1 cup	240	80	230	9	10	4.7	2.9	1.3	24	26	199	182	1.0	139	730	260	72	0.12	0.24	1.0	Tr
From home recipe[38]	1 cup	200	58	430	17	22	9.8	7.4	3.6	44	40	362	322	1.8	240	1,086	860	232	0.20	0.40	1.8	1
Quiche Lorraine, 1/8 of 8-in diam. quiche[51]	1	176	47	600	13	48	23.2	17.8	4.1	285	29	211	276	1.0	283	653	1,640	454	0.11	0.32	Tr	Tr
Spaghetti (enriched) in tomato sauce with cheese																						
Canned	1 cup	250	80	190	6	2	0.4	0.4	0.5	3	39	40	88	2.8	303	955	930	120	0.35	0.28	4.5	10
From home recipe	1 cup	250	77	260	9	9	3.0	3.6	1.2	8	37	80	135	2.3	408	955	1,080	140	0.25	0.18	2.3	13
Spaghetti (enriched) with meatballs and tomato sauce																						
Canned	1 cup	250	78	260	12	10	2.4	3.9	3.1	23	29	53	113	3.3	245	1,220	1,000	100	0.15	0.18	2.3	5
From home recipe	1 cup	248	70	330	19	12	3.9	4.4	2.2	89	39	124	236	3.7	665	1,009	1,590	159	0.25	0.30	4.0	22
Fast food entrees																						
Cheeseburger																						
Regular	1	112	46	300	15	15	7.3	5.6	1.0	44	28	135	174	2.3	219	672	340	65	0.26	0.24	3.7	1
4 oz patty	1	194	46	525	30	31	15.1	12.2	1.4	104	40	236	320	4.5	407	1,224	670	128	0.33	0.48	7.4	3
Chicken, fried. See Poultry and Poultry Products.																						
Enchilada	1	230	72	235	20	16	7.7	6.7	0.6	19	24	97	198	3.3	653	1,332	2,720	352	0.18	0.26	Tr	Tr
English muffin, egg, cheese, and bacon	1	138	49	360	18	18	8.0	8.0	0.7	213	31	197	290	3.1	201	832	650	160	0.46	0.50	3.7	1
Fish sandwich																						
Regular, with cheese	1	140	43	420	16	23	6.3	6.9	7.7	56	39	132	223	1.8	274	667	160	25	0.32	0.26	3.3	2
Large, without cheese	1	170	48	470	18	27	6.3	8.7	9.5	91	41	61	246	2.2	375	621	110	15	0.35	0.23	3.5	1

Food	Amount																				
Hamburger																					
Regular	1	98	46	245	12	11	4.4	5.3	0.5	32	28	56	107	2.2	202	463	80	14	0.23	0.24	3.8	1
4 oz patty	1	174	50	445	25	21	7.1	11.7	0.6	71	38	75	225	4.8	404	763	160	28	0.38	0.38	7.8	1
Pizza, cheese, 1/8 of 15-in diam. pizza[51]	1	120	46	290	15	9	4.1	2.6	1.3	56	39	220	216	1.6	230	699	750	106	0.34	0.29	4.2	2
Roast beef sandwich	1	150	52	345	22	13	3.5	6.9	1.8	55	34	60	222	4.0	338	757	240	32	0.40	0.33	6.0	2
Taco	1	81	55	195	9	11	4.1	5.5	0.8	21	15	109	134	1.2	263	456	420	57	0.09	0.07	1.4	1

POULTRY AND POULTRY PRODUCTS

Food	Amount																				
Chicken																					
Fried, flesh, with skin[53]																					
Batter dipped																					
Breast, 1/2 breast (5.6 oz with bones)	4.9 oz	140	52	365	35	18	4.9	7.6	4.3	119	13	28	259	1.8	281	385	90	28	0.16	0.20	14.7	0
Drumstick (3.4 oz with bones)	2.5 oz	72	53	195	16	11	3.0	4.6	2.7	62	6	12	106	1.0	134	194	60	19	0.08	0.15	3.7	0
Flour coated																					
Breast, 1/2 breast (4.2 oz with bones)	3.5 oz	98	57	220	31	9	2.4	3.4	1.9	87	2	16	228	1.2	254	74	50	15	0.08	0.13	13.5	0
Drumstick (2.6 oz with bones)	1.7 oz	49	57	120	13	7	1.8	2.7	1.6	44	1	6	86	0.7	112	44	40	12	0.04	0.11	3.0	0
Roasted, flesh only																					
Breast, 1/2 breast (4.2 oz with bones and skin)	3.0 oz	86	65	140	27	3	0.9	1.1	0.7	73	0	13	196	0.9	220	64	20	5	0.06	0.10	11.8	0
Drumstick, (2.9 oz with bones and skin)	1.6 oz	44	67	75	12	2	0.7	0.8	0.6	41	0	5	81	0.6	108	42	30	8	0.03	0.10	2.7	0
Stewed, flesh only, light and dark meat, chopped or diced	1 cup	140	67	250	38	9	2.6	3.3	2.2	116	0	20	210	1.6	252	98	70	21	0.07	0.23	8.6	0
Chicken liver																					
Cooked	1	20	68	30	5	1	0.4	0.3	0.2	126	Tr	3	62	1.7	28	10	3,270	983	0.03	0.35	0.9	3
Duck																					
Roasted, flesh only	½	221	64	445	52	25	9.2	8.2	3.2	197	0	27	449	6.0	557	144	170	51	0.57	1.04	11.3	0
Turkey																					
Roasted, flesh only																					
Dark meat, piece, 2½ by 1⅝ by ¼ in	4	85	63	160	24	6	2.1	1.4	1.8	72	0	27	173	2.0	246	67	0	0	0.05	0.21	3.1	0
Light meat, piece, 4 by 2 by ¼ in	2	85	66	135	25	3	0.9	0.5	0.7	59	0	16	186	1.1	259	54	0	0	0.05	0.11	5.8	0
Light and dark meat																					
Chopped or diced	1 cup	140	65	240	41	7	2.3	1.4	2.0	106	0	35	298	2.5	417	98	0	0	0.09	0.25	7.6	0
Pieces (1 slice white meat, 4 by 2 by ¼ in and 2 slices dark meat, 2½ by 1⅝ by ¼ in)	3	85	65	145	25	4	1.4	0.9	1.2	65	0	21	181	1.5	253	60	0	0	0.05	0.15	4.6	0

Appendix 1 (Continued)
Nutritive Value of the Edible Part of Food*

Item	Foods, Approximate Measures, Units, and Weight (Weight of Edible Portion Only)	Weight (g)	Water (%)	Food Energy (kcal)	Protein (g)	Fat (g)	Fatty Acids Saturated (g)	Monounsaturated (g)	Polyunsaturated (g)	Cholesterol (mg)	Carbohydrate (g)	Calcium (mg)	Phosphorus (mg)	Iron (mg)	Potassium (mg)	Sodium (mg)	Vitamin A Value (IU)	Vitamin A Value (RE)	Thiamine (mg)	Riboflavine (mg)	Niacin (mg)	Ascorbic Acid (mg)
Poultry food products																						
Chicken																						
Canned, boneless	5 oz	142	69	235	31	11	3.1	4.5	2.5	88	0	20	158	2.2	196	714	170	48	0.02	0.18	9.0	3
Frankfurter (10 per 1-lb pkg)	1	45	58	115	6	9	2.5	3.8	1.8	45	3	43	48	0.9	38	616	60	17	0.03	0.05	1.4	0
Roll, light (6 slices per 6 oz pkg)	2	57	69	90	11	4	1.1	1.7	0.9	28	1	24	89	0.6	129	331	50	14	0.04	0.07	3.0	0
Turkey																						
Gravy and turkey, frozen	5 oz	142	85	95	8	4	1.2	1.4	0.7	26	7	20	115	1.3	87	787	60	18	0.03	0.18	2.6	0
Ham, cured turkey thigh meat (8 slices per 8-oz pkg)	2	57	71	75	11	3	1.0	0.7	0.9	32	Tr	6	108	1.6	184	565	0	0	0.03	0.14	2.0	0
Loaf, breast meat (8 slices per 6-oz pkg)	2	42	72	45	10	1	0.2	0.2	0.1	17	0	3	97	0.2	118	608	0	0	0.02	0.05	3.5	0
Patties, breaded, battered, fried (2.25 oz)	1	64	50	180	9	12	3.0	4.8	3.0	40	10	9	173	1.4	176	512	20	7	0.06	0.12	1.5	0
Roast, boneless, frozen, seasoned, light and dark meat, cooked	3 oz	85	68	130	18	5	1.6	1.0	1.4	45	3	4	207	14	253	578	0	0	0.04	0.14	5.3	0
SOUPS, SAUCES, AND GRAVIES																						
Soups																						
Canned, condensed																						
Prepared with equal volume of milk																						
Clam chowder, New England	1 cup	248	85	165	9	7	3.0	2.3	1.1	22	17	186	156	1.5	300	992	160	40	0.07	0.24	1.0	3
Cream of chicken	1 cup	248	85	190	7	11	4.6	4.5	1.6	27	15	181	151	0.7	273	1,047	710	94	0.07	0.26	0.9	1
Cream of mushroom	1 cup	248	85	205	6	14	5.1	3.0	4.6	20	15	179	156	0.6	270	1,076	150	37	0.08	0.28	0.9	2
Tomato	1 cup	248	85	160	6	6	2.9	1.6	1.1	17	22	159	149	1.8	449	932	850	109	0.13	0.25	1.5	68

Prepared with equal volume of water

Food	Measure																				
Bean with bacon	1 cup	253	84	170	8	6	1.5	2.2	1.8	3	23	81	132	2.0	402	951	890	89	0.09	0.03	0.6	2
Beef broth, bouillon, consomme	1 cup	240	98	15	3	1	0.3	0.2	Tr	Tr	Tr	14	31	0.4	130	782	0	0	Tr	0.05	1.9	0
Beef noodle	1 cup	244	92	85	5	3	1.1	1.2	0.5	5	9	15	46	1.1	100	952	630	63	0.07	0.06	1.1	Tr
Chicken noodle	1 cup	241	92	75	4	2	0.7	1.1	0.6	7	9	17	36	0.8	55	1,106	710	71	0.05	0.06	1.4	Tr
Chicken rice	1 cup	241	94	60	4	2	0.5	0.9	0.4	7	7	17	22	0.7	101	815	660	66	0.02	0.02	1.1	Tr
Clam chowder, Manhattan	1 cup	244	90	80	4	2	0.4	0.4	1.3	2	12	34	59	1.9	261	1,808	920	92	0.06	0.05	1.3	3
Cream of chicken	1 cup	244	91	115	3	7	2.1	3.3	1.5	10	9	34	37	0.6	88	986	560	56	0.03	0.06	0.8	Tr
Cream of mushroom	1 cup	244	90	130	2	9	2.4	1.7	4.2	2	9	46	49	0.5	100	1,032	0	0	0.05	0.09	0.7	1
Minestrone	1 cup	241	91	80	4	3	0.6	0.7	1.1	2	11	34	55	0.9	313	911	2,340	234	0.05	0.04	0.9	1
Pea, green	1 cup	250	83	165	9	3	1.4	1.0	0.4	0	27	28	125	2.0	190	988	200	20	0.11	0.07	1.2	2
Tomato	1 cup	244	90	85	2	2	0.4	0.4	1.0	5	17	12	34	1.8	264	871	690	69	0.09	0.05	1.4	66
Vegetable beef	1 cup	244	92	80	6	2	0.9	0.8	0.1	5	10	17	41	1.1	173	956	1,890	189	0.04	0.05	1.0	2
Vegetarian	1 cup	241	92	70	2	2	0.3	0.8	0.7	0	12	22	34	1.1	210	822	3,010	301	0.05	0.05	0.9	1

Dehydrated

Unprepared

| Bouillon | 1 pkt | 6 | 3 | 15 | 1 | 1 | 0.3 | 0.2 | Tr | 1 | 1 | 4 | 19 | 0.1 | 27 | 1,019 | Tr | Tr | Tr | 0.01 | 0.3 | 0 |
| Onion | 1 pkt | 7 | 4 | 20 | 1 | Tr | 0.1 | 0.2 | Tr | Tr | 4 | 10 | 23 | 0.1 | 47 | 627 | Tr | Tr | 0.02 | 0.04 | 0.4 | Tr |

Prepared with water

Chicken noodle	1 pkt (6 fl oz)	188	94	40	2	1	0.2	0.4	0.3	2	6	24	24	0.4	23	957	50	5	0.05	0.04	0.7	Tr
Onion	1 pkt (6 fl oz)	184	96	20	1	Tr	0.1	0.2	0.1	0	4	9	22	0.1	48	635	Tr	Tr	0.02	0.04	0.4	Tr
Tomato vegetable	1 pkt (6 fl oz)	189	94	40	1	1	0.3	0.2	0.1	0	8	6	23	0.5	78	856	140	14	0.04	0.03	0.6	5

Sauces

From dry mix

Cheese, prepared with milk	1 cup	279	77	305	16	17	9.3	5.3	1.6	53	23	569	438	0.3	552	1,565	390	117	0.15	0.56	0.3	2
Hollandaise, prepared with water	1 cup	259	84	240	5	20	11.6	5.9	0.9	52	14	124	127	0.9	124	1,564	730	220	0.05	0.18	0.1	Tr
White sauce, prepared with milk	1 cup	264	81	240	10	13	6.4	4.7	1.7	34	21	425	256	0.3	444	797	310	92	0.08	0.45	0.5	3

From home recipe

| White sauce, medium[55] | 1 cup | 250 | 73 | 395 | 10 | 30 | 9.1 | 11.9 | 7.2 | 32 | 24 | 292 | 238 | 0.9 | 381 | 888 | 1,190 | 340 | 0.15 | 0.43 | 0.8 | 2 |

Ready to serve

| Barbecue | 1 tbsp | 16 | 81 | 10 | Tr | Tr | Tr | 0.1 | 0.1 | 0 | 2 | 3 | 3 | 0.1 | 28 | 130 | 140 | 14 | Tr | Tr | 0.1 | 1 |
| Soy | 1 tbsp | 18 | 68 | 10 | 2 | 0 | 0.0 | 0.0 | 0.0 | 0 | 2 | 3 | 38 | 0.5 | 64 | 1,029 | 0 | 0 | 0.01 | 0.02 | 0.6 | 0 |

Gravies

Canned

Beef	1 cup	233	87	125	9	5	2.7	2.3	0.2	7	11	14	70	1.6	189	1,305	0	0	0.07	0.08	1.5	0
Chicken	1 cup	238	85	190	5	14	3.4	6.1	3.6	5	13	48	69	1.1	259	1,373	880	264	0.04	0.10	1.1	0
Mushroom	1 cup	238	89	120	3	6	1.0	2.8	2.4	0	13	17	36	1.6	252	1,357	0	0	0.08	0.15	1.6	0

From dry mix

| Brown | 1 cup | 261 | 91 | 80 | 3 | 2 | 0.9 | 0.8 | 0.4 | 2 | 14 | 66 | 47 | 0.2 | 61 | 1,147 | 0 | 0 | 0.04 | 0.09 | 0.9 | 0 |
| Chicken | 1 cup | 260 | 91 | 85 | 3 | 2 | 0.5 | 0.9 | 0.4 | 3 | 14 | 39 | 47 | 0.3 | 62 | 1,134 | 0 | 0 | 0.05 | 0.15 | 0.8 | 3 |

SUGARS AND SWEETS

Candy

| Caramels, plain or chocolate | 1 oz | 28 | 8 | 115 | 1 | 3 | 2.2 | 0.1 | 0.1 | 1 | 22 | 42 | 35 | 0.4 | 54 | 64 | Tr | Tr | 0.01 | 0.05 | 0.1 | Tr |

(continued)

Appendix 1 (Continued)
Nutritive Value of the Edible Part of Food*

Item	Foods, Approximate Measures, Units, and Weight (Weight of Edible Portion Only)	Weight (g)	Water (%)	Food Energy (kcal)	Protein (g)	Fat (g)	Fatty Acids Saturated (g)	Monounsaturated (g)	Polyunsaturated (g)	Cholesterol (mg)	Carbohydrate (g)	Calcium (mg)	Phosphorus (mg)	Iron (mg)	Potassium (mg)	Sodium (mg)	Vitamin A Value (IU)	(RE)	Thiamine (mg)	Riboflavine (mg)	Niacin (mg)	Ascorbic Acid (mg)
Chocolate																						
Milk, plain	1 oz	28	1	145	2	9	5.4	3.0	0.3	6	16	50	61	0.4	96	23	30	10	0.02	0.10	0.1	Tr
Milk, with almonds	1 oz	28	1	150	3	10	4.8	4.1	0.7	5	15	65	77	0.5	125	23	30	8	0.02	0.12	0.2	Tr
Milk, with peanuts	1 oz	28	1	155	4	11	4.2	3.5	1.5	5	13	49	83	0.4	138	19	30	8	0.07	0.07	1.4	Tr
Milk, with rice cereal	1 oz	28	2	140	2	7	4.4	2.5	0.2	6	18	48	57	0.2	100	46	30	8	0.01	0.08	0.1	Tr
Semisweet, small pieces (60 per oz)	1 cup or 6 oz	170	1	860	7	61	36.2	19.9	1.9	0	97	51	178	5.8	593	24	30	3	0.10	0.14	0.9	Tr
Sweet (dark)	1 oz	28	1	150	1	10	5.9	3.3	0.3	0	16	7	41	0.6	86	5	10	1	0.01	0.04	0.1	Tr
Fondant, uncoated (mints, candy corn, other)	1 oz	28	3	105	Tr	0	0.0	0.0	0.0	0	27	2	Tr	0.1	1	57	0	0	Tr	Tr	Tr	0
Fudge, chocolate, plain	1 oz	28	8	115	1	3	2.1	1.0	0.1	1	21	22	24	0.3	42	54	Tr	Tr	0.01	0.03	0.1	Tr
Gum drops	1 oz	28	12	100	Tr	Tr	Tr	Tr	0.1	0	25	2	Tr	0.1	1	10	0	0	0.00	Tr	Tr	0
Candy																						
Hard	1 oz	28	1	110	0	0	0.0	0.0	0.0	0	28	Tr	2	0.1	1	7	0	0	0.00	0.00	0.0	0
Jelly beans	1 oz	28	6	105	Tr	Tr	Tr	Tr	0.1	0	26	1	1	0.3	11	7	0	0	0.00	Tr	Tr	0
Marshmallows	1 oz	28	17	90	1	Tr	0.0	0.0	0.0	0	23	1	2	0.5	2	25	Tr	Tr	0.00	Tr	Tr	0
Custard																						
Baked	1 cup	265	77	305	14	15	6.8	5.4	0.7	278	29	297	310	1.1	387	209	530	146	0.11	0.50	0.3	1
Gelatin dessert																						
Prepared with gelatin dessert powder and water	½ cup	120	84	70	2	0	0.0	0.0	0.0	0	17	2	23	Tr	Tr	55	0	0	0.00	0.00	0.0	0
Honey																						
Strained or extracted	1 cup	339	17	1,030	1	0	0.0	0.0	0.0	0	279	17	20	1.7	173	17	0	0	0.02	0.14	1.0	3
	1 tbsp	21	17	65	Tr	0	0.0	0.0	0.0	0	17	1	1	0.1	11	1	0	0	Tr	0.01	0.1	Tr
Jams and preserves	1 tbsp	20	29	55	Tr	Tr	Tr	Tr	Tr	0	14	4	2	0.2	18	2	Tr	Tr	Tr	0.01	Tr	Tr
	1 packet	14	29	40	Tr	Tr	0.0	Tr	Tr	0	10	3	1	0.1	12	2	Tr	Tr	Tr	Tr	Tr	Tr
Jellies	1 tbsp	18	28	50	Tr	Tr	Tr	Tr	Tr	0	13	2	Tr	0.1	16	5	Tr	Tr	Tr	0.01	Tr	1
	1 packet	14	28	40	Tr	Tr	Tr	Tr	Tr	0	10	1	Tr	Tr	13	4	Tr	Tr	Tr	Tr	Tr	1
Popsicle																						
3-fl-oz size	1	95	80	70	0	0	0.0	0.0	0.0	0	18	0	0	Tr	4	11	0	0	0.00	0.00	0.0	0

Puddings

Canned

Food	Measure																					
Chocolate	5 oz	142	68	205	3	11	9.5	0.5	0.1	1	30	74	117	1.2	254	285	100	31	0.04	0.17	0.6	Tr
Tapioca	5 oz	142	74	160	3	5	4.8	Tr	Tr	Tr	28	119	113	0.3	212	252	Tr	Tr	0.03	0.14	0.4	Tr
Vanilla	5 oz	142	69	220	2	10	9.5	0.2	0.1	1	33	79	94	0.2	155	305	Tr	Tr	0.03	0.12	0.6	Tr

Dry mix, prepared with whole milk

Chocolate

Food	Measure																					
Instant	½ cup	130	71	155	4	4	2.3	1.1	0.2	14	27	130	329	0.3	176	440	130	33	0.04	0.18	0.1	1
Regular (cooked)	½ cup	130	73	150	4	4	2.4	1.1	0.1	15	25	146	120	0.2	190	167	140	34	0.05	0.20	0.1	1
Rice	½ cup	132	73	155	4	4	2.3	1.1	0.1	15	27	133	110	0.5	165	140	140	33	0.10	0.18	0.6	1
Tapioca	½ cup	130	75	145	4	4	2.3	1.1	0.1	15	25	131	103	0.1	167	152	140	34	0.04	0.18	0.1	1

Vanilla

Food	Measure																					
Instant	½ cup	130	73	150	4	4	2.2	1.1	0.2	15	27	129	273	0.1	164	375	140	33	0.04	0.17	0.1	1
Regular (cooked)	½ cup	130	74	145	4	4	2.3	1.0	0.1	15	25	132	102	0.1	166	178	140	34	0.04	0.18	0.1	1

Sugars

Food	Measure																					
Brown, pressed down	1 cup	220	2	820	0	0	0.0	0.0	0.0	0	212	187	56	4.8	757	97	0	0	0.02	0.07	0.2	0
White Granulated	1 cup	200	1	770	0	0	0.0	0.0	0.0	0	199	3	Tr	0.1	7	5	0	0	0.00	0.00	0.0	0
	1 tbsp	12	1	45	0	0	0.0	0.0	0.0	0	12	Tr	Tr	Tr	Tr	Tr	0	0	0.00	0.00	0.0	0
	1 packet	6	1	25	0	0	0.0	0.0	0.0	0	6	Tr	Tr	Tr	Tr	Tr	0	0	0.00	0.00	0.0	0
Powdered, sifted, spooned into cup	1 cup	100	1	385	0	0	0.0	0.0	0.0	0	100	1	Tr	Tr	4	2	0	0	0.00	0.00	0.0	0

Syrups

Chocolate-flavored syrup or topping

Food	Measure																					
Thin type	2 tbsp	38	37	85	1	Tr	0.2	0.1	0.1	0	22	6	49	0.8	85	36	Tr	Tr	0.02	0.02	0.1	0
Fudge type	2 tbsp	38	25	125	2	5	3.1	1.7	0.2	0	21	38	60	0.5	82	42	40	13	0.02	0.08	0.1	0
Molasses, cane, blackstrap	2 tbsp	40	24	85	0	0	0.0	0.0	0.0	0	22	274	34	10.1	1,171	38	0	0	0.04	0.08	0.8	0
Table syrup (corn and maple)	2 tbsp	42	25	122	0	0	0.0	0.0	0.0	0	32	1	4	Tr	7	19	0	0	0.00	0.00	0.0	0

VEGETABLES AND VEGETABLE PRODUCTS

Alfalfa seeds

Food	Measure																					
Sprouted, raw	1 cup	33	91	10	1	Tr	Tr	Tr	0.1	0	1	11	23	0.3	26	2	50	5	0.03	0.04	0.2	3

Artichokes

Food	Measure																					
globe or French, cooked, drained	1	120	87	55	3	Tr	Tr	Tr	0.1	0	12	47	72	1.6	316	79	170	17	0.07	0.06	0.7	9

Asparagus

Green

Cooked, drained — From raw

Food	Measure																					
Cuts and tips	1 cup	180	92	45	5	1	0.1	Tr	0.2	0	8	43	110	1.2	558	7	1,490	149	0.18	0.22	1.9	49
Spears, ½-in diam. at base	4	60	92	15	2	Tr	Tr	Tr	0.1	0	3	14	37	0.4	186	2	500	50	0.06	0.07	0.6	16

(continued)

Appendix 1 (Continued)
Nutritive Value of the Edible Part of Food*

Item	Foods, Approximate Measures, Units, and Weight (of Edible Portion Only)	Weight (g)	Water (%)	Food Energy (kcal)	Protein (g)	Fat (g)	Saturated (g)	Monounsaturated (g)	Polyunsaturated (g)	Cholesterol (mg)	Carbohydrate (g)	Calcium (mg)	Phosphorus (mg)	Iron (mg)	Potassium (mg)	Sodium (mg)	Vitamin A Value (IU)	Vitamin A Value (RE)	Thiamine (mg)	Riboflavin (mg)	Niacin (mg)	Ascorbic Acid (mg)
From frozen																						
Cuts and tips	1 cup	180	91	50	5	1	0.2	Tr	0.3	0	9	41	99	1.2	392	7	1,470	147	0.12	0.19	1.9	44
Spears, ½-in diam. at base	4	60	91	15	2	Tr	0.1	Tr	0.1	0	3	14	33	0.4	131	2	490	49	0.04	0.06	0.6	15
Canned, spears, ½-in diam. at base	4	80	95	10	1	Tr	Tr	Tr	0.1	0	2	11	30	0.5	122	[56]278	380	38	0.04	0.07	0.7	13
Bamboo shoots																						
Canned, drained	1 cup	131	94	25	2	1	0.1	Tr	0.2	0	4	10	33	0.4	105	9	10	1	0.03	0.03	0.2	1
Beans																						
Lima, immature seeds, frozen, cooked, drained																						
Thick-seeded types (Ford-hooks)	1 cup	170	74	170	10	1	0.1	Tr	0.3	0	32	37	107	2.3	694	90	320	32	0.13	0.10	1.8	22
Thin-seeded types (baby limas)	1 cup	180	72	190	12	1	0.1	Tr	0.3	0	35	50	202	3.5	740	52	300	30	0.13	0.10	1.4	10
Snap																						
Cooked, drained																						
From raw (cut and French style)	1 cup	125	89	45	2	Tr	0.1	Tr	0.2	0	10	58	49	1.6	374	4	[57]830	[57]83	0.09	0.12	0.8	12
From frozen (cut)	1 cup	135	92	35	2	Tr	Tr	Tr	0.1	0	8	61	32	1.1	151	18	710	[58]71	0.06	0.10	0.6	11
Canned, drained solids (cut)	1 cup	135	93	25	2	Tr	Tr	Tr	0.1	0	6	35	26	1.2	147	[59]339	[58]470	[60]47	0.02	0.08	0.3	6
Beans, mature. See Beans, dry and Black-eyed peas, dry.																						
Bean sprouts (mung)																						
Raw	1 cup	104	90	30	3	Tr	Tr	Tr	0.1	0	6	14	56	0.9	155	6	20	2	0.09	0.13	0.8	14
Cooked, drained	1 cup	124	93	25	3	Tr	Tr	Tr	Tr	0	5	15	35	0.8	125	12	20	2	0.06	0.13	1.0	14
Beets																						
Cooked, drained																						
Diced or sliced	1 cup	170	91	55	2	Tr	Tr	Tr	Tr	0	11	19	53	1.1	530	83	20	2	0.05	0.02	0.5	9
Whole beets, 2-in diam.	2	100	91	30	1	Tr	Tr	Tr	Tr	0	7	11	31	0.6	312	49	10	1	0.03	0.01	0.3	6
Canned, drained solids, diced or sliced	1 cup	170	91	55	2	Tr	Tr	Tr	0.1	0	12	26	29	3.1	252	[61]466	20	2	0.02	0.07	0.3	7

Fatty Acids

(continued)

Food	Measure	Grams	Water (%)	Calories	Protein	Fat	Sat. fat	Mono	Poly	Cholesterol	Carbohydrate	Calcium	Phosphorus	Iron	Potassium	Sodium	Vit. A (IU)	Vit. A (RE)	Thiamin	Riboflavin	Niacin	Ascorbic acid
Beet greens Leaves and stems, cooked, drained	1 cup	144	89	40	4	Tr	Tr	0.1	0.1	0	8	164	59	2.7	1,309	347	7,340	734	0.17	0.42	0.7	36
Black-eyed peas Immature seeds, cooked and drained																						
From raw	1 cup	165	72	180	13	1	0.3	0.1	0.6	0	30	46	196	2.4	693	7	1,050	105	0.11	0.18	1.8	3
From frozen	1 cup	170	66	225	14	1	0.3	0.1	0.5	0	40	39	207	3.6	638	9	130	13	0.44	0.11	1.2	4
Broccoli Raw	1	151	91	40	4	1	0.1	Tr	0.3	0	8	72	100	1.3	491	41	2,330	233	0.10	0.18	1.0	141
Cooked, drained From raw																						
Spear, medium	1	180	90	50	5	1	0.1	Tr	0.2	0	10	82	86	2.1	293	20	2,540	254	0.15	0.37	1.4	113
Spears, cut into ½-in pieces	1 cup	155	90	45	5	Tr	0.1	Tr	0.2	0	9	71	74	1.8	253	17	2,180	218	0.13	0.32	1.2	97
From frozen Piece, 4½ to 5 in long	1 piece	30	91	10	1	Tr	Tr	Tr	Tr	0	2	15	17	0.2	54	7	570	57	0.02	0.02	0.1	12
Chopped	1 cup	185	91	50	6	Tr	0.1	Tr	0.1	0	10	94	102	1.1	333	44	3,500	350	0.10	0.15	0.8	74
Brussels sprouts, cooked, drained From raw, 7–8 sprouts, 1¼ to 1½-in diam.	1 cup	155	87	60	4	1	0.2	0.1	0.4	0	13	56	87	1.9	491	33	1,110	111	0.17	0.12	0.9	96
From frozen	1 cup	155	87	65	6	1	0.1	Tr	0.3	0	13	37	84	1.1	504	36	910	91	0.16	0.18	0.8	71
Cabbage Common varieties Raw, coarsely shredded or sliced	1 cup	70	93	15	1	Tr	Tr	Tr	0.1	0	4	33	16	0.4	172	13	90	9	0.04	0.02	0.2	33
Cooked, drained	1 cup	150	94	30	1	Tr	Tr	Tr	0.2	0	7	50	38	0.6	308	29	130	13	0.09	0.08	0.3	36
Cabbage, Chinese Pak-choi, cooked, drained	1 cup	170	96	20	3	Tr	Tr	Tr	0.1	0	3	158	49	1.8	631	58	4,370	437	0.05	0.1	0.7	44
Pe-tsai, raw, 1-in pieces	1 cup	76	94	10	1	Tr	Tr	Tr	0.1	0	2	59	22	0.2	181	7	910	91	0.03	0.04	0.3	21
Cabbage, red Raw, coarsely shredded or sliced	1 cup	70	92	20	1	Tr	Tr	Tr	0.1	0	4	36	29	0.3	144	8	30	3	0.04	0.02	0.2	40
Cabbage, savoy Raw, coarsely shredded or sliced	1 cup	70	91	20	1	Tr	Tr	Tr	Tr	0	4	25	29	0.3	161	20	700	70	0.05	0.02	0.2	22
Carrots *Raw, without crowns and tips, scraped* Whole, 7½ by 1⅛ in, or strips, 2½ to 3 in long	1 carrot or 18 strips	72	88	30	1	Tr	Tr	Tr	0.1	0	7	19	32	0.4	233	25	20,250	2,025	0.07	0.04	0.7	7
Grated	1 cup	110	88	45	1	Tr	Tr	Tr	0.1	0	11	30	48	0.6	355	39	30,940	3,094	0.11	0.06	1.0	10
Cooked, sliced, drained From raw	1 cup	156	87	70	2	Tr	0.1	Tr	0.1	0	16	48	47	1.0	354	103	38,300	3,830	0.05	0.09	0.8	4
From frozen	1 cup	146	90	55	2	Tr	Tr	Tr	0.1	0	12	41	38	0.7	231	86	25,850	2,585	0.04	0.05	0.6	4

Appendix 1 (Continued)
Nutritive Value of the Edible Part of Food*

Item	Foods, Approximate Measures, Units, and Weight (Weight of Edible Portion Only)	Weight (g)	Water (%)	Food Energy (kcal)	Protein (g)	Fat (g)	Fatty Acids Saturated (g)	Monounsaturated (g)	Polyunsaturated (g)	Cholesterol (mg)	Carbohydrate (g)	Calcium (mg)	Phosphorus (mg)	Iron (mg)	Potassium (mg)	Sodium (mg)	Vitamin A Value (IU)	Vitamin A Value (RE)	Thiamine (mg)	Riboflavin (mg)	Niacin (mg)	Ascorbic Acid (mg)
Canned, sliced, drained solids	1 cup	146	93	35	1	Tr	Tr	Tr	0.1	0	8	37	35	0.9	261	[62]352	20,110	2,110	0.03	0.04	0.8	4
Cauliflower																						
Raw, (flowerets)	1 cup	100	92	25	2	Tr	Tr	Tr	0.1	0	5	29	46	0.6	355	15	20	2	0.06	0.06	0.6	72
Cooked, drained																						
From raw (flowerets)	1 cup	125	93	30	2	Tr	Tr	Tr	0.1	0	6	34	44	0.5	404	8	20	2	0.06	0.07	0.7	69
From frozen (flowerets)	1 cup	180	94	35	3	Tr	0.1	Tr	0.2	0	7	31	43	0.7	250	32	40	4	0.07	0.10	0.6	56
Celery, pascal type																						
Raw																						
Stalk, large outer, 8 by 1½ in (at root end)	1	40	95	5	Tr	Tr	Tr	Tr	Tr	0	1	14	10	0.2	114	35	50	5	0.01	0.01	0.1	3
Pieces, diced	1 cup	120	95	20	1	Tr	Tr	Tr	0.1	0	4	43	31	0.6	341	106	150	15	0.04	0.04	0.4	8
Collards																						
Cooked, drained																						
From raw (leaves without stems)	1 cup	190	96	25	2	Tr	0.1	Tr	0.2	0	5	148	19	0.8	177	36	4,220	422	0.03	0.08	0.4	19
From frozen (chopped)	1 cup	170	88	60	5	1	0.1	0.1	0.4	0	12	357	46	1.9	427	85	10,170	1,017	0.08	0.20	1.1	45
Corn																						
Sweet																						
Cooked, drained																						
From raw, ear 5 by 1¾ in	1	77	70	85	3	1	0.2	0.3	0.5	0	19	2	79	0.5	192	13	[63]170	[63]17	0.17	0.06	1.2	5
From frozen																						
Ear, trimmed to about 3½ in long	1	63	73	60	2	Tr	0.1	0.1	0.2	0	14	2	47	0.4	158	3	[63]130	[63]13	0.11	0.04	1.0	3
Kernels	1 cup	165	76	135	5	Tr	Tr	Tr	0.1	0	34	3	78	0.5	229	8	[63]410	[63]41	0.11	0.12	2.1	4
Canned																						
Cream style	1 cup	256	79	185	4	1	0.2	0.3	0.5	0	46	8	131	1.0	343	[64]730	[63]250	[63]25	0.06	0.14	2.5	12
Whole kernel, vacuum pack	1 cup	210	77	165	5	1	0.2	0.3	0.5	0	41	11	134	0.9	391	[65]571	[63]510	[63]51	0.09	0.15	2.5	17
Cowpeas																						
See Black-eyed peas, immature, mature.																						

Cucumber																						
With peel, slices, 1/8 in thick (large, 2 1/8-in diam.; small, 1 3/4-in diam.)	6 large or 8 small slices	28	96	5	Tr	Tr	Tr	Tr	Tr	0	1	4	5	0.1	42	1	10	1	0.01	0.01	0.1	1
Dandelion greens																						
Cooked, drained	1 cup	105	90	35	2	1	0.1	Tr	0.3	0	7	147	44	1.9	244	46	12,290	1,229	0.14	0.18	0.5	19
Eggplant																						
Cooked, steamed	1 cup	96	92	25	1	Tr	Tr	Tr	0.1	0	6	6	21	0.3	238	3	60	6	0.07	0.02	0.6	1
Endive																						
Curly (including escarole), raw, small pieces	1 cup	50	94	10	1	Tr	Tr	Tr	Tr	0	2	26	14	0.4	157	11	1,030	103	0.04	0.04	0.2	3
Jerusalem-artichoke																						
Raw, sliced	1 cup	150	78	115	3	Tr	0.0	Tr	Tr	0	26	21	117	5.1	644	6	30	3	0.30	0.09	2.0	6
Kale																						
Cooked, drained																						
From raw, chopped	1 cup	130	91	40	2	1	0.1	Tr	0.3	0	7	94	36	1.2	296	30	9,620	962	0.07	0.09	0.7	53
From frozen, chopped	1 cup	130	91	40	4	1	0.1	Tr	0.3	0	7	179	36	1.2	417	20	8,260	826	0.06	0.15	0.9	33
Kohlrabi																						
Thickened bulb-like stems, cooked, drained, diced	1 cup	165	90	50	3	Tr	Tr	Tr	0.1	0	11	41	74	0.7	561	35	60	6	0.07	0.03	0.6	89
Lettuce																						
Raw																						
Butterhead, as Boston types																						
Head, 5-in diam	1	163	96	20	2	Tr	Tr	Tr	0.2	0	4	52	38	0.5	419	8	1,580	158	0.10	0.10	0.5	13
Leaves	1 outer or 2 inner leaves	15	96	Tr	Tr	Tr	Tr	Tr	Tr	0	Tr	5	3	Tr	39	1	150	15	0.01	0.01	Tr	1
Crisphead, as iceberg																						
Head, 6-in diam	1	539	96	70	5	1	0.1	Tr	0.5	0	11	102	108	2.7	852	49	1,780	178	0.25	0.16	1.0	21
Wedge, 1/4 of head	1	135	96	20	1	Tr	Tr	Tr	0.1	0	3	26	27	0.7	213	12	450	45	0.06	0.04	0.3	5
Pieces, chopped or shredded	1 cup	55	96	5	1	Tr	Tr	Tr	0.1	0	1	10	11	0.3	87	5	180	18	0.03	0.02	0.1	2
Looseleaf (bunching varieties including romaine or cos), chopped or shredded pieces	1 cup	56	94	10	1	Tr	Tr	Tr	0.1	0	2	38	14	0.8	148	5	1,060	106	0.03	0.04	0.2	10
Mushrooms																						
Raw, sliced or chopped	1 cup	70	92	20	1	Tr	Tr	Tr	0.1	0	3	4	73	0.9	259	3	0	0	0.07	0.31	2.9	2
Cooked, drained	1 cup	156	91	40	3	1	0.1	Tr	0.3	0	8	9	136	2.7	555	3	0	0	0.11	0.47	7.0	6
Canned, drained solids	1 cup	156	91	35	3	Tr	0.1	Tr	0.2	0	8	17	103	1.2	201	663	0	0	0.13	0.03	2.5	0
Mustard greens																						
Without stems and midribs, cooked, drained	1 cup	140	94	20	3	Tr	Tr	0.2	0.1	0	3	104	57	1.0	283	22	4,240	424	0.06	0.09	0.6	35
Okra pods																						
3 by 5/8 in, cooked	8	85	90	25	2	Tr	Tr	Tr	Tr	0	6	54	48	0.4	274	4	490	49	0.11	0.05	0.7	14
Onions																						
Raw																						
Chopped	1 cup	160	91	55	2	Tr	0.1	0.1	0.2	0	12	40	46	0.6	248	3	0	0	0.10	0.02	0.2	13
Sliced	1 cup	115	91	40	1	Tr	0.1	Tr	0.1	0	8	29	33	0.4	178	2	0	0	0.07	0.01	0.1	10
Cooked (whole or sliced), drained	1 cup	210	92	60	2	Tr	0.1	Tr	0.1	0	13	57	48	0.4	319	17	0	0	0.09	0.02	0.2	12

(continued)

Appendix 1 (Continued)
Nutritive Value of the Edible Part of Food*

Item	Foods, Approximate Measures, Units, and Weight (Weight of Edible Portion Only)	Weight (g)	Water (%)	Food Energy (kcal)	Protein (g)	Fat (g)	Saturated (g)	Monounsaturated (g)	Polyunsaturated (g)	Cholesterol (mg)	Carbohydrate (g)	Calcium (mg)	Phosphorus (mg)	Iron (mg)	Potassium (mg)	Sodium (mg)	Vitamin A Value (IU)	Vitamin A Value (RE)	Thiamine (mg)	Riboflavin (mg)	Niacin (mg)	Ascorbic Acid (mg)
Onions, spring																						
Raw, bulb (⅜-in diam.) and white portion of top	6	30	92	10	1	Tr	Tr	Tr	Tr	0	2	18	10	0.6	77	1	1,500	150	0.02	0.04	0.1	14
Onion rings																						
Breaded, par-fried, frozen, prepared	2	20	29	80	1	5	1.7	2.2	1.0	0	8	6	16	0.3	26	75	50	5	0.06	0.03	0.7	Tr
Parsley																						
Raw	10 sprigs	10	88	5	Tr	Tr	Tr	Tr	Tr	0	1	13	4	0.6	54	4	520	52	0.01	0.01	0.1	9
Freeze-dried	1 tbsp	0.4	2	Tr	Tr	Tr	Tr	Tr	Tr	0	Tr	1	2	0.2	25	2	250	25	Tr	0.01	Tr	1
Parsnips																						
Cooked (diced or 2 in lengths), drained	1 cup	156	78	125	2	Tr	0.1	0.2	0.1	0	30	58	108	0.9	573	16	0	0	0.13	0.08	1.1	20
Peas, edible pod																						
Cooked, drained	1 cup	160	89	65	5	Tr	0.1	Tr	0.2	0	11	67	88	3.2	384	6	210	21	0.20	0.12	0.9	77
Peas, green																						
Canned, drained solids	1 cup	170	82	115	8	1	0.1	0.1	0.3	0	21	34	114	1.6	294	[66]372	1,310	131	0.21	0.13	1.2	16
Frozen, cooked, drained	1 cup	160	80	125	8	Tr	0.1	Tr	0.2	0	23	38	144	2.5	269	139	1,070	107	0.45	0.16	2.4	16
Peppers																						
Hot chili, raw	1	45	88	20	1	Tr	Tr	Tr	Tr	0	4	8	21	0.5	153	3	[67]4,840	[67]484	0.04	0.04	0.4	109
Sweet (about 5 per lb, whole), stem and seeds removed																						
Raw	1	74	93	20	1	Tr	Tr	Tr	0.2	0	4	4	16	0.9	144	2	[68]390	[68]39	0.06	0.04	0.4	[68]95
Cooked, drained	1	73	95	15	Tr	Tr	Tr	Tr	0.1	0	3	3	11	0.6	94	1	[70]280	[70]28	0.04	0.03	0.3	[71]81
Potatoes																						
Cooked																						
Baked (about 2 per lb, raw)																						
With skin	1	202	71	220	5	Tr	0.1	Tr	0.1	0	51	20	115	2.7	844	16	0	0	0.22	0.07	3.3	26
Flesh only	1	156	75	145	3	Tr	Tr	Tr	0.1	0	34	8	78	0.5	610	8	0	0	0.16	0.03	2.2	20
Boiled (about 3 per lb, raw)																						
Peeled after boiling	1	136	77	120	3	Tr	Tr	Tr	0.1	0	27	7	60	0.4	515	5	0	0	0.14	0.03	2.0	18
Peeled before boiling	1	135	77	115	2	Tr	Tr	Tr	0.1	0	27	11	54	0.4	443	7	0	0	0.13	0.03	1.8	10

Fatty Acids

(continued)

Food	Measure	Grams	Water (%)	Food energy (cal)	Protein (g)	Fat (g)	Saturated (g)	Monounsaturated (g)	Polyunsaturated (g)	Cholesterol (mg)	Carbohydrate (g)	Calcium (mg)	Phosphorus (mg)	Iron (mg)	Potassium (mg)	Sodium (mg)	Vitamin A (IU)	Vitamin A (RE)	Thiamin (mg)	Riboflavin (mg)	Niacin (mg)	Ascorbic acid (mg)
French fried, strip, 2 to 3½ in long, frozen																						
Oven heated	10	50	50	110	2	4	2.1	1.8	0.3	0	17	5	43	0.7	229	16	0	0	0.06	0.02	1.2	5
Fried in vegetable oil	10	50	50	160	2	8	2.5	1.6	3.8	0	20	10	47	0.4	366	108	0	0	0.09	0.01	1.6	5
Potato products																						
Prepared																						
Au gratin																						
From dry mix	1 cup	245	79	230	6	10	6.3	2.9	0.3	12	31	203	233	0.8	537	1,076	520	76	0.05	0.20	2.3	8
From home recipe	1 cup	245	74	325	12	19	11.6	5.3	0.7	56	28	292	277	1.6	970	1,061	650	93	0.16	0.28	2.4	24
Hashed brown, from frozen	1 cup	156	56	340	5	18	7.0	8.0	2.1	0	44	23	112	2.4	680	53	53	0	0.17	0.03	3.8	10
Mashed																						
From home recipe																						
Milk added	1 cup	210	78	160	4	1	0.7	0.3	0.1	4	37	55	101	0.6	628	636	40	12	0.18	0.08	2.3	14
Milk and margarine added	1 cup	210	76	225	4	9	2.2	3.7	2.5	4	35	55	97	0.5	607	620	360	42	0.18	0.08	2.3	13
From dehydrated flakes (without milk), water, milk, butter, and salt added	1 cup	210	76	235	4	12	7.2	3.3	0.5	29	32	103	118	0.5	489	697	380	44	0.23	0.11	1.4	20
Potato salad																						
Made with mayonnaise	1 cup	250	76	360	7	21	3.6	6.2	9.3	170	28	48	130	1.6	635	1,323	520	83	0.19	0.15	2.2	25
Scalloped																						
From dry mix	1 cup	245	79	230	5	11	6.5	3.0	0.5	27	31	88	137	0.9	497	835	360	51	0.05	0.14	2.5	8
From home recipe	1 cup	245	81	210	7	9	5.5	2.5	0.4	29	26	140	154	1.4	926	821	330	47	0.17	0.23	2.6	26
Potato chips	10	20	3	105	1	7	1.8	1.2	3.6	0	10	5	31	0.2	260	94	0	0	0.03	Tr	0.8	8
Pumpkin																						
Cooked from raw, mashed	1 cup	245	94	50	2	Tr	0.1	Tr	Tr	0	12	37	74	1.4	564	2	2,650	265	0.08	0.19	1.0	12
Canned	1 cup	245	90	85	3	1	0.4	0.1	Tr	0	20	64	86	3.4	505	12	54,040	5,404	0.06	0.13	0.9	10
Radishes																						
Raw, stem ends, rootlets cut off	4	18	95	5	Tr	Tr	Tr	Tr	Tr	0	2	4	3	0.1	42	4	Tr	Tr	Tr	0.01	0.1	4
Sauerkraut																						
Canned, solids and liquid	1 cup	236	93	45	2	Tr	0.1	Tr	0.1	0	10	71	47	3.5	401	1,560	40	4	0.05	0.05	0.3	35
Seaweed																						
Kelp, raw	1 oz	28	82	10	Tr	Tr	0.1	Tr	Tr	0	3	48	12	0.8	25	66	30	3	0.01	0.04	0.1	[1]
Spirulina, dried	1 oz	28	5	80	16	2	0.8	0.2	0.6	0	7	34	33	8.1	386	297	160	16	0.67	1.04	3.6	3
Southern peas																						
See Black-eyed peas, immature.																						
Spinach																						
Raw, chopped	1 cup	55	92	10	2	Tr	0.1	Tr	0.1	0	2	54	27	1.5	307	43	3,690	369	0.04	0.10	0.4	15
Cooked, drained																						
From raw	1 cup	180	91	40	5	Tr	0.1	Tr	0.1	0	7	245	101	6.4	839	126	14,740	1,474	0.17	0.42	0.9	18
From frozen (leaf)	1 cup	190	90	55	6	Tr	0.1	Tr	0.2	0	10	277	91	2.9	566	163	14,790	1,479	0.11	0.32	0.8	23
Canned, drained solids	1 cup	214	92	50	6	1	0.2	Tr	0.4	0	7	272	94	4.9	740	683[7]	18,780	1,878	0.03	0.30	0.8	31
Spinach souffle	1 cup	136	74	220	11	18	7.1	6.8	3.1	184	3	230	231	1.3	201	763	3,460	675	0.09	0.30	0.5	3

Appendix 1 (Continued)
Nutritive Value of the Edible Part of Food*

Item / Foods, Approximate Measures, Units, and Weight (Weight of Edible Portion Only)	Weight (g)	Water (%)	Food Energy (kcal)	Protein (g)	Fat (g)	Saturated (g)	Monounsaturated (g)	Polyunsaturated (g)	Cholesterol (mg)	Carbohydrate (g)	Calcium (mg)	Phosphorus (mg)	Iron (mg)	Potassium (mg)	Sodium (mg)	Vitamin A Value (IU)	Vitamin A Value (RE)	Thiamine (mg)	Riboflavine (mg)	Niacin (mg)	Ascorbic Acid (mg)
Squash																					
Cooked																					
Summer (all varieties), sliced, drained · 1 cup	180	94	35	2	1	0.1	Tr	0.2	0	8	49	70	0.6	346	2	520	52	0.08	0.07	0.9	10
Winter (all varieties), baked, cubes · 1 cup	205	89	80	2	1	0.3	0.1	0.5	0	18	29	41	0.7	896	2	7,290	729	0.17	0.05	1.4	20
Sunchoke																					
See Jerusalem artichoke																					
Sweet potatoes																					
Cooked (raw, 5 by 2 in; about 2½ per lb)																					
Baked in skin, peeled · 1	114	73	115	2	Tr	Tr	Tr	0.1	0	28	32	63	0.5	397	11	24,880	2,488	0.08	0.14	0.7	28
Boiled, without skin · 1	151	73	160	2	Tr	Tr	Tr	0.2	0	37	32	41	0.8	278	20	25,750	2,575	0.08	0.21	1.0	26
Candied, 2½ by 2-in piece · 1	105	67	145	1	3	1.4	0.7	0.2	8	29	27	27	1.2	198	74	4,400	440	0.02	0.04	0.4	7
Canned																					
Solid pack (mashed) · 1 cup	255	74	260	5	1	0.1	Tr	0.2	0	59	77	133	3.4	536	191	38,570	3,857	0.07	0.23	2.4	13
Vacuum pack, piece 2¾ by 1 in · 1	40	76	35	1	Tr	Tr	Tr	Tr	0	8	9	20	0.4	125	21	3,190	319	0.0	0.02	0.3	11
Tomatoes																					
Raw, 2⅗-in diam (3 per 12 oz pkg) · 1	123	94	25	1	Tr	Tr	Tr	0.1	0	5	9	28	0.6	255	10	1,390	139	0.07	0.06	0.7	22
Canned, solids and liquid · 1 cup	240	94	50	2	1	0.1	0.1	0.2	0	10	62	46	1.5	530	[73]391	1,450	145	0.11	0.07	1.8	36
Tomato juice																					
Canned · 1 cup	244	94	40	2	Tr	Tr	Tr	0.1	0	10	22	46	1.4	537	[74]881	1,360	136	0.11	0.08	1.6	45
Tomato products																					
Canned																					
Paste · 1 cup	262	74	220	10	2	0.3	0.4	0.9	0	49	92	207	7.8	2,442	[75]170	6,470	647	0.41	0.50	8.4	111
Puree · 1 cup	250	87	105	4	Tr	Tr	Tr	0.1	0	25	38	100	2.3	1,050	[76]50	3,400	340	0.18	0.14	4.3	88
Sauce · 1 cup	245	89	75	3	Tr	Tr	0.1	0.2	0	18	34	78	1.9	909	[77]1,482	2,400	240	0.16	0.14	2.8	32
Turnips																					
Cooked, diced · 1 cup	156	94	30	1	Tr	Tr	Tr	0.1	0	8	34	30	0.3	211	78	0	0	0.04	0.04	0.5	18

Turnip greens

Food	Measure	Grams	Water (%)	Calories	Protein (g)	Fat (g)	Saturated (g)	Monounsaturated (g)	Polyunsaturated (g)	Carbohydrate (g)	Calcium (mg)	Phosphorus (mg)	Iron (mg)	Potassium (mg)	Sodium (mg)	Vitamin A (IU)	Vitamin A (RE)	Thiamin (mg)	Riboflavin (mg)	Niacin (mg)	Ascorbic acid (mg)
Turnip greens Cooked, drained																					
From raw (leaves and stems)	1 cup	144	93	30	2	Tr	0.1	Tr	0.1	6	197	42	1.2	292	42	7,920	792	0.06	0.10	0.6	39
From frozen (chopped)	1 cup	164	90	50	5	1	0.2	Tr	0.3	8	249	56	3.2	367	25	13,080	1,308	0.09	0.12	0.8	36
Vegetable juice cocktail Canned	1 cup	242	94	45	2	Tr	Tr	Tr	0.1	11	27	41	1.0	467	883	2,830	283	0.10	0.07	1.8	67
Vegetables, mixed																					
Canned, drained solids	1 cup	163	87	75	4	Tr	0.1	Tr	0.2	15	44	68	1.7	474	243	18,990	1,899	0.08	0.08	0.9	8
Frozen, cooked, drained	1 cup	182	83	105	5	Tr	0.1	Tr	0.1	24	46	93	1.5	308	64	7,780	778	0.13	0.22	1.5	6
Water chestnuts Canned	1 cup	140	86	70	1	Tr	Tr	Tr	Tr	17	6	27	1.2	165	11	10	1	0.02	0.03	0.5	2
Baking powders for home use Sodium aluminum sulfate																					
With monocalcium phosphate monohydrate	1 tsp	3	2	5	0	0	0.0	0.0	0.0	1	58	87	0.0	5	329	0	0	0.00	0.00	0.0	0
With monocalcium phosphate monohydrate, calcium sulfate	1 tsp	2.9	1	5	Tr	0	0.0	0.0	0.0	1	183	45	0.0	4	290	0	0	0.00	0.00	0.0	0
Straight phosphate	1 tsp	3.8	2	5	Tr	0	0.0	0.0	0.0	1	239	359	0.0	6	312	0	0	0.00	0.00	0.0	0
Low sodium	1 tsp	4.3	1	5	Tr	0	0.0	0.0	0.0	1	207	314	0.0	891	Tr	0	0	0.00	0.00	0.0	0
Catsup	1 cup	273	69	290	5	1	0.2	0.2	0.4	69	60	137	2.2	991	2,845	3,820	382	0.25	0.19	4.4	41
	1 tbsp	15	69	15	Tr	Tr	Tr	Tr	Tr	4	3	8	0.1	54	156	210	21	0.01	0.01	0.2	2
Celery seed	1 tsp	2	6	10	1	1	Tr	0.3	0.3	1	35	11	0.9	28	3	Tr	Tr	0.01	0.01	0.1	Tr
Chili powder	1 tsp	2.6	8	10	Tr	Tr	0.1	Tr	0.1	1	7	8	0.4	50	26	910	91	0.01	0.02	0.2	2
Chocolate																					
Bitter or baking	1 oz	28	2	145	3	15	9.0	4.9	0.5	8	22	109	1.9	235	1	10	1	0.01	0.07	0.4	0
Semisweet, see Candy.																					
Cinnamon	1 tsp	2.3	10	5	Tr	Tr	Tr	Tr	Tr	2	28	1	0.9	12	1	10	1	Tr	Tr	Tr	1
Curry powder	1 tsp	2	10	5	Tr	Tr	(¹)	(¹)	(¹)	1	10	7	0.6	31	1	20	2	Tr	0.01	0.1	Tr
Garlic powder	1 tsp	2.8	6	10	Tr	Tr	Tr	Tr	Tr	2	2	12	0.1	31	1	0	0	0.01	Tr	Tr	Tr
Gelatin Dry	1 envelope	7	13	25	6	Tr	Tr	Tr	Tr	0	1		0.0	2	6	0	0	0.00	0.00	0.0	0
Mustard Prepared, yellow	1 tsp or individual packet	5	80	5	Tr	Tr	Tr	0.2	Tr	Tr	4	4	0.1	7	63	0	0	Tr	0.01	Tr	Tr
Olives Canned																					
Green	4 medium or 3 extra large	13	78	15	Tr	2	0.2	1.2	0.1	Tr	8	2	0.2	7	312	40	4	Tr	Tr	Tr	0
Ripe, Mission, pitted	3 small or 2 large	9	73	15	Tr	2	0.3	1.3	0.2	Tr	10	2	0.2	2	68	10	1	Tr	Tr	Tr	0
Onion powder	1 tsp	2.1	5	5	Tr	Tr	Tr	Tr	Tr	2	8	7	0.1	20	1	Tr	Tr	0.01	Tr	Tr	0
Oregano	1 tsp	1.5	7	5	Tr	Tr	Tr	0.1	0.1	1	24	3	0.7	25	Tr	100	10	0.01	Tr	0.1	1
Paprika	1 tsp	2.1	10	5	Tr	Tr	Tr	0.2	0.2	1	4	7	0.5	49	1	1,270	127	0.01	0.04	0.3	1
Pepper, black	1 tsp	2.1	11	5	Tr	Tr	Tr	Tr	Tr	1	9	4	0.6	26	Tr	Tr	Tr	Tr	0.01	Tr	0

(continued)

Appendix 1 (Continued)
Nutritive Value of the Edible Part of Food*

Item (Foods, Approximate Measures, Units, and Weight of Edible Portion Only)		Weight (g)	Water (%)	Food Energy (kcal)	Protein (g)	Fat (g)	Fatty Acids Saturated (g)	Monounsaturated (g)	Polyunsaturated (g)	Cholesterol (mg)	Carbohydrate (g)	Calcium (mg)	Phosphorus (mg)	Iron (mg)	Potassium (mg)	Sodium (mg)	Vitamin A Value (IU)	Vitamin A Value (RE)	Thiamine (mg)	Riboflavin (mg)	Niacin (mg)	Ascorbic Acid (mg)
Pickles																						
Cucumber																						
Dill, medium, whole, 3¾-in long, 1¼-in diam.	1 pickle	65	93	5	Tr	Tr	Tr	Tr	0.1	0	1	17	14	0.7	130	928	70	7	Tr	0.01	Tr	4
Fresh-pack, slices 1½-in diam., ¼-in thick	2 slices	15	79	10	Tr	Tr	Tr	Tr	Tr	0	3	5	4	0.3	30	101	20	2	Tr	Tr	Tr	1
Sweet, gherkin, small, whole, about 2½ in long, ¾-in diam.	1 pickle	15	61	20	Tr	Tr	Tr	Tr	Tr	0	5	2	2	0.2	30	107	10	1	Tr	Tr	Tr	1
Popcorn																						
See Grain Products																						
Relish																						
Finely chopped, sweet	1 tbsp	15	63	20	Tr	Tr	Tr	Tr	Tr	0	5	3	2	0.1	30	107	20	2	Tr	Tr	0.0	1
Salt	1 tsp	5.5	0	0	0	0	0.0	0.0	0.0	0	0	14	3	Tr	Tr	2,132	0	0	0.00	0.00	0.0	0
Vinegar																						
Cider	1 tbsp	15	94	Tr	Tr	0	0.0	0.0	0.0	0	1	1	1	0.1	15	Tr	0	0	0.00	0.00	0.0	0
Yeast																						
Baker's, dry, active	1 pkg	7	5	20	3	Tr	Tr	0.1	Tr	0	3	3	90	1.1	140	4	Tr	Tr	0.16	0.38	2.0	Tr
Brewer's, dry	1 tbsp	8	5	25	3	Tr	Tr	Tr	0.0	0	3	[7,8]17	140	1.4	152	10	Tr	Tr	1.25	0.34	3.0	Tr

Fatty Acids

* Tr indicates nutrient present in trace amount.
[1] Value not determined.
[2] Mineral content varies depending on water source.
[3] Blend of aspartame and saccharin; if only sodium saccharin is used, sodium is 75 mg, if only aspartame is used, sodium is 23 mg.
[4] With added ascorbic acid.
[5] Vitamin A value is largely from beta-carotene used for coloring.
[6] Yields 1 qt of fluid milk when reconstituted according to package directions.
[7] With added vitamin A.
[8] Carbohydrate content varies widely because of amount of sugar added and amount and solids content of added flavoring. Consult the label if more precise values for carbohydrate and calories are needed.
[9] For salted butter, unsalted butter contains 12 mg sodium per stick, 2 mg per tbsp, or 1 mg per pat.
[10] Values for vitamin A are year-round average.
[11] For salted margarine.
[12] Based on average vitamin A content of fortified margarine Federal specifications for fortified margarine require a minimum of 15,000 IU per pound.
[13] Fatty acid values apply to product made with regular margarine.
[14] Dipped in egg, milk, and breadcrumbs; fried in vegetable shortening.
[15] If bones are discarded, value for calcium will be greatly reduced.
[16] Dipped in egg, breadcrumbs, and flour, fried in vegetable shortening.
[17] Made with drained chunk light tuna, celery, onion, pickle relish, and mayonnaise-type salad dressing.

18 Sodium bisulfite used to preserve color; unsulfited product would contain less sodium.
19 Also applies to pasteurized apple cider.
20 Without added ascorbic acid. For value with added ascorbic acid, refer to label.
21 With added ascorbic acid.
22 For white grapefruit; pink grapefruit have about 310 IU or 31 RE.
23 Sodium benzoate and sodium bisulfite added as preservatives.
24 Egg bagels have 44 mg cholesterol and 22 IU or 7 RE vitamin A per bagel.
25 Made with vegetable shortening.
26 Made with white cornmeal. If made with yellow cornmeal, value is 32 IU or 3 RE.
27 Nutrient added.
28 Cooked without salt. If salt is added according to label recommendations, sodium content is 540 mg.
29 For white corn grits. Cooked yellow grits contain 145 IU or 14 RE.
30 Value based on label declaration for added nutrients.
31 For regular and instant cereal. For quick cereal, phosphorus is 102 mg and sodium is 142 mg.
32 Cooked without salt if salt is added according to label recommendations, sodium content is 390 mg.
33 Cooked without salt. If salt is added according to label recommendations, sodium content is 324 mg.
34 Cooked without salt. If salt is added according to label recommendations, sodium content is 374 mg.
35 Excepting angel food cake, cakes were made from mixes containing vegetable shortening and frostings were made with margarine.
36 Made with vegetable oil.
37 Cake made with vegetable shortening; frosting with margarine.
38 Made with margarine.
39 Crackers made with enriched flour except for rye wafers and whole-wheat wafers.
40 Made with lard.
41 Cashews without salt contain 21 mg sodium per cup or 4 mg per oz.
42 Cashews without salt contain 22 mg sodium per cup or 5 mg per oz.
43 Macadamia nuts without salt contain 9 mg sodium per cup or 2 mg per oz.
44 Mixed nuts without salt contain 3 mg sodium per oz.
45 Peanuts without salt contain 22 mg sodium per cup or 4 mg per oz.
46 Outer layer of fat was removed to within approximately 1/2 inch of the lean Deposits of fat within the cut were not removed.
47 Fried in vegetable shortening.
48 Value varies widely.
49 Contains added sodium ascorbate. If sodium ascorbate is not added, ascorbic acid content is negligible.
50 One patty (8 per pound) of bulk sausage is equivalent to 2 links.
51 Crust made with vegetable shortening and enriched flour.
52 Made with corn oil.
53 Fried in vegetable shortening
54 If sodium ascorbate is added, product contains 11 mg ascorbic acid.
55 Made with enriched flour, margarine, and whole milk.
56 For regular pack; special dietary pack contains 3 mg sodium.
57 For green varieties; yellow varieties contain 101 IU or 10 RE.
58 For green varieties, yellow varieties contain 151 IU or 15 RE.
59 For regular pack; special dietary pack contains 3 mg sodium.
60 For green varieties; yellow varieties contain 142 IU or 14 RE.
61 For regular pack; special dietary pack contains 78 mg sodium.
62 For regular pack; special dietary pack contains 61 mg sodium.
63 For yellow varieties, white varieties contain only a trace of vitamin A.
64 For regular pack, special dietary pack contains 8 mg sodium.
65 For regular pack; special dietary pack contains 6 mg sodium.
66 For regular pack, special dietary pack contains 3 mg sodium.
67 For red peppers; green peppers contain 350 IU or 35 RE.
68 For green peppers, red peppers contain 4,220 IU or 422 RE.
69 For green peppers; red peppers contain 141 mg ascorbic acid.
70 For green peppers; red peppers contain 2,740 IU or 274 RE.
71 For green peppers, red peppers contain 121 mg ascorbic acid.
72 With added salt; if none is added, sodium content is 58 mg.
73 For regular pack; special dietary pack contains 31 mg sodium.
74 With added salt; if none is added, sodium content is 24 mg.
75 With no added salt; if salt is added, sodium content is 2,070 mg.
76 With no added salt; if salt is added, sodium content is 998 mg.
77 With salt added.
78 Value may vary from 6 to 60 mg.
(United States Dept. of Agriculture, Human Nutrition Information Service Nutritive value of foods Washington, DC US Government Printing Office, 1991 Home and Garden bulletin 72.)

769

Appendix 2
Food and Nutrition Board, National Academy of Sciences—National Research Council Recommended Dietary Allowances,* Revised 1989

Designed for the maintenance of good nutrition of practically all healthy people in the United States

Category	Age (years) or Condition	Weight (kg)	Weight (lb)	Height (cm)	Height (in)	Protein (g)	Fat-Soluble Vitamins				Water-Soluble Vitamins							Minerals						
							Vitamin A (μg R.E.)‡	Vitamin D (μg)§	Vitamin E (mg α-T.E.)‖	Vitamin K (μg)	Vitamin C (mg)	Thiamin (mg)	Riboflavin (mg)	Niacin (mg N.E.)¶	Vitamin B₆ (mg)	Folate (μg)	Vitamin B₁₂ (μg)	Calcium (mg)	Phosphorus (mg)	Magnesium (mg)	Iron (mg)	Zinc (mg)	Iodine (μg)	Selenium (μg)
INFANTS	0.0–0.5	6	13	60	24	13	375	7.5	3	5	30	0.3	0.4	5	0.3	25	0.3	400	300	40	6	5	40	10
	0.5–1.0	9	20	71	28	14	375	10	4	10	35	0.4	0.5	6	0.6	35	0.5	600	500	60	10	5	50	15
CHILDREN	1–3	13	29	90	35	16	400	10	6	15	40	0.7	0.8	9	1.0	50	0.7	800	800	80	10	10	70	20
	4–6	20	44	112	44	24	500	10	7	20	45	0.9	1.1	12	1.1	75	1.0	800	800	120	10	10	90	20
	7–10	28	62	132	52	28	700	10	7	30	45	1.0	1.2	13	1.4	100	1.4	800	800	170	10	10	120	30
MALES	11–14	45	99	157	62	45	1,000	10	10	45	50	1.3	1.5	17	1.7	150	2.0	1,200	1,200	270	12	15	150	40
	15–18	66	145	176	69	59	1,000	10	10	65	60	1.5	1.8	20	2.0	200	2.0	1,200	1,200	400	12	15	150	50
	19–24	72	160	177	70	58	1,000	10	10	70	60	1.5	1.7	19	2.0	200	2.0	1,200	1,200	350	10	15	150	70
	25–50	79	174	176	70	63	1,000	5	10	80	60	1.5	1.7	19	2.0	200	2.0	800	800	350	10	15	150	70
	51+	77	170	173	68	63	1,000	5	10	80	60	1.2	1.4	15	2.0	200	2.0	800	800	350	10	15	150	70
FEMALES	11–14	46	101	157	62	46	800	10	8	45	50	1.1	1.3	15	1.4	150	2.0	1,200	1,200	280	15	12	150	45
	15–18	55	120	163	64	44	800	10	8	55	60	1.1	1.3	15	1.5	180	2.0	1,200	1,200	300	15	12	150	50
	19–24	58	128	164	65	46	800	10	8	60	60	1.1	1.3	15	1.6	180	2.0	1,200	1,200	280	15	12	150	55
	25–50	63	138	163	64	50	800	5	8	65	60	1.1	1.3	15	1.6	180	2.0	800	800	280	15	12	150	55
	51+	65	143	160	63	50	800	5	8	65	60	1.0	1.2	13	1.6	180	2.0	800	800	280	10	12	150	55
PREGNANT						60	800	10	10	65	70	1.5	1.6	17	2.2	400	2.2	1,200	1,200	320	30	15	175	65
LACTATING	1st 6 months					65	1,300	10	12	65	95	1.6	1.8	20	2.1	280	2.6	1,200	1,200	355	15	19	200	75
	2nd 6 months					62	1,200	10	11	65	90	1.6	1.7	20	2.1	260	2.6	1,200	1,200	340	15	16	200	75

(Reprinted with permission from the National Academy of Sciences, Washington, DC.)

*The allowances, expressed as average daily intake over time, are intended to provide for individual variations among most normal persons as they live in the United States under usual environmental stresses. Diets should be based on a variety of common foods in order to provide other nutrients for which human requirements have been less well defined.

† Weights and heights of Reference Adults are actual medians for the U.S. population of the designated age, as reported by NHANES II. The use of these figures does not imply that the height-to-weight ratios are ideal.

‡ Retinol equivalents. 1 retinol equivalent = 1 μg retinol or 6 μg β-carotene.

§ As cholecalciferol. 10 μg cholecalciferol = 400 I.U. of vitamin D.

‖ α-Tocopherol equivalents. 1 mg d-α tocopherol = 1 α-T.E.

¶ 1 N.E. (niacin equivalents) is equal to 1 mg of niacin or 60 mg of dietary tryptophan.

Appendix 3
Estimated Safe and Adequate Daily Dietary Intakes of Selected Vitamins and Minerals*

		Vitamins		Trace Elements†					
Category	Age (years)	Biotin (µg)	Pantothenic Acid (mg)	Copper (mg)	Manganese (mg)	Fluoride (mg)	Chromium (µg)	Molybdenum (µg)
INFANTS	0–0.5	10	2	0.4–0.6	0.3–0.6	0.1–0.5	10–40	15–30
	0.5–1	15	3	0.6–0.7	0.6–1.0	0.2–1.0	20–60	20–40
CHILDREN AND	1–3	20	3	0.7–1.0	1.0–1.5	0.5–1.5	20–80	25–50
ADOLESCENTS	4–6	25	3–4	1.0–1.5	1.5–2.0	1.0–2.5	30–120	30–75
	7–10	30	4–5	1.0–2.0	2.0–3.0	1.5–2.5	50–200	50–150
	11+	30–100	4–7	1.5–2.5	2.0–5.0	1.5–2.5	50–200	75–250
ADULTS		30–100	4–7	1.5–3.0	2.0–5.0	1.5–4.0	50–200	75–250

(Food and Nutrition Board, National Research Council. Recommended Dietary Allowances, 10th ed. Washington DC: National Academy Press, 1989)

*Because there is less information on which to base allowances, these figures are not given in the main table of RDA and are provided here in the form of ranges of recommended intakes.

†Since the toxic levels for many trace elements may be only several times usual intakes, the upper levels for the trace elements given in this table should not be habitually exceeded.

Appendix 4
Estimated Sodium, Chloride, and Potassium Minimum Requirements of Healthy Persons*

Age	Weight (kg)*	Sodium (mg)*†	Chloride (mg)*†	Potassium (mg)‡
MONTHS				
0–5	4.5	120	180	500
6–11	8.9	200	300	700
YEARS				
1	11.0	225	350	1,000
2–5	16.0	300	500	1,400
6–9	25.0	400	600	1,600
10–18	50.0	500	750	2,000
>18§	70.0	500	750	2,000

(Food and Nutrition Board, National Research Council. Recommended Dietary Allowances, 10th ed. Washington DC: National Academy Press, 1989)
* No allowance has been included for large, prolonged losses from the skin through sweat.
† There is no evidence that higher intakes confer any health benefit.
‡ Desirable intakes of potassium may considerably exceed these values (~3,500 mg for adults).
§ No allowance included for growth. Values for those below 18 years assume a growth rate at the 50th percentile reported by the National Center for Health Statistics and averaged for males and females.

Appendix 5
Diet and Drugs

Many drugs have the potential to affect, and be affected by, nutrition. Sometimes, drug-nutrient interactions are the intended action of the drug; at other times, alterations in nutrient intake, metabolism, or excretion may be an unfortunate side effect of drug therapy.

Although well-nourished individuals on short-term drug therapy may easily withstand the negative effects of drug-nutrient interactions, malnourished clients or clients on long-term drug regimens may experience significant nutrient deficiencies and decreased tolerance to drug therapy. Although potential and actual drug-nutrient interactions vary considerably among specific drugs, clients at greatest risk for developing drug-induced nutrient deficiencies include those

- Whose diets are chronically inadequate.
- Who have increased nutritional needs, such as infants, adolescents, and pregnant and lactating women.
- Who are elderly.
- Who have chronic illnesses.
- On long-term or multiple drug regimens.
- Who self-medicate.
- Who are substance abusers.

The mechanisms by which drugs can affect food and nutrients are listed below.

Mechanism: Altered Food Intake Related to the Following:

Increased Appetite: The following drugs may stimulate appetite:

- Antihistamines: cyproheptadine hydrochloride
- Psychotropic drugs: chlorpromazine, chlordiazepoxide, diazepam, meprobamate
- Some mild tranquilizers with antiemetic and antihistaminic properties (however, the elderly may experience decreased appetite and weight loss when given tranquilizers)
- Tricyclic antidepressants: amitriptyline hydrochloride
- Steriods: anabolic steroids like testosterone; glucocorticoids like prednisone

Anorexia: The following drugs may cause anorexia:

- Amphetamines
- Alcohol
- Anticancer agents: 5-fluorouracil, methotrexate
- Antihypertensives: captopril, enalapril, rauwolfia
- Cardiac drugs: amiodarone, digoxin, encainide, procainamide

Increased Satiety Caused by Delayed Gastric Emptying: Delayed gastric emptying may be caused by

- Beta-adrenergic stimulant: salbutamol
- Dopamine precursor: levodopa

Changes in the Sense of Taste or Smell: The following drugs may alter taste or smell sensations:

- Local anesthetics: benzocaine, cocaine, procaine
- Antibiotics: amphotericin B, ampicillin, griseofulvin, lincomycin, strepto-mycin, tetracyclines
- Anticancer agents: methotrexate, doxorubicin hydrochloride
- Anticoagulant: phenindione
- Antihistamine: chlorpheniramine maleate
- Antihypertensive agents: captopril, diazoxide, ethacrynic acid
- Anti-infectious agent: metronidazole
- Chelating agent: d-penicillamine
- Cholesterol-lowering agent: clofibrate
- Diuretics
- Hypoglycemia agent: glipizide
- Psychoactive agents: carbamazepine, lithium carbonate, phenytoin, amphetamines
- Toothpaste ingredient: sodium lauryl sulfate

Nausea or Vomiting

- Almost all drugs have the potential to induce nausea and vomiting, depending on the dosage and length of time used.
- Nausea and vomiting are often the major side effects of anticancer drugs, such as alkylating agents, antimetabolites, and natural and synthetic agents.

Inflammation of the Mouth: Sores in the mouth may be attributed to the use of:

- Anticancer agents: mechlorethamine, mercaptopurine, methotrexate, bleomycin, vinblastine sulfate
- Antiprotozoal: sulfadoxine + pyrimethamine

Mechanism: Altered Nutrient Absorption Related to the Following:

Changes in the pH of the GI Tract: The following drugs can change the GI pH:

- Antacids increase the pH of the GI tract and may thereby decrease the absorption of thiamine, folic acid, iron (carbonate antacids), phosphate (aluminum antacids), or vitamin A (aluminum hydroxide).
- Potassium supplements can decrease the absorption of vitamin B_{12} by lowering ileal pH.

Increased GI motility

- Laxatives like bisacodyl, senna, and phenolphthalein speed the passage of food through the GI tract and thereby reduce the time available for nutrient absorption.

Damage to the Intestinal Mucosa: Drugs that can damage the intestinal mucosa include:

- Alcohol → malabsorption of vitamin B_{12} and folic acid
- Antibiotic: neomycin → malabsorption of fat, vitamin B_{12}, nitrogen, lactose, sucrose, sodium, potassium, iron, and calcium
- Antigout: colchicine → malabsorption of fat, vitamin B_{12}, carotene, lactose, sodium, and potassium
- Antimetabolite: methotrexate → malabsorption of calcium
- Non-narcotic analgesics: chronic use of aspirin and other salicylates can erode the lining of the stomach and intestine, leading to blood loss and iron deficiency.

Binding Agents or Physical Barriers that Prevent Absorption: Binding agents or barriers include:

- Antacids: aluminum hydroxide antacids bind with phosphate or iron to prevent its absorption.
- Anti-inflammatory: salicylazosulfapyridine blocks the absorption of folic acid.
- Antituberculosis agent: para-aminosalicylic acid blocks the absorption of vitamin B_{12}.
- Chelating agent: penicillamine binds with copper, iron, and zinc.
- Laxatives: mineral oil blocks the absorption of the fat-soluble vitamins.

Mechanism: Altered Nutrient Metabolism Related to the Following:

Drugs That Function as Nutrient Antagonists

- Folic acid antagonists include: methotrexate, pyrimethamine, triamterene, trimethoprim.
- Vitamin B_6 antagonists include: isoniazid, hydralazine, cycloserine, levodopa, penicillamine
- Vitamin B_{12} antagonist: nitrous oxide
- Vitamin K antagonists include coumarin anticoagulants.

Altered Enzyme Systems That Metabolize Nutrients

- Anticonvulsants: phenobarbital and phenytoin can cause vitamin D deficiency by altering enzyme systems that increase the inactivation of vitamin D.
- Antimalarial: pyrimethamine inhibits enzymes necessary for normal folic acid metabolism.

Increased/Decreased Nutrient Degradation

- Antacid: aluminum hydroxide destroys thiamine.

Mechanism: Altered Nutrient Excretion Related to the Following:

Altered Renal Reabsorption

- Alcohol increases the excretion of magnesium and zinc.
- Antigout: probenecid decreases urinary excretion of pantothenic acid.
- Diuretics generally may increase urinary thiamine, vitamin B_6, calcium, magnesium, potassium, phosphate, and zinc. Specifically
    Acetazolamide increases urinary calcium and potassium.
    Chlorthalidone increases urinary zinc and potassium.
    Ethacrynic acid and furosemide increase urinary calcium, magnesium, and potassium.
    Mercurials increase urinary thiamine, magnesium, and calcium.
    Spironolactone increases urinary calcium and magnesium.
    Thiazides increase urinary potassium, magnesium, zinc, and riboflavin.
    Triamterene may increase urinary calcium.

Just as drugs can alter nutrients, food and nutrients can alter drug absorption, metabolism, and excretion. Specific mechanisms are listed below.

Mechanism: Altered Drug Absorption Related to the Following:

Altered Secretion of Digestive Juices

Altered GI Motility

Food-Drug Binding, Which Renders the Drug Incapable of Being Absorbed

Examples of drugs whose absorption is delayed by the presence of food include[3]

- Acetaminophen (pectin)
- Amoxicillin
- Aspirin
- Cephaloxin
- Cephradine
- Digoxin
- Erythromycin
- Furosemide
- Sulfadiazine
- Sulfamethoxazole
- Sulfamethoxypridazine
- Sulfanilamide
- Sulfisoxazole

Examples of drugs whose absorption is increased by the presence of food include

- Diazepam
- Griseofulvin (fat)
- Hydrochlorothiazide
- Metoprolol
- Nitrofurantoin
- Propranolol
- Riboflavin

Examples of drugs whose absorption is decreased by the presence of food include

- Amoxicillin
- Ampicillin
- Aspirin
- Demethylchlortetracycline
- Doxycycline
- Isoniazid
- Levodopa (protein, amino acids)
- Methacycline
- Methyldopa (protein, amino acids)
- Oxytetracycline
- Penicillamine
- Penicillin G
- Penicillin V (K)
- Phenethicillin
- Phenobarbital
- Propantheline
- Rifampin
- Tetracycline

Mechanism: Food May Alter Drug Metabolism By the Following:

Interfering With the Action of a Drug: Examples:

- A large intake of coffee, tea, or other caffeine-containing beverages may enhance the side effects of theophylline.
- Large amounts of natural licorice, which tends to increase potassium excretion and sodium retention, may interfere with the action of antihypertensive agents and diuretics. Clients who take digitalis and who experience licorice-induced hypokalemia are at increased risk of digitalis toxicity.
- A high-salt (sodium) intake reduces the therapeutic response to lithium; a low-salt diet may enhance drug activity.
- A high intake of vitamin K-rich vegetables (broccoli, turnip greens, lettuce, cabbage) may inhibit the action of the anticoagulant warfarin.

Contributing Pharmacologically Active Substances: Example:

- Monoamine oxidase inhibitors (MAOIs) are antidepressants that potentiate the cardiovascular effect of tyramine and other vasoactive amines in food. A hypertensive crisis may occur within several hours after foods containing tyramine are ingested with MAOIs. Signs and symptoms include increased blood pressure, headache, pallor, nausea, vomiting, restlessness, dilated pupils, sweating, palpitations, angina, and fever. Death caused by intracranial bleeding occurs rarely. Tyramine-containing foods that are contraindicated during MAOI therapy include[1] the following:

> All aged and mature cheese, such as bleu, Boursault, brick, brie, Camembert, cheddar, emmentdaler, gruyère, mozzarella, parmesan, processed American, provolone, romano, roquefort, stilton
>
> Aged, dried, fermented, salted, smoked and pickled meat and fish, including processed meats and luncheon meats such as bacon, sausage, liverwurst and hot dogs, corned beef, pepperoni, salami, bologna, and ham
>
> Fermented soybean products (miso, some tofu products)
>
> Broad beans and pods
>
> Overripe and spoiled fruit
>
> Sauerkraut
>
> Some alcoholic beverages: Beer, chianti wine, burgundy, sherry, vermouth, ale
>
> Sour dough and homemade yeast breads
>
> Yeast extracts and meat extracts, which can be found in soups, gravies, stews, and sauces

The following foods should be limited to one item per day of ½ cup, 4 oz or less, during MAOI therapy:

> Buttermilk
>
> Yogurt
>
> Sour cream
>
> Caviar
>
> Soy sauce, teriyaki sauce
>
> Excessive caffeine (>2 cups coffee/day)
>
> Certain fruits: bananas, avocados, canned figs, raisins, red plums, raspberries
>
> Other wines and distilled spirits
>
> Chocolate and products containing chocolate

Mechanism: Food May Alter Drug Excretion by the Following:

Changing Urinary pH: Example:

- An excess intake of citrus juices may increase the pH of the urine, and therefore increase blood levels of quinidine.

Bibliography

1. American Dietetic Association: Manual of Clinical Dietetics. Developed by The Chicago Dietetic Association and The South Suburban Dietetic Association, 1992
2. Skidmore-Roth, L. Mosby's 1995 Nursing Drug Reference. St Louis: Mosby, 1995
3. Williams, S. Nutrition and Diet Therapy (7th ed) St. Louis: Mosby, 1993

Appendix 6
Test Diets

Test diets vary among facilities, based on the laboratory's policies. Dietary modifications for common test diets are listed below:

Test	Purpose	Dietary Modifications
Fecal fat determination	To diagnose steatorrhea. Fecal fat in excess of 7g/24 hr indicates steatorrhea	100 g of fat/day (ie, a high-fat diet) is consumed for 3 days before stool collection. Recommended intake includes at least the following foods or their equivalent: 2 c whole milk 8 oz lean meat 1 egg 5 or more servings of fruits and vegetables 6 or more servings of bread and cereals 10 tsp fat (ie, butter, mayonnaise, oil)
Glucose tolerance test	To diagnose diabetes mellitus	A diet adequate to maintain weight that provides at least 150 g CHO/d is consumed for 3 days prior to the test. A fasting period precedes the actual glucose load; coffee, tea, and physical exertion are avoided.
Calcium test	To diagnose hypercalciuria, which is detectable only at moderately high calcium intakes	An intake of 1000 mg of calcium is recommended. Of that, 400 mg is apt to be from dietary sources and the remaining 600 mg obtained from supplements.
Serotonin test (5 HIAA or 4 hydrosyindoleacetic acid)	To determine the metabolite of malignant tumors of the intestinal tract: carcinoid tumors secrete serotonin, which metabolizes into 5 HIAA. 5 HIAA is measured in the urine.	Eliminate the following foods for at least 24 hours before the test: alcohol, butternuts, eggplant, hickory nuts, kiwi fruit, pecans, walnuts, bananas, plantains, avocados, tomatoes, plums, pineapples, pineapple juice

Source: American Dietetic Association: Manual of Clinical Dietetics. Developed by The Chicago Dietetic Association and the South Suburban Dietetic Association, 1992.

Appendix 7
Selected Adult Enteral Formulas and Supplements

I. INTACT NUTRIENT FORMULAS

Section A: Standard Tube Feeding Formulas

Provide approximately 1.0–1.2 cal/ml and 14%–16% total calories from protein. Low in residue; lactose free. Intended for routine tube feedings; some are also routinely used as oral supplements.

Product	Manufacturer	Form	Composition	Nutritional Considerations	Volume to Meet 100% USRDA Vit/Min
Attain	Sherwood Medical	Liquid	Protein sodium and calcium caseinates CHO: maltodextrin Fat: Corn oil, MCT oil	1.0 cal/ml 40 g pro/1000 cal 300 mOsm	1250
Ensure	Ross Products	Liquid	Protein: Sodium and calcium caseinates, soy protein isolates CHO: Corn syrup, sucrose Fat: Corn oil	1.06 cal/ml 35.2 g pro/1000 cal 450 mOsm Used as oral supplement	1887 ml
Isocal	Mead Johnson	Liquid	Protein: Calcium and sodium caseinates, soy protein isolates CHO: Maltodextrin Fat: Soy oil, MCT	1.06 cal/ml 32 g pro/1000 cal 270 mOsm Low sodium	1890 ml
Isolan	Elan Pharma	Liquid	Protein: Caseinates CHO: Maltodextrin Fat: Corn oil, MCT oil	1.06 cal/ml 38 g pro/1000 cal 300 mOsm	1250 ml
Isosource Standard	Sandoz	Liquid	Protein: Sodium and calcium caseinates, soy protein isolates CHO: Hydrolyzed cornstarch Fat: MCT (50% of fat calories), canola oil	1.2 cal/ml 35.7 g pro/1000 cal 360 mOsm	1500 ml
Nutren 1.0 Diet	Clintec	Liquid	Protein: Calcium–potassium caseinate CHO: Maltodextrin, corn syrup solids Fat: Canola oil, MCT oil, corn oil, soy lecithin	1.0 cal/ml 40 g pro/1000 cal 300–350 mOsm	1500 ml
Osmolite	Ross Products	Ready to use	Protein: Sodium and calcium caseinates, soy protein isolate CHO: Hydrolyzed cornstarch Fat: MCT, corn oil, soy oil	1.06 cal/ml 35.2 g pro/1000 cal 290 mOsm	1887 ml
Resource Standard	Sandoz Nutrition	Ready to use	Protein: Sodium and calcium caseinates, soy protein isolate CHO: Hydrolyzed cornstarch, sucrose Fat: Corn oil	1.06 cal/ml 35 g pro/1000 cal 430 mOsm Used as oral supplement	1890 ml

Section B: High Protein Formulas

Provide 1.0–2.0 cal/ml and more than 16% total calories from protein. Low in residue.
Intended for clients with high protein requirements; some are also used as oral supplements.

Product	Manufacturer	Form	Composition	Nutritional Considerations	Volume to Meet 100% USRDA Vit/Min
Ensure HN	Ross Products	Liquid	Protein: Sodium and calcium caseinates, soy protein isolate CHO: Corn syrup, sucrose Fat: Corn oil	1.06 cal/ml 42 g pro/1000 cal 470 mOsm Used as oral supplement	1321 ml
Entrition HN	Clintec	Liquid	Protein: Sodium and calcium caseinate CHO: Maltodextrin Fat: Corn oil, soy lecithin	1.0 cal/ml 44 g pro/1000 cal 300 mOsm	1300 ml
Isocal HN	Mead Johnson	Liquid	Protein: Calcium and sodium caseinates CHO: Maltodextrin Fat: Soybean oil, MCT	1.06 cal/ml 42 g pro/1000 cal 270 mOsm	1180 ml
Isosource HN	Sandoz	Liquid	Protein: Sodium and calcium caseinates, soy protein isolate CHO: Hydrolyzed corn starch Fat: MCT oil, canola oil, soy lecithin	1.2 cal/ml 44 g/1000 cal 330 mOsm	1500 ml
NuBasics VHP	Clintec	Liquid	Protein: Calcium and potassium caseinate CHO: Corn syrup solids, sucrose Fat: Canola oil, corn oil, soy lecithin	1.0 cal/ml 62.5 g pro/1000 cal 460 mOsm Intended as oral supplement	2000 ml
Osmolite HN	Ross Products	Liquid	Protein: Sodium and calcium caseinates, soy protein isolate CHO: Hydrolyzed cornstarch Fat: MCT, corn oil, soy oil	1.06 cal/ml 42 g pro/1000 cal 300 mOsm	1320 ml
Promote	Ross Products	Liquid	Protein: Sodium and calcium caseinates, soy protein isolate CHO: Hydrolyzed cornstarch, sucrose Fat: High oleic safflower oil, canola oil, MCT oil	1.0 cal/ml 62.5 g pro/1000 cal. 330 mOsm May be used as oral supplement	1250 ml
Replete	Clintec	Liquid	Protein: Calcium and potassium caseinate CHO: Corn syrup solids Fat: Canola oil, MCT oil, soy lecithin	1.0 cal/ml 62.5 g pro/1000 cal 300 mOsm	1000 ml
Sustacal Liquid	Mead Johnson	Liquid	Protein: Sodium and calcium caseinate, soy protein isolate CHO: Sugar, corn syrup Fat: Partially hydrogenated soy oil	1.0 cal/ml 61 g pro/1000 cal 6.50 mOsm May be used as oral supplement	1060 ml

(continued)

Appendix 7 (Continued)
Selected Adult Enteral Formulas and Supplements

Section C: High Calorie Formulas

Provide 1.5–2.0 cal/ml and 14%–17% total calories from protein. Lactose free.

Intended for clients who require volume and/or fluid restrictions, or weight gain.

Product	Manufacturer	Form	Composition	Nutritional Considerations	Volume to Meet 100% USRDA Vit/Min
Comply	Sherwood Medical	Liquid	Protein: Sodium, calcium caseinates CHO: Maltodextrin Fat: Corn oil, MCT oil	1.5 cal/ml 40 g pro/1000 cal 410 mOsm	1000 ml
Deliver 2.0	Mead Johnson	Liquid	Protein: Sodium and calcium caseinate CHO: Corn syrup Fat: Soy oil, MCT oil	2.0 cal/ml 38 g pro/1000 cal 640 mOsm	1000 ml
Ensure Plus	Ross Products	Liquid	Protein: Sodium and calcium caseinates, soy protein isolate CHO: Corn syrup, sucrose Fat: Corn oil	1.5 cal/ml 36.6 g pro/1000 cal 690 mOsm May be used orally	1420 ml
Ensure Plus HN	Ross Products	Liquid	Protein: CHO: } Same as Ensure Plus Fat:	1.5 cal/ml 41.7 g pro/1000 cal 650 mOsm May be used orally	947 ml
Magnacal	Sherwood Medical	Liquid	Protein: Calcium and sodium caseinates CHO: Maltodextrin, sucrose Fat: Partially hydrogenated soy oil	2.0 cal/ml 35 g pro/1000 cal 590 mOsm	1000 ml
Nutren 2.0	Clintec	Liquid	Protein: Calcium–potassium caseinate CHO: Corn syrup solids, maltodextrin Fat: MCT oil, canola oil	2.0 cal/ml 40 g pro/1000 cal 720 mOsm	750 ml
Resource Plus	Sandoz	Liquid	Protein: Sodium calcium caseinates, soy protein isolate CHO: Hydrolyzed cornstarch, sugar Fat: Corn oil	1.5 cal/ml 37 g pro/1000 cal 600 mOsm May be used orally	1400 ml
Sustacal Plus	Mead Johnson	Liquid	Protein: Calcium and sodium caseinates CHO: Corn syrup, solids sugar Fat: Corn oil, soy lecithin	1.52 cal/ml 40 g pro/1000 cal 630 mOsm May be used orally	1180 ml
TwoCal HN	Ross Products	Liquid	Protein: Sodium calcium caseinate CHO: Hydrolyzed cornstarch, sucrose Fat: Corn oil, MCT oil	2.0 cal/ml 41.7 g pro/1000 cal 690 mOsm	947 ml

Section D. Formulas Containing Fiber

Provide 1.0–1.5 cal/ml and 14%–17% calories from protein. Lactose free.

Intended as tube feedings for clients who experience diarrhea or constipation from low residue formulas; some are appropriate for oral use.

Product	Manufacturer	Form	Composition	Nutritional Considerations	Volume to Meet 100% USRDA Vit/Min
Ensure with Fiber	Ross Laboratories	Liquid	Protein: Sodium and calcium caseinates, soy protein isolate CHO: Hydrolyzed cornstarch, sucrose, soy fiber (fiber source) Fat: Corn oil	1.1 cal/ml 36 g pro/1000 cal 480 mOsm 13.1 g fiber/1000 cal; 3.4 g fiber/8 g Used as oral supplement	1530
Fibersource	Sandoz	Liquid	Protein: Sodium and calcium caseinates CHO: Hydrolyzed cornstarch, soy fiber Fat: MCT (50% of fat calories), canola oil	1.2 cal/ml 36 g pro/1000 cal 390 mOsm 8 g fiber/1000 cal	1500 ml
Fibersource HN	Sandoz	Liquid	Protein: ⎫ CHO: ⎬ Same as above Fat: ⎭	1.2 cal/ml 45 g pro/1000 cal 390 mOsm 6 g fiber/1000 cal	1500 ml
Jevity	Ross Products	Liquid	Protein: Sodium and calcium caseinates CHO: Hydrolyzed cornstarch, soy fiber Fat: MCT (50% of fat calories), corn oil, soy oil	1.06 cal/ml 42 g pro/1000 cal 300 mOsm 13.6 g fiber/1000 cal	1321 ml
Nutren 1.0 with Fiber Diet	Clintec	Liquid	Protein: Calcium and potassium caseinates CHO: Maltodextrin, corn syrup solids Fat: Canola oil, MCT oil, corn oil, soy lecithin	1.0 cal/ml 40 g pro/1000 cal 310–370 mOsm 14 g fiber/1000 cal	1500 ml
Profiber	Sherwood Medical	Liquid	Protein: Sodium, calcium caseinates CHO: Maltodextrin Fat: MCT oil, corn oil	1.0 cal/ml 40 g pro/1000 cal 300 mOsm 12 g fiber/1000 cal	1250 ml
Sustacal with Fiber	Mead Johnson	Liquid	Protein: Sodium and calcium caseinates, soy protein isolate CHO: Maltodextrin, sugar Fat: Corn oil	1.06 cal/ml 43 g pro/1000 cal 480 mOsm 10 g fiber/1000 cal Used as oral supplement	1420 ml
Ultracal	Mead Johnson	Liquid	Protein: Sodium and calcium caseinates CHO: Maltodextrin, oat fiber, soy fiber Fat: Soy oil, MCT	1.06 cal/ml 42 g pro/1000 cal 310 mOsm 13.6 g fiber/1000 cal	1180 ml

(continued)

Section E. Blenderized Formulas

Provide approximately 1.0 cal/ml and 16% total calories from protein. Made from blended mixture of regular foods; may contain lactose. Tube feeding use only.

Product	Manufacturer	Form	Composition	Nutritional Considerations	Volume to Meet 100% USRDA Vit/Min
Compleat Regular Formula	Sandoz, Nutrition	Liquid	Protein: Beef, nonfat milk CHO: Fruits, vegetables, maltodextrin, nonfat milk Fat: Beef, corn oil	1.07 cal/ml 40 g pro/1000 cal 450 mOsm Contains lactose	1500 ml
Compleat Modified Formula	Sandoz Nutrition	Liquid	Protein: Beef, calcium caseinate CHO: Maltodextrin, fruits, vegetables Fat: Beef, corn oil	1.07 cal/ml 40 g pro/1000 cal 300 mOsm Lactose free	1500 ml
Vitaneed	Sherwood Medical	Liquid	Protein: Beef, sodium and calcium caseinates CHO: Maltodextrin, puréed fruit and vegetables Fat: Soy oil, beef	1.0 cal/ml 35 g pro/1000 cal 310 mOsm Lactose free	2000 ml

Section F. Specialty Formulas

Formulated for specific diseases or medical conditions. Made from intact nutrients, except where indicated.

Half-strength Formulas.

Used as introductory tube feeding or in place of standard formulas when low calorie intake is desired.

Provide approximately 0.5 cal/ml and 14%–17% calories from protein.

Product	Manufacturer	Form	Composition	Nutritional Considerations	Volume to Meet 100% USRDA Vit/Min
Entrition 0.5	Clintec	Liquid	Protein: Sodium–calcium caseinate CHO: Maltodextrin Fat: Corn oil, soy lecithin	0.5 cal/ml 35 g pro/1000 cal 120 mOsm	4000 ml
Introlite	Ross Products	Liquid	Protein: Sodium and calcium caseinate, soy protein isolate CHO: Hydrolyzed cornstarch Fat: MCT oil, corn oil, soy oil	0.53 cal/ml 42 g pro/1000 cal 220 mOsm	1321 ml

Low Carbohydrate/High Fat Formulas
For clients with pulmonary disease/impaired respiratory function. Designed to reduce carbon dioxide production.

Product	Manufacturer	Form	Composition	Nutritional Considerations	Volume to Meet 100% USRDA Vit/Min
NutriVent Diet	Clintec	Liquid	Protein: Calcium and potassium caseinate CHO: Maltodextrin Fat: Canola oil, MCT oil, corn oil, soy lecithin	1.5 cal/ml 45 g pro/1000 cal 330–465 mOsm 55% cal from fat	1000 ml
Pulmocare	Ross Products	Liquid	Protein: Sodium and calcium caseinates CHO: Sucrose, hydrolyzed cornstarch Fat: Canola oil, MCT oil, corn oil, high-oleic safflower oil	1.5 cal/ml 41.7 g pro/1000 cal 475 mOsm 55.1% calories from fat	947 ml
Respalor	Mead Johnson	Liquid	Protein: Calcium and sodium caseinate CHO: Corn syrup, sugar Fat: Canola oil, MCT oil	1.5 cal/ml 50 g pro/1000 cal 580 mOsm 41% calories from fat	1422 ml

Renal Formulas
For clients with impaired renal function. Low in fluid and electrolytes; protein content varies.

Product	Manufacturer	Form	Composition	Nutritional Considerations	Volume to Meet 100% USRDA Vit/Min
AminAid Instant Drink	R&D Laboratories	Powder	Protein: Free essential amino acids plus histidine CHO: Maltodextrin, sucrose Fat: soybean oil	2.0 cal/ml 10 g pro/1000 cal 700 mOsm	N/A (Incomplete formula; does not provide vitamins or minerals)
Nepro	Ross Products	Liquid	Protein: Magnesium, calcium, and sodium caseinates CHO: Hydrolyzed cornstarch, sucrose Fat: High-oleic safflower oil, soy oil	2.0 cal/ml 34.9 g pro/1000 cal 635 mOsm For clients on dialysis	947 ml
RenalCal Diet	Clintec	Liquid	Protein: Essential l-amino acids, select nonessential amino acids, whey protein concentrate CHO: Maltodextrin, modified cornstarch Fat: MCT oil, canola oil, corn oil, soy lecithin	2.0 cal/ml 17.2 g pro/1000 cal 600 mOsm 67% essential amino acids	N/A (Does not provide fat-soluble vitamins)
Suplena	Ross Products	Liquid	Protein: Sodium, calcium caseinates CHO: Hydrolyzed cornstarch, sucrose Fat: High-oleic safflower oil, soy oil	2.0 cal/ml 15 g pro/1000 cal 600 mOsm For non-dialyzed clients with renal failure	947 ml

(continued)

Appendix 7 (Continued)
Selected Adult Enteral Formulas and Supplements

Abnormal Glucose Tolerance/Diabetes Formulas

Low-to-moderate carbohydrate, high fiber formulas. Contain higher-than-normal levels of monounsaturated fat.

Name	Manufacturer	Form	Composition	Volume
Choice DM	Mead Johnson	Liquid	Protein: Milk protein concentrate CHO: Maltodextrin, sucrose, microcrystalline cellulose, soy fiber Fat: Canola oil, high-oleic sunflower oil, corn oil, MCT oil	1.06 cal/ml 42.4 g pro/1000 cal 300–440 mOsm 43% cal from fat 13.6 g fiber/1000 cal 1000 ml
Glytrol	Clintec	Liquid	Protein: Calcium and potassium caseinate CHO: Maltodextrin, cornstarch, fructose Fat: Canola oil, high-oleic safflower oil, MCT oil, soy lecithin	1.0 cal/ml 45 g pro/1000 cal 380 mOsm 42% cal from fat 15 g fiber/1000 cal 1400 ml
Glucerna	Ross Products	Liquid	Protein: Sodium and calcium caseinate CHO: Hydrolyzed cornstarch, soy fiber, fructose Fat: High-oleic safflower oil, soy oil, soy lecithin	1.0 cal/ml 41.8 g pro/1000 cal 375 mOsm 50% cal from fat 14.4 g fiber/1000 cal 1422 ml

Formulas for Immunocompromised Clients

High-protein, low-fat formulas; some enriched with selected ingredients that have been shown to improve immune function. Intended for clients with HIV/AIDS.

Name	Manufacturer	Form	Composition	Volume
Advera	Ross Products	Liquid	Protein: Soy protein hydrolysate, sodium caseinate CHO: Maltodextrin, sugar, soy fiber Fat: Canola oil, MCT oil, deodorized sardine oil	1.28 cal/ml 46.8 g pro/1000 cal 680 mOsm 15.8% cal from fat May be used as oral supplement 1184 ml
Immun-Aid	McGaw	Powder	Protein: Lactalbumin, arginine, glutamine, branched chain amino acids CHO: Maltodextrins Fat: Canola oil, MCT oil	1.0 cal/ml 37 g pro/1000 cal 460 mOsm 2000 ml
Impact	Sandoz	Liquid	Protein: Sodium and calcium caseinates, l-arginine CHO: Hydrolyzed corn starch Fat: Structured lipid, menhaden oil	1.0 cal/ml 56 g pro/1000 cal 375 mOsm 1500 ml

MCT-based Formula

High calorie, low residue; 85% of fat from MCT oil. Intended for clients with fat malabsorption (ie, inflammatory bowel disease, cystic fibrosis, HIV infection).

Lipisorb Liquid	Mead Johnson	Liquid	Protein: Calcium and sodium caseinates CHO: Maltodextrin, sugar Fat: MCT oil, soy oil	1.35 cal/ml 42 g pro/1000 cal 630 mOsm	1180 ml

Hepatic Disease Formulas

Low fat, high in branched chain amino acids, low in aromatic amino acids.

Hepatic-Aid II Instant Drinks	McGaw	Powder	Protein: L-amino acids (46% branch chain amino acids) CHO: Maltodextrin, sucrose Fat: Soybean oil, lecithin	1.2 cal/ml 38 g pro/1000 cal 560 mOsm May be taken via tube or orally; flavored	n/a (Contains negligible quantities of electrolytes and no vitamins)
NutriHep Diet	Clintec	Liquid	Protein: L-amino acids, whey protein (50% branched chain amino acids) CHO: Maltodextrin Fat: MCT oil, canola oil, soy lecithin, corn oil	1.5 cal/ml 26.7 g pro/1000 cal 690 mOsm	1000 ml

Metabolic Stress Formulas

Provide 1.0–1.5 cal/ml and 20%–25% calories from protein.

Perative	Ross	Liquid	Protein: Partially hydrolyzed sodium caseinate, lactalbumin hydrolysate, L-arginine CHO: Hydrolyzed cornstarch Fat: canola oil, MCT oil, corn oil	1.3 cal/ml 51.2 g pro/1000 cal 385 mOsm	1155 ml
TraumaCal	Mead Johnson	Liquid	Protein: Calcium and sodium caseinates CHO: Corn syrup, sugar Fat: Soy oil, MCT oil	1.5 cal/ml 55 g pro/1000 cal 490 mOsm	2000 ml

(continued)

Appendix 7 (Continued)
Selected Adult Enteral Formulas and Supplements

II. ELEMENTAL FORMULAS

Provide approximately 1.0–1.5 cal/ml and 8%–17% of total calories from protein. Made from partially or fully hydrolyzed nutrients; are lactose-free, low residue. Most have high osmolality. Intended as tube feedings for clients with altered digestion and/or absorption.

Product	Manufacturer	Form	Composition	Nutritional Considerations	Volume to Meet 100% USRDA Vit/Min
Alitraq	Ross Products	Powder	Protein: Soy hydrolysate, whey protein concentrate; lactalbumin hydrolysate, free amino acids CHO: Hydrolyzed cornstarch, sucrose, fructose Fat: MCT oil, safflower oil	1.0 cal/ml 52.5 g pro/1000 cal 575 mOsm	1500 ml
Criticare HN	Mead Johnson	Liquid	Protein: Enzymatically hydrolyzed casein CHO: Maltodextrin, modified cornstarch Fat: Safflower oil, soy oil	1.06 cal/ml 36 g pro/1000 cal 650 mOsm	1890 ml
Peptamen	Clintec	Liquid	Protein: Enzymatically hydrolyzed whey CHO: Maltodextrin, corn starch Fat: MCT oil, sunflower oil, soy lecithin	1.0 cal/ml 40 g pro/1000 cal 270–380 mOsm	1500 ml
Reabilan	Clintec	Liquid	Protein: Enzymatically hydrolyzed casein and whey (small peptides) CHO: Maltodextrin, tapioca starch Fat: MCT oil, canola oil, soy lecithin	1.0 cal/ml 31.5 g pro/1000 cal 350 mOsm	2000 ml
Reabilan HN	Clintec	Liquid	Protein: Enzymatically hydrolyzed casein and whey (small peptides) CHO: Maltodextrin, tapioca starch Fat: MCT, soy oil, Canola oil, soy lecithin	1.33 cal/ml 44 g pro/1000 cal 490 mOsm	1500 ml
SandoSource Peptide	Sandoz	Liquid	Protein: Casein hydrolysate, free amino acids, sodium caseinate CHO: Hydrolyzed corn starch Fat: MCT oil, soybean oil	1.0 cal/ml 50 g pro/1000 cal 500 mOsm	1750 ml
Tolerex	Sandoz	Powder	Protein: Free amino acids CHO: Maltodextrin Fat: Safflower oil	1.0 cal/ml 21 g pro/1000 cal 550 mOsm	3160 ml
Vital HN	Ross Products	Powder	Protein: Peptides from partially hydrolyzed whey, soy, and meat protein, with added free essential amino acids CHO: Hydrolyzed cornstarch, sucrose Fat: Safflower oil, MCT	1.0 cal/ml 41.7 g pro/1000 cal 500 mOsm	1500 ml

(continued)

					Volume to Meet 100% USRDA Vit/Min
Vivonex Plus	Sandoz	Powder	Protein: Free amino acids CHO: Maltodextrin, modified starch Fat: Soybean oil	1.0 cal/ml 45 g pro/1000 cal 650 mOsm	1800 ml
Vivonex T.E.N.	Sandoz Nutrition	Powder	Protein: Free amino acids (33% branched-chain amino acids) CHO: Maltodextrins, modified starch Fat: Safflower oil	1.0 cal/ml 38 g pro/1000 cal 630 mOsm	2000 ml

III. MILK-BASED ORAL SUPPLEMENTS

High-protein, flavored drinks for clients able to tolerate lactose.

Product	Manufacturer	Form	Composition	Nutritional Considerations	Volume to Meet 100% USRDA Vit/Min
Carnation Instant Breakfast	Clintec	Powder	Protein: Nonfat milk, fluid milk used to mix powder CHO: Maltodextrin, sugar, lactose Fat: Butterfat from milk used to mix powder	0.93 cal/ml 48 g pro/1000 cal 661–747 mOsm	1065 ml
Carnation Instant Breakfast Ready-to-Drink	Clintec	Liquid	Protein: Nonfat milk, milk protein CHO: Sugar, lactose, dextrose Fat: Corn oil	0.67 cal/ml 63 g pro/1000 cal 510 mOsm	1200 ml
Delmark Instant Breakfast	Sandoz	Powder	Protein: Nonfat milk, fluid milk used to mix powder CHO: Dextrose, sugar, lactose Fat: Butterfat from milk used to mix powder	1.22 cal/ml 52 g pro/1000 cal 796 mOsm	n/a
Forta Shake	Ross Products	Powder	Protein: Nonfat milk, fluid milk used to mix powder CHO: Sucrose, lactose Fat: Butterfat from milk used to mix powder	1.2 cal/ml 59 g pro/1000 cal	948 ml
Great Shake	Menu Magic	Liquid	Protein: Skim milk, nonfat milk solids CHO: Corn syrup, high fructose corn syrup Fat: Partially hydrogenated soybean oil	1.67 cal/ml 30 g pro/1000 cal	900 ml
Sustacal Powder	Mead Johnson	Powder; mixes with milk or water	Protein: Nonfat milk, whole milk CHO: Sugar, corn syrup solids, lactose Fat: Butterfat	3 cal/ml 58 g pro/1000 cal 1.09 cal/ml (prepared with skim milk) 1% cal from fat	1160 ml

Appendix 7 (Continued)
Selected Adult Enteral Formulas and Supplements

	Manufacturer	Form	Composition	Nutritional Considerations	Volume to Meet 100% USRDA Vit/Min
Sustagen	Mead Johnson	Powder	Protein: milk, calcium caseinate CHO: Corn syrup solids, lactose, dextrose Fat: Butterfat	1.9 cal/ml 61 g pro/1000 cal 1130 mOsm 8% cal from fat	1030 ml

IV. CLEAR LIQUID SUPPLEMENTS

Low-fat, minimal residue formulas appropriate as protein +/or calorie supplement for clients on clear liquid diets.

Product	Manufacturer	Form	Composition	Nutritional Considerations	Volume to Meet 100% USRDA Vit/Min
Citrotein	Sandoz Nutrition	Powder	Protein: Egg white solids CHO: Sucrose, maltodextrin Fat: Partially hydrogenated soybean oil	0.66 cal/ml 62 g pro/1000 cal 2% cal from fat	n/a
Forta Drink	Ross Products	Powder	Protein: Whey protein CHO: Sucrose Fat: Negligible	0.56 cal/ml 59 g pro/1000 cal	n/a

V. MODULAR PRODUCTS—INCOMPLETE DIET SUPPLEMENTS

Intended for oral use; may be mixed with food or enteral formulas.

Protein Modules

	Manufacturer	Form	Ingredients	Nutritional Considerations
Casec	Mead Johnson	Powder	Calcium caseinate	88 g protein/100 g powder
ProMod	Ross Products	Powder	D-Whey protein concentrate and soy lecithin	75 g protein/100 g powder

CHO Modules

	Manufacturer	Form	Ingredients	Nutritional Considerations
Moducal	Mead Johnson	Powder	100% Maltodextrin	3.75 cal/g powder
Polycose	Ross Products	Powder	Glucose polymers derived from starch hydrolysis	94 g CHO/100 g powder
Polycose	Ross Products	Liquid	Glucose polymers derived from starch hydrolysis	50 g CHO/100 ml liquid

Fat Modules

MCT Oil	Mead Johnson	Liquid	Medium chain triglycerides	8.3 cal/g 116 cal/1 tbsp (14 g)

VI. OTHER SUPPLEMENTS

Biocare Drink Mix	Food Sciences Corporation	200 cal/8 oz prepared 10 g protein/serving 2 flavors For clients with altered taste perception	
Biocare Pudding Mix	Food Sciences Corporation	260 cal/1/2 c prepared 10 g protein/serving 3 flavors Lactose-free	
Ensure Pudding	Ross Products	250 cal/5 oz 6.8 g pro/5 oz 4 flavors Pre-prepared	
NuBasics Complete Nutrition Bar	Clintec	125 cal/bar 4.4 g pro/bar 2 flavors	
NuBasics Complete Nutrition Soup	Clintec	250 cal/serving 8.75 g pro/serving 2 flavors Mixes with hot water	
Sustacal Pudding	Mead Johnson	240 cal/5 oz 6.8 g pro/5 oz Various flavors Pre-prepared	

Appendix 8
Caffeine Content of Selected Beverages and Foods

Source	Average mg of Caffeine
COFFEE (6 OZ CUP)	
Brewed	103
Instant	57
FLAVORED COFFEE FROM INSTANT MIXES (6 OZ)	
Cafe amaretto	60
Cafe francais	53
Cafe vienna	56
Irish mocha mint	27
Orange cappuncino	71
Suisse mocha	41
COFFEE, INSTANT DRY POWDER (1 TEASPOON)	
Regular	57
Coffee with chicory	38
Decaffeinated	2
TEA BEVERAGE	
Brewed black, 3 min (6 fl oz)	36
Instant powder (1 tsp)	31
SOFT DRINKS CONTAINING CAFFEINE (12 FL OZ)	
Cherry, Coca-Cola	46
Coca-Cola	46
Cola soda, decaffeinated	tr
Diet Coke	46
Diet RC	48
Mountain Dew	54
Mr. Pibb	40
Mello Yello	52
Pepsi Cola	38
Diet Pepsi	36
RC Cola	18
7 Up Gold	46
CHOCOLATE PRODUCTS	
Baking chocolate, 1 oz unsweetened	58
Chocolate frozen pudding pop with chocolate coating, 1 pop	7
Chocolate milk, 8 fl oz	8
Chocolate Nestle Crunch candy bar, 1.4 oz	10
Chocolate powder for milk, 1 T	8
Chocolate syrup, 2 T	5
Chocolate pudding, from instant mix ½ c	5
Cocoa beverage, 6 fl oz	4
Cocoa unsweetened, dry powder, 1 T	12
Milk chocolate chips, 1 cup	43

Source: Pennington JAT: Bowes and Church's Food Values of Portions Commonly Used, 16th. Philadelphia: JB Lippincott, 1994

Appendix 9
NCHS Percentile Growth Charts

GIRLS: BIRTH TO 36 MONTHS
PHYSICAL GROWTH
NCHS PERCENTILES*

NAME_____ RECORD #_____

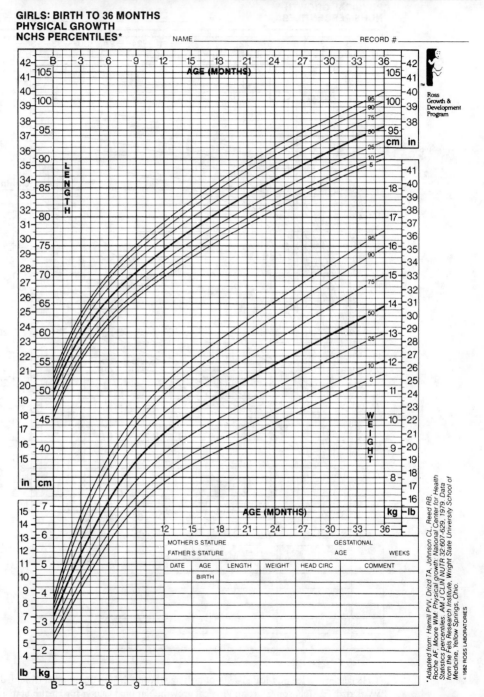

NCHS percentiles for physical growth of girls aged from birth to 36 months. (Adapted from Hamill PVV, Drizd TA, Johnson CL et al: Physical growth: National Center for Health Statistics percentiles. *Am J Clin Nutr* 32:607, 1979. Data from the Fels Research Institute, Wright State University School of Medicine, Yellow Springs, Ohio.)

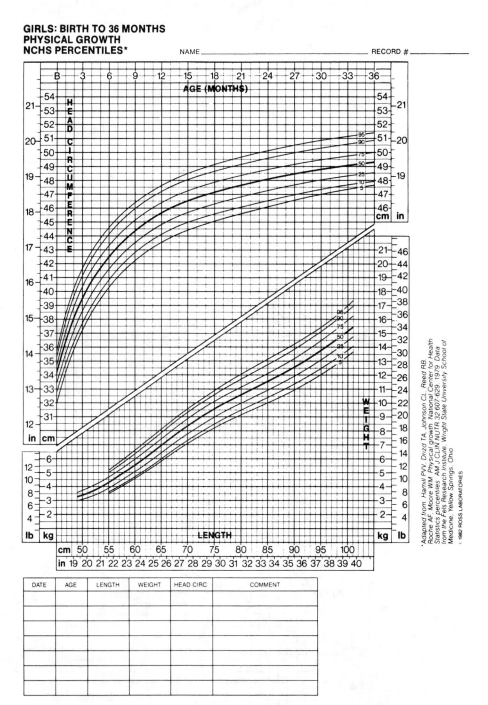

NCHS percentiles for physical growth of girls aged from birth to 36 months. (Adapted from Hamill PVV, Drizd TA, Johnson CL et al: Physical growth: National Center for Health Statistics percentiles. *Am J Clin Nutr* 32:607, 1979. Data from the Fels Research Institute, Wright State University School of Medicine, Yellow Springs, Ohio.)

**GIRLS: PREPUBESCENT
PHYSICAL GROWTH
NCHS PERCENTILES***

NAME_____ RECORD #_____

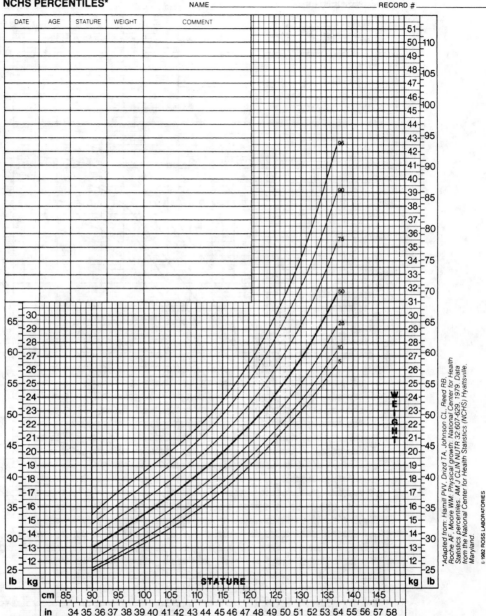

NCHS percentiles for physical growth of prepubescent girls. (Adapted from Hamill PVV, Drizd TA, Johnson CL et al: Physical growth: National Center for Health Statistics percentiles. *Am J Clin Nutr* 32:607, 1979. Data from the National Center for Health Statistics, Hyattsville, Maryland.)

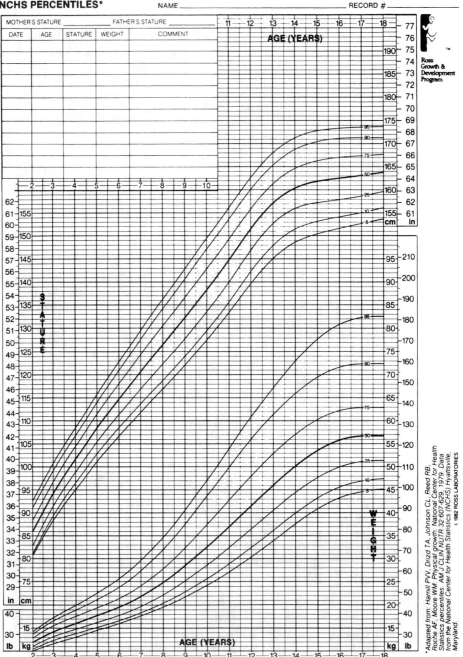

**GIRLS: 2 TO 18 YEARS
PHYSICAL GROWTH
NCHS PERCENTILES***

NCHS percentiles for physical growth of girls aged from 2 to 18 years. (Adapted from Hamill PVV, Drizd TA, Johnson CL et al: Physical growth: National Center for Health Statistics percentiles. *Am J Clin Nutr* 32:607, 1979. Data from the National Center for Health Statistics, Hyattsville, Maryland.)

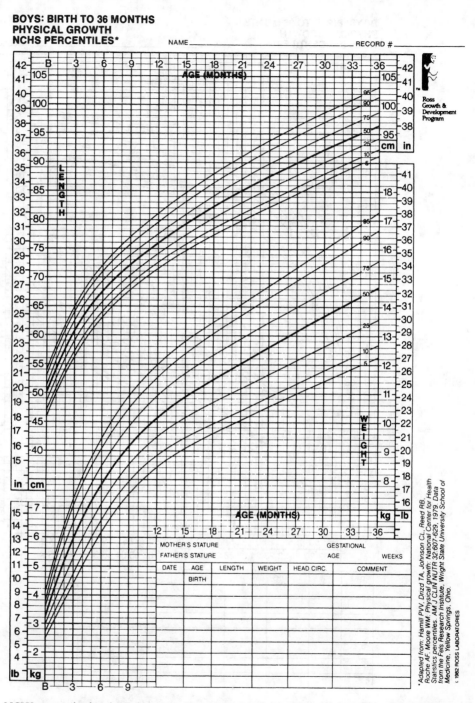

NCHS percentiles for physical growth of boys aged from birth to 36 months. (Adapted from Hamill PVV, Drizd TA, Johnson CL et al: Physical growth: National Center for Health Statistics percentiles. *Am J Clin Nutr* 32:607, 1979. Data from the Fels Research Institute, Wright State University School of Medicine, Yellow Springs, Ohio.)

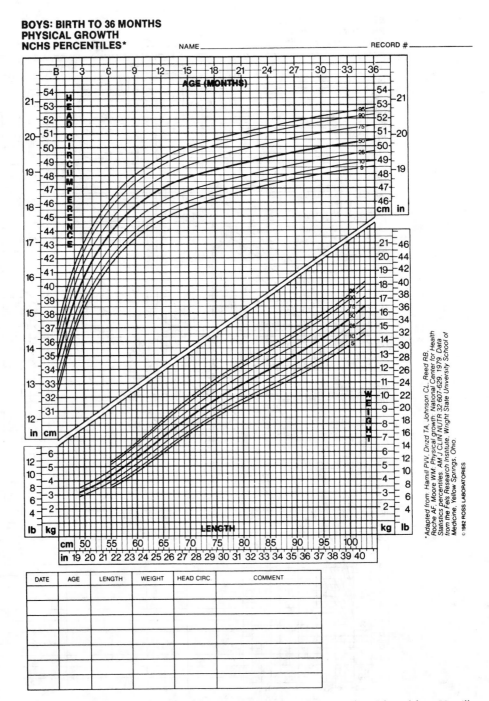

BOYS: BIRTH TO 36 MONTHS
PHYSICAL GROWTH
NCHS PERCENTILES*

NCHS percentiles for physical growth of boys aged from birth to 36 months. (Adapted from Hamill PVV, Drizd TA, Johnson CL et al: Physical growth: National Center for Health Statistics percentiles. *Am J Clin Nutr* 32:607, 1979. Data from the Fels Research Institute, Wright State University School of Medicine, Yellow Springs, Ohio.)

**BOYS: PREPUBESCENT
PHYSICAL GROWTH
NCHS PERCENTILES***

NAME _____ RECORD # _____

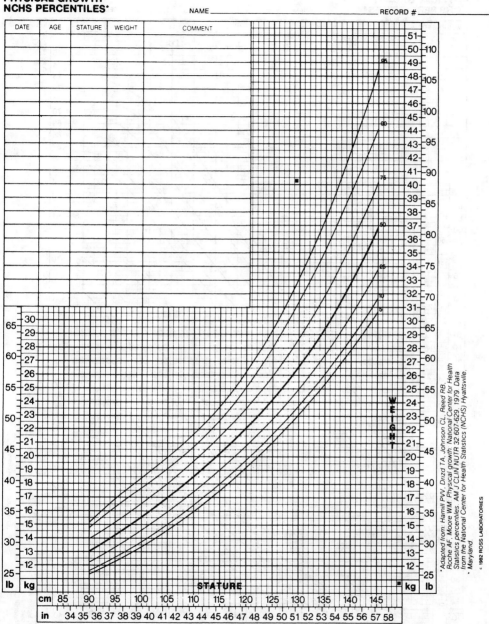

NCHS percentiles for physical growth of prepubescent boys. (Adapted from Hamill PVV, Drizd TA, Johnson CL et al: Physical growth: National Center for Health Statistics percentiles. *Am J Clin Nutr* 32:607, 1979. Data from the National Center for Health Statistics, Hyattsville, Maryland.)

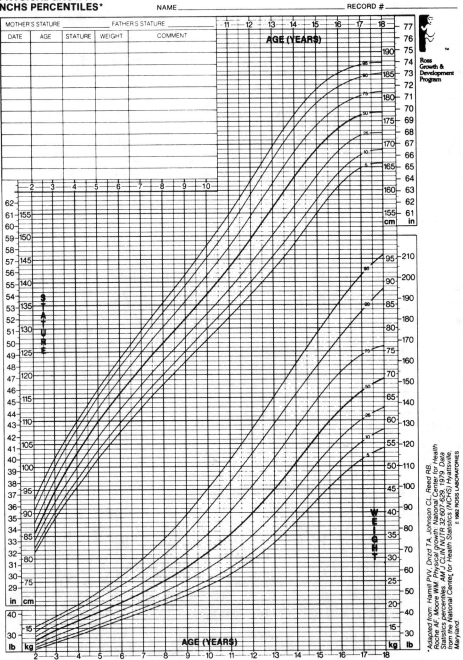

NCHS percentiles for physical growth of boys aged from 2 to 18 years. (Adapted from Hamill PVV, Drizd TA, Johnson CL et al: Physical growth: National Center for Health Statistics percentiles. *Am J Clin Nutr* 32:607, 1979. Data from the National Center for Health Statistics, Hyattsville, Maryland.)

Appendix 10
Two Methods for Determining Calorie Requirements

Method I.

Using BEE (basal energy requirements)

$$\text{BEE for men} = 66 + [13.7 \times \text{wt (kg*)}] + [5 \times \text{ht (cm)}] - [6.8 \times \text{age (years)}]$$

$$\text{BEE for women} = 655.1 + [9.65 \times \text{wt (kg*)}] + [1.7 \times \text{ht (cm)}] - [4.7 \times \text{age (years)}]$$

For people who weight >125% of ideal body weight, use adjusted body weight instead of actual body weight in the above equation (because only approximately 25% of body fat issue is metabolically active).

$$\text{Adjusted body weight} = (\text{Actual body weight} - \text{IBW}) \times .25 + \text{IBW}$$

For Weight Maintenance:

$$\text{BEE} \times 1.2 - 1.3 = \text{total calories needed/day to maintain weight}$$

For Weight Loss:

$$(\text{BEE} \times 1.2) - 500 = \text{total calories needed/day to lose 1 pound/week}$$

For Weight Gain:

$$(\text{BEE} \times 1.2) + 500 = \text{total calories needed/day to gain 1 pound/week}$$

Method II.

Using current body weight,* estimation of weight status, and level of physical activity

To maintain weight: multiply weight in kg by the appropriate factor, based on weight status and activity:

	Sedentary	Moderate	Active
Overweight	20–25 cal/kg	30 cal/kg	35 cal/kg
Normal weight	30 cal/kg	35 cal/kg	40 cal/kg
Underweight	30 cal/kg	40 cal/kg	45–50 cal/kg

* If actual weight is >125% IBW, use adjusted body weight. Adjusted body weight = (actual body weight − IBW) × .25 + IBW.

Appendix 11
Exchange Lists for Meal Planning*

CARBOHYDRATE LISTS

Starch List

One starch exchange equals 15 grams carbohydrate, 3 grams protein, 0–1 grams fat, and 80 calories.

BREAD

Bagel	½ (1 oz)	Pita, 6 in. across	½
Bread, reduced-calorie	2 slices (1½ oz)	Roll, plain, small	1 (1 oz)
Bread, white, whole-wheat, pumpernickel, rye	1 slice (1 oz)	Raisin bread, unfrosted	1 slice (1 oz)
		Tortilla, corn, 6 in. across	1
Bread sticks, crisp, 4 in. long × ½ in	2 (⅔ oz)	Tortilla, flour, 7–8 in. across	1
English muffin	1/2	Waffle, 4½ in. square, reduced-fat	1
Hot dog or hamburger bun	½ (1 oz)		

CEREALS AND GRAINS

Bran cereals	½ cups	Millet	¼ cup
Bulgur	½ cup	Muesli	¼ cup
Cereals	½ cup	Oats	½ cup
Cereals, unsweetened, ready-to-eat	¾ cup	Pasta	½ cups
Cornmeal (dry)	3 Tbsp	Puffed cereal	1½ cups
Couscous	⅓ cup	Rice milk	½ cups
Flour (dry)	3 Tbsp	Rice, white or brown	⅓ cup
Granola, low-fat	¼ cup	Shredded Wheat	½ cup
Grape-Nuts	¼ cup	Sugar-frosted cereal	½ cup
Grits	½ cup	Wheat germ	3 Tbsp
Kasha	½ cup		

STARCHY VEGETABLES

Baked beans	⅓ cup	Plantain	½ cup
Corn	½ cup	Potato, baked or boiled	1 small (3 oz)
Corn on cob, medium	1 (5 oz)	Potato, mashed	½ cup
Mixed vegetables with corn, peas, or pasta	1 cup	Squash, winter (acorn, butternut)	1 cup
Peas, green	½ cup	Yam, sweet potato, plain	½ cup

CRACKERS AND SNACKS

Animal crackers	8	Pretzels	¾ oz
Graham crackers, 2½ in. square	3	Rice cakes, 4 in. across	2
Matzoh	¾ oz	Saltine-tye crackers	6
Melba toast	4 slices	Snack chips, fat-free (tortilla, potato)	15–20 (¾ oz)
Oyster crackers	24	Whole-wheat crackers, no fat added	2–5 (¾ oz)
Popcorn (popped, no fat added or low-fat microwave)	3 cups		

* = 400 mg or more sodium per exchange.

DRIED BEANS, PEAS, AND LENTILS

(Count as 1 starch exchange, plus 1 very lean meat exchange.)

Beans and peas (garbanzo, pinto, kidney, white, split, black-eyed)	½ cup	Lima beans	⅔ cup
		Lentils	½ cup
		Miso*	3 Tbsp

STARCHY FOODS PREPARED WITH FAT

(Count as 1 starch exchange, plus 1 fat exchange.)

Biscuit, 2½ in. across	1	Pancake, 4 in. across	2
Chow mein noodles	½ cup	Popcorn, microwave	3 cups
Corn bread, 2 in. cube	1 (2 oz)	Sandwich crackers, cheese or peanut butter filling	3
Crackers, round butter type	6		
Croutons	1 cup	Stuffing, bread (prepared)	⅓ cup
French-fried potatoes	16–25 (3 oz)	Taco shell, 6 in. across	2
Granola	¼ cup	Waffle, 4½ in. square	1
Muffin, small	1 (1½ oz)	Whole-wheat crackers, fat added	4–6 (1 oz)

Fruit List

One fruit exchange equals 15 grams carbohydrate and 60 calories. The weight includes skin, core, seeds, and rind.

FRUIT

Apple, unpeeled, small	1 (4 oz)	Kiwi	1 (3½ oz)
Applesauce, unsweetened	½ cup	Mandarin oranges, canned	¾ cup
Apples, dried	4 rings	Mango, small	½ fruit (5½ oz) or ½ cup
Apricots, fresh	4 whole (5½ oz)		
Apricots, dried	8 halves	Nectarine, small	1 (5 oz)
Apricots, canned	½ cup	Orange, small	1 (6½ oz)
Banana, small	1 (4 oz)	Papaya	½ fruit (8 oz) or 1 cup cubes
Blackberries	¾ cup		
Blueberries	¾ cup	Peach, medium, fresh	1 (6 oz)
Cantaloupe, small	⅓ melon (11 oz) or 1 cup cubes	Peaches, canned	½ cup
		Pear, large, fresh	½ (4 oz)
Cherries, sweet, fresh	12 (3 oz)	Pears, canned	½ cup
Cherries, sweet, canned	½ cup	Pineapple, fresh	¾ cup
Dates	3	Pineapple, canned	½ cup
Figs, fresh	1½ large or 2 medium (3½ oz)	Plums, small	2 (5 oz)
		Plums, canned	½ cup
Figs, dried	1½ cup	Prunes, dried	3
Fruit cocktail	½ cup	Raisins	2 Tbsp
Grapefruit, large	½ (11 oz)	Raspberries	1 cup
Grapefruit sections, canned	¾ cup	Strawberries	1¼ cup whole berries
Grapes, small	17 (3 oz)	Tangerines, small	2 (8 oz)
Honeydew melon	1 slice (10 oz) or 1 cup cubes	Watermelon	1 slice (13½ oz) or 1¼ cup cubes

FRUIT JUICE

Apple juice/cider	½ cup	Grapefruit juice	½ cup
Cranberry juice cocktail	⅓ cup	Orange juice	½ cup
Cranberry juice cocktail, reduced-calorie	1 cup	Pineapple juice	½ cup
Fruit juice blends, 100% juice	⅓ cup	Prune juice	⅓ cup
Grape juice	⅓ cup		

Milk List

One milk exchange equals 12 grams carbohydrate and 8 grams protein.

SKIM AND VERY LOW-FAT MILK (0–3 GRAMS FAT PER SERVING)

Skim milk	1 cup	Nonfat dry milk	⅓ cup dry
½% milk	1 cup	Plain nonfat yogurt	¾ cup
1% milk	1 cup	Nonfat or low-fat fruit-flavored yogurt	
Nonfat or low-fat buttermilk	1 cup	sweetened with aspartame or with a	
Evaporated skim milk	½ cup	nonnutritive sweetener	1 cup

LOW-FAT (5 GRAMS FAT PER SERVING)

2% milk	1 cup	Sweet acidophilus milk	1 cup
Plain low-fat yogurt	¾ cup		

WHOLE MILK (8 GRAMS FAT PER SERVING)

Whole milk	1 cup	Goat's milk	1 cup
Evaporated whole milk	½ cup	Kefir	1 cup

Other Carbohydrates List

One exchange equals 15 grams carbohydrate, or 1 starch, or 1 fruit, or 1 milk.

Food	Serving Size	Exchanges Per Serving
Angel food cake, unfrosted	1/12th cake	2 carbohydrates
Brownie, small, unfrosted	2 in. square	1 carbohydrate, 1 fat
Cake, unfrosted	2 in. square	1 carbohydrate, 1 fat
Cake, frosted	2 in square	2 carbohydrates, 1 fat
Cookie, fat-free	2 small	1 carbohydrate
Cookie or sandwich cookie with creme filling	2 small	1 carbohydrate, 1 fat
Cupcake, frosted	1 small	2 carbohydrates, 1 fat
Cranberry sauce, jellied	¼ cup	2 carbohydrates
Doughnut, plain cake	1 medium (1½ oz)	1½ carbohydrates, 2 fats
Doughnut, glazed	3¾ in. across (2 oz)	2 carbohydrates, 2 fats
Fruit juice bars, frozen, 100% juice	1 bar (3 oz)	1 carbohydrate
Fruit snacks, chewy (pureed fruit concentrate)	1 roll (¾ oz)	1 carbohydrate
Fruit spreads, 100% fruit	1 Tbsp	1 carbohydrate
Gelatin, regular	½ cup	1 carbohydrate
Gingersnaps	3	1 carbohydrate
Granola bar	1 bar	1 carbohydrate, 1 fat
Granola bar, fat-free	1 bar	2 carbohydrates
Hummus	⅓ cups	1 carbohydrate, 1 fat
Ice cream	½ cup	1 carbohydrate, 2 fats
Ice cream, light	½ cup	1 carbohydrate, 1 fat
Ice cream, fat-free, no sugar added	½ cup	1 carbohydrate
Jam or jelly, regular	1 Tbsp	1 carbohydrate
Milk, chocolate, whole	1 cup	2 carbohydrates, 1 fat

Food	Serving Size	Exchanges Per Serving
Pie, fruit, 2 crusts	⅙ pie	3 carbohydrates, 2 fats
Pie, pumpkin or custard	⅛ pie	1 carbohydrate, 2 fats
Potato chips	12–18 (1 oz)	1 carbohydrate, 2 fats
Pudding, regular (made with low-fat milk)	½ cup	2 carbohydrates
Pudding, sugar-free (made with low-fat milk)	½ cup	1 carbohydrate
Salad dressing, fat-free*	¼ cup	1 carbohydrate
Sherbert, sorbet	½ cup	2 carbohydrates
Spaghetti or pasta sauce, canned*	½ cup	1 carbohydrate, 1 fat
Sweet roll or Danish	1 (2½ oz)	2½ carbohydrates, 2 fats
Syrup, light	2 Tbsp	1 carbohydrate
Syrup, regular	1 Tbsp	1 carbohydrate
Syrup, regular	¼ cup	4 carbohydrates
Tortilla chips	6–12 (1 oz)	1 carbohydrate, 2 fats
Yogurt, frozen, low-fat, fat-free	⅓ cup	1 carbohydrate, 0–1 fat
Yogurt, frozen, fat-free, no sugar added	½ cup	1 carbohydrate
Yogurt, low-fat with fruit	1 cup	3 carbohydrates, 0–1 fat
Vanilla wafers	5	1 carbohydrate, 1 fat

Vegetable List

One vegetable exchange equals 5 grams carbohydrate, 2 grams protein, 0 grams fat, and 25 calories.
In general, one vegetable exchange is ½ cup cooked vegetables or vegetable juice or 1 cup raw vegetables.

Artichoke	Celery	Mushrooms	Spinach
Artichoke hearts	Cucumber	Okra	Summer squash
Asparagus	Eggplant	Onions	Tomato
Beans (green, wax, Italian)	Green onions or scallions	Pea pods	Tomatoes, canned
Bean sprouts	Greens (collard, kale,	Peppers (all varieties)	Tomato sauce*
Beets	mustard, turnip)	Radishes	Tomato/vegetable juice*
Broccoli	Kohlrabi	Salad greens (endive,	Turnips
Brussels sprouts	Leeks	escarole, lettuce,	Watercress
Cabbage	Mixed vegetables (without	romaine, spinach)	Zucchini
Carrots	corn, peas, or pasta)	Sauerkraut*	
Cauliflower			

MEAT AND MEAT SUBSTITUTES LIST

Very Lean Meat and Substitutes List

One exchange equals 0 grams carbohydrate, 7 grams protein, 3 grams fat, and 55 calories. One very lean meat exchange is equal to any one of the following items:

Poultry: Chicken or turkey (white meat, no skin), Cornish hen (no skin)   1 oz

Fish: Fresh or frozen cod, flounder, haddock, halibut, trout; tuna fresh or canned water   1 oz

Shellfish: Clams, crab, lobster, scallops, shrimp, imitation shellfish   1 oz

Game: Duck or pheasant (no skin), venison, buffalo, ostrich   1 oz

Cheese with 1 gram or less fat per ounce:
   Nonfat or low-fat cottage cheese   ¼ cup
   Fat-free cheese   1 oz

* = 400 mg or more sodium per exchange.

Other: Processed sandwich meats with 1 gram or less fat per ounce, such as deli thin, shaved meats, chipped beef,* turkey ham ... 1 oz

Egg whites ... 2

Egg substitutes, plain ... ¼ cup

Hot dogs with 1 gram or less fat per ounce* ... 1 oz

Kidney (high in cholesterol) ... 1 oz

Sausage with 1 gram or less fat per ounce ... 1 oz

Count as one very lean meat and one starch exchange.

Dried beans, peas, lentils (cooked) ... ½ cup

Lean Meat and Substitutes List

One exchange equals 0 grams carbohydrate, 7 grams protein, 3 grams fat, and 55 calories. One lean meat exchange is equal to any one of the following items:

Beef: USDA Select or Choice grades of lean beef trimmed of fat, such as round, sirloin, and flank steak; tenderloin; roast (rib, chuck, rump); steak (T-bone, porterhouse, cubed), ground round ... 1 oz

Pork: Lean pork, such as fresh ham; canned, cured, or boiled ham; Canadian bacon;* tenderloin, center loin chip ... 1 oz

Lamb: Roast, chop, leg ... 1 oz

Veal: Lean chop, roast ... 1 oz

Poultry: Chicken, turkey (dark meat, no skin), chicken white meat (with skin), domestic duck or goose (well-drained of fat, no skin) ... 1 oz

Fish:

Herring (uncreamed or smoked) ... 1 oz

Oysters ... 6 medium

Salmon (fresh or canned), catfish ... 1 oz

Sardines (canned) ... 2 medium

Tuna (canned in oil, drained) ... 1 oz

Game: Goose (no skin), rabbit ... 1 oz

Cheese:

4.5%-fat cottage cheese ... ¼ cup

Grated Parmesan ... 2 Tbsp

Cheese with 3 grams or less fat per ounce ... 1 oz

Other:

Hot dogs with 3 grams or less fat per ounce* ... 1½ oz

Processed sandwich meat with 3 grams or less fat per ounce, such as turkey pastrami or kielbasa ... 1 oz

Liver, heart (high in cholesterol) ... 1 oz

Medium-Fat Meat and Substitutes List

One exchange equals 0 grams carbohydrate, 7 grams protein, 5 grams fat, and 75 calories. One medium-fat meat exchange is equal to any one of the following items:

Beef: Most beef products fall into this category (ground beef, meatloaf, corned beef, short ribs, Prime grades of meat trimmed of fat, such as prime rib) ... 1 oz

Pork: Top loin, chip, Boston butt, cutlet ... 1 oz

Lamb: Rib roast, ground ... 1 oz

Veal: Cutlet (ground or cubed, unbreaded) ... 1 oz

Poultry: Chicken dark meat (with skin), ground turkey or ground chicken, fried chicken (with skin) ... 1 oz

Fish: Any fried fish product ... 1 oz

* = 400 mg or more sodium per exchange.

Cheese: With 5 grams or less fat per ounce

Feta	1 oz
Mozzarella	1 oz
Ricotta	¼ cup (2 oz)

Other:

Egg (high in cholesterol, limit to 3 per week)	1
Sausage with 5 grams or less fat per ounce	1 oz
Soy milk	1 cup
Tempeh	¼ cup
Tofu	4 oz or ½ cup

High-Fat Meat and Substitutes List

One exchange equals 0 grams carbohydrate, 7 grams protein, 8 grams fat, and 100 calories.

Remember these items are high in saturated fat, cholesterol, and calories and may raise blood cholesterol levels if eaten on a regular basis. One high-fat meat exchange is equal to any one of the following items.

Pork: Spareribs, ground pork, pork sausage	1 oz
Cheese: All regular cheeses, such as American,* cheddar, Monterey jack, Swiss	1 oz

Other: Processed sandwich meats with 8 grams or less fat per ounce, such as

bologna, pimento loaf, salami	1 oz
Sausage, such as bratwurst, Italian, knockwurst, Polish, smoked	1 oz
Hot dog (turkey or chicken)*	1 (10/lb)
Bacon	3 slices (20 slices/lb)

Count as one high-fat meat plus one fat exchange.

Hot dog (beef, pork, or combination)*	1 (10/lb)
Peanut butter (contains unsaturated fat)	2 Tbsp

FAT LIST

Monounsaturated Fats List

One fat exchange equals 5 grams fat and 45 calories.

Avocado, medium	⅛ (1 oz)	mixed (50% peanuts)	6 nuts
Oil (canola, olive, peanut)	1 tsp	peanuts	10 nuts
Olives: ripe (black)	8 large	pecans	4 halves
green, stuffed*	10 large	Peanut butter, smooth or crunchy	2 tsp
Nuts		Sesame seeds	1 Tbsp
almonds, cashews	6 nuts	Tahini paste	2 tsp

Polyunsaturated Fats List

One fat exchange equals 5 grams fat and 45 calories.

Margarine: stick, tub, or squeeze	1 tsp	Salad dressing: regular*	1 Tbsp
lower-fat (30% to 50% vegetable oil)	1 Tbsp	reduced-fat	2 Tbsp
Mayonnaise: regular	1 tsp	Miracle Whip Salad Dressing: regular	2 tsp
reduced-fat	1 Tbsp	reduced-fat	1 Tbsp
Nuts, walnuts, English	4 halves	Seeds: pumpkin, sunflower	1 Tbsp
Oil (corn, safflower, soybean)	1 tsp		

* = 400 mg or more sodium per exchange.

Saturated Fats List†

One fat exchange equals 5 grams of fat and 45 calories.

Bacon, cooked	1 slice (20 slices/lb)	Cream, half and half	2 Tbsp
Bacon, grease	1 tsp	Cream cheese: regular	1 Tbsp (½ oz)
Butter: stick	1 tsp	reduced-fat	2 Tbsp (1 oz)
whipped	2 tsp	Fatback or salt pork, see below‡	
reduced-fat	1 Tbsp	Shortening or lard	1 tsp
Chitterlings, boiled	2 Tbsp (½ oz)	Sour cream: regular	2 Tbsp
Coconut, sweetened, shredded	2 Tbsp	reduced-fat	3 Tbsp

FREE FOOD LISTS

A *free food* is any food or drink that contains less than 200 calories or less than 5 grams of carbohydrate per serving. Foods with a serving size listed should be limited to three servings per day. Be sure to spread them out throughout the day. If you eat all three servings at one time, it could affect your blood glucose level. Food listed without a serving size can be eaten as often as you like.

Fat-Free or Reduced-Fat Foods

Cream cheese, fat-free	1 Tbsp	Miracle Whip®, reduced-fat	1 tsp
Creamers, nondairy, liquid	1 Tbsp	Nonstick cooking spray	
Creamers, nondairy, powdered	2 tsp	Salad dressing, fat-free	1 Tbsp
Mayonnaise, fat-free	1 Tbsp	Salad dressing, fat-free, Italian	2 Tbsp
Mayonnaise, reduced-fat	1 tsp	Salsa	¼ cup
Margarine, fat-free	4 Tbsp	Sour cream, fat-free, reduced-fat	1 Tbsp
Margarine, reduced-fat	1 tsp	Whipped topping, regular or light	1 Tbsp
Miracle Whip®, nonfat	1 Tbsp		

Sugar-Free or Low-Sugar Foods

Candy, hard, sugar-free	1 candy	Jam or jelly, low-sugar or light	2 tsp
Gelatin dessert, sugar-free		Sugar substitutes§	
Gelatin, unflavored		Syrup, sugar-free	2 Tbsp
Gum, sugar-free			

Drinks

Bouillon, broth, consomme*		Club soda	
Bouillon or broth, low-sodium		Diet soft drinks, sugar-free	
Carbonated or mineral water		Drink mixes, sugar-free	
Cocoa powder, unsweetened	1 Tbsp	Tea	
Coffee		Tonic water, sugar-free	

* = 400 mg or more of sodium per choice.

† Saturated fats can raise blood cholesterol levels.

‡ Use a piece 1 in. × 1 in. × ¼ in. if you plan to eat the fatback cooked with vegetables. Use a piece 2 in. × 1 in. × ½ in. when eating only the vegetables with the fatback removed.

§ Sugar substitutes, alternatives, or replacements that are approved by the Food and Drug Administration (FDA) are safe to use. Common brand names include:

Equal (aspartame)
Sprinkle Sweet (saccharin)
Sweet One (acesulfame K)
Sweet-10 (saccharin)
Sugar Twin (saccharin)
Sweet 'n Low (saccharin)

Condiments

Catsup	1 Tbsp	Pickles, dill*	1½ large
Horseradish		Soy sauce, regular or light*	
Lemon juice		Taco sauce	1 Tbsp
Lime juice		Vinegar	
Mustard			

Seasonings

Be careful with seasonings that contain sodium or are salts, such as garlic or celery salt, and lemon pepper.

Flavoring extracts	Pimento	Tabasco or hot pepper	Wine, used in cooking
Garlic	Spices	sauce	Worcestershire sauce
Herbs, fresh or dried			

COMBINATION FOODS LIST

Many of the foods we eat are mixed together in various combinations. These combination foods do not fit into any one exchange list. Often it is hard to tell what is in a casserole dish or baked food item. This is a list of exchanges for some typical combination foods. This list will help you fit these food meal plan. Ask your dietitian for information about any combination foods you would like to eat.

Food	Serving Size	Exchanges Per Serving
ENTREES		
Tuna noodle casserole, lasagna, spaghetti with meatballs, chili with beans, macaroni and cheese*	1 cup (8 oz)	2 carbohydrates, 2 medium-fat meats
Chow mein (without noodles or rice)	2 cups (16 oz)	1 carbohydrate, 2 lean meats
Pizza, cheese, thin crust*	¼ of 10 in. (5 oz)	2 carbohydrates, 2 medium-fat meats, 1 fat
Pizza, meat topping, thin crust*	¼ of 10 in. (5 oz)	2 carbohydrates, 2 medium-fat meats, 1 fat
Pizza, meat topping, thin crust*	¼ of 10 in. (5 oz)	2 carbohydrates, 2 medium-fat meats, 2 fats
Pot pie*	1 (7 oz)	2 carbohydrates, 1 medium-fat meat, 4 fats
FROZEN ENTREES		
Salisbury steak with gravy, mashed potato*	1 (11 oz)	2 carbohydrates, 3 medium-fat meats, 3–4 fats
Turkey with gravy, mashed potato, dressing*	1 (11 oz)	2 carbohydrates, 2 medium-fat meats, 2 fats
Entree with less than 300 calories*	1 (8 oz)	2 carbohydrates, 3 lean meats
SOUPS		
Bean*	1 cup	1 carbohydrate, 1 very lean meat
Cream (made with water)*	1 cup (8 oz)	1 carbohydrate, 1 fat
Split pea (made with water)*	½ cup (4 oz)	1 carbohydrate
Tomato (made with water)*	1 cup (8 oz)	1 carbohydrate
Vegetable beef, chicken noodle, or other broth-type*	1 cup (8 oz)	1 carbohydrate

* = 400 mg or more sodium per exchange.

FAST FOODS†

Food	Serving Size	Exchanges Per Serving
Burritos with beef*	2	4 carbohydrates, 2 medium-fat meats, 2 fats
Chicken nuggets*	6	1 carbohydrate, 2 medium-fat meats, 1 fat
Chicken breast and wing, breaded and fried*	1 each	1 carbohydrate, 4 medium-fat meats, 2 fat
Fish sandwich/tartar sauce*	1	3 carbohydrates, 1 medium-fat meat, 3 fats
French fries, thin	20–25	2 carbohydrates, 2 fats
Hamburger, regular	1	2 carbohydrates, 2 medium-fat meats
Hamburger large*	1	2 carbohydrates, 3 medium-fat meats, 1 fat
Hot dog with bun*	1	1 carbohydrate, 1 high-fat meat, 1 fat
Individual pan pizza*	1	5 carbohydrates, 3 medium-fat meats, 3 fats
Soft-serve cone	1 medium	2 carbohydrates, 1 fat
Submarine sandwich*	1 sub (6 in.)	3 carbohydrates, 1 vegetable, 2 medium-fat meats, 1 fat
Taco, hard shell*	1 (6 oz)	2 carbohydrates, 2 medium-fat meats, 2 fats
Taco, soft shell*	1 (3 oz)	1 carbohydrate, 1 medium-fat meat, 1 fat

* = 400 mg or more of sodium per exchange.
† Ask your fast-food restaurant for nutrition about your favorite fast foods.

The Exchange Lists are the basis of a meal planning system designed by a committee of the American Diabetes Association and The American Dietetic Association. While designed primarily for people with diabetes and others who must follow special diets, the Exchange Lists are based on principles of good nutrition that apply to everyone. © 1995 American Diabetes Association, Inc., The American Dietetic Association.

Appendix 12
Calcium and Phosphorus Content of Selected Foods

Item	Amount	Calcium (mg)	Phosphorus (mg)
MILK AND MILK BEVERAGES			
Skim	1 cup	302	247
1%	1 cup	300	235
2%	1 cup	297	232
Whole	1 cup	291	228
Goat milk	1 cup	326	270
Chocolate milk (with 1% milk)	1 cup	287	256
YOGURT			
Plain low-fat with nonfat dry milk	1 cup	415	326
Plain whole milk	1 cup	274	215
Low-fat fruit-flavored	1 cup	314	247
CHEESE			
Cheddar	1 oz	214	145
Cottage cheese, lowfat	½ cup	78	170
Mozarella	1 oz	147	105
Ricotta, part skim	½ cup	337	226
Swiss	1 oz	272	171
Processed American	1 oz	184	211
American cheese food	1 oz	163	130
DESSERTS			
Ice cream, chocolate	1 cup	186	168
Ice cream, vanilla, reg	1 cup	176	134
Ice milk, vanilla	1 cup	176	129
Ice milk, vanilla soft serve	1 cup	274	202
Pudding, instant vanilla from skim milk	½ cup	157	314
Orange sherbet	1 cup	103	74
FISH AND SHELLFISH			
Oysters	¾ cup	129	204
Salmon, chinook, cnd	⅔ cup	154	289
Sardines, cnd in brine	3½ oz	303	354
Scallops, steamed	3½ oz	115	338
Shrimp, cnd, dry pack	3½ oz	115	263
Tuna, cnd, in oil	6½ oz	61	3
"GREENS"			
Collard	½ cup	179	50
Dandelion	½ cup	147	44
Turnip	½ cup	134	27
Mustard	½ cup	97	23
Spinach	½ cup	84	34

Index

Page numbers followed by *f* indicate figures; those followed by *t* indicate tabular material.
Page numbers followed by *b* indicate boxed material.

Phytochemicals
  sources and functions of, 89b
Pica, 322
  in iron deficiency anemia, 589
  during pregnancy, 280b–281b
Pinch test for body fat, 390b
Plaques, 545–546
Polydextrose, 81b
Polysaccarides (complex carbohydrates)
  classification of, 4–5
Polysaccharides (complex carbohydrates), 9t, 9–11
  classification of, 4–5
  composition of, 9t, 27
  digestion of, 14f
  sources of, 9, 9t
Polyunsaturated fats, 63t, 64, 66, 68
Portal systemic encephalopathy. See Hepatic systemic encephalopathy
Potassium. See also Hyperkalemia; Hypokalemia
  absorption of, 158
  deficiency of, 160
  drug interactions with, 161–162
  drug interaction with, 371b
  effect on blood pressure, 159
  excess of, 160–161
  excretion of, 158
  fluid balance and, 151
  functions of, 154t, 158
  for hypokalemia, 166
  intake of
    in hypertension, 584–585
    minimum estimated, 154t
    recommended and average, 154t, 159–160
    in renal failure, 646t, 648, 654, 659
  RDA of
    for adults, 159
  serum
    altered, 160, 161
    normal, 160
  sources of, 575b
    food, 154t, 158
    salt substitutes, 158, 159b
  supplemental, 159b
    postintestinal bypass, 475b
    side effects of, 161, 586b
    with sodium-restricted diets, 581
Potassium chloride
  effect on vitamin B$_{12}$, 120
Poultry
  cooking of, 219b

exchange lists for, 77b
intake of
  guide to, 205t
  suggested, 199b–200b
  nutritive attributes of, 204b
Prealbumin (PAB), 249t, 249–250
Prednisone
  effect of
    on appetite, 486b
  problems/interventions with, 674b
Preeclampsia, 282b
Pregnancy
  adolescent, 286–287, 335
    counseling in, 287
    diet counseling in, 287
    nutrition in, 286
    nutrition problems in, 286
    required nutrients in, 286–287
  anemia in, 264t, 278b, 280b
  anthropometric data and, 274b
  assessment in, 273–277
    criteria for, 274b
  blood volume changes in, 264t
  calories in, 265, 266t, 267t
  client teaching in, 284–285
  complications of
    diabetes, 281b–282b
    hypertension, 282b
    medical, 278b, 281b–282b
    nutritional, 278b–281b
  constipation in, 275, 278b
  daily food guide for, 267–268, 269t
  diabetes mellitus in, 281b–282b
  diagnosis in: Health Seeking Behaviors, as evidenced by a lack of knowledge of diet for lactation and a desire to learn, 277
  dietary management of, 267–268, 271–273
    daily food guide in, 267–268, 269t
    Food Guide Pyramid in, 267–268
    goals in, 283–284
    monitoring of, 285
  folic acid in, 268f
  gastrointestinal effects of, 264t, 275, 278b
  heartburn in, 264t, 278b
    interventions for, 278b
  hypertension in, 282b
  iron-deficiency anemia in, 271, 278b, 280b
    iron supplements for, 271, 272t, 285b

lactose or milk intolerance in, 285
medico-socioeconomic data in, 274t
metabolism in
  altered, 264
myths in, 283b
nausea and vomiting in, 278b
nutrition in
  risk factors for poor, 274b
phenylketonuria in, 281b
physiologic changes during, 264t
pica in, 280, 281b
problems in
  nutrition-related, 278b–282b
RDA for, 265, 265t, 267
vegetarian diet and, 280b
vitamin supplements in, 271, 272t, 276
weight gain in, 263–264, 268, 270–271, 284
  excessive, 279b–280b
  inadequate, 266, 270, 278b–279b
  for normal weight women, 275f
  for overweight women, 270–271, 277f
  recommended ranges, 270, 270t
  for underweight women, 270, 276f
Pregnancy-induced hypertension, 282b
Preschooler nutrition
  assessment in, 322
  diagnosis in: Health Seeking Behaviors as evidenced by a lack of knowledge of age-appropriate behavior COMPLETE AT END, 323
  eating behaviors in, 325–326
  feeding problems in, 323
  Food Guide Pyramid in, 308t
  good eating habits for, 326–327
  growth characteristics and nutritional implications of, 322
  heart-healthy diet for, 323–324
  monitoring of, 327
  problems and interventions in, 304b–307b
  teaching in, 325–326
Preterm infant
  feeding of, 312b–314b
  nutritional needs of, 312b–313b
  requirements of, 312b–313b
  vitamins for, 102

movement across cell mem-
branes, 152b
output of, 149f, 149–150
percentage in selected foods,
150t
RDA of
for adults, 151
for infants, 151
in saliva, 173t
sources of
beverages, 148–149
bottled, 150b
intravenous solutions, 149,
153
isotonic saline solutions, 149,
153
in wound healing and surgery,
477t
Water balance, 148–150, 149f
Water intoxication, 155
Water-soluble vitamins. *See*
Vitamin(s), water-soluble
Weight. *See also* Weight reduction
assessment of
in lactation, 293
changes in
interpretation of, 242
in elderly, 358
energy intake for, 381, 382t
gain in
age-based, 303t
with insulin therapy, 623b
with oral hypoglycemics,
623b
during pregnancy, 264–264,
268, 270–271, 276,
278–280, 284. *See also*
Pregnancy, weight gain in
healthy, 383t
ideal, 382–384, 382–385
loss of
in cancer, 699
in COPD, 486
drug-induced, 371b
in elderly, 357–358
institutionalized, 368
in HIV/AIDS, 711b, 714
postoperative, 472

measurement of
adult, 241
infants and children, 240–241
interpretation of adult,
241–242
Metropolitan Life Insurance
tables for, 384, 385t
Weight reduction. *See also* Obesity;
Overweight
assessment for, 406–407
behavior modification in, 396,
397b
diets for
balance in, 408
1200 calorie, 398, 408
1500 calorie, 401t, 408
evaluation for, 399b
management of, 409
in moderate to severe obesity,
402–403
in overweight to mild obesity,
398–401
very-low-calorie, 402–403
exercise in, 395–396
fasting for
total, 403
fat intake in, 409
gimmicks in, 401
goals in, 408
in gout, 678
in hypertension, 584
monitoring in, 411
in noninsulin-dependent diabetes,
609
in osteoarthritis, 673, 675–676
planning and implementation in,
407
programs for, 400
social support for, 395
surgical procedures for, 403–404
teaching in, 409–411
Weight Watchers, 396, 400
White fat, 62
Wines
calorie, carbohydrate, alcohol
content of, 26t
Wound healing
nutrients for, 477t

X
Xylitol
sources of, 7t

Y
Yeast-free diet
in HIV/AIDS, 715b
Yersinia enterocolitica, 221

Z
Zen-macrobiotic diet, 715b
Zinc
absorption of, 142
from breast milk, 290b
deficiency of, 143
with high-fiber diet, 506b
immune response and, 709b
populations at risk for, 143
in renal failure, 649–650
signs of, 136t, 143
elemental
for taste abnormalities, 705t
excretion of, 143
function of, 136t, 142
homeostasis of, 143
intake of
in children, 329
estimated average, 136t
nutrient/drug interactions with,
143–144
RDA of
for adults, 136t
for children, 307t
for infants, 307t
for men, 143
during pregnancy, 265t
for women, 143
sources of
food, 136t, 142
supplemental
during pregnancy, 272t
toxicity of, 143
signs of, 136t
in wound healing and surgery,
477t